Sports Neurology
Second Edition

Sports Neurology
Second Edition

Editors

Barry D. Jordan, M.D.
Instructor in Neurology
Reed Neurological Research Center
UCLA School of Medicine
Los Angeles, California

Adjunct Associate Professor of Psychiatry
Biobehavioral Research Center
Charles Drew University
Los Angeles, California

Former Medical Director, New York State Athletic Commission

Peter Tsairis, M.D.
Director of Neurology, Emeritus
Attending Neurologist
The Hospital for Special Surgery
New York, New York

Associate Professor of Neurology
Cornell Medical College
New York, New York

Russell F. Warren, M.D.
Surgeon-in-Chief
The Hospital for Special Surgery
New York, New York

Professor of Orthopaedic Surgery
Cornell Medical Center
New York, New York

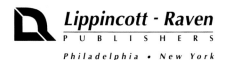
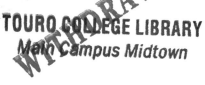
Lippincott - Raven
PUBLISHERS
Philadelphia • New York

Midterm

Acquisitions Editor: Danette Knopp
Developmental Editor: Juleann Sattinger
Manufacturing Manager: Kevin Watt
Production Manager: Kathleen Bubbeo
Production Editor: Tony DeGeorge
Cover Designer: Patricia Gast
Indexer: Leon Kremzner
Compositor: Circle Graphics
Printer: Kingsport Press

Printed in the United States of America

9 8 7 6 5 4 3 2 1

Library of Congress Cataloging-in-Publication Data
Sports neurology / editors, Barry D. Jordan, Peter Tsairis, Russell F.
  Warren. — 2nd ed.
      p.   cm.
   Includes bibliographical references and index.
   ISBN 0-397-51629-0
   1. Nervous system—Wounds and injures.   2. Sports injuries.
 I. Jordan, Barry D.   II. Tsairis, Peter.   III. Warren, Russell F.
   [DNLM: 1. Brain Injuries.   2. Athletic Injuries.   3. Spinal Cord
Injuries.   4. Sports Medicine.   WL 354 S764 1998]
RD593.S68   1998
617.4′8044—dc21
DNLM/DLC
for Library of Congress   98-23250
                                                                     CIP

3/19/99
Phys. Asst.

Contents

Contributors

Brian R. Apatoff, M.D., Ph.D.
Multiple Sclerosis Clinical Care and Research Center
Department of Neurology & Neuroscience
The New York Hospital/Cornell Medical Center
525 East 68th Street
New York, New York 10021

Julian E. Bailes, M.D.
Division of Neurosurgery
Osceola Regional Medical Center
Orlando, Florida 32801

Ronnie P. Barnes, M.S., A.T.C.
Head Athletic Trainer
New York Football Giants
Giants Stadium
East Rutherford, New Jersey 07073

Richard D. Birrer, M.D., M.P.H.
Associate Professor
Department of Family and Emergency Medicine
Catholic Medical Center of Brooklyn and Queens, Inc.
88-25 153 Street
Jamaica, New York 11432

Doris M. Bixby-Hammett, M.D.
103 Surrey Road
Waynesville, North Carolina 28786

William H. Brooks, M.D.
Neurosurgeon
Neurosurgical Associates
1401 Harrodsburg Road, Suite B485
Lexington, Kentucky 40504; and
Chairman
United States Pony Club, Safety Committee; and
Former President
American Medical Equestrian Association

Janny Dwyer Brust, M.P.H.
Director of Research
Allina Health System
Allina Foundation
5601 Smetana Drive
Minneapolis, Minnesota 55440

Sheldon Burns, M.D.
Minneapolis Sports Medicine Center
720 Washington Avenue South
Edina, Minnesota 55435

Frank P. Cammisa, Jr., M.D.
Assistant Professor of Surgery
Cornell University Medical College; and
Chief, Spine Service
The Hospital for Special Surgery
535 East 70th Street
New York, New York 10021

Robert C. Cantu, M.D., F.A.C.S., F.A.C.S.M.
Director
Service of Sports Medicine and
Chief, Neurosurgery Service
Emerson Hospital
Concord, Massachusetts; and
Medical Director
National Center for Catastrophic Sports Injury
Research; and
Neurological Surgery, Inc.
John Cuming Building
Suite 820
Concord, Massachusetts 01742

John J. Caronna, M.D.
Professor of Clinical Neurology and
Vice Chairman, Department of Neurology
Cornell University Medical College
520 East 70th Street
New York, New York 10021

Yasoma B. Challenor, M.D.
Clinical Professor Emerita
Physical Medicine & Rehabilitation
Columbia University, College of Physicians and
Surgeons
630 West 168th Street
New York, New York 10032

Kenneth S. Clarke
27751 Calle Rabano
Sun City, California 92585

Steven B. Cohen, B.A.
Robert Wood Johnson Medical School
University of Medicine and Dentistry of New Jersey
675 Hoes Lane
Piscataway, New Jersey 08903

Orrin Devinsky, M.D.
Professor of Neurology, Neurosurgery, and
*   Psychiatry*
Department of Neurology
New York University School of Medicine
301 East 17th Street
New York, New York 10003

Joseph H. Feinberg, M.D.
Director
Sports Medicine
Kessler Institute for Rehabilitation
1199 Pleasant Valley Way
West Orange, New Jersey 07052

William E. Garrett, Jr., M.D., Ph.D.
Professor of Orthopaedic Surgery
Duke University Medical Center
Science Drive
Durham, North Carolina 27710

Susan Goodwin Gerberich, Ph.D., M.S.P.H.
Associate Professor and Director
Regional Injury Prevention Research Center and
*   Center for Violence Prevention and Control*
Division of Environmental and Occupational Health
University of Minnesota School of Public Health
Box 807-UMHC
420 Delaware Street SE
Minneapolis, Minnesota 55455

Peter G. Gerbino II, M.D.
Instructor in Orthopaedic Surgery
Department of Orthopaedic Surgery
Division of Sport Medicine
Harvard Medical School
Children's Hospital
300 Longwood Avenue
Boston, Massachusetts 02115

Barth A. Green, M.D.
Professor and Chairman
Department of Neurological Surgery
President and Co-Founder
The Miami Project to Cure Paralysis
University of Miami School of Medicine
P.O. Box 016960 (M813)
Miami, Florida 33101

Hugh D. Greer III, M.D.
Santa Barbara Medical Foundation Clinic
P.O. Box 1200
Santa Barbara, California 93102

Ludwig Gutmann, M.D.
Professor and Chairman
Department of Neurology
West Virginia University Health Sciences Center
P.O. Box 9180
Morgantown, West Virginia 26505-9180

Brian Hainline, M.D.
Clinical Associate Professor of Neurology
New York University School of Medicine; and
Chief
Neurology and Pain Management
ProHEALTH Care Associates
2800 Marcus Avenue
Lake Success, New York 11042

Mark Hallett, M.D.
Clinical Director
National Institute of Neurological Disorders and
*   Stroke*
National Institutes of Health
Building 10, Room 5N226
10 Center Drive, MSC 1428
Bethesda, Maryland 20892-1428

Carl Heise, M.D.
Department of Neurology
Hospital for Special Surgery
535 East 70th Street
New York, New York 10021

Edward G. Hixon, M.D., F.A.C.S.,
*   **F.A.C.S.M.***
Adirondack Surgical Group
R.F.D. Box 410B
Lake Colby Drive
Lake Saranac, New York 12983

Arnold M. Illman, M.D.
Associate Professor Orthopedic Surgery
Stonybrook Medical School
Nassau County Medical Center
2201 Hempstead Turnpike
East Meadow, New York 11554

Beth Johnson, B.A.
4260 Pleasant Avenue South
Minneapolis, Minnesota 55409

Barry D. Jordan, M.D., M.P.H.
Instructor in Neurology
Reed Neurological Research Center
UCLA School of Medicine
710 Westwood Plaza
Los Angeles, California 90095-1769; and
Adjunct Associate Professor of Psychiatry
Biobehavioral Research Center
Charles Drew University; and
Former Medical Director
New York State Athletic Commission

Donald T. Kirkendall, Ph.D.
Clinical Assistant Professor
Department of Orthopaedic Surgery and
Department of Physical and Occupational
*   Therapy*
Duke University Medical Center
Box 3435
Durham, North Carolina 27710

Thomas T. Lee, M.D.
Department of Neurological Surgery
University of Miami School of Medicine
P.O. Box 016960 (M813)
Miami, Florida 33101

A. J. Lees, M.D., F.R.C.P.
Consultant Neurologist
National Hospital for Neurology &
*   Neurosurgery*
Queen Square
London WC1N 3BG
United Kingdom

Boris Leybel, M.D.
Fellow
New York Headache Center
State University of New York, HSCB
30 East 76th Street
New York, New York 10021

Baron S. Lonner, M.D.
Assistant Professor
Department of Orthopaedic Surgery
Albert Einstein College of Medicine;
Director
Spine and Scoliosis Service
Long Island Jewish Medical Center
Schneider Children's Hospital
270-05 76th Avenue
New Hyde Park, New York 11040

Daniel MacGowan, M.D.
253 W. 73rd Street
Apartment 3E
New York, New York 10023

Glen R. Manzano, B.S.
Senior Staff Assistant
Department of Neurological Surgery
University of Miami School of Medicine
P.O. Box 01690 (M813)
Miami, Florida 33101

Erik J. T. Matser, M.D.
Neuropsychologist
Department of Neuropsychology
St. Anna Hospital, Geldrop
Postbox 90
5660 AB Geldrop
The Netherlands

Alexander Mauskop, M.D., F.A.A.N.
Associate Professor of Clinical Neurology
State University of New York, HSCB; and
Director
New York Headache Center
30 East 76th Street
New York, New York 10021

Paul McCrory, M.B.B.S., F.R.A.C.P.,
**   F.A.C.S.P., F.A.S.M.F.**
Department of Neurology
Austin & Repatriation Medical Centre
Studley Road
Heidelberg, Victoria 3084
Australia; and
Chairman
Department of Neurology
Olympic Park Sports Medicine Centre
Swan Street, Melbourne 3004
Australia

Salah M. Mesad, M.D.
Senior Clinical Neurophysiology Fellow
Department of Neurology
New York University, Hospital for Joint
*   Diseases*
301 East 17th Street
New York, New York 10003

Lyle J. Micheli, M.D.
Associate Clinical Professor
Department of Orthopaedic Surgery
Harvard Medical School; and
Director
Division of Sports Medicine
Children's Hospital
319 Longwood Avenue
Boston, Massachusetts 02115

Patrick F. O'Leary, M.D.
Clinical Associate Professor
Department of Surgery
Cornell University Medical College; and
Chief
Spine Service
Lenox Hill Hospital; and
Attending Physician
The Hospital for Special Surgery
535 East 70th Street
New York, New York 10021

Stephen E. Olvey, M.D.
Associate Professor of Clinical Neurological
   Surgery; and
Director
Neurosurgical Intensive Care
University of Miami School of Medicine
1501 NW 9th Avenue
Miami, Florida 33136

Louis H. Rappoport, M.D.
Orthopaedic Spine Surgeon
Arizona Spine Consultants, Ltd.
6036 North 19th Avenue, Suite 306
Phoenix, Arizona 85015

Ruth Solomon, B.A.
Professor of Theatre Arts and Dance
Dance Theater Program
University of California, Santa Cruz
Santa Cruz, California 95064

Bradford A. Stephens, M.D.
Lake Placid Sports Medicine Center
P.O. Box 790
Lake Placid, New York 12946

Charles H. Tator, M.D., M.A., Ph.D.,
   F.R.C.S.C., F.A.C.S.
Professor and Chair
Division of Neurosurgery; and
President
SportSmart Canada
Toronto Hospital and University of Toronto
399 Bathurst Street
Toronto, Ontario M5T 2S8
Canada

Peter Tsairis, M.D.
Director of Neurology, Emeritus
Attending Neurologist
The Hospital for Special Surgery; and
Associate Professor of Neurology
Cornell Medical College
535 East 70th Street
New York, New York 10021

Russell F. Warren, M.D.
Surgeon-in-Chief
The Hospital for Special Surgery; and
Professor of Orthopaedics
Cornell Medical Center
535 East 70th Street
New York, New York 10021

Robert G. Watkins, M.D.
501 East Hardy Street, #300
Inglewood, California 90301

Stuart M. Weinstein, M.D.
Clinical Assistant Professor
Department of Rehabilitation Medicine
University of Washington; and
Puget Sound Sports and Spine Physicians, P.S.
1600 East Jefferson Street, Suite 401
Seattle, Washington 98122-5647

Robert D. Zimmerman, M.D.
Professor, Director of MRI, and
   Associate Chair for Education
Department of Radiology
The New York and Presbyterian Hospital
525 East 68th Street
New York, New York 10021

Preface

The first edition of *Sports Neurology,* published in 1989, established sports neurology as a distinct medical subspecialty. Since the late 1980s, sports neurology has grown as a discipline and its clinical importance has become increasingly apparent. Over the past decade several sports neurology programs have emerged worldwide. In addition, sports neurology has been a focus of several national and international conferences, including those sponsored by the American Academy of Neurology, the American College of Sports Medicine, and the World Congress of Neurology.

Several clinical and scientific advances have contributed to the growth of sports neurology. First, the growing public health concern regarding concussion in sports served as an impetus for the American Academy of Neurology to establish consensus guidelines for the evaluation and management of concussion in sports. This document has been endorsed by several medical societies and organizations. In addition, neuropsychology has emerged as an important neurodiagnostic tool in the evaluation of neurocognitive impairment associated with traumatic brain injury in sports. Neuropsychological testing has been utilized in several sports, including boxing, football, soccer, rugby, ice hockey, and auto racing. Furthermore, neuropsychological testing is currently being utilized to establish recovery curves from concussion in sports and criteria for return to competition. Currently, the National Football League and the National Hockey League have instituted programs to utilize neuropsychological testing in the evaluation of concussion. Other advances in the field of sports neurology include an increased awareness of the second impact syndrome and its pathobiology and neurodiagnostic approaches in the evaluation of transient neurapraxia to the cervical spinal cord.

Probably the most exciting and landmark scientific discovery within sports neurology has been advancement of our understanding of the neurobiology of chronic traumatic brain injury in boxing (i.e., dementia pugilistica) and its neuropathological similarities with Alzheimer's disease. Recent studies have suggested that dementia pugilistica and Alzheimer's disease may involve similar pathogenic mechanisms.

The second edition of *Sports Neurology* includes several new chapters. There has been an expansion of athletic injuries to the spine as well as a chapter on the functional anatomy and biomechanics of the spine. Also, other neurologic disorders including multiple sclerosis and movement disorders have been added. The section on sport-specific neurologic injuries has been expanded to include auto racing, dance, cycling, and rugby. The second edition of *Sports Neurology* should continue to serve as a reference text for health care professionals involved in the treatment of athletes with neurological injuries and/or disorders.

Preface to the First Edition

Injury to the nervous system can occur in almost any sport and may involve any level of the nervous system. Certain sports, such as boxing, football, equestrian sports, ice hockey, rugby, and the martial arts, are often associated with an increased risk of neurologic injury compared to other sports, such as basketball, archery, and other noncontact sports. Injuries involving the central nervous system (i.e., the brain or spinal cord) are often associated with significant morbidity and mortality, whereas injuries to the peripheral nervous system (i.e., the peripheral nerves or muscle) are often much less devastating but can result in prolonged disability.

Traditionally, sports medicine and neurology have been recognized as two distinct and unrelated subspecialties of medicine. The potential for catastrophic neurologic injury in sports, however, requires the mutual consideration of these distinct medical subspecialties. Because most sports medicine personnel are not sufficiently trained in neurologic care, and because most neurologists and neurosurgeons are not formally trained in sports medicine, the management of the neurologically injured or disabled athlete can be problematic. Accordingly, neurologic aspects of sports medicine require special attention.

This book is designed to assist the health care professional in recognizing and managing neurologic problems encountered by the athlete. The contents will help prepare team physicians or trainers to deal with neurologic injuries and to familiarize themselves with the potential neurologic hazards of various sports. Furthermore, the book can serve as a reference for the neurologist or neurosurgeon involved with the treatment of a neurologically impaired athlete.

The first section discusses some general concepts of sports neurology, including psychological and behavioral aspects of sports and the influence of drugs on the nervous system. The roles of neuroradiology and electrophysiology in diagnosing neurologic injuries and the rehabilitation of the neurologically impaired athlete are also discussed. The second section addresses the diagnosis and treatment of major neurologic disorders that may be encountered in the athlete, and the third section elaborates on the neurologic injuries that occur in specific sports.

Acknowledgments

The editors would like to thank Danette Knopp and Juleann Sattinger for their assistance and inexhaustible efforts in bringing the second edition of *Sports Neurology* to fruition.

PART I

General Concepts

Sports Neurology, Second Edition,
edited by Barry D. Jordan.
Lippincott–Raven Publishers, Philadelphia © 1998.

1

Sports Neuroepidemiology

Kenneth S. Clarke and *Barry D. Jordan

*27751 Calle Rabano, Sun City, California 92585; °Reed Neurological Research Center,
UCLA School of Medicine, 710 Westwood Plaza, Los Angeles, California 90095-1769*

Sports neuroepidemiology is concerned with delineating the distribution and dynamics of neurologic injury within sports. Its method is to follow frequencies and patterns of injuries in the search for causative agents (determinants) or risk factors. Its goals are to remove or negate the influence of an alleged determinant and then to observe whether the distribution or frequency of the injury is altered accordingly. While addressing cause and effect, the epidemiologic model must deal with associations. A documented association between a hypothesized determinant (e.g., a defective helmet design) and a particular type of injury (e.g., cerebral neurotrauma) does not constitute proof of cause and effect. A stable leavening of the problem after removing the alleged agent is strong confirmation of a hypothesis, but a more powerful argument obtained with epidemiologic data is that of disconfirmation. If, for example, a particular helmet is alleged to be the cause of serious cerebral neurotrauma because of its defective design, a strong association between the use of that helmet and such injuries must be found or the cause–effect relationship is disconfirmed.

METHODOLOGIC CONSIDERATIONS

To evaluate injury patterns (frequencies and association), a comparison must be made. Whether the comparison is year to year, sport to sport, squad to squad, helmet to helmet, or male to female, one must have both a reasonable rationale and sufficient data to permit a fair comparison.

The epidemiologic model requires a merging of population data, injury data, and athletic exposure data to delineate the risk of injury in a particular sport.

Population Data

In order to establish accurate injury rates, the investigator must identify the population at risk (i.e., the number of participants in the particular sport of interest). Documenting the absolute number of injuries without acknowledging the denominator or number of participants does not afford the opportunity to calculate injury rates that can be compared between sports, leagues, or competition levels. For example, 20 neurologic injuries in an athletic or sporting activity that has 50 participants (i.e., 40 injuries per 100 athletes) represent a more serious health concern than 20 neurologic injuries in an activity in which 1000 athletes participate (i.e., 2 injuries per 100 athletes). Accordingly, in order to make comparisons or document the health burden of a particular sport, the population at risk must be identified.

The identification of the population at risk enables the clinical investigator to identify the population not at risk. This "not at risk" cohort could potentially serve as a control group for the population "at risk." However, the selection of a control group for the population at risk should be carefully conducted. The control group should be devoid of any inherent biases that may influence the validity and interpretability of the collected data. For example, if an investigator was attempting to determine whether American football was associated with an increased rate of neurologic injury, it would be inappropriate to utilize rugby players as a control group. The rugby athletes would be an inappropriate control group because that sport has an injury profile similar to that of American football. Accordingly, a more appropriate control group would be athletes in a noncontact sport (e.g., track and field).

Injury Data

In sports neuroepidemiology, proper identification of a case requires an accurate diagnosis and classification of the injury. Any injury that is documented should be correctly diagnosed. In addition, the definition or classification of injuries is extremely important. For example, traumatic brain injuries should be classified according to the specific type of brain injury (e.g., concussion, intracranial hemorrhage) and not classified as head injuries. Head injuries may also include injuries to the eyes, ears, nose, or mouth that are not associated with any brain injury. Accordingly, in the epidemiologic investigation of neurologic injuries in sport, special attention should be paid to the accuracy of the diagnosis and the definition or classification of neurologic disease.

Documentation of Exposure

The documentation of athletic exposure represents a vital methodologic concern in sports neuroepidemiology. Athletic exposure documentation can be reported in various ways and is dependent on the sport of interest. When comparing injury rates between sports, one must recognize that athletic exposures may not be identical. For example, in baseball or American football, an athlete's exposure may be a game (i.e., 2 or more hours), whereas in boxing it may be a competitive bout (less than 1 hour). Furthermore, the time associated with an athletic exposure within a sport may also vary. For example, in American football, the athletic exposure of a starting quarterback may be considerably longer than the exposure of a football player on special

teams (e.g., punt, kickoff). The astute epidemiologist must be cognizant of these variances when interpreting injury data in sport.

The calculation of injury rates is dependent on the documentation of athletic exposure. Although injury rates can be calculated by dividing the number of injuries by the number of participants (e.g., 7.5 concussions per 1000 athletes), this statistic may be less informative than calculating injuries per athlete-exposure. For example, 50 athletes attending 5 games would constitute 250 athlete-exposures. If 2 athletes were injured, the rate would be 2 cases per 250 athlete-exposures or 8 cases per 1000 athlete-exposures. This rate would be preferable than simply stating 2 cases or injuries per 50 athletes, because the former statistic takes into account the exposure an athlete experiences. This is particularly the case because athletes on the same team or in the same sport may not share similar exposures.

MORTALITY

Although fatal injuries can occur in any sport or athletic activity, accurate mortality rates in sports are limited. Table 1 presents the relative risk of fatality in various competitive sports where the denominator (i.e., the number of participants) was available. Although the majority of fatal athletic accidents are usually attributable to either cardiac or neurologic etiologies, the percentage of fatalities associated with neurologic causes is unknown. As expected, however, high-velocity racing events are associated with higher fatality rates.

Football is the only high school and college sport for which sufficient mortality incidence

TABLE 1. *Average annual fatality rates in selected competitive sports, 1960–1964*

Sport	Fatalities	Fatality rate per 100,000 participants
Football	26	3.9
Power boating	1	16.7
Automobile racing	30	120.0
Horse racing	2	133.3
Motorcycling	5	178.6

From ref. 2, with permission.

data are available (since 1931) (1). The data first received epidemiologic treatment in the mid-1960s (2). In that study, the football fatality data had been reported by the Metropolitan Life Insurance Company (3). From 1964 to the present, there was a significant reduction in deaths attributable to football. In high school and college football one fatality was experienced in the fall of 1964 for every 1.5 million athlete-exposures. By 1974, it had improved to one fatality for every 6 million athlete-exposures (4). Since 1977, it has been about one fatality for every 10 million athlete-exposures. From the 1950s through the present, nine of every ten football deaths resulting from traumatic injury have involved the head or neck. Moreover, when distinguishing between head and neck injuries, different frequency patterns are seen (Fig. 1). The development of the modern helmet and face mask in the 1950s and 1960s was associated with changes in blocking and tackling techniques (i.e., the helmeted head was brought into contact more purposefully). It is apparent that these changes were accompanied by a substantial increase in deaths resulting from head injuries, whereas death from cervical spinal cord injury remained infrequent yet persistent over the years. The trend in head-related fatalities was reversed not only by the "infrequent yet persistent" level of neck injuries. Several determinants were responsible.

In the late 1960s the National Operating Committee for Safety in Athletic Equipment (NOCSAE) was established initially to develop impact standards against which all football helmet models were to be tested successfully before being marketed. By 1974, these standards were adopted by the National Federation of State High School Athletic Associations (NFSHSA) and the National Collegiate Athletic Association (NCAA) and were utilized by all manufacturers, even though wearing helmets that passed NOCSAE standards did not become mandatory until 1978 at the college level and 1980 at the high school level. NOCSAE has since broadened its attention to baseball helmets and has future interests in boxing, cycling, and hockey headgear.

In addition, by the late 1960s an educational campaign against spear tackling had been intensified by the American Medical Association, NFSHSA, NCAA, and others (5). Then in January 1976, high school rules and coaching ethics were formally adopted to prohibit tackling–blocking techniques in which the helmeted head received the brunt of the initial impact. The primary reason for these rules (NCAA rule 9-1-2-n and NFSHSA rule 9-3-1) was the vulnerability of the athlete's cervical spine when he struck his opponent with the top or the crown of the helmet. The phrasing and intent, however, were also intended to preclude the deliberate use (and teaching) of face mask and brow content (NCAA rule 9-1-2-1 and NFSHSA rule 9-3-2-k). The contention was that in leading with the head, the player cannot al-

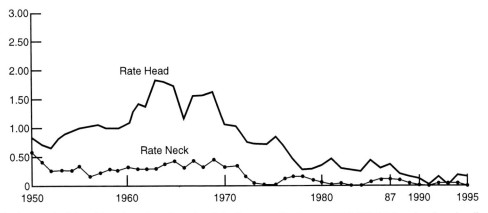

FIG. 1. Football fatalities, head and neck related, respectively, per 100,000 high school and college players combined, smoothed (average of previous, current, and subsequent years' rates).

ways be sure of achieving the desired football position of "head up, eyes forward, neck bulled" at the moment of contact and that improper execution could put the player's head or neck in a vulnerable position. When the player was not leading with the head, improper execution was not considered potentially devastating, and the rule was thereby adopted. In 1978, an organized approach to the coach's education of the athlete, concerning the latter's shared responsibility in this regard, was initiated by the NCAA (6). By 1980, the NFSHSA and football helmet manufacturers had created posters for locker rooms with the same message.

To sum up, several observations can be made with respect to fatalities:

1. Football is the only sport for which sufficient fatality data for epidemiologic analysis are available.
2. The advent of conscious attention to helmet standards in the late 1960s and early 1970s was associated with a distinct decrease in deaths related to head injuries.
3. The advent of rule changes in 1976 that prohibited leading with the head for contact was associated with another distinct drop in deaths related to head injuries.
4. The emergence of the face mask in the 1950s and its subsequent continuous use were not accompanied by a sustained increase in the relative frequency of deaths related to neck injuries.

MORBIDITY

Brain Injury

Since 1975, the National Athletic Injury/Illness Reporting System (NAIRS) has been following all athletic injuries in various sports, including concussions, with the support of two grants from the U.S. Consumer Product Safety Commission (7). The frequency of the more potentially catastrophic intracranial hemorrhage was far too low for the NAIRS sample to yield interpretable data on that level of injury. However, the registry of Torg et al. (8) has been able to obtain information about the annual incidence of intracranial hemorrhage.

In the NAIRS system, a reportable concussion is any incident of disorientation caused by trauma that requires cessation of play to examine the athlete, no matter how momentary the symptoms and no matter what the subsequent disposition of the athlete with respect to participation. The rate of reportable concussions among the collegiate athletes followed by NAIRS is given in Table 2. By both population and exposure, football is clearly the sport most frequently associated with these injuries. Adjusted for exposure, however, the data reveal a difference between spring football and fall football. They also show strikingly uniform rates among the other sports. NAIRS was also able to retrieve injury data by degree of severity. Customarily, preference for analysis is given to the significant injury (i.e., one keeping the athlete out of participation for at least 1 week) because it is considered the most reliable and meaningful. Table 3 reveals that the year-to-year rates of both reportable and significant concussions in football were stable. Since the 1976 rule changes, however, the proportion of significant concussions resulting from tackling has dropped steadily.

Although cerebral concussion is an infrequent occurrence in football, the next concern is whether particular helmets may contribute to more than their share of these injuries. If a par-

TABLE 2. *Average annual incidence of reportable concussions in selected college sports, 1975–1978*

Sports	Average number of teams	Cases per 10,000 athlete-exposures	Cases per 100 athletes
Football, spring	26	11.1	2.2
Football, fall	49	7.3	6.1
Lacrosse	5	4.1	1.9
Ice hockey	8	3.5	3.7
Softball (women)	10	3.5	1.7
Wrestling	20	3.0	2.5
Basketball (women)	21	2.7	2.2
Soccer	13	2.7	1.6

From National Athletic Injury Reporting System, Pennsylvania State University, 1979.

TABLE 3. *Average annual rate (cases per 100 athletes) of concussions in collegiate football accompanied by proportion of significant concussions associated with tackling*

Concussions	1975	1976	1977	1978
Reportable	5.8	6.4	6.0	7.0
Significant	0.6	0.7	0.6	0.6
(while tackling)	58%	40%	30%	23%

From National Athletic Injury/Illness Reporting System, Pennsylvania State University, 1979.

TABLE 5. *Annual rate (cases per 1000 athlete-exposures) of significant concussions by type of playing surface in college football, 1975–1977*

Surface	1975	1976	1977
Natural grass			
Athlete-exposures	171,386	157,665	318,040
Concussion rate	0.1	0.1	0.1
Astroturf			
Athlete-exposures	95,803	87,382	155,027
Concussion rate	0.0	0.1	0.1
Tartanturf			
Athlete-exposures	35,300	28,652	43,161
Concussion rate	0.0[a]	0.1	0.1

[a] Not zero but less than 0.05.
From ref. 9, with permission.

ticular helmet is sufficiently defective in design to account for a disproportionate number of these injuries, the rate of concussions would be lowered if that helmet were removed from use.

NAIRS data were examined for this possibility; Table 4 displays the findings for significant concussions per 1000 athlete-exposures per type and brand of helmet for the seasons 1975 through 1977 (7). Clearly, these injuries were distributed randomly through the population in proportion to the frequency of use of each helmet.

NAIRS data also made it possible to examine the influence of the playing surface on the incidence of selected injuries in college football (9). The results clearly reveal no undue association of any playing surface with significant concussions when analyzed on an equivalent exposure basis (Table 5).

Overall, the exact incidence of traumatic brain injury related to sports can only be estimated. Worldwide estimates of the incidence of traumatic brain injuries of all causes range from 152 to 430 cases per 100,000 population per year (10). The percentage of brain injuries related to sports ranges anywhere from 3% to 25% (10). Utilizing these figures, the rates of sports-related brain injuries could theoretically range from 4.6 to 67.5 cases per 100,000 population per annum. This estimate may be conservative if one includes bicycle and motorcycle injuries.

Spinal Cord Injury

Data on the incidence of spinal cord injury in sport are vaguely delineated with the exception of a few sports (e.g., football, gymnastics). The worldwide incidence of all spinal cord injuries ranges from 150 to 500 cases per 100,000 population. The percentage of spinal cord injuries related to recreational and sporting activities ranges from 3% to 19% (10). Accordingly, the frequency of sports-related spinal cord injuries could range from 4.5 to 95 cases per 100,000 population.

TABLE 4. *Average annual rate (cases per 1000 athlete-exposures) of significant concussions by type and brand of helmet in high school and college football, 1975–1977*

Parameter	All helmets	Helmet style												
		1	2	3	4	5	6	7	8	9	10	11	12	13
Rate	0.1	0.1	0.1	0.1	0.1	0.1	0.1	0.1	0.0	0.1	0.0	0.0	0.1	0.0
Number of cases	92	7	19	6	24	2	5	19	0	3	3	0	3	0
Percentage use	100	6.5	22.7	9.9	15.2	2.7	5.8	19.7	3.2	2.7	5.9	0.1	2.1	0.5

In 1977, Clarke (11) surveyed retrospectively (1973 to 1975) spinal cord injuries in the varsity programs of all high schools and colleges in the nation and found that gymnastics had the highest average annual injury rate of all sports (Table 6). Of the others, only football and wrestling showed an annual persistence of such injuries. Of these three sports, only gymnastics and football displayed describable patterns. The patterns of injury among all gymnastic events revealed that permanent spinal cord injuries were associated primarily with the trampoline (as a training device) but not to the exclusion of other gymnastic apparatuses (Table 7). The vast majority of these injuries occurred when the athlete came down incorrectly on the trampoline. This finding, coupled with a subsequent finding that the injured trampolinist had invariably been attempting a somersault, resulted in national consensus guidelines in 1978 on the controlled use of the trampoline and minitrampoline (12,13).

Another offshoot of this survey was the advent, in July 1978, of a National Registry of Gymnastic Catastrophic Injuries patterned after the American Football Coaches Association (AFCA) Football Fatality Report (14). In its first 4 years (through June 1982), 20 gymnastics-related injuries that resulted in serious cervical neurotrauma occurred across the nation: 17 athletes developed permanent quadriplegia, and 3 died. As shown in Table 8, most injuries were incurred by skilled performers while practicing; most of the injuries did not occur under conditions of organized sport. As was found earlier, the trampoline and minitrampoline, although associated with many of these cases, are not the

TABLE 7. *Adjusted proportion of permanent spinal cord injuries by type of event in high school– and college-sponsored gymnastics, 1973–1975*

Event	Men (%)	Women (%)
Trampoline	33	71
Minitrampoline	11	
Horizontal bar	22	
Rings	11	
Floor exercise	22	14
Uneven parallel bars		14

From ref. 11, with permission.

only apparatuses in gymnastics that can lead to serious neurotrauma if used improperly. Also as found earlier, safety in gymnastics is a feasible expectation if reasonable controls and supervision are in place. The results of the first 4 years of the study indicate that catastrophic injuries in gymnastics have lessened substantially since the mid-1970s as a result of increased compliance with recommended controls.

In the fall of 1975, while Clarke was preparing the retrospective survey of spinal cord injuries in school sports and physical education, Torg et al. (15) were establishing a National Football Head and Neck Injury Registry patterned after the clinical case finding method used by Schneider (16) in 1963. Initially, Torg et al. solicited retrospective documentation of catastrophic causes experienced during the 1971 through 1975 seasons to have a 5-year period comparable with that of Schneider's survey (1959 through 1963). In cooperation with the AFCA program, Torg continued to maintain the registry as a continuous surveillance system for catastrophic injuries other than fatalities. In 1985, Torg completed a survey review of the status of all athletes in the registry and made some (minor) changes in the original data published earlier.

Tables 9 and 10 compare the findings of Torg et al. for catastrophic injury patterns in football during 1971 through 1975 with Clarke's findings for 1973 through 1975. The degree of comparability lends credence to the principal injury scenario of a defensive back coming up to make an open-field tackle.

Tables 11 and 12 display the different patterns of serious neurotrauma in high school and col-

TABLE 6. *Average annual incidence of spinal cord injury in high school– and college-sponsored sports, 1973–1975*

Sport	Athletes per case	Programs per case
Gymnastics, men	7,000	281
Gymnastics, women	24,000	1,113
Football	28,000	403
Wrestling	62,000	1,781
Baseball	177,000	6,254
Basketball, men	793,000	23,024

From ref. 11, with permission.

TABLE 8. *National incidence of gymnastics-related catastrophic injuries, July 1978 through June 1982*

Event	Sex of participant	Characteristics of participant	Circumstances	Injury
Trampoline	M	Skilled teenager	Practice, gymnastic club	Quadriplegia
Trampoline	M	Young boy	Backyard recreation	Death
Trampoline	M	Skilled young adult	Backyard game of "horse"	Quadriplegia
Trampoline	M	Advanced beginner teen	Military base recreation	Quadriplegia
Trampoline	M	College assistant instructor	Class demonstration	Quadriplegia
Minitrampoline	M	College cheerleader	Warm-up for football game	Quadriplegia
Minitrampoline	M	High school gymnast	Practice for pep rally	Quadriplegia
Tumbling	F	High school cheerleader	Cheerleader practice	Death
Trampoline	M	College gymnast	Practice high-bar dismount	Quadriplegia
Uneven parallel bars	F	High school gymnast	Practicing routine	Quadriplegia
Minitrampoline	F	College cheerleader	Unscheduled practice	Quadriplegia
Minitrampoline	F	High school	Practice for competition	Quadriplegia
Trampoline	M	Skilled young adult	Backyard recreation	Quadriplegia
Minitrampoline	M	Skilled college student	Intramural activity	Quadriplegia
Uneven parallel bars	M	College gymnast	Practice for competition	Quadriplegia
Trampoline	M	College physical education assistant	Demonstration in class	Quadriplegia
Vault	F	Unskilled high school student	Physical education class	Quadriplegia
Trampoline	M	College student	Physical education class	Quadriplegia
Uneven parallel bars	F	Unskilled junior high school student	Physical education class	Death
Rings	M	Semiskilled high school student	Physical education class	Quadriplegia

From ref. 14, with permission.

lege football during 1959 through 1963 and 1971 through 1975. Essentially, both the frequency of and mortality from serious cerebral injuries had decreased. Serious cervical cord injuries, on the other hand, had increased (unless they were disguised by Schneider's 60% response rate). Their predominantly nonfatal nature had precluded detection of this trend through the annual fatality report.

As seen in Fig. 2, however, the registry of Torg et al. (8) reveals a distinct drop in quadri-

plegia after 1976, confirming the wisdom of the nature of the rule changes that had been adopted. Because the rule changes in 1976 required profound adjustments of athlete, coach, and official to new expectations and different techniques, the 1-year lag in their impact was not unexpected. In fact, the continued lowering of the incidence of

TABLE 9. *Proportion of quadriplegic cases in high school and college football associated with tackling*

Level	Torg (%, 1971–1975)	Clarke (%, 1973–1975)
High school	72	83
College	78	83

From refs. 11 and 15, with permission.

TABLE 10. *Proportion of quadriplegic cases in high school and college football associated with selected positions*

Position	Torg (%, 1971–1975)	Clarke (%, 1973–1975)
Defensive back		
High school	52	50
College	73	67
Linebacker		
High school	10	29
College	0	0

From refs. 11 and 15, with permission.

TABLE 11. *Comparison of permanent cerebral injuries nationally in high school and college football*

Statistic	Schneider (1959–1963)	Torg (1971–1975)
Total cases reported	112	72
High school and college cases	87 (estimated)	65
Average annual incidence per 100,000 athletes	2.6 (estimated)	1.0
Fatal cases	41%	81%

From refs. 15 and 16, with permission.

football-related quadriplegia after 1980 may be attributable to the extension of widespread educational efforts and broader acceptance of the rule changes. It must be remembered that the "face-into-the-number" technique for blocking and tackling was considered the proper football position before 1976, that there was great resistance to compliance until the epidemiologic data had covered a sufficient number of years to prove the point, and that it took years for that technique to be "unlearned" by the players who had participated in football prior to 1976.

Calculated as rates, the incidence of permanent cervical cord injury, nonfatal and fatal combined, 1 per 100,000 athletes in 1977 and 1978, had returned to roughly the same value as the incidence during the 1960 period of Schneider's study (Table 12).

Thus the various efforts in the late 1960s to develop mandatory helmet standards and the teaching and practice of blocking and tackling tech-

TABLE 12. *Comparison of permanent cervical spinal cord injuries nationally in high school and college football*

Statistic	Schneider (1959–1963)	Torg (1971–1975)
Total cases reported	38	99
High school and college cases	35 (estimated)	95
Average annual incidence per 100,000 athletes	1.0 (estimated)	1.5
Fatal cases	42%	8%

From refs. 15 and 16, with permission.

niques eventually resulted in a decline in the frequency of both fatal and nonfatal catastrophic neurotrauma. This does not mean that all helmets in use at the time were substandard; it means that all helmet models being sold had not yet been subjected to performance tests that would provide confidence that they were not substandard. Similarly, this does not mean that coaches were necessarily teaching an improper technique; it means that improper execution of certain techniques constituted a highly serious hazard.

The comparison of the data of Torg et al. (15) and Schneider (16) initially suggested that a trade-off was occurring; the request for helmet standards was associated with both lowered cerebral injury frequencies and increased cervical cord injuries. To some this meant that the modern helmet was literally causing these injuries (i.e., the back of the helmet was forcibly impinging on the spine), instead of, or in addition to, prompting the well-protected athlete to "stick his head and neck in places where he never used to." Nevertheless, the distinct drop in the frequency of cervical cord injuries since 1976 disconfirms the implication of the helmets as causative agents. The premise for the 1976 rule changes was that helmets can neither cause nor prevent serious neck injuries; it is principally a matter of the blocking and tackling technique. The available epidemiologic data remain consistent with that contention.

As was the case for fatalities alone, the trends in relative frequency of all cervical neurotrauma, which by 1978 had returned to that of 1960, do not support an indictment of the face mask as a causative agent.

Peripheral Nerve Injury

The incidence of injury to peripheral nerve in sports is largely unknown. Peripheral nerve injuries in sports are relatively uncommon and are not typically detected by injury surveillance systems interested in more severe or catastrophic injury. Concern regarding the frequency of peripheral nerve injury in sport arose primarily from football. With the rule changes in 1976 requiring a return to shoulder-blocking and tackling techniques, concern was frequently expressed about an increase in brachial plexus injuries resulting

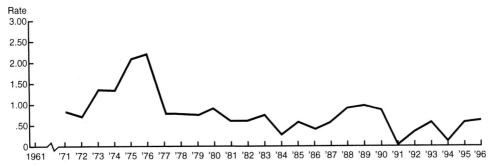

FIG. 2. Football permanent quadriplegic injuries, per 100,000 high school and college players combined.

from these changes. The potential for this had been acknowledged by those encouraging the 1976 changes, but the trade-off between "burners" and quadriplegia presented no argument.

Interestingly, NAIRS data reveal no shift in frequency of reportable or significant brachial plexus injuries after 1976 (Table 13). The slight rise in 1978 is currently not significant (i.e., is well within the range of normal variation). Table 13 also permits examination of this concern on the basis of the proportion of such injuries resulting from tackling (the principal activity associated with this injury). A steady increase in this association is seen among significant brachial plexus injuries from 1975 to 1977 (31% to 47%). In 1978, however, this trend was clearly reversed. It is plausible to assume that the new coaching techniques for tackling have evolved into improved methods or that better neck-conditioning practices have been implemented.

PREVENTION

Much attention has been given in this chapter to the capability of epidemiologic information to spot areas in which preventive measures could be effective and then to confirm or disconfirm whether those measures were indeed effective. Helmet standards, skill techniques, and supervisory expectation were among the preventive measures. Relevant to both football and the trampoline has been the affixing of a warning label as a necessary adjunctive preventive measure, the contention being that the label would

not just advise the athlete that he or she could be hurt if the equipment is used improperly but also help instruct on the method of preventing serious neurotrauma.

Trampoline manufacturers began adding warning labels to trampoline beds in the mid-1970s, and football helmet manufacturers began adding warning labels to helmets in the early 1980s (in addition to implementing other educational measures). How much these actions were undertaken because of legal prudence (to avoid lawsuits filed only because of the absence of warning labels) cannot be determined from the literature. No epidemiologic information is available to support that intervention as an effective and thereby necessary deterrent to injury, however. Furthermore, the existing research literature on the effectiveness of warning labels in any arena of consumer product use definitely does not support the use of warning labels as a preventive measure in society or sport.

TABLE 13. *Rate (cases per 100 athletes) of brachial plexus injuries in collegiate football accompanied by proportion of such injuries associated with tackling*

Parameter	1975	1976	1977	1978
Reportable cases	2.2	2.2	2.2	2.4
(while tackling)	45%	47%	43%	38%
Significant cases	0.5	0.5	0.5	0.7
(while tackling)	31%	40%	47%	27%

From National Athletic Injury/Illness Reporting System, Pennsylvania State University, 1979.

After reviewing 400 articles covering this topic, McCarthy et al. (17) reported to the Human Factors Society in 1984, citing some revealing studies for illustration, that "We have yet to identify a product that, when evaluated in an unbiased manner, clearly demonstrates the utility of any warning label which was placed on the product. . . . In the face of evidence that warning labels do not positively impact safety, use of on product warning labels must be judged at best an ineffective safety measure and potentially a misallocation of safety resources."

Horst et al. (18) updated this review 2 years later, commenting further that "From a Human Factors perspective, excessive warnings are as bad as insufficient warnings. People become accustomed to the warnings and tend to ignore them. Warnings should be reserved for high-probability events. . . . Attention to the presentation and format of safety messages is not sufficient to change safety-related behavior."

DISCUSSION

Catastrophic neurotrauma in organized sports is infrequent yet consistently associated with gymnastics, football, and wrestling. Such injuries occur periodically in other active sports, such as baseball and basketball, but not with the persistence that would enable epidemiologic analysis.

From the catastrophic data at hand, for fatal and nonfatal injuries, the definitive measures adopted by those sharing responsibility for school and college sports have been followed by a substantial lessening of the problems that were identified.

1. The clarification of guidelines for the controlled use of the trampoline and minitrampoline in high school and college programs has been followed (to date) by a drop in catastrophic injuries resulting from these activities.

2. The decision to promulgate uniform testing standards for football helmets in the late 1960s was accompanied by a downward trend in serious cerebral trauma.

3. The decision, in 1976, to outlaw by rule and ethic the use of the helmeted head as the initial point of contact in blocking and tackling was followed by both another drop in fatal cerebral injuries and a substantial drop in fatal cervical spinal cord injuries. Moreover, the latter changes have not caused (to date) an anticipated increase in another type of neurologic injury, that to the brachial plexus.

In addition, analysis of epidemiologic data disconfirmed the possibility that a particular type or brand of helmet or playing surface was a determinant in cerebral injuries in football. Furthermore, continuous use of the face mask during the period of evaluation was not associated with any trends that would suggest its involvement as a determinant in serious neck injuries related to hyperextension and impingement on the cervical vertebrae. This has since been corroborated by clinical and biomechanical studies.

In football, as in gymnastics and probably wrestling and other sports for which reliable data are not available, the problem of neurotrauma is principally a matter of player technique, equipment standards, and supervision. Education of coaches, athletes, and officials about the catastrophic hazards of improper techniques should continue to be emphasized in preventive efforts.

A catastrophic injury, however, is only one outcome on an injury spectrum of graded severity stemming from a particular etiologic mechanism. It is advisable to monitor continuously any injury pattern that is associated with the threat of permanent impairment.

REFERENCES

1. Blyth C, Arnold D. *The forty-seventh annual football fatality report.* Chapel Hill, NC: American Football Coaches Association, 1979.
2. Clarke K. Calculated risk of sports fatalities. *JAMA* 1966;197:894.
3. Competitive sports and their hazards. *Stat Bull Metrop Life Insur Co* 1965;461:1.
4. Clarke K., Braslow A. Football fatalities in actuarial perspective. *Med Sci Sports* 1979;10:94.
5. AMA Committee on the Medical Aspects of Sports. Spearing and football. In: *Tips on athletic training*, vol 10. Chicago: American Medical Association, 1968:6–7.
6. *Shared responsibility for sports safety. A statement of the Committee of Competitive Safeguards and Medical As-*

pects of Sports. Shawnee Mission, KS: National Collegiate Athletic Association, 1978.

7. Clarke K, Powell J. Football helmets and neurotrauma—an epidemiological overview of three seasons. *Med Sci Sports* 1979;11:138.

8. Torg J, Vegso JJ, Sennelt B, Das M. The National Football Head and Neck Injury Registry, 14-year report on cervical quadriplegia, 1971 through 1984. *JAMA* 1985; 254:3439–3443.

9. Clarke K, Alles W, Powell J. An epidemiological examination of the association of selected products with related injuries in football, 1975–77. Final report, US Consumer Product Safety Commission (contract CPSC-C-77-0039), 1978.

10. Kraus JF. Epidemiologic features of injuries to the central nervous system. In: Anderson DW, ed. *Neuroepidemiology, a tribute to Bruce Schoenberg.* Boca Raton, FL: CRC Press, 1991:333–357.

11. Clarke K. Survey of spinal cord injuries in schools and college sports, 1973–75. *J Safety Res* 1977;9:140.

12. The use of the trampoline for the development of competitive skills: a policy statement of the American Al-liance for Health, Physical Education, Recreation, and Dance. Washington, DC, 1978.

13. The use of the trampoline for the development of competitive skills: a policy statement of the National Collegiate Athletic Association Committee on Competitive Safeguards and Medical Aspects of Sports. Shawnee Mission, KS: National Collegiate Athletic Association; 1978.

14. Christensen C, Clarke K, et al. Fourth Annual Gymnastics Catastrophic Injury Report (1979–82). Washington, DC: US Gymnastics Safety Association, 1984.

15. Torg J, Truex R Jr, Quedenfeld TC, Burstein A, Spealman A, Nichols C 3d. The National Football Head and Neck Injury Registry. Report and conclusions, 1978. *JAMA* 1979;241:1477.

16. Schneider, R. Serious and fatal neurosurgical football injuries. *Clin Neurosurg* 1965;12:226.

17. McCarthy R, et al. Product information presentation, user behavior, and safety. *Proc Hum Factor Soc* 1984: 81–85.

18. Horst, DP, et al. Safety information presentation: factors influencing the potential for changing behavior. *Proc Hum Factors Soc* 1986:111–115.

Sports Neurology, Second Edition,
edited by Barry D. Jordan.
Lippincott–Raven Publishers, Philadelphia © 1998.

2

Sports Neuropsychology

Erik J. T. Matser

Department of Sports Neurology, St. Anna Hospital, 5660 AB Geldrop, The Netherlands

This chapter deals with an Achilles dilemma variant. Young athletes perform in heroic circumstances, celebrating wins and not realizing real losses. For some athletes, at the end of the career, their fit body will become their dead, worn-out changed enemy.

In thinking about sports neuropsychology and writing this chapter, I realized that there is no uniformity in the treatment of brain-injured athletes and no uniformity in "return to play" regulations (1–5). It is notable that millions of athletes incur concussions annually and that there is no uniformity in classifying these concussions.

Injury to the brain is one of the leading causes of disability in the industrialized nations (6,7). A significant part of these injuries are incurred in sports; 4% to 22% of all traumatic brain injury (TBI) treated in hospitals are sports related (8–11).

TBIs incurred in sports can have devastating effects on cognitive functioning and social behavior. Coaches may not be aware of the impact of TBIs on cognition and emotional behavior (12–15). Frequently, an athlete's physical recovery from a TBI creates expectations for adequate functioning. However, a normal physical appearance can severely mask underlying cognitive and social deficits associated with the TBI.

In this chapter the term head injury refers to any traumatic injury to the head and face. These injuries are frequently accompanied by cervical injury. The brain may be, but is not necessarily, injured. Damage may be restricted to soft tissue, vasculature, and peripheral nerves. Head injury should not be used interchangeably with traumatic brain injury because head injury, by definition, does not imply damage to the brain.

TBI is a consequence of head injury in which damage to the head results in damage to the brain. Damage may result in symptoms that are transient or permanent. Long-term impairment may be absent, trivial, or severe (16).

TBI incurred in sports has been the focus of increasing attention. Two articles have been published in which a neurologist and a neuropsychologist working with athletes provided information about treatment of brain-injured athletes (17,18). In these articles the authors showed their concern about treatment and follow-up of athletes who sustained TBI and who are at risk for severe brain injuries.

The articles highlighted three main issues that should be addressed by any guidelines for the management of TBI in sport: (a) appropriate management of the injured athlete at the time of injury, (b) prevention of a catastrophic outcome related to acute brain swelling, and (c) avoidance of cumulative brain injury caused by repeated concussions and the accumulations of trivial traumas.

TBI incurred in sports is caused by a single heavy blow to the head or cumulations of mild traumatic brain injury (MTBI). Matser (19) showed that the number of "headers" in professional soccer and the number of professional soccer training sessions had a negative association with memory and planning capacity.

Deficits in attention and concentration, memory, planning, executive functions, speed of information processing, and visual spatial and visuual perceptual processing are the most frequently reported cognitive sequelae of TBIs in both adults and children (20–33).

As memory, speed of information processing, planning, and attention are critical for adequate functioning in even the most basic aspects of everyday life, deficits in these processes often contribute to disability after TBI (29).

Psychopathologic factors are highly correlated with TBI. Affective disorders in particular are found to be substantially involved in the sequelae of TBI (34). Anxiety and a depressed mood are common but poorly substantiated and documented. Deterioration of quality of life, duration of illness, response to intellectual and cognitive impairments, and perception of discrepancy between a normal lifestyle and a lifestyle with shortcomings and physical disability are risk factors for developing such outcomes (35).

CAUSES OF TRAUMATIC BRAIN INJURIES IN SPORTS

Initial Mechanical Damaging Factors

A change in the velocity of the brain caused by a blow to the cranium can produce linear and rotational movements of the brain within the skull (36). When the skull and the brain within it are accelerated in a straight-line direction, coup–contrecoup injuries can occur. The bruise spots at the impact side are called coup lesions; contrecoup lesions are bruise spots to the brain in the area opposite the blow (37).

After a rapid rotation of the head (for example, when an athlete is hit by a head blow coming in at an angle) diffuse axonal injury (DAI) and stretching and snapping of blood vessels may occur. The rotation of the brain within the cranial vault tends to be delayed relative to the initiating change in velocity, because of the brain's intrinsic inertia. This lagging movement of the brain leads to stretching and shearing forces on the fibers (DAI) and blood vessels (38–45).

The brain can also be injured when the moving head suddenly stops as in falls or collisions. The moving head and the brain within it are stopped, which is followed by a sudden deceleration until the brain's movement stabilizes. Coup–contrecoup injuries and shearing injuries can result. Falls on the back of the head may result in fracture of the skull and contrecoup contusions on the orbital surface of the frontal lobes and the tips of the temporal lobes. Furthermore, the accelerating–decelerating brain slides around within the cranial cavity. This can result in small hemorrhages in both the cortical gray matter and subcortical white matter (46). In general, TBI is often a result of an interaction between linear and rotational forces and is seldom due to a pure rotational or linear acceleration (47).

Brain damage can also be induced by hypoxia. Martial arts strangulation techniques, for example, in which the blood supply to the brain is blocked by pressure on the carotid arteries, can produce hypoxia and unconsciousness if the victim fails to submit (48).

Secondary Damaging Factors

TBI occurs in different ways, involves different mechanisms, and results in different types of clinical disorders. The speed, localization, and direction of mechanical force at impact are factors that contribute to the pattern of neuropsychologic alterations.

Most TBI is not immediate; brain damage should be seen as a process and not as an event (38). The sequelae of TBI depend not only on the primary mechanical damage but also on the pre-existent functions and the complex interaction of pathophysiologic events that follow the initial distortion of brain tissue (38,49–58).

CONCUSSIONS

Concussions are often incurred in sports. Kelly and Rosenberg (17) define concussion as a trauma-induced alteration in mental status that may or may not involve loss of consciousness.

Some frequently observed features of concussion are vacant stare, inability to focus attention, disorientation (walking in the wrong direction, being unaware of time, data, place), slurred or incoherent speech, incoordination, emotional lability, memory deficits, problems with abstract reasoning, slowed reaction time, slowed mental and motor speed, problems with planning and judgment, and difficulties in processing novel or complex visual spatial stimuli (32,34,39,44,60–71).

Symptoms of concussion can be classified as early and late. Early symptoms (minutes to hours after injury) are headache, dizziness or vertigo, lack of awareness of surroundings, nausea, and vomiting. Late symptoms (days to weeks after injury) are persistent low-grade headache, lightheadedness, poor attention and concentration, memory dysfunction, easy fatigability, irritability and low frustration tolerance, intolerance of bright lights or difficulty focusing vision, intolerance of loud noises, sometimes ringing in the ears, anxiety and depressed mood, sleep disturbances, memory problems, inefficient information processing, inadequate perceptual processing, problems with planning, and slowed reaction time (17,70,72,73).

Case

A 12-year-old girl visited the department of sports neurology. She fell from a horse and hit a wooden fence. She lost consciousness for several minutes and was dazed for some hours. She was not able to go to school for some weeks because of headaches, nausea, and dizziness. After she went back to school, her school performance significantly deteriorated. Neuropsychologic examination 8 months after the injury showed problems in memory, attention, planning, speed of information processing, impulsiveness, and emotional lability.

Cumulative effects of concussion—that is, disabling headache, classic migraine, and delayed recovery of brain function (after a second concussion)—have been reported in studies of MTBI (74,75). Gronwall and Wrightson (32) found that deficits in information storage and retrieval were exacerbated by successive injuries.

Case

A 30-year-old professional soccer player visited the department of sports neurology. He complained of severe headaches, memory problems, difficulty in doing two things at a time, and irritability. At the interview, he told the neuropsychologist that he had lost consciousness twice during the season and was stunned by a collision once. Neuropsychologic testing showed selective and sustained attention and concentration problems, verbal retrieval problems, and fatigue, and the player complained of increasing headaches after performing tests of a long duration. After cessation of soccer for 6 months, the headaches disappeared and the cognitive dysfunction dissipated.

To sustain a repeated concussion when someone is still symptomatic can be life threatening (see Chapter 17). The second impact syndrome is thought to be the result of a second concussion occurring while the individual is still symptomatic from an earlier concussion. In second-impact syndrome the athlete suffers from brain swelling and marked increase in intracranial pressure. Animal research has shown that this type of brain swelling is difficult to control (17).

WHIPLASH

Acceleration and deceleration of the cervical spine may result in a postwhiplash syndrome. During whiplash the head is subject to acceleration forces that result in bending of the neck. Although classically described in association with movements in the saggital plane, it is clear that a whiplash injury may also follow lateral and frontal impacts (76).

Patients who suffered concussions and victims of whiplash injury of the cervical spine may share common neuropsychologic symptoms (77). Torres and Shapiro (78) compared 45 patients suffering from whiplash injuries and 45 suffering from MTBIs and found similar symptoms in the two groups. Headaches, nervousness, tenseness, restlessness, vertigo, and difficulty in concentrating were common in both groups.

From reviews of emergency room records, it is evident that cervical spine injuries commonly accompany head injuries. The energy transfer in the fall or hit does not need to be of great magnitude to produce a cervical injury, and this should be taken into account when taking care of an injured athlete who suffers a head injury.

Case

A 31-year-old rugby player complained of neck and shoulder pain, headaches, and cognitive deficits after he was hit in the back during a jump. There was no head impact. The day after the match his shoulders and neck were stiff and he was dizzy and lightheaded. For a period of 3 months the rugby player was easily fatigued, could not concentrate properly, and complained of planning and memory problems. He had to perform tasks one after another and he had a limited amount of energy. During the day the fatigue increased and in the evening he was worn out. Even sleep disturbances were reported.

The neuropsychologic tests (6 weeks after the impact) revealed visual memory problems, difficulties regarding divided and sustained attention, and lessened cognitive flexibility. The rugby player reported more neckaches and headaches after tests with a long duration. Three months after the injury he was able to join his team for training.

FRONTAL LOBE DAMAGE

The functions of the frontal lobes, particularly the prefrontal areas, are among neuropsychology's greatest mysteries. Famous researchers in neuroscience describe the frontal lobes as a riddle, as the youngest and most complex and the least studied portion of the cerebral hemisphere, or as the most mystifying of the major subdivisions of the cerebral cortex (79–82).

The frontal cortex can be divided into regions. Damasio and Anderson (83) divided the frontal cortex into the precentral (motor)–premotor cortex, the prefrontal cortex, and the limbic cortex. Milner (84) subdivided the prefrontal cortex into two functional areas: dorsolateral and orbital. Others (85) subdivided it into three areas; dorsolateral, orbital, and

medial. Still others (86) identify basal medial, dorsolateral, mesial, and orbital areas.

Depending on the cause and location, a variety of frontal lobe symptoms can appear. Social and behavioral changes, affective changes, and cognitive changes can be the result of frontal lobe damage (13).

Personality changes, including changes in social behavior, impulsiveness, and deterioration of cognitive processing that regulates planning and decision making, are the most disabling and characteristic changes that sometimes result from frontal lobe damage (87). Lack of foresight, tact, and concern and inability to plan ahead or judge the consequences of actions can result from frontal lobe damage (86,88,89). This may lead to antisocial conduct and conflicts with the law.

Cognitive frontal lobe problems are characterized by difficulties in cognitive flexibility, memory, planning, initiation, and attention and poor judgment and impulse control (86). Frontal deficits affect memory and other cognitive processes through poor organization, inability to use effective strategies, and susceptibility to interference (90).

Cognitive flexibility refers to the ability to switch lines of thought. It is essential for adaptation to novelty (91). Perseverations may be seen as the converse of flexibility. An example of perseveration of thought is demonstrated in the next case.

Case

A soccer player with a right-sided frontal lobe injury caused by a collision with a soccer goalkeeper visited the department of sports neurology. On verbal tests, the athlete had to name words beginning with the letter N. After he named Dutch cities starting with "new," we asked him to name other words starting with the letter N. He produced "new bike" and "new car."

WHITE MATTER INJURIES

Brain functioning depends on cerebral white matter, which facilitates network communication (92). White matter disorders can impair cognitive functioning with effects ranging from inattention and memory disturbance to severe dementia or persistent vegetative state (93). Research data show increasingly clearly that deficits in the speed of information processing, attention and concentration, memory retrieval, and abstract reasoning are associated with white matter abnormalities as seen on magnetic resonance imaging (MRI) (94–97). Deficits of this sort appear only when a certain threshold of white matter involvement is reached (98). It is conceivable that some of the posttraumatic neuropsychologic changes (e.g., cognitive slowing, memory and concentration problems) may be due to in part to changes in cerebral white matter (99). Affective disorders and psychosis, as a result of white matter damage, may also occur (100).

TRAUMATIC BRAIN INJURIES
IN SPORTS

In almost any sport, cranial injuries and TBI occur (101). Of all TBI cases, 4% to 22% treated in hospitals are incurred in sports (8–11). TBI in sports is not limited to adults; the rate of TBI in children (0 to 15 years old) caused by sporting activities and treated in hospitals is 11% (51).

In some sports the head is the target. In other sports, such as soccer, the head is an element of playing the game ("heading" balls). The brain can also be injured in sports by accidents such as collisions or by tools used in play (e.g., sticks). It is obvious that in almost any sport, there is a risk for sustaining a TBI or accumulations of TBIs.

TBI incurred in sports is caused not only by prolonged participation in a single sport with well-known risks for head injury but also by concurrent participation by an athlete in a number of sports, all of which result in blows to the head, a concept termed sports synergy (9,10).

The most common TBI in sports is a concussion, estimated to occur in the United States at a rate of 250,000 per year in American football alone (61,102,103). It can also result from falls in all forms of athletic activity and from collisions (17,104). Concussions may occur without the athletes ever suffering loss of conciousness. For that reason it is difficult to recognize a sports-related concussion.

Severe brain injury incurred in sports is fortunately relatively rare. Certain sports by their design (punches, collisions, headers, high speed) are more likely to result in the occurrence of severe TBI. These include the contact sports such as football, boxing, ice hockey, rugby, soccer, and the martial arts (105). In recreational athletic activities, severe TBIs occur at one of the highest rates in downhill skiing. Many of these serious injuries occur as a result of high-speed falls and collisions with trees and other skiers (106).

Athletes can even develop a severe chronic progressive traumatic encephalopathy (dementia pugilistica) after being exposed to a cumulation of mild traumatic brain injuries. The syndrome follows a three-stage clinical pattern (107–110). The first stage is manifested by affective disturbances and mild motor incoordination. In the second stage, affective symptoms increase; paranoid ideas and mild dysarthria and tremor may appear. The third stage is characterized by a decrease in general cognitive functions (memory deficits, dysarthria, motor incoordination), impaired hearing, hyperreflexia, and intention tremor. Furthermore, dementia, personality change (immaturity, aggressiveness, suspiciousness), and social instability have been described.

Some athletes receive several thousand head blows during a career (46). As the effects of repeated MTBI may be cumulative (32,111–113), it has been suggested that an encephalopathy similar to that seen in boxing (107–109,114) may also occur in other sports. In 1976 Corsellis (115) asked 165 British neurologists if they had encountered a condition resembling the "punch drunk" state among either boxers or athletes of any category. Professional soccer was mentioned five times.

NEUROPSYCHOLOGIC ASSESSMENT

In the 1940s a science called neuropsychology separated itself from the disciplines of neurology and psychology. An important component of neuropsychologic evaluation is that of providing descriptions (quantitative and qualitative measurements of behavior) of the extent to which individuals manifest specific cognitive, sensory, emotional, and social characteristics. These

TABLE 1. *Sports neuropsychologic assessment procedures*

Sports battery used by Matser
Sports population: boxers and soccer players

History taking
Raven Progressive Matrices
Paced Auditory Serial Addition Task
California verbal word learning task
Wechsler Memory Scale Revised
Figure of Rey
  Copy
  Immediate recall
  Delayed recall
Trailmaking Test forms A and B
Stroop Test
  Card I (words)
  Card II (colors)
  Card III (interference)
Bourdon–Wiersma test (sustained attention task)
The Symbol Digits Modalities Test
Figure Detection
The Puncture Test
Benton Facial Recognition Task
Wisconsin Card Sorting Task
Beck's Questionnaire

Sports battery used by Julian Bailes
Sports population: professionals of
  National Football League

Orientation questionnaire
Digit Span Test
Stroop Test
Trailmaking Test forms A and B
Symbol Digits Modalities
Controlled Oral Word Association test
Hopkins Verbal Learning Task
Grooved Pegboard Task

Sports battery used by Wayne Alves
Sports population: university football players

Smith's Symbol Digit Test
Paced Auditory Serial Addition Task
Ammon's Quick Test
Psychiatric Research Epidemiology Interview (Peri)
Anxiety Scale (six-item questionnaire)
Sadness Scale (four-item questionnaire)
Enervation Scale (six-item questionnaire)
Insomnia Scale (three-item questionnaire)
Confused Thinking Scale (four-item questionnaire)
Other questionaire items
Symptoms and complaints
Previous athletic experience
Medical history of head injury
Injury event and details
Problems with school, family, and other domains

Sports battery used in the Johns Hopkins Study
Sports population: U.S. amateur boxers

Digit Symbol Modalities
Digit Span Forward
Digit Span Backward
Rey Auditory Verbal Learning Test
Rey Complex Figure
  Copy
  Immediate recall
Block Design (subtest, Wechsler Adult
  Intelligence Scale)
Grooved Pegboard for Left and Right Hand
Sharpened Romberg
Beam Eyes Opened
Beam Eyes Closed

characteristics can reflect abnormalities in brain–behavior associations (116). Qualitative measurements rely more on careful intensive observations of the abnormal or normal responses and behavior of the individual. An accurate assessment methodology should incorporate both quantitative and qualitative measurements.

In the past decade, neuropsychologic assessment entered the arena of sports medicine. The sports neuropsychologist assesses brain function by studying athletes' cognitive, sensory, motor, emotional, and social behavior. Neuropsychologic tests and observations of the subject enable the neuropsychologist to measure, quantify, and qualify declines of mental, cognitive, and social functioning associated with TBI in athletes.

There are several sports neuropsychologic assessment procedures (Table 1), and, strikingly, there is no uniform concept in these procedures. Some test batteries have their focus mainly on neuropsychiatric changes and others have a more cognitive focus.

WHY NEUROPSYCHOLOGY IN SPORTS MEDICINE? (Figs. 1–3)

Continued neuropsychologic follow-up of athletes and sideline testing shortly after injury are informative about whether symptoms of TBI are present, lessened, transient, or progressive. With a neuropsychologic assessment procedure athletes can be tested or retested during a season (e.g., after a TBI or suspicion of one). Annual baseline testing (done in the preseason) and sideline testing (examination shortly after injury) should have high priority.

A

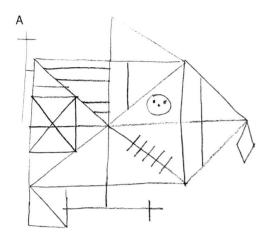

B

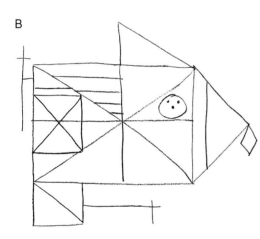

C

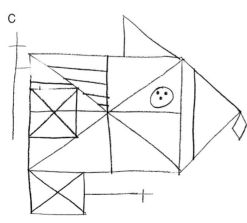

FIG. 1. Control group, 27 years, no head injury.
A: Copy of the Figure of Rey. **B:** Immediate recall. **C:** Delayed recall.

Example: incorporated baseline and sideline testing in the Philips Soccer Team Eindhoven

All the players of the professional Philips Soccer Team Eindhoven (PSV) are tested annually by a neurologist and a neuropsychologist (preseason). The team physician performs sideline testing when a TBI is suspected after a head blow or collision. If the results of sideline testing are positive, the player is sent to the department of sports neurology for neurologic and neuropsychologic examinations. After the player has recovered to his previous neurologic and cognitive baseline level, he can return to competition.

The diagnosis and demonstration of decline in mental status are valuable for the athlete, team physicians, trainers, coaches, officials, and relatives of the athlete. They can obtain insight into and understanding of the extent and improvement of the injury.

In addition, computed tomography and MRI often do not show evidence of morphologic abnormalities after MTBI and the neurologic evaluation is often within normal limits. However, the neuropsychologic examination can provide useful information and detect mild cognitive abnormalities consistent with TBI.

Effective neuropsychologic testing in athletes must cover cognitive and emotional problems, be reproducible, and be somewhat tailored for the examination. In research and baseline testing, test batteries can be advised. However, in some cases, rigid use of test batteries in these circumstances can be questioned. In some professional sports large numbers of athletes with different cultural backgrounds play on the same team, and invalid results, for example, in fluency tasks, may be due to cultural differences. After an athlete incurs a severe TBI the neuropsychologist should select tests that are sensitive to the problems the athlete is complaining of, as in normal practice.

POPULATION OF PATIENTS IN SPORTS NEUROPSYCHOLOGY

The Assessment Process

In this section tests and assessment techniques are presented for most neuropsychologic assessment

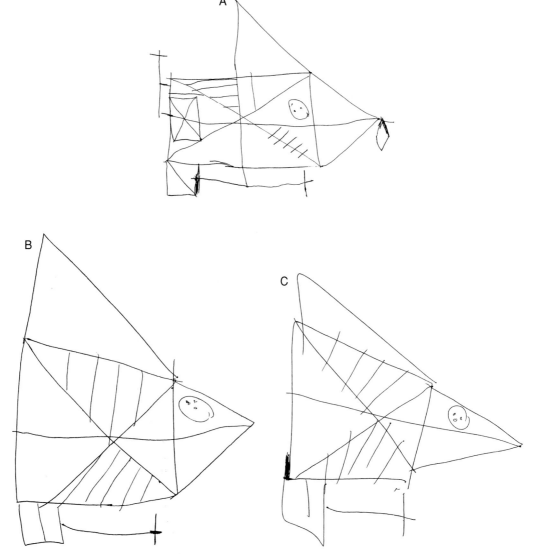

FIG. 2. Professional boxer, 28 years, 22 professional bouts. **A:** Copy of the Figure of Rey. **B:** Immediate recall. **C:** Delayed recall.

purposes in an athlete population. The tests used for athletes should include a wide range of tests of cognitive functions. History taking and questionnaires should be added to detect cognitive, emotional, and social deviations. In a battery developed for athletes, concentration, reaction time, mental and motor speed, new learning (memory), planning, sequencing abilities, and judgment should have high priority. These cognitive func-

tions are most prone to deteriorate after MTBI and the accumulation of trivial traumata (19–33,117,118).

The neuropsychologic test procedure usually starts with an interview (history taking). The athlete's behavior during the interview can add information about cognitive and emotional disturbances (35). Detailed history taking is essential for neuropsychologic evaluation; it gives the neuropsy-

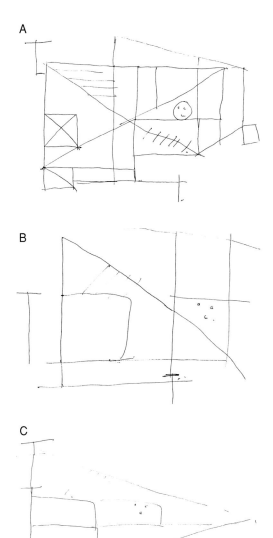

FIG. 3. Retired soccer player, defense position, 12 years professional soccer. **A:** Copy of the Figure of Rey. **B:** Immediate recall. **C:** Delayed recall.

ring to abstract reasoning, concept formation, planning, memory, attention and concentration, visual perception (spatial processes and object identification), fine motor behavior, language, executive functions, and emotional status. The test scores, test performance, and emotional status provide information about cognitive status and severity of injury.

Return to Play

There are no uniform guidelines for return to play. The American Academy of Neurology suggested guidelines for return to play after concussion (Table 2). Matser uses cognitive test scores as a guideline for return to play. An athlete is suspended from competition after sustaining TBI and can return to competition only when the athlete's cognitive status is normalized to the baseline level. The threshold for a stop is 1 or 1.5 standard deviations below the athlete's intrapersonal norm score. Return to play is permitted only when an athlete is within the limit of 0.5 standard deviation from his or her intrapersonal norm. McCrory et al. (3) advocate that players who are concussed and have convulsions can return within 2 weeks after the incident and that prohibition from collision sports is unwarranted.

CONCLUDING REMARKS

The neuropsychologic evaluation of athletes can add valuable information for the neurologic diagnosis, especially when there is suspicion of chronic TBI, MTBI or deleterious effects of cumulations of MTBI. The neuropsychologic evaluation can be of importance for the athlete and coach regarding return to play and health considerations.

Acknowledgment

When starting a sports neuropsychology practice in The Netherlands, Professor Muriel D. Lezak (Oregon Health Science University, Portland) was helpful with advice and support. Several ideas in this chapter are derived from her personally and from her outstanding book *Neuropsychological Assessment,* 3rd edition.

chologist useful information for a correct diagnosis and the impact of the disorder on daily life (116).

After the interview, cognitive tests and questionnaires are administered to detect intact and disturbed cognitive functions and emotional status. The neuropsychologist can select tests refer-

TABLE 2. *American Academy of Neurology guidelines for the management of concussion in sports*

Grade	Recommendations
Grade 1: Transient confusion; no loss of consciousness; concussion symptoms or mental status abnormalities that resolve in less than 15 min	1. Remove from contest. 2. May return to contest if mental status abnormalities or postconcussive symptoms clear within 15 min.
Grade 2: Transient confusion; no loss of consciousness; concussion symptoms or mental status abnormalities that last more than 15 min	1. Remove from contest and disallow return that day. 2. May return to play after 1 full asymptomatic week at rest and with exertion.
Grade 3: Any loss of consciousness either brief (seconds) or prolonged (minutes)	1. Transport the athlete to the nearest emergency room if the athlete is still unconscious or if worrisome signs are detected. 2. May return to competition if asymptomatic for 1 week (brief) or 2 weeks (prolonged).

REFERENCES

1. American Academy of Neurology. Practice parameter: the management of concussion in sports (summary statement). *Neurology* 1997;49:581–585.
2. Cantu RC. Guidelines for return to contact sports after a cerebral concussion. *Physician Sport Med* 1996; 14(19):86–92.
3. McCrory PM, Bladin PF, Berkovic SF. Retrospective study of convulsions in elite Australian rules and rugby league footballers: phenomenology, aetiology and outcome. *Br Med J* 1997;314:171–174.
4. Putukian M, Echemendia RJ. Managing successive minor head injuries: which tests guide return to play? *Physician Sports Med* 1996;24:25–38.
5. Hugenholtz H, Richard MT. Return to athletic competition after concussion. *Can Med Assoc* 1982; 127:827–829.
6. Goldstein M. Traumatic brain injury: a silent epidemic. *Ann Neurol* 1990;27:327.
7. Johnson DA. Head injured children and education: a need for greater delineation and understanding. *Br J Educ Psychol* 1992;62:404–409.
8. Frenquelli A, Ruscito P, Sicciolo G, Rizzo S, Massarelli N. Head and neck trauma in sporting activities. Review of 208 cases. *J Craniomaxillofac Surg* 1991;19(4):178–181.
9. Lehman LB, Nervous system sports-related injuries. *Am J Sports Med* 1987;15:494–499.
10. Lehman LB. Reducing neurologic trauma in sports. *NY State J Med* 1988;84:15–17.
11. Hitchcock ER, Karmi MZ. Sports injuries to the central nervous system. *J R Coll Surg Edinb* 1982;27:46–49.
12. Brooks N. Closed head injury: Psychological, social, and family consequences. Oxford: Oxford University Press, 1984.
13. Grafman J, Vance SC, Weingartner H, Salazar AM, Amin D. The effects of lateralized frontal lesions on mood regulation. *Brain* 1986;109:1127–1148.
14. Gronwal D. Cumulative and persisting effects on concussion on attention and cognition. In: Levin HS, Eisenberg HM, Benton AL, eds. *Mild head injury.* New York: Oxford University Press, 1989:153–162.
15. Evans RW. The post concussion syndrome and the sequelae of mild head injury. *Neurol Clin* 1992;10: 815–847.
16. Kay T, Newman B, Cavallo M, Ezrachi O, Resnick M. Toward a neuropsychological model of functional disability after mild traumatic brain injury. *Neuropsychology* 1992;6:371–384.
17. Kelly JP, Rosenberg JH. Diagnosis and management of concussion in sports. *Neurology* 1997;48:575–580.
18. McCrea M. Use of standardized assessment of concussion (SAC) in the immediate sideline examination of football players. Abstract, Sports Related Concussion and Nervous System Injuries Symposium, Orlando, Feb 8–10, 1997.
19. Matser JT. Traumatic brain injuries in professional soccer players. Presented at the Sports Related Concussion and Nervous System Injuries Symposium, Orlando, Feb 8–10, 1997.
20. Bohnen N, Jolles J, Twijnstra A. Neuropsychological deficits in patients with persistent symptoms six months after mild head injury. *Neurosurgery* 1992;30:692–696.
21. Bohnen N, Twijnstra A, Jolles J. Persistence of postconcussional symptoms in uncomplicated mildly head-injured patients: A prospective cohort study. *Neuropsychiatry Neuropsychol Behav Neurol* 1993; 6(3):193–200.
22. Bohnen NI, Jolles J, Twijnstra A, Mellink R, Wijnen G. Late neuro-behavioral symptoms after mild head injury. *Brain Injury* 1995;9(1):27–33.
23. Dalby PR, Obrzut HE. Epidemiological characteristics and sequelae of closed head injured children and adolescents. A review. *Dev Neuropsychol* 1991;7(1): 35–68.
24. Beers SR. Cognitive effects of mild head injury in children and adolescents. *Neuropsychol Rev* 1992;3(4): 281–320.
25. Binder LM. Persisting symptoms after mild head injury. A review of the postconcussive syndrome. *J Clin Exp Neuropsychol* 1986;8:323–346.
26. Donders J. Memory functioning after traumatic brain injury in children. *Brain Injury* 1993;7:431–437.
27. Kauffmann PM, Fletcher JM, Levin HS, Miner ME. Attentional disturbances after pediatric closed head injury. *J Child Neurol* 1993;8:348–353.

28. Levin HS, High W, Ewing-Cobbs L, et al. Memory functioning during the first year after closed head injury in children and adolescents. *Neurosurgery* 1988;22:1043–1052.

29. Ewing-Cobbs L, Fletcher JM, Levin HS. Neuropsychological sequelae following pediatric head injury. In: M. Ylvisaker M, ed. *Head injury rehabilitation: children and adolescents.* San Diego: College-Hill, 1985:71–89.

30. Lehr E. *Psychological management of traumatic brain injuries in children and adolescents.* Rockville, MD: Aspen Publishers, 1990.

31. Mattson AJ, Levin HS, Breitmeyer B. Visual information processing after severe closed head injury. Effects of forward and backward masking. *J Neurol Neurosurg Psychiatry* 1994;57:818–824.

32. Gronwall D, Wrightson P. Cumulative effect of concussion. *Lancet* 1975;2:995–997.

33. Parasuraman R, Mutter SA, Molloy R. Sustained attention following mild closed head injury. *J Clin Exp Neuropsychol* 1991;13:789–811.

34. Arcia E, Gualtiery CT. Association between patient report of symptoms after mild head injury and neurobehavioral performance. *Brain Injury* 1993;7:481–489.

35. Lezak MD. *Neuropsychological assessment,* 3rd ed. New York: Oxford University Press, 1995.

36. Holbourn AHC. Mechanics of head injuries. *Lancet* 1943;2:438–441.

37. Zoomeren AH van, van den Burg W. Residual complaints of patients two years after severe head injury. *J Neurol Neurosurg Psychiatry* 1985;48:21–28.

38. Gennarelli TA. The Pathobiology of Traumatic Brain Injury. *Neuroscientist* 1997;3(1):73–80.

39. Lampert PW, Hardman JM. Morphological changes in brains of boxers, *JAMA* 1984;251:2676–2679.

40. Strich SJ. Shearing of nerve fibers as a cause of brain damage due to head injury. A pathological study of twenty cases. *Lancet* 1961;2:443–448.

41. Perez G. La Boxe est-elle dangereuse, Abstract AIBA meeting, Paris Faculte de Medecine Pitie-Salpetiere. 1989.

42. Denny-Brown D, Russell WR. Experimental cerebral concussion. *Brain* 1941;64:93–164.

43. Yarnell B, Ommaya AH. Experimental cerebral concussion in the rhesus monkey. *Bull N Y Acad Sci* 1969;45:39–45.

44. Ommaya AK, Gennarelli TA. Cerebral concussion and traumatic unconsciousness, correlation of experimental and clinical observations of blunt head injuries. *Brain* 1974;97:633–654.

45. Adams JH, Mitchell ED, Graham DJ, Doule D. Diffuse brain damage of immediate impact type: its relation to primary brain stem damage in head injury. *Brain* 1979;100:489–502.

46. Tysvaer AT, Storli O. Soccer injuries to the brain. A neurologic and electroencephalographic study of active football players. *Am J Sports Med* 1989;17:573–578.

47. Jordan BD. Neurologic aspects of boxing. *Arch Neurol* 1987;44:453–459.

48. Owens RG, Ghadiali EJ. Judo as a possible cause of anoxic brain damage, *J Sports Med Phys Fitness* 1991;31:627–628.

49. Povlishock JT, Christman CW. The pathobiology of traumatically induced axonal injury in animals and humans: a review of current thoughts. *J Neurotrauma* 1995;12:555–564.

50. Bruce DA, Alavi A, Biloniuk L, et al. Diffuse cerebral swelling following head injuries in children: the syndrome of malignant brain edema. *J Neurosurg* 1981;54:170–178.

51. Hansen TB, Pless S, Bravvers M. Cranial injuries among children in the county of Ringkobing, *Ugeskr Laeg* 1991;154:2947–2949.

52. Graham DJ, Ford I, Adams J, et al. Ischaemic brain damage is still common in fatal nonmissile head injury. *J Neurol Neurosurg Psychiatry* 1989;52:346–350.

53. Ikeda Y, Long DM. The molecular basis of brain injury and brain edema: the role of oxygen free radicals. *Neurosurgery* 1990;27:1–11.

54. Fineman I, Hovda DA, Smith M, et al. Concussive brain injury is associated with a prolonged accumulation of calcium; a Ca autoradiographic study. *Brain Res* 1993;624:94–102.

55. Jiang JY, Lyeth BG, Delahunty T, et al. Muscarinic cholinergic receptor binding in rat brain at 15 days following traumatic brain injury. *Brain Res* 1994;651:123–128.

56. Hall ED, Braughler JM. In: Waxman SG, ed. *Molecular and cellular approaches to the treatments of neurological disease.* New York: Raven Press, 1993:81–105.

57. Soares HD, Hicks RR, Smith DH, McIntosh TK. Inflammatory leukocytic recruitment and diffuse neuronal degeneration are separate pathological processess resulting from traumatic brain injury. *J Neurosci* 1995;15:8223–8233.

58. Bazan MG, Rodriguez de Turco EB, Allan G. Mediators of injury in neurotrauma: intracellular signal transduction and gene expression. *J Neurotrauma* 1995; 12:791–814.

59. Jordan BD. Neurologic injuries in boxing, In: Jordan BD, Tsairis P, Warren RF, eds. *Sports Neurology.* Rockville, MD: Aspen Publishers, 1989:219–227.

60. Dencker SV. A follow up study of 128 closed head injuries in twins using co-twins as controls. *Acta Psychiatr Neurol Scan* 1958;33:123–125.

61. Alves WM, Jane JA. Mild brain injury, Damage and Outcome. In: Beck DP, Povlishock JT, eds. *Central nervous system trauma status report.* Washington, DC: National Institutes of Health, 1985.

62. Adams JH, Graham DI, Gennarelli TA. Axonal degeneration induced by experimental non-invasive minor head injury. *J Neurosurg* 1985;62:96–100.

63. Levin HS, Gary HE, High WM, et al. Minor head injuries and post concussion syndrome: methodological issues in outcome studies. In: Levin HS, Grafman J, Eisenberg HM, eds. *Neurobehavioral recovery from head injury.* New York: Oxford University Press, 1987.

64. Carlsson GS, Svardsudd K, Welin L. Long term effects of head injury sustained during life in three male populations. *J Neurosurg* 1987;67:197–205.

65. Jacobsen J, Baadsgaard SE, Thomsen S, Henriksen PB. Prediction of post concussional sequelae by reaction time test. *Acta Neurol Scand* 1987;75:341–345.

66. Alexander MP. Mild traumatic brain injury: pathophysiology, natural history and clinical management. *Neurology* 1995;45:1253–1260.

67. Gualtieri TC. Pharmacotherapy and the neurobehavioral sequelae of traumatic brain injury. *Brain Injury* 1988;2:101–129.

68. Gennarelli TA. Head injury mechanisms. In: Torg JS, ed. *Athletic injuries to the face and neck.* Philadelphia: Lea & Febiger, 1982.

69. Gennarelli TA. Head injury in man and experimental animals—clinical aspects. *Acta Neurochir Suppl* 1983; 32:1–13. Gennarelli, T.A. (1987). Cerebral concussion and diffuse brain injuries. In: Cooper PR ed. *Head Injury,* Baltimore: Willieams and Wilkins: 108–124.

70. Rimel RW, Giordani B, Barth JT, Boll TJ, Jane JA. Disability caused by minor head injury. *Neurosurgery* 1981;9:221–228.

71. King NS. Emotional, neuropsychological and organic factors: their use in the prediction of persisting post-concussion symptoms after moderate and mild head injuries. *J Neurol Neurosurg Psychiatry* 1996;61: 75–81.

72. Klein M. Cognitive aging, attention and mild traumatic brain injury. Thesis, Department of Neuropsychology University of Maastricht, 1997.

73. De Kruijk JR, Twijnstra A, Leffers P. Geen uniformiteit in radiodiagnostiek en adviezen van Nederlandse neurologen bij patienten met licht hersenletsel. *Ned Tijdschr Geneesk* 1996;140:1763–1765.

74. Rutherford WH, Merret JD, McDonald JR. Symptoms at one year follwing concussion from head injuries. *Injury* 1979;10:225–230.

75. Wrightson P, Gronwall D. Time off work and symptoms after minor head injury. *Injury* 1980;12:445–454.

76. Barnsley L, Lord S, Bogduk N. Whiplash injury. *Pain* 1994;58:283–307.

77. Kischka U, Ettlin TM, Heim S, Schmid G. Cerebral symptoms following whiplash injury. *Eur Neurol* 1991; 31:136–140.

78. Torres F, Shapiro SK. Electro-encephalograms in whiplash injury. *Arch Neurol* 1961;5:28–35.

79. Teuber HL. The riddle of frontal lobe function in man. In: Warren JM, Akert K, eds. *The frontal granular cortex and behavior.* New York: McGraw-Hill, 1964:16–48.

80. Benton AL. Differential behavioral effect in frontal lobe disease. *Neuropsychologia* 1968;6:53–60.

81. Luria AR. *Higher cortical functions in man,* 2nd ed. New York: Basic Books, 1980.

82. Nauta WJH. The problem of frontal lobe: a reinterpretation. *J Psychiatr Res* 1971;8:167–187.

83. Damasio A, Anderson SW. The frontal lobes. In: Heilman KM, Valenstein E, eds. *Clinical neuropsychology.* New York: Oxford University Press, 1993: 409–460.

84. Milner B. Some cognitive effects of frontal-lobe lesions in man. *Trends Neurosci* 1982;7:403–407.

85. Kolb B, Whishaw IQ. *Fundamentals of human neuropsychology,* 3rd ed. New York: WH Freeman, 1990.

86. Stuss D, Benson D. Neuropsychological studies of the frontal lobes. *Psychol Bull* 1984;95(1):3–28.

87. Damasio AR, Tranel D, Damasio H. Individuals with sociopathic behavior caused by frontal damage fail to respond autonomically to social stimuli. *Behav Brain Res* 1990;41:81–94.

88. Blumer D, Benson DF. Personality changes with frontal and temporal lesions. In: Benson DF, Blumer D, eds. *Psychiatric aspects of neurological disease.* New York: Grune & Stratton, 1975:151–169.

89. Stuss D, Gow C, Hetherington C. 'No longer Gage': frontal lobe dysfunction and emotional changes. *J of Consult Clin Psychol* 1992; 60:349–359.

90. Mayes AE. The memory problems caused by frontal lobe lesions. In: Mayes AE, ed. *Human organic memory disorders.* Cambridge: Cambridge University Press, 1988:102–123.

91. Goldberg E. Varieties of perseveration: a comparison of two taxonomies. *J Clin Exp Neuropsychol* 1986; 8:710–726.

92. Fletcher JM, Bohan TP, Brandt ME, et al. Cerebral white matter and cognition in hydrocephalic children. *Arch Neurol* 1992;49:818–824.

93. Jennett B, Bond M. Assessment of outcome after severe brain damage. *Lancet* 1975;1:480–484.

94. Franklin GM, Heaton RK, Nelson LM. Correlations of neuropsychological and MRI findings in chronic/ progressive multiple sclerosis. *Neurology* 1988;38: 1826–1829.

95. Rao SM, Leo GJ, Haughton VM, et al. Correlations of magnetic resonance imaging with neuropsychological testing in multiple sclerosis. *Neurology* 1989;39: 161–166.

96. Yikoski R, Yikoski A, Erkinjutti T, Sukova R, Raininko R, Tilvis R. White matter changes in healthy elderly persons correlate with speed of information processing. *Arch Neurol* 1993;50:818–824.

97. Junque C, Pujol J, Vendrel P, et al. Leuko-ariosis on MRI and speed of mental processing. *Arch Neurol* 1990;47:151–156.

98. Swirsky-Sacchetti T, Mitchel DR, Seward J, et al. Neuropsychological and structural brain damage in multiple sclerosis: a regional analysis. *Mov Disord* 1995;10:418–423.

99. Aston-Jones G, Rogers J, Shaver RD, Dinan TG, Moss DE. Age-impaired impulse flow from nucleus basalis to cortex. *Nature* 1985;318:462–464.

100. Becker T, Retz W, Hofmann E, Becker G, Teichmann G, Gsell W. Some methodological issues in neuroradiological research in psychiatry. *J Neural Transm Gen Sect* 1995;99(1–3):7–54.

101. Jordan BD. Head injury in sports. In: *Sportsneurology.* Rockville, MD: Aspen Publishers, 1989.

102. Cantu C. When to return to contact sports after cerebral concussion. *Sports Med Dig* 1988;10:1–2.

103. Torg JS, Vegso JJ, Sennet B, et al. The national football head and neck injury registry. *JAMA* 1985;254: 3429–3443.

104. Hawkins RD, Fuller CW. Risk assessment in professional football: an examination of accidents and incidents in the 1994 World Cup finals. *Br J Sports Med* 1996;30(2):165–170.

105. Bailes J. Abstract, Sports Related Concussion and Nervous System Injuries Conference, Orlando, Feb 8–10, 1997.

106. Harris JB. Neurological injuries in winter sports. *Phys Sportsmed* 1982;11(1):110–122.

107. Burns S, Koppenberg R, McKenna A, Wood C. Brain injury: personality, psychopathology and neuropsychology. *Brain Inj* 1994;8:413–427.

108. Robberts AH. *Brain damage in boxers.* London: Pittman Medical and Scientific, 1969.

109. Robberts GW, Allsop D, Bruton CJ. The occult aftermath of boxing. *J Neurol Neurosurg Psychiatry* 1990; 53:221–228.

110. Hollnagel P. Punch drunk syndrome. *Ugeskr Laeg* 1974;136:2871–2874.

111. Windle WF, Groat RA, Fox CA. Experimental structural alteration in the brain during and after concussion. *Surg Gynaecol Obstet* 1994;79:561–572.

112. Symonds C. Concussion and its sequelae. *Lancet* 1962;1:1–5.

113. Corsellis, JA, Bruton CJ, Freeman-Brown D. Aftermath of boxing. *Psychol Med* 1973;3:270–303.

114. Johnson J. Organic psychosyndrome due to boxing. *Br J Psychiatry* 1969;115:45–63.

115. Corsellis JA. Brain damage in sport. *Lancet* 1976; 1:401–402. CPSC report. Injuries associated with soccer goalposts, United States. *JAMA* 1994;271: 1233–1234.

116. Howieson DB, Lezak MD, Yudofsky SC, Hales RE. The neuropsychological evaluation. In: *The American textbook of neuropsychiatry*. Washington, DC: American Psychiatric Press, 1992:127–151.

117. Levin HS, Mattis S, Ruff RM, et al. Neurobehavioral outcome following minor head injury: a three center study. *J Neurosurg* 1987;66:234–243.

118. Matser JT, de Bijl MAO, Luytelaar G. Is amateur boxing dangerous? *Dev Psychology* 1992;12:515–521.

Sports Neurology, Second Edition,
edited by Barry D. Jordan.
Lippincott–Raven Publishers, Philadelphia © 1998.

3

Drug Use in Sports

Brian Hainline

ProHEALTH Care Associates, Lake Success, New York 11042

Drug use has been documented in athletic competition since the third century B.C. when the Greeks ingested mushrooms to improve athletic performance (1). In the nineteenth century, athletes began to experiment with alcohol, caffeine, nitroglycerin, opium, and strychnine (1,2). The first recorded fatality from drug use in sports occurred in 1886, when an English cyclist died from an overdose of trimethyl (3).

Drug use continues to be a well-documented problem in high school, college, and professional athletics. There are some encouraging trends. In the 1993 National Study of the Substance Use and Abuse Habits of College Student-Athletes, Anderson et al. (4) noted that use of performance-enhancing drugs in men's sports was uniformly down compared with 1985 and 1989 statistics. The same trend was not observed in women's sports, where drug use was noted to be increased in several sports for different performance-enhancing drugs. In the same study, the use of social drugs in men's sports was generally down or about the same when compared with 1985 and 1989. A notable exception was an increase in the use of smokeless tobacco among male tennis players. In women's sports, the trend for social drug use was generally downward or about the same. Again, a notable exception occurred among women tennis players, in whom there was an increase in the use of alcohol, marijuana or hashish, and smokeless tobacco.

Drug use in sports is a multifaceted problem. Athletes are at least as vulnerable to drug use and abuse as are other members of society (5).

Furthermore, athletes are significantly exposed to therapeutic drugs as well as performance-enhancing agents (ergogenic drugs).

Categories of drugs used in sports include

- Therapeutic: drugs for specific medical indications in accordance with standards of good medical practice
- Recreational: drugs used to alter mood and perception
- Performance-enhancing (ergogenic): drugs used for the purpose of gaining athletic advantage

A neat division does not exist among the categories of drug use in sport. For example, human growth hormone is clearly therapeutic when administered to children deficient in this hormone but is abused by some athletes for its ergogenic properties. This chapter is a brief survey of the epidemiology, rationale for use, and pharmacology of drug use in sport (Table 1). Individuals entrusted with the care of athletes should be aware of the various drugs often used and abused in sports. For a comprehensive discussion of drug use in sport, the reader is referred to *Drugs and the Athlete* (6).

ANABOLIC–ANDROGENIC STEROIDS

Pharmacology

Testosterone is the principal anabolic–androgenic steroid found in the plasma of males, and dihydrotestosterone is the principal intracellular

TABLE 1. *Drug use in sports*

Anabolic steroids	Miscellaneous
Stimulants	β-blockers
Amphetamines	Amino acids
Cocaine	Diuretics
Caffeine	Nonsteroidal
Look-alikes	antiinflammatory
Sedative-hypnotics	drugs
Alcohol	Bicarbonate doping
Barbiturates	Phosphate loading
Benzodiazepines	Vitamins
Narcotics	Carnitine
Blood doping and	Nicotine
erythropoietin	Marijuana
Human growth	Glucocorticosteroids
hormone	Masking drugs

mediator of hormonal action. Intracellularly, testosterone first binds to cytoplasmic receptors, which results in a biochemical transformation (7). The transformed complex binds to chromatin receptor sites, resulting in protein synthesis. The limiting factor with respect to the action of testosterone appears to be the number of existing receptor sites (7).

Laboratory modification of the testosterone molecule has made possible the synthesis of both oral and parenteral testosterone-like drugs. These drugs are referred to as anabolic–androgenic steroids or simply anabolic steroids. To date, efforts to dissociate the androgenic or masculinizing effects of these agents from the tissue-building effects have been largely unsuccessful (8).

Anabolic–androgenic steroids come in both oral and parenteral preparations. Alkylation of the 17-A position of testosterone prevents significant liver metabolism, allowing the oral preparation to be effective. Oral preparations are associated with an increase in liver toxicity and have a shorter half-life than parenteral anabolic steroids. For the athlete, this means that more frequent dosing is required to obtain the desired effect. Parenteral anabolic–androgenic steroids are made through esterification of the 17-B hydroxyl group of testosterone with a variety of carboxylic acids. These preparations are given less frequently because of the long half-life. Athletes who try to avoid detection of anabolic–androgenic steroid use often use the oral preparations closer to the time of competition.

Use in Sports

In the 1993 National Study of the Substance Use and Abuse Habits of College Student-Athletes (4), the reported use of anabolic–androgenic steroids was down compared with surveys performed in 1985 and 1989. Two and a half percent of student athletes reported the use of anabolic–androgenic steroids in the previous 12 months. Student athletes who use anabolic–androgenic steroids also report use of other ergogenic substances that have effects complementary to those of anabolic–androgenic steroids, including the following: epitestosterone (21.4%), clenbuterol (25.0%), human growth hormone (11.1%), erythropoietin (7.65%), amino acids (53.3%). The majority of student athletes who use anabolic–androgenic steroids obtain them from a friend or relative (37.1%), dealer (22.9%), teammate or other athlete (17.1%), or other physician (14.3%). Most student athletes who use anabolic–androgenic steroids do so to improve athletic performance (64.7%). Other reasons for using these drugs include improved appearance (14.7 %), nonsport injury (11.8%), and sport injury (8.8%). The majority of student athletes who take anabolic–androgenic steroids began such use in high school (40.0%). In men's college sports, football players use anabolic–androgenic steroids more than participants in other sports studied, including baseball, basketball, tennis, and track and field. In women's college sports, tennis players and track and field participants reported using anabolic–androgenic steroids more than participants in other sports.

Anabolic–androgenic steroid use is prominent among both athletes and nonathletes throughout the United States. Yesalis et al. (9) performed a cross-sectional study using data from the national household survey on drug abuse. This study demonstrated that there are more than 1 million current or former anabolic–androgenic steroid users in this country, with more than half of the lifetime user population being 26 years of age or older. More than 300,000 individuals used anabolic–androgenic steroids in the past year. The median age of first use of anabolic–androgenic steroids for this study population was 18 years. Anabolic–androgenic steroid use was significantly and positively associated with the use of other illicit drugs and alcohol. For 12- to 17-year-old children, anabolic–androgenic steroid use was significantly and positively associated with the use of cigarettes. DuRant et al. (10) reported that among ninth grade students, 5.4% of boys and 1.5% of girls use anabolic–androgenic steroids. Among users, 25% reported sharing needles to inject drugs. The frequency of anabolic–androgenic steroid use was significantly associated with use in the previous 30 days of cocaine, injectable drugs, alcohol, marijuana, cigarettes, and smokeless tobacco.

Athletes use anabolic–androgenic steroids for two primary reasons:

1. To increase muscle bulk and strength
2. To shorten recovery time after intense training and workouts

Shortened recovery time may be the primary ergogenic benefit of anabolic–androgenic steroid use. Although there is a popular myth that anabolic–androgenic steroids increase muscle bulk and strength, this may be of limited benefit in certain sports. However, the ability to shorten recovery time between intense workouts, thereby allowing the athlete to train more intensely, may well be an understated but primary beneficial effect of anabolic–androgenic steroid use. With this in mind, anabolic–androgenic steroid use is not ergogenic when taken just before an athletic event.

The skeletal muscle response to anabolic–androgenic steroids includes the following:

- Increased amino acid uptake
- Increased amino acid incorporation into skeletal muscle protein
- Increased nucleic acid synthesis, especially messenger RNA and ribosomal RNA
- Decreased amino acid and protein catabolism

The ability of athletes who use anabolic steroids to train more intensely is secondary to an anticatabolic affect. Intense training is associated with skeletal muscle and body catabolism, which is mediated in part by glucocorticosteroids. The skeletal muscle response to glucocorticosteroids includes the following (11):

- Decreased amino acid uptake
- Decreased amino acid incorporation into skeletal muscle protein
- Decreased DNA and RNA synthesis
- Increased protein catabolism

Therefore, use of anabolic–androgenic steroids may result in glucocorticosteroid receptor antagonism, thereby curtailing a physiologic catabolic response to intense training.

No beneficial effect of anabolic–androgenic steroids has ever been shown on aerobic metabolism or an individual's maximal venous oxygen capacity (12). Even with regard to bulk and strength, some controversy exists. Ryan (13) stated that anabolic–androgenic steroids do not contribute significantly to gains in lean muscle bulk or muscle strength in healthy young adults. Haupt and Rovere (12), on the other hand, stated that anabolic–androgenic steroid use consistently results in increased muscle strength under specific conditions, which include the following:

1. Athletes must train intensively in weight lifting before and after beginning the steroid regimen.
2. A high-protein diet must be maintained.
3. Changes in strength must be measured by the single repetition–maximal weight techniques for the exercises with which the athlete trains.

Much of the controversy regarding anabolic–androgenic steroid effects on performance results from retrospective efforts to compare different studies using different study designs. Furthermore, the standard for assessing the efficacy of anabolic–androgenic steroids has been their effect on an ability to increase the maximal weight lifted in a single repetition of a lifting exercise (maximal voluntary isometric contraction). How this benchmark correlates with actual performance in various competitive sports remains speculative.

The physiologic and ergogenic responses to anabolic–androgenic steroids in women and hypogonadic males are more pronounced because of low endogenous testosterone levels and the high number of unsaturated testosterone

TABLE 2. *Some side effects of anabolic–androgenic steroids*

Liver function abnormalities
Benign and malignant liver tumors
Rare systemic tumors
Testicular atrophy
Enlarged breasts
Feminization
Hypercholesterolemia
Behavior changes
Psychiatric disorders
Acne
Premature epiphyseal closure in adolescents

receptors in the skeletal muscle (8). Strauss et al. (14) reported that ten women athletes noted a significant increase in muscle size, muscle strength, and performance when they first started using anabolic–androgenic steroids.

Side effects of anabolic–androgenic steroids (Table 2) have not been well studied in athletes (6,15,16). Reported side effects are derived primarily from studies of patients taking these drugs in therapeutic doses for medical indications. Potential future side effects in young athletes taking megadoses of anabolic–androgenic steroids remain speculative and a genuine cause of concern.

STIMULANTS

The major stimulants used in athletic competition include amphetamines, cocaine, caffeine, and the "look-alikes."

Amphetamines

Pharmacology

Amphetamines have powerful central and peripheral nervous system effects. Peripherally, they act indirectly by releasing endogenous norepinephrine and directly as agonists, thereby causing the sympathetic effects. Centrally, amphetamines are psychomotor stimulants. They cause an increase in the concentrations of both norepinephrine and dopamine through synaptic reuptake blockade and act directly as central nervous system agonists. Amphetamines also augment synaptic catecholamine release (17). Most

of the pleasant psychomotor effects are probably mediated through the mesolimbic system (18). The main psychic effects of amphetamine include wakefulness, alertness, decreased sense of fatigue, elevation of mood, increased initiative, and increased self-confidence (18).

Benzedrine is the racemic isomer of amphetamine, and Dexedrine is the D-isomer. Both are available in 5- and 10-mg tablets. Methamphetamine is primarily a centrally acting drug.

Amphetamines are rapidly absorbed, and clinical effects can appear within ½ hour and last in excess of 3 hours. The plasma half-life is about 2 hours, and most amphetamine is excreted unchanged in the urine. Amphetamines are not metabolized by catechol O-methyltransferase or monoamine oxidase.

Use in Sports

In the 1993 National Study of the Substance Use and Abuse Habits of College Student–Athletes (4), 2.1% of student-athletes reported the use of amphetamines in the previous 12 months. In men's and women's sports, the highest use of amphetamines was by women softball athletes (4%). The majority of athletes who use amphetamines obtain them from a friend or relative (44%) or from a teammate or other athlete (28%). Among student athletes who use amphetamines, the majority do so to improve athletic performance (42.9%). Other reasons for use of amphetamines include the following: to increase energy (20.0%), social or personal reasons (17.1%), nonsport injury (5.7%), sport injury (2.9%), appetite suppressant (2.9%), other reasons (8.6%).

Amphetamines delay the point of fatigue during sustained intense exercise (19), and their most dramatic effects occur when performance has been reduced by fatigue and lack of sleep, a principle widely exploited by students and truck drivers.

In 1959, Smith and Beecher (20) published a classic paper on amphetamines and athletic performance. Amphetamine, in doses of 14 mg per 70 kg of body weight, improved the performance of the majority (75%) of athletes. The subjects consisted of highly trained runners, swimmers, and throwers. This paper demonstrated an improvement in sports requiring a maximal exertional effort but did not consider other factors such as eye–hand coordination, judgment, timing, stance stability, and hand–arm steadiness.

Subsequent studies have demonstrated positive effects of amphetamines with regard to these other factors. Low doses of amphetamines can improve performance in tasks requiring prolonged attention, even in a nonfatigued condition (21). Although it is widely believed that amphetamines cause jitteriness and anxiety—symptoms that should interfere with fine motor coordination—direct study contradicts this assumption. Hand–arm steadiness, resting tremor, stability of stance, and tasks of precision-hole steadiness do not differ significantly between subjects treated with amphetamines and those given a placebo (22,23). No difference in maximal venous oxygen capacity is observable in subjects treated with amphetamines compared with placebo, but anaerobic capacity and time to exhaustion increase after dextroamphetamine ingestion (24).

Side effects of amphetamines are related primarily to central and peripheral nervous system stimulation (6,17), but chronic exposure may cause a vasculitis, peripheral neuropathy, and severe psychiatric abnormalities (25–29) (Table 3).

TABLE 3. *Some side effects of amphetamines*

Central nervous system stimulation
  Restlessness
  Irritability
  Insomnia
  Confusion
  Delirium
  Hallucinations
  Convulsions
  Cerebrovascular accident, hemorrhage
  Coma, death
Peripheral stimulation
  Hypertension
  Tachycardia
  Cardiac arrythmias
  Angina, myocardial infarction
Chronic exposure
  Vasculitis
  Neuropathy
  Addiction
  Dyskinesias
  Paranoia

Cocaine

Pharmacology

Cocaine is an ecgonine alkaloid obtained from the leaf of the plant *Erythroxylon coca* and related species. Cocaine exerts complex physiologic effects on the brain and shares similarities with other stimulants such as amphetamines and caffeine. The psychic effects are in many ways similar to those of amphetamines and mediated through the reward or reinforcing circuitry of the mesolimbic system and the dopaminergic synapses of the nucleus accumbens (18).

Cocaine has been shown to increase the neurotransmitter concentrations of both norepinephrine and dopamine synapses by blocking reuptake of neurotransmitter. Cocaine potentiates the response of sympathetically innervated organs to norepinephrine, sympathetic nerve stimulation, and, to a lesser degree, epinephrine. Only Freud's 1884 self-experimentation with cocaine (30) supports the claim of muscle strength increases while an individual is under the influence of this drug.

The effects of cocaine are related to both the amount taken and the route of administration. Cocaine can be absorbed by the oral route, with more subtle and enduring effects. In the United States most cocaine is taken through nasal inhalation ("snorting"). In this fashion, blood concentration increases rapidly for 20 minutes, peaks at 60 minutes, and then gradually returns to baseline. Brain levels may increase more rapidly, however, because physiologic and subjective effects peak after 5 to 15 minutes (31). With intravenous cocaine, specific effects begin within 30 seconds. Vaporized cocaine base ("crack") may have an even more intense psychic effect than intravenous cocaine because large quantities of the drug can be quickly absorbed thorough the vascular bed of the lungs.

Use in Sports

In the 1993 National Study of the Substance Use and Abuse Habits of College Student-Athletes (4), 1.1% of student athletes reported the use of cocaine or crack in the previous 12 months. Male basketball players used cocaine more than other athletes (2.5%). Of athletes who used cocaine, 63.2% did so for recreational or social reasons and 36.8% used the drug because "it makes me feel good." No athletes reported that cocaine use improved athletic performance. This is consistent with other studies that indicated that cocaine is used primarily for recreational purposes and not for ergogenic purposes. In this regard, cocaine is a dangerous drug. In addition to its physiologic toxicity, cocaine use is associated with 26.7% of all New York City residents receiving a fatal injury.

No evidence suggests that, aside from potential effects on endurance and the generation of a sense of enhanced mental prowess, cocaine enhances athletic performance in a sustained fashion. Nevertheless, its similarity to amphetamines suggests that there may be certain performance-enhancing attributes at a narrow dose range. On the other hand, Gold (32) observed an impairment of eye–hand coordination in baseball, football, and basketball players who use cocaine. According to Czechowitz (32), coaches reported that an early clue to cocaine abuse is a distortion of a sense of time; athletes showed up either early or late to practice.

Kelly et al. (33) studied the physiologic effects of cocaine and exercise in rats. Cocaine-conditioned rats were compared with cocaine-naive rats after administration of cocaine, and a controlled group was also studied. Both chronically and acutely cocaine-exposed rats had higher lactate values during exercise than control animals. Both groups also had greater reductions in the glycogen content of the white and red vastus muscles and an increase in corticosterone compared with the controlled group. Cocaine-conditioned rats had a greater rise in norepinephrine and epinephrine in response to exercise than did rats acutely exposed to cocaine.

Side effects of cocaine are virtually indistinguishable from those of amphetamines (6) (see Table 3). However, cocaine is frequently taken in large doses, especially in the form of crack, and considerable risk exists of severe acute central and peripheral nervous system complications secondary to the stimulatory effects (34).

Caffeine

Pharmacology

Caffeine, a methylated xanthine, originates naturally in 63 species of plants (35). Peripheral effects in muscle are mediated primarily by an increase in the permeability of the sarcoplasmic reticulum to calcium, thereby increasing the amount of intracellular calcium available for muscle contraction. This may strengthen the force of muscular contraction (36). Caffeine also increases cellular cyclic adenosine monophosphate (AMP), resulting in increased glycogenolysis (increased blood sugar) and increased lipolysis (increased free fatty acids) (37). The latter in particular gives rise to increased energy and work output in long-term exercise (36,38).

The stimulant effects of caffeine may result from sensitization of central catecholamine postsynaptic receptors, possible alternation of acetylcholine and serotonin turnover and receptor functions, and opiate receptor antagonist activity (35,39). Caffeine is readily absorbed, and peak blood levels are reached in 60 minutes. The half-life is 2 to 12 hours.

Use in Sports

Caffeine has long been consumed by athletes in the belief that it enhances performance (40). A distinction must be made, however, between caffeine's effect on high-intensity, short-duration activities and its effect on endurance activities (41).

Caffeine enhances skeletal muscle contraction in situ when low-frequency electrical stimulation is given (42); this effect is mediated through intracellular calcium transport. No enhancing effect on fatigued or resting muscle is observed with high-frequency electrical stimulation, which is analogous to maximal voluntary contraction (36).

No firm conclusions can be drawn with regard to caffeine's effect on the oxygen transport system (36,38). Endurance-enhancing effects have been observed with a dose of 250 mg of caffeine given 1 hour before the endurance exercise. This is attributable to muscle glycogen sparing secondary to caffeine's lipolytic effect, whereby free fatty acids become an alternative substrate

TABLE 4. *Some side effects of caffeine*

Nervousness
Irritability
Insomnia
Gastrointestinal distress
Peptic ulcer
Cardiac arrythmias
Following massive doses:
   Delirium
   Seizures
   Coma, death

for aerobic metabolism (43). Tarnopolsky et al. (44) studied the physiologic responses to caffeine during endurance running and in habitual caffeine users. Caffeine administration 60 minutes prior to exercise significantly increased plasma free fatty acid levels both prior to and during exercise. Caffeine administration did not alter Vo_2; heart rate; respiratory exchange ratio; perceived exertion; plasma levels of glucose, lactate, epinephrine, or norepinephrine; or measures of neuromuscular function. However, when Arogyasami et al. (45,46) studied the effects of caffeine on glycogenolysis during exercise and in endurance-trained rats, no changes were noted in free fatty acid levels, endurance run time, glucose, lactate, or muscle glycogen.

Contradictory data exist with regard to caffeine's effect on concentration and psychomotor performance (21,47,48). In addition, conflicting data regarding hand–arm steadiness and precision–coordination tasks make it difficult to assess caffeine's effect on performance in these realms (21,23,49).

Side effects of caffeine are related to its excitatory properties but, in doses commonly used, are generally mild (6,50). Taken in massive doses, caffeine can be fatal (51) (Table 4).

The "Look-Alikes"

Pharmacology

Phenylpropanolamine and ephedrine are sympathomimetic amines that may be used in combination with caffeine to produce "look-alikes"—drugs that mimic the action of amphetamines (52). Phenylpropanolamine and ephedrine are less lipid soluble than amphetamines, so their central stimulatory effects are less than those of amphetamines (18). Even with extremely high doses of phenylpropanolamine and ephedrine, significantly less depletion of central monoamines occurs than with amphetamines, and significantly less potency with regard to locomotor activity and stereotyped behavior is observed. Phenylpropanolamine and ephedrine exert indirect effects on the sympathetic nervous system by displacing norepinephrine and other monoamine transmitters from their storage sites. In addition, they may have some direct effect on alpha and beta receptors of the sympathetic nervous system (52).

Blood levels of phenylpropanolamine and ephedrine peak in 1 to 2 hours, and most of the drug is excreted unchanged in the urine. The plasma half-life of phenylpropanolamine and ephedrine is about 2 hours. Clinical effects appear as early as 30 minutes and last up to 3 hours.

Use in Sports

No epidemiologic data are available regarding the use of the look-alikes in sports. In the 1972 Olympic Games, Rick DeMont, an American swimmer with asthma, was disqualified for taking medication containing ephedrine. Sidney and Lefcoe (53) performed the only prospective study to examine the possible ergogenicity of the look-alikes, and they reported no physical or mental performance enhancement when therapeutic doses of ephedrine were taken prior to submaximal and maximal exercise testing.

Sympathomimetic drugs are often combined with antihistamines to treat upper respiratory symptoms. Montgomery and Deuster (54,55) studied the effects of antihistamine ingestion on exercise performance, muscle strength, and endurance. Antihistamine ingestion (diphenhydramine hydrochloride and terfenadine) neither compromises nor improves aerobic glycolytic work performance, nor is there a significant effect on muscle endurance or maximal peak torque at a variety of velocities.

The significance in sports of the look-alikes is severalfold. Theoretically, they may be performance enhancing in ways similar to amphetamines when taken in certain combinations or in very large doses. Phenylpropanolamine is often used by athletes for weight control purposes. Even though phenylpropanolamine and ephedrine are over-the-counter drugs, side effects may include a dangerous increase in blood pressure, especially when they are used in combination with nonsteroidal antiinflammatory drugs (56). In addition, the look-alikes produce many side effects identical to those of amphetamines (6) (see Table 3), including central nervous system vasculitis and cerebrovascular accidents (57,58).

SEDATIVE-HYPNOTICS

Alcohol

Pharmacology

The central nervous system is the primary target for the clinical manifestation of alcohol. Alcohol is a central nervous system depressant, affecting both excitatory and inhibitory postsynaptic potentials. Acute administration of low doses may increase neuronal excitability secondary to depression of inhibitory cortical mechanisms and consequent increased circulatory catecholamines (59).

On the average, one drink (3 ounces of wine, 12 ounces of beer, 1 ounce of whiskey) results in a maximal blood concentration of 25 mg per 100 mL. In nonalcoholics, impairment of sensory perception, cognitive functions, and motor coordination occurs with ethanol concentrations of 31 to 65 mg per 100 mL. Blood ethanol levels decline at an average rate of 10 to 20 mg per 100 mL per hour (60).

Use in Sports

In the 1993 National Study of the Substance Use and Abuse of College Student-Athletes (4), 88.2% of student athletes reported the use of alcohol in the previous 12 months. Among men, baseball and tennis players used alcohol more frequently than basketball, football, or track and field athletes. Among women, tennis athletes used alcohol more commonly than basketball, softball, swimming, and track and field athletes. Among users, 17.7% of students have three to five drinks once per week, 11.6% of students

have three to five drinks twice per week, and 13.3% of students have six to nine drinks per week. Of the student athletes polled, 82.6% used alcohol for recreational or social reasons and 0.3% used alcohol to improve athletic performance. The majority of student athletes (62.4%) began alcohol use during high school.

Aside from caffeine, by far the most commonly used mind-altering drug in the United States is alcohol. About 100,000,000 Americans—that is, nearly half the population older than 12 years—drink alcohol regularly. Ten percent of those who drink alcohol are alcoholics (6). Social consequences are profound. In addition to the effects on relationships and medical adverse effects, the risk of dying is considerable. Nearly half of the roughly 35,000 fatal automobile accidents in the United States each year are alcohol related. Arrests for driving while intoxicated increase the risk of eventual death in an alcohol-related crash (62).

Alcohol is not perceived as an ergogenic drug because of its known effects on motor coordination and cognition. The possibility exists, however, that a finely titrated low dose of alcohol may be ergogenic. Low doses of alcohol may facilitate short-term memory (63), and anxiolytic effects may occur. Alcohol is effective in controlling postural essential tremor (64), and for this reason its effect may be ergogenic for athletes participating in sports such as riflery, where hand steadiness is essential. Data conflict regarding change in muscular strength after alcohol use (65,66). Aerobic capacity, maximal oxygen uptake, and oxygen consumption are unaffected by alcohol administration (67–69). Motor–visual coordination, balance, and reaction times are all adversely affected with low to moderate doses of alcohol (70–72). Of relevance to the athlete is that the social use of alcohol the evening prior to competition may have deleterious effects on performance. Airline pilots tested 14 hours after achieving a blood alcohol level of 100 to 125 mg/dl performed significantly worse in tasks requiring attention and visual–motor skills (73).

Side effects of alcohol are considerable and can include every organ system in the body (74). Acute side effects are usually related to impaired judgment and unfortunately are a major cause of

TABLE 5. *Some chronic side effects of alcohol*

Neurologic
  Wernicke-Korsakoff syndrome
  Cerebellar degeneration
  Dementia
  Peripheral neuropathy
  Muscle wasting (atrophy) ± myoglobinuria
Cardiac
  Cardiomyopathy
Gastrointestinal
  Hepatitis, cirrhosis
  Pancreatitis
  Esophagitis
  Peptic ulcer disease
Hematologic
  Pancytopenia
  Folate vitamin B_{12} deficiency

motor vehicle accidents and death (75). Chronic side effects are related to long-term nutritional and direct toxic insults to the various organs (Table 5). In addition, alcohol is addicting, and discontinuation can cause a life-threatening withdrawal syndrome.

Barbiturates

Pharmacology

Barbiturates depress the activity of all excitable central nervous system activity and particularly the reticular and vestibular systems (76). Inhibitory effects are exerted in two ways: (a) by facilitation of synaptic actions of the inhibitory transmitter γ-*aminobutyric* acid and (b) by general cortical suppression unrelated to the former (77). As a result of the general cortical suppressant effect, any anxiolytic actions of the barbiturates are usually associated with sedation.

None of the barbiturates available for oral use in the United States for hypnosis has a sufficiently short half-life to ensure complete elimination in 24 hours; this results in accumulation with repetitive dosing (78).

Use in Sports

In the 1993 National Study of the Substance Use and Abuse of College Student-Athletes (4), 1.4% of athletes reported the use of barbiturates or tranquilizers in the previous 12 months. Four percent of women tennis players reported using these

drugs in the previous year, which is a considerably higher percentage than in all other men's and women's sports studied. Seventy-five percent of respondents began use of barbiturates or tranquilizers in high school and 25% began such use during the freshman year of college. Of the student athletes, 44.4% use these drugs for social or personal reasons, 22.2% for a sport injury, 22.2% for a nonsport injury, and 11.1% to improve athletic performance. Therefore, although barbiturates or sedatives may not be commonly viewed as ergogenic drugs, it is clear from this study that athletes are using these drugs both to recover from injuries and to improve athletic performance.

Barbiturates are somewhat similar to alcohol both from an ergogenic perception viewpoint and in their effects on reaction time and coordination. Reaction time, cognitive function, and visual tracking are all diminished with barbiturates in doses equivalent to 100 mg of secobarbital (79–81). In one subgroup of weight throwers in the study by Smith and Beecher (20), however, improvement in total distance was demonstrated after administration of 50 mg of secobarbital per 70 kg. No other study has demonstrated a significant effect on strength or endurance after administration of barbiturates. Even though judgment and performance may be impaired or not improved, athletes may subjectively feel better and perceive their performance as superior while under the influence of secobarbital (82). Barbiturates are often used to treat essential tremor (83) and in this regard may be used by the athlete in sports such as riflery, which require hand steadiness.

Side effects of barbiturates are related to the central nervous system sedative effects (6) (Table 6). In addition, barbiturates are addicting, and discontinuation can cause a withdrawal syndrome that in some cases can be life threatening.

TABLE 6. *Some side effects of barbiturates*

Sedation
Decreased attention
Poor balance
Impaired memory
Respiratory depression
In massive doses: stupor, coma, death

Benzodiazepines

Pharmacology

Benzodiazepine receptors are located in the brain and are coupled with γ-aminobutyric acid receptors at the molecular level. The receptors are particularly prominent in the limbic system and in subcortical–cortical projections, and their activation results in the inhibition of pathways related to anxiety-induced responses. In contradistinction to the barbiturates, benzodiazepines have self-limited neuronal depressive effects because their actions depend on the availability of the endogenous inhibitory transmitter γ-aminobutyric acid (78). Benzodiazepines are lipid soluble, and plasma concentrations may reach their peak in 30 minutes. The biologic half-life of the benzodiazepines varies widely among the various preparations and is largely influenced by the presence of biologically active metabolites.

Use in Sports

Benzodiazepines may theoretically alleviate anxiety without diminishing motor performance, but relevant data for athletes are often contradictory (6). Benzodiazepines are commonly prescribed in anxiety disorders. A generalized anxiety disorder is characterized by unrealistic or excessive anxiety and worry about life circumstances (84). Up to 15% of adults in the United States have a 1-year prevalence of anxiety. Although athlete-specific data are unavailable, it is highly unlikely that the athlete is immune to this widespread syndrome. Several symptoms of a generalized anxiety disorder—motor tension, autonomic hyperactivity, and vigilance and scanning—can be detrimental to athletic performance. Benzodiazepines may thus be perceived as ergogenic to athletes suffering from a generalized anxiety disorder.

Benzodiazepines may reduce tremor amplitude, particularly for individuals requiring intermittent therapy (85), which is analogous to the situation of the athlete wishing to steady his or her hand for a particular event. Athletes may be susceptible to benzodiazepine use because the potential calming effect may be sought in anticipation of athletic competition. In addition, athletes using stimulants may use benzodiazepines to counteract the stimulant effect.

Collomp (86) studied the effects of benzodiazepines using a Wingate test, which consists of 30 seconds of supramaximal cycling against resistance determined relative the subject's body weight. Performance and metabolic parameters were studied after ingestion of placebo, lorazepam, or lorazepam plus caffeine. Subjects who ingested lorazepam had a significant decrease in peak power, with a significant increase in maximal blood lactate and end-exercise epinephrine. Caffeine ingestion antagonized the lactate and epinephrine effects but had no effect on performance. Therefore, acute benzodiazepine ingestion has a detrimental affect on peak power in aerobic activity.

Side effects of benzodiazepines are generally similar to those of barbiturates (6) (see Table 6), although milder in therapeutic doses. As with barbiturates, benzodiazepines are addictive and discontinuation can cause a withdrawal syndrome. Fatal reactions resulting from massive quantities of benzodiazepines occur less frequently than with barbiturates.

NARCOTICS

Pharmacology

Morphine is representative of the narcotic analgesics. The primary effects of morphine are directed at the central nervous system and the gastrointestinal tract; both pathways are mediated through specific opioid receptors. Morphine-like drugs take advantage of innate central nervous system mechanisms that modulate pain, emotions, and other functions.

Morphine and the opioids do not alter the threshold of responsivity of afferent peripheral nerve endings to noxious stimuli; rather, alterations probably occur at the various levels of sensory integration, beginning in the spinal cord. Through receptor binding, the central release of neurotransmitters can be altered, with subsequent attenuation of pain perception (87). The primary effects of morphine and other narcotics include analgesia, euphoria, drowsiness, mental clouding.

In the narcotics more commonly used for mild to moderate pain, the time of peak analgesia ranges from 1 to 2 hours, and the duration of action is generally from 3 to 6 hours.

Use in Sports

In the 1993 National Study of the Substance Use and Abuse Habits of College Student-Athletes (4), 30.1% of student athletes reported using major pain medications in the previous 12 months. Thirty-four percent of male football players used major pain medications during the previous year, more than in any other men's or women's sport. The vast majority of students obtained major pain medications from either another physician (41.9%) or a team physician (31.6%). Of the respondents, 71.9% used major pain medications for a sport injury, 23.1% for a nonsport injury, 3.6% for social or personal reasons, and 1.3% to improve athletic performance.

Narcotics are not generally perceived as ergogenic drugs, but their potential for misuse in sports may be high because of pressures on the athlete to perform competitively despite musculoskeletal injuries. In the acute setting, especially in naive subjects, narcotics may cause sedation, drowsiness, clouding of the sensorium, difficulty in mentation, reduced visual acuity, nausea, and vomiting (88,89). However, the available evidence suggests that chronic narcotic use does not necessarily impair skills of relevance to the athlete. In several studies, no significant difference has been observed between addicts and age-matched control subjects with regard to motor strength, rapid alternating eye movements, eye–hand coordination, visual perception, and cognitive skills (90–92). The effect of narcotics on endurance has not been assessed.

Narcotics may be administered intraarticularly (93) and may produce a potent antinociceptive effect by interacting with local opioid receptors and inflamed peripheral tissue. Such administration decreases central side effects of opiods but is potentially dangerous to the athlete in that the significance of damaged tissue may not be appreciated during athletic competition.

TABLE 7. *Some side effects of narcotics*

Dizziness
Mental clouding
Euphoria, dysphoria
Nausea, vomiting
Constipation

Narcotic dependence and addiction are unlikely after short-term use in the management of pain. The issues of tolerance and dependency may be obviated by the use of equianalgesic doses of nonsteroidal antiinflammatory drugs for the treatment of musculoskeletal pain (94,95).

Side effects of narcotics are related to the sedative and mood-changing properties resulting from central nervous system receptor binding and constipation from gastrointestinal receptor binding (Table 7). Chronic narcotic use causes tolerance and addiction, and discontinuation of a drug can cause a severe, but generally not fatal, withdrawal syndrome.

BLOOD DOPING AND ERYTHROPOIETIN

Blood Doping

Blood doping refers to the practice of intravenously infusing blood into an individual to increase the hemoglobin and hematrocrit above normal baseline levels. Autologous (one's own blood) doping is more commonly done in sports than homologous (donated blood) doping. Blood doping is used by athletes engaged in aerobic activities in an attempt to increase total aerobic power by increasing the amount of oxygen available to the working muscle.

The maximal benefit from blood doping occurs if the following conditions are met (96):

- Two units of blood are removed from the athlete 4 to 8 weeks prior to the anticipated athletic event.
- The red blood cells are preserved by glycerol freezing.
- The athlete retrains to full aerobic capacity post phlebotomy.

• Reinfusion of the stored red blood cells is done 1 to 7 days prior to the athletic event.

Immediately after blood doping, blood volume is restored to normal because of compensatory physiologic shifts of plasma from the intravascular to the extravascular space (97). No change in the affinity of the red blood cell for oxygen occurs, and cardiac output is not significantly changed (90). Robertson et al. (99) have demonstrated that both the volume of oxygen delivered by the left ventricle and the volume of oxygen actually used during maximal exercise are significantly increased after blood doping.

Erythropoietin

The rate of formation of red blood cells is determined primarily by erythropoietin. Recombinant human erythropoietin is now available through the technique of genetic engineering, and this substance has been proved to be efficacious in increasing the hematocrit of patients who suffer chronic anemia secondary to chronic renal failure (100,101).

Use in Sports

No data are available regarding the incidence of blood doping in sports, although anecdotal stories of runners and cyclists utilizing this technique are plentiful (102). Erythropoietin doping by athletes has not been reported, but speculation has surfaced about its potential abuse (103).

If the proper technical conditions for blood doping are met, this technique clearly improves performance for endurance events. Statistically significant differences in racing time have been documented when the athlete acts as his or her own control (98). Subcutaneous erythropoietin administration results in a slow increase of hemoglobin, but the increase in Vo$_2$max is similar to the acute increase in hemoglobin as a result of red blood cell reinfusion (104).

Homologous blood transfusions carry a 3% risk of immune-related side effects; viral infection such as hepatitis and the acquired immunodeficiency syndrome (AIDS) occur less commonly but may be fatal. Autologous blood transfusions are safe when performed by trained personnel for appropriate medical indications. Any flaw in technique may lead to potentially severe complications ranging from infections to fatal reactions due to blood mislabeling. No serious toxic effects have been reported with recombinant erythropoietin under medical supervision in patients with chronic renal failure. Any form of induced erythrocythemia carries with it the potential medical complications of polycythemia, including cerebrovascular accidents, tissue hypoxia, and blood clotting (105).

HUMAN GROWTH HORMONE

Pharmacology

Growth hormone is secreted by the somatotrophs of the anterior pituitary, and the episodic secretion of growth hormone is under hypothalamic control. Metabolic effects are divided into acute and delayed (106). Acute effects of growth hormone secretion are insulin-like and include (107)

1. Increased amino acid uptake and incorporation into protein in muscle and liver
2. Stimulation of glucose uptake in muscle and adipose tissue
3. Antilipolytic effects in adipose tissue

Delayed effects of human growth hormone include

1. Increased mobilization of free fatty acids from adipose tissue secondary to triglyceride lipolysis
2. Increased sensitivity to the lipolytic effects of catecholamines
3. Inhibition of glucose uptake and utilization

Nearly every organ is dependent on growth hormone for proper growth and development (6). Exogenous human growth hormone administration causes more normal skeletal growth in hormone-deficient children. Accelerated growth occurs in normal children, but it is not known whether the final height obtained exceeds that which would have occurred without exogenous growth hormone administration (108–110).

Growth hormone is now available as a biologically active agent produced by recombinant DNA technology. The half-life of growth hormone varies from 17 to 45 minutes and is unchanged by exercise.

Use In Sports

In the 1993 National Study of the Substance Use and Abuse of College Student-Athletes (4), the general use of human growth hormone was not specifically studied. However, among users and nonusers of anabolic–androgenic steroids, questions were asked regarding human growth hormone use. Among anabolic–androgenic steroid users, 11.1% of student athletes reported using human growth hormone. Among nonusers of anabolic steroids, 0.8% of respondents indicated they had used human growth hormone during the previous year. Therefore, human growth hormone is used as a supplement to anabolic–androgenic steroids by some athletes.

Growth hormone has been demonstrated to produce anticatabolic affect in patients suffering with catabolic illness (111), with uncertain implications for the training athlete. In rat studies, growth hormone administration led to an increase in both size and strength of atrophied muscles. The effects on contractile elements and functional performance in normal muscles are less clear (112,113).

MISCELLANEOUS

β-Blockers

β-blockers are a group of drugs that produce blockade of the β-adrenergic receptors. Nonselective β-blockers produce blockade of both β_1- and β_2-receptors, whereas the selective β-blocking drugs block only β_1-receptors. Peripheral inhibition of β_1-receptors results in bradycardia; β_2-blockade inhibits bronchodilatation and peripheral vascular vasodilatation.

Aerobic endurance, maximal oxygen capacity, and anaerobic endurance are all significantly decreased with β-blockade (114). The anxiolytic and antitremor effects of β-blockers have become the basis for their use in sports. Thus, β-blockers may be ergogenic in sports such as riflery and archery (115).

In hypertensive patients, physician should follow traditional guidelines for treating athletes. However, given the choice, β-blockers might impede performance compared with other antihypertensive agents such as clonidine, prazosin, and diltiazem (116,117). If β-blockers are used, patients with coronary artery disease are still capable of deriving the expected enhancement of cardiorespiratory fitness during training. In general, β_1-selective blockers are preferable to nonselective agents in patients engaged in exercise training. Nonselective β-blockers may increase a predisposition to exertional hyperthermia (118).

Adverse effects of β-blockers occur because of the receptor blockade. In patients with pre-existing cardiac dysfunction, congestive heart failure may occur. Nonselective β-blockers are contraindicated for asthmatics because of the likelihood of precipitating bronchospasm, but at moderate to high doses even β_1-selective drugs may be problematic (119).

Amino Acids

Amino acids are utilized by the body for protein synthesis, neurotransmitter function, and energy production. Proteins are enzymatically hydrolyzed to amino acids after ingestion. Amino acids may also be ingested in commercially produced pills or tablets. Amino acids can be divided into two groups: Essential amino acids are not synthesized in the body and must be ingested; nonessential amino acids can be made within the body from carbon and nitrogen precursors (6). Amino acids are popular supplements to other anabolic agents and are sometimes taken without such agents in an effort to increase muscle strength, bulk, and stamina (120, 121). However, no evidence supports ergogenicity after amino acid drug use. Some athletes may use amino acids to supplement protein intake. Although it is controversial, most authors agree that the protein needs of strength and endurance athletes do not differ from those of nonathletes. A diet containing 15% of its total energy as protein can easily provide the needs of the athlete (121–123).

Excessive amino acid intake may cause dehydration, gout, liver damage, kidney damage, loss of urinary calcium, and impairment of other essential amino acid absorption (6). Ingestion of commercially produced tryptophan may cause eosinophilia–myalgia syndrome (124).

Diuretics

Diuretics are drugs that increase the rate of urine formation. Athletes use diuretics for the following reasons: (a) to achieve rapid weight loss in sports such as wrestling or horse racing; (b) to dilute the urine, thereby reducing the concentration of banned drugs and decreasing the likelihood of a positive urine test; (c) to decrease extracellular fluid when taking other drugs such as anabolic steroids, which cause fluid retention; and (d) to reduce extracellular fluid around the time of menstruation (125,126). Taken before competition, diuretics may cause performance impairment by reducing maximal venous oxygen capacity and workload during maximal exercise (127). Acute weight loss is sometimes achieved among wrestlers by diuretic administration. Webster et al. (128) have demonstrated that this deleteriously affects strength, anaerobic power, anaerobic capacity, lactate threshold, and aerobic power.

Diuretics should be taken only under medical supervision. Dehydration, hypovolemia, and muscle cramps are potential complications of forced diuresis. Hypokalemia can develop and in severe cases is life threatening (6).

Nonsteroidal Antiinflammatory Drugs

Nonsteroidal antiinflammatory drugs (NSAIDs) have analgesic, antiinflammatory, and antipyretic properties. They are the mainstay of pharmacologic therapy for the treatment of soft tissue athletic injuries. Athletes use NSAIDs primarily under the following conditions: (a) the treatment of acute injuries such as ligament and muscle strains and cartilage damage; (b) the treatment of chronic injuries such as tendinitis, bursitis, fasciitis, and stress fractures; and (c) the treatment of arthritis (129). NSAIDs may be ergogenic in that performance is less pain limited after taking

these drugs (6). Prophylactic use of nonsteroidal antiinflammatory drugs (ibuprofen) does not prevent creatine kinase release from muscle but does decrease muscle soreness perception and may assist in restoring muscle function (130).

Gastric upset and occasional upper gastrointestinal bleeding occur frequently after NSAID use, especially when such use becomes chronic. NSAID therapy may worsen preexisting acute soft tissue bleeding, and a minimum of 24 hours should elapse before these drugs are given under such circumstances (6).

Bicarbonate Doping

Bicarbonate doping refers to the practice of ingesting sodium bicarbonate (baking soda) before an athletic event. The rationale for such a practice is to reduce muscle lactic acidosis, thereby delaying muscle fatigue. No evidence supports an ergogenic effect of bicarbonate doping before aerobic events. There is a possibility that bicarbonate doping may improve athletic performance under specific anaerobic circumstances. Wilkes et al. (131) demonstrated improved 800-m running times when athletes ingested sodium bicarbonate 30 minutes before race time. However, when equivalent amounts of sodium in the form of sodium chloride are administered to exercising subjects and compared with sodium bicarbonate administration, no change in performance is noted. Therefore, it is possible that the intravascular volume expansion with sodium bicarbonate rather than the increase in blood buffer capacity may underlie the apparent benefit in exercise performance (132).

Large quantities of sodium bicarbonate can cause diarrhea or gastric distress, and chronic use can cause disturbances in body sodium and water balance (6).

Phosphate Loading

Phosphate loading refers to the practice of ingesting phosphate 1 week before an athletic event in an attempt to improve oxygen delivery. Levels of 2,3-diphosphoglycerate may increase after phosphate supplementation, although this is not uniformly observed (133). Maximal oxygen uptake and ventilatory threshold are beneficially influenced among athletes ingesting phosphate, but functional affects on athletic performance are less clear (134). Adverse affects of short-term phosphate loading are unknown.

Vitamins

Vitamins are essential for the maintenance of normal metabolic functions within the cell, but they are not synthesized in the body. Vitamins have never been shown to enhance performance when taken in quantities greater than the recommended daily allowance (135). A daily multivitamin is recommended to avoid the development of a deficiency state when individuals are not eating regular well-balanced meals.

Vitamins are by no means innocuous (136). Large doses of vitamin A can cause dangerous increases in intracranial pressure, bone resorption, cirrhosis, and hypercalcemia. Vitamin D abuse can cause hypercalcemia, apathy, headache, anorexia, and bone pain. Vitamin E, in doses greater than 150 mg daily, can lead to weakness, fatigue, headache, nausea, diarrhea, and phlebitis. Vitamin B_6 (pyridoxine), in doses as low as 200 mg daily, can cause a progressive sensory neuropathy (137). Niacin use is associated with flushing, urticaria, and bronchospasm. Vitamin C, taken in quantities greater than 2000 mg daily, can cause diarrhea and nausea and may lead to destruction of endogenous vitamin B_{12}.

Carnitine

The primary function of L-carnitine appears to be as a carrier molecule of long-chain fatty acids into the mitochondria. Lipid storage myopathies have been associated with lower than normal levels of carnitine (138). Extrapolating from these data, endurance athletes have taken carnitine supplements in efforts to enhance their performance by enhancing the metabolism of fatty acids. Carnitine administration does not result in an increase in muscle carnitine content, nor does it alter lipid oxidation in exercising athletes. This suggests that there is an adequate amount of carnitine present within the mitochondria to support lipid oxidation (139). During submaximal exer-cise after depletion of muscle glycogen, overall metabolism is not influenced by L-carnitine administration (140). Ingestion of D,L-carnitine may produce a myopathy (141).

Nicotine

Nicotine, a potent alkaloid found in smoking and chewing tobacco, has both stimulant and depressant effects in the neuromuscular system. Small doses can facilitate the transmission of autonomic ganglionic impulses, stimulate the adrenal medulla to release catecholamines, and cause central nervous system stimulation secondary to norepinephrine and dopamine release (142). Nicotine administration increases anaerobic energy production and produces an increased tachycardic response to submaximal workload (143). Perception of exertion during low-intensity physical exercise or physical activity is not altered by nicotine administration (144). Nicotine users perform better than nonusers when having to react to cognitively challenging task situations (145). Facilitation of memory and attention (146), euphorigenic effects similar to those seen after morphine and amphetamine administration (147), and a general calming effect (148) may be observed following nicotine use. Nicotine ergogenicity has not been clearly established in humans, although athletes may use the drug, primarily in the form of smokeless tobacco, for both its stimulatory and its calming effects (142).

The side effects of smoking and smokeless tobacco are considerable, and the interested reader is referred to *Drugs and the Athlete* for a more detailed discussion (6). Every day another 3000 young people become regular tobacco smokers (149). Smoking tobacco is the chief single avoidable cause of death in our society (150), primarily because of its relationship to lung cancer, chronic obstructive pulmonary disease, and cardiovascular disease. Of concern, but less publicized, are the side effects of smokeless (chewing) tobacco, which is becoming more popular among the young. Severe periodontal disease, including oral cancer, may occur with chronic use of chewing tobacco (151).

Marijuana

Marijuana is derived from the herbaceous plant *Cannabis sativa,* and the principal active constituent is Δ^9-tetrahydrocannabinol. Diverse neurochemical changes have been described after marijuana use, and associated behavioral changes include decreased attention span, euphoria, excitement, dissociation of ideas, relaxation, and a decrement in psychomotor performance (152).

Marijuana is the most widely used of all illicit drugs, and its acute effects are deleterious to athletic performance because of the psychomotor changes. Furthermore, Yesavage et al. (153) demonstrated impairment in flying skills for as long as 24 hours after marijuana intoxication, despite the fact that the subjects did not perceive any impairment. This study casts doubt on the commonly held belief that the social use of marijuana the evening before an athletic event does not affect performance.

"Health aspects of cannabis" (154) is an excellent review of the side effects of marijuana, which are beyond the scope of this chapter. Aside from the acute behavioral changes, the potential user should bear in mind that potential contaminants of marijuana may have more deleterious health effects than the cannabinoids themselves (154).

Glucocorticosteroids

The adrenocortex produces both glucocorticosteroids and adrogens. Glucocorticosteroids are not stored in the adrenocortex. The amount of biosynthesis and the rate of secretion parallel each other. Glucocorticosteroid synthesis and secretion are under hormonal control, specifically by adrenocorticotropic hormone (ACTH). Glucocorticosteroids, like anabolic–androgenic steroids, act by controlling the rate of biosynthesis of proteins. Glucocorticosteroids react with receptor proteins in the cytoplasm of cells to form a steroid–receptor complex. These receptors have been identified in many tissues. Following modification, the steroid–receptor complex moves into the nucleus, where it binds to chromatin. This then directs protein synthesis (155).

Glucocorticosteroids have a widespread affect in the body, influencing body metabolism, cardiovascular and nervous system function, electrolyte balance, carbohydrate and protein metabolism, lipid metabolism, and inflammatory and immune responses. Glucocorticosteroids may be administered orally or parenterally. Cortisone was the first glucocorticosteroid used for its antiinflammatory affects. Many other glucocorticosteroids are available, and they all vary with regard to relative antiinflammatory potency, sodium-retaining potency, duration of action, absorption, and potency. Physicians administering glucocorticosteroids must be aware of the relative potency and pharmacologic affects of the different types of drugs available (156).

The incidence of glucocorticosteroid use in sports is not known. However, their use in sports medicine in general is widespread, especially in injectable form (155). Glucocorticosteroids are used almost exclusively for their antiinflammatory and antiswelling effects in sport injuries. Glucocorticosteroid administration can reverse pain and swelling that result from an acute inflammatory response. Because of their potency, glucocorticosteroids can mask potentially serious causes of acute pain, inflammation, and swelling, with potentially devastating consequences. In the athlete, a premature return to play after glucocorticosteroid use may result in more serious injury, including tendon rupture.

Glucocorticosteroids are given primarily in injectable form for athletic injuries. It is critical that a specific diagnosis first be made and that a rehabilitation program be in place. Glucocorticosteroids do not replace the principles of rest and rehabilitation. They should be used only as an adjunct in treatment. The risk of tendon ruptures is especially high if glucocorticosteroids are administered indiscriminately and return to play by the athlete is hastened (156).

In addition to the risk of tendon rupture, glucocorticosteroids have several other side effects, but these result primarily from prolonged use. Chronic administration results in adrenal suppression, making patients susceptible to acute adrenal insufficiency upon withdrawal of medication. Other chronic side effects include, but are not limited to, hyperglycemia, susceptibility to infections, peptic ulcer disease, osteoporosis, myopathy, Cushing's syndrome, and behavioral changes (155).

Masking Drugs

Masking drugs are agents without any perceived performance-enhancing effect that may mask the presence of other drugs being tested for in the urine. Examples of masking agents are probenecid, diuretics, and sulfinpyrazone.

DRUG TESTING

Drug testing for athletes did not begin until the 1960s. Prompted by the amphetamine-related death of two cyclists, the Medical Commission of the International Olympic Commission published a list of banned drugs for the 1968 Winter Olympics (157). Although the principal intent of drug testing is to eliminate any competitive advantage, other factors such as general health and safety, role model perception, deterrence, and minimizing criminality are often considered as well (158). The method of drug testing has a significant bearing on the results; therefore, the intent of a given drug-testing program must be well defined beforehand (6).

The sensitivity and specificity of methods may vary considerably. Thin-layer chromatography is inexpensive and rather insensitive and non-specific. Radioimmunoassay and enzyme immunoassay are immunologic techniques that are more sensitive and specific than thin-layer chromatography, but neither differentiates between specific drugs within a class of drugs and both may yield false-positive results in athletes taking nonsteroidal antiinflammatory drugs. Gas chromatography–mass spectrometry is the most sensitive and accurate technique currently available in the field of drug testing. Because of its sensitivity, low levels of drugs can be detected in the urine many days after drug use. Because of its specificity, gas chromatography–mass spectrometry is used to confirm positive test results obtained by other techniques (6).

REFERENCES

1. Puffer F. The use of drugs in swimming. *Clin Sports Med* 1986;5:77–89.
2. Burks TF. Drug use in athletics. *Fed Proc* 1981; 40:2680–2681.
3. Dyment PG. Drugs and the adolescent athlete. *Pediatr Ann* 1984;13:602–604.
4. Anderson WA, Albrecht RR, McKeag DB. Second replication of a National Study of the Substance Use and Abuse Habits of College Student-Athletes. Presented to the National Collegiate Athletic Association, Overland Park, KS, July 30, 1993.
5. Ryan AJ. Causes and remedies of drug misuse and abuse by athletes. *JAMA* 1984;252;517–519.
6. Wadler GI, Hainline B. *Drugs and the athlete.* Philadelphia: FA Davis Co, 1989.
7. Hickson RC, Kurowski TG. Anabolic steroids and training. *Clin Sports Med* 1986;5:461–469.
8. Wilson JD. Androgens. In: Gilman AG, Goodman LS, Rall YW, et al., eds. *The pharmacological basis of therapeutics,* 8th ed. New York: Macmillan, 1993: 1413–1430.
9. Yesalis CE III, Kennedy NJ, Kopstein AN, Bahrke MS. Anabolic-androgenic steroid use in the United States. *JAMA* 1993;270:1217–1221.
10. DuRant RH, Rickert VI, Ashworth CS, Newman C, Slavens G. Use of multiple drugs among adolescents who use anabolic steroids. *N Engl J Med* 1993; 328:922–926.
11. Hickson RC, Czerwinski SM, Falduto MT, Young AP, Glucocorticoid antagonism by exercise and androgenic–anabolic steroids. *Med Sci Sports Exerc* 1990;22:331–340.
12. Haupt HA, Rovere GD. Anabolic steroids: a review of the literature. *Am J Sports Med* 1984;12:469–484.
13. Ryan AJ. Anabolic steroids are fool's gold. *Fed Proc* 1981;40:2682–2688.
14. Strauss RH, Liggett MT, Lanese RR. Anabolic steroid use and perceived effects in ten weight-trained women athletes. *JAMA* 1985;253:2871–2873.
15. Position Stand: *Anabolic steroids and athletes.* Indianapolis: American College of Sports Medicine, 1987.
16. Pope HG, Katz DL. Affective and psychotic symptoms associated with anabolic steroid use. *Am J Psychiatry* 1988;145:487–490.
17. Wise RA. Neural mechanisms of the reinforcing action of cocaine. In: Gragowski J, ed. *Cocaine: pharmacology, effects, and treatment of abuse* (NIDA Research Monograph 50). Rockville, MD: National Institute on Drug Abuse, 1984:15–33.
18. Hoffman BB, Lefkowitz RJ. Catecholamines and sympathomimetic drugs. In: Gilman AG, ed: *The Pharmacological Basis of Therapeutics,* 8th ed. New York: Macmillan, 1993:187–220.
19. Langston JW, Langston EB. Neurological consequences of drug abuse. In: Asbury AK, McKhann GM, McDonald WI, eds. *Diseases of nervous system— clinical neurobiology.* Philadelphia: WB Saunders, 1986:1333–1340.
20. Smith GM, Beecher HK. Amphetamine sulfate and athletic performance: objective effects. *JAMA* 1959; 170:542–557.
21. Blum B, Stern M. A comparative evaluation of the action of depressant and stimulant drugs on human performance. *Psychopharmacology* 1964;6:173–177.
22. Domino EF, Albers JW, Potvin AR, Repa BS, Tourtellotte WW. Effects of D-amphetamine on quantitative measures of motor performance. *Clin Pharmacol Ther* 1972;13:251–257.
23. Lovingood B. Effects of D-amphetamine sulfate, caffeine and high temperature on human performance. *Res Q* 1965;38:64–71.

24. Chandler J, Blair S. The effect of amphetamines on selected physiological components related to athletic success. *Med Sci Sports Exerc* 1980;12:65–69.
25. Citron B, Halpern M, McCarron M, et al. Necrotizing angiitis associated with drug abuse. *N Engl J Med* 1970;2873:1003–1011.
26. Bostwick D. Amphetamine induced cerebral vasculitis. *Hum Pathol* 1981;12:1031–1033.
27. Stafford CR, Bogdanoff BM, Green L, Spector HB. Mononeuropathy multiplex as a complication of amphetamine angiitis. *Neurology* 1975;25:570–575.
28. Caplan JR, Hier DB, Banks G. Current concepts of cerebrovascular disease—stroke: stroke and drug abuse. *Stroke* 1982;13:869–874.
29. Fischman MW. Cocaine and the amphetamine. In: Meltzer HY, ed. *Psychopharmacology: the third generation progress.* New York: Raven Press, 1987:1543–1551.
30. Freud S. *Cocaine papers.* New York: Stonehill, 1974:97–104.
31. Resnick RB, Resnick EB. Cocaine abuse and its treatment. *Psychiatr Clin North Am* 1984;7:713–729.
32. Cited in Kirkman D. Experts: coke even hurts best athletes. *Newsday* 1986 April, 24:64.
33. Kelly KP, Han DH, Fellingham GW, Winder WW, Conlee RK. Cocaine and exercise: physiological responses of cocaine-conditioned rats. *Med Sci Sports Exerc* 1995;27:65–72.
34. Lowenstein DH, Massa SM, Rowbotham MC, Collins SD, McKinney HE, Simon RP. Acute neurologic and psychiatric complications associated with cocaine abuse. *Am J Med* 1987;83:841–846.
35. Greden JF. Caffeine and tobacco dependence. In: Kaplan HL, Sadock BJ, eds. *Comprehensive textbook of psychiatry,* 4th ed. Baltimore: Williams & Wilkins, 1985;4:1026–1033.
36. Powers SK, Dodd S. Caffeine and endurance performance. *J Sports Med* 1985;2:165–174.
37. Curatolo PW, Roberton D. The health consequences of caffeine. *Ann Intern Med* 1983;2:165–174.
38. Toner MM, Kirkendall DT, Delio DJ. Metabolic and cardiovascular responses to exercise with caffeine. *Ergonomics* 1982;25:1175–1183.
39. Boublik JH, Quinn MJ, Clements JA, Herington AC, Wynne KN, Funder JW. Coffee contains potent opiate receptor–binding activity. *Nature* 1983;301:246.
40. Delbeke FT, Debackere M. Caffeine: use and abuse in sports. *Int J Sports Med* 1984;5:179–182.
41. Eichner ER. The caffeine controversy: effects on endurance and cholesterol. *Phys Sportsmed* 1986;14:124–132.
42. Lopes JM, Aubier M, Jardim J, Aranda JV, Macklem PT. Effect of caffeine on skeletal muscle function before and after fatigue. *J Appl Physiol* 1983;54:1303–1305.
43. Ivy JL, Costill DL, Fink WJ, Lower RW. Influence of caffeine and carbohydrate feedings on endurance performance. *Med Sci Sports* 1979;11:6–11.
44. Tarnopolsky MA, Alkinson SA, MacDougall JD, Sale DG, Sutton JR. Physiological responses to caffeine during endurance running in habitual caffeine users. *Med Sci Sports Exerc* 1989;21:418–424.
45. Arogyasami J, Yang HT, Winder WW. Effect of intravenous caffeine on muscle glycogenolysis in fasted exercising rats. *Med Sci Sports Exerc* 1989;21:167–172.
46. Arogyasami J, Yang HT, Winder WW. Effect of caffeine on glycogenolysis during exercise in endurance trained rats. *Med Sci Sports Exerc* 1989;21:173–177.
47. Holliday A, Devery W. Effects of drugs on the performance of a task in fatigued subjects. *Clin Pharmacol Ther* 1982;3:5–15.
48. Goldstein A, Kaizer S, Warren R. Psychotropic effects of caffeine in man: alertness, psychomotor coordination, and mood. *J Pharmacol Exp Ther* 1965;150:146–151.
49. Franks HM, Hagedorn H, Hensley VR, Hensley WJ, Starmer GA. The effect of caffeine on human performance alone and in combination with ethanol. *Psychopharmacology* 1975;45:177–181.
50. Curatolo PW, Robertson D. The health consequences of caffeine. *Ann Intern Med* 1983;98:641–653.
51. Alsott RL, Miller AJ, Forney RB. Report of a human fatality due to caffeine. *J Forensic Sci* 1973;18:135–136.
52. Lake CR, Quirk RS. CNS stimulants and the look-alike drugs. *Psychiatr Clin North Am* 1984;7:689–701.
53. Sidney KH, Lefcoe NM. The effects of ephedrine on the physiological and psychological responses to submaximal and maximal exercise in man. *Med Sci Sports* 1977;9:95–99.
54. Montgomery LC, Deuster PA. Acute antihistamine ingestion does not affect muscle strength and endurance. *Med Sci Sports Exerc* 1991;23:1016–1019.
55. Montgomery LC, Deuster PA. Ingestion of an antihistamine does not affect exercise performance. *Med Sci Sports Exerc* 1992;24:383–388.
56. Johnson DA, Etter HS, Reeves DM. Stroke and phenylpropanolamine use. *Lancet* 1983;2:970. Letter.
57. Wooten MR, Khangure MD, Murphy MJ. Intracerebral hemorrhage and vasculitis related to ephedrine abuse. *Ann Neurol* 1983;13:337–340.
58. Kase CS, Foster TE, Reed JE, Spatz EL, Girgis GN. Intracerebral hemorrhage and phenylpropanolamine use. *Neurology* 1987;37:399–404.
59. Eisenhofer G. Lambie D, Johnson R. Effects of ethanol on plasma catecholamines and norepinephrine clearance. *Clin Pharmacol Ther* 1983;34:143–147.
60. Baselt RC. *Disposition of toxic drugs and chemicals in man,* 2nd ed. Davis, CA: Biomedical Publishing, 1982:299–303.
61. Angell M, Kassirer JP. Alcohol and other drugs—toward a more rational and consistent policy. *N Engl J Med* 1994;331:537–539.
62. Brewer RD, Morris PD, Cole TB, Watkins S, Patetta MJ, Popkin C. The risk of dying in alcohol-related automobile crashes among habitual drunk drivers. *N Engl J Med* 1994;331:513–517.
63. Ryback R. Facilitation and inhibition of learning and memory by alcohol. *Ann N Y Acad Sci* 1973;215:187–194.
64. Koller WC, Biary N. Effect of alcohol on tremors: comparison with propranolol. *Neurology* 1984;34:221–222.
65. Hebbelinck M. The effects of a moderate dose of alcohol on a series of functions of physical performance in man. *Acta Int Pharmacol* 1959;120:402–405.
66. Williams M. Effect of selected doses of alcohol on fatigue parameters of the forearm flexor muscles. *Res Q* 1969;40:832–840.
67. Bobo W. Effects of alcohol upon maximum oxygen uptake, lung ventilation and heart rate. *Res Q* 1972;43:1–6.

68. Bond V, Franks B, Hawsley E. Effects of small and moderate doses of alcohol on submaximal cardiorespiratory function, perceived exertion and endurance performance in abstainers and moderate drinkers. *J Sports Med* 1983;23:221–228.

69. Blonquist G, Saltin B, Mitchell J. Acute effects of ethanol ingestion on the response to submaximal and maximal exercise in man. *Circulation* 1970; 42:463–470.

70. Gustafson R. Alcohol and vigilance performance: effect of small doses of alcohol on simple visual reaction time. *Percept Motor Skills* 1986;62:951–955.

71. Moskowitz H, Burns M. Effects of alcohol on the psychological refractory period. *Q J Stud Alcohol* 1971;32:782–790.

72. Rundell O, Williams H. Alcohol and speed accuracy trade-off. *Hum Factors* 1979;21:433–436.

73. Yesavage JA, Leirer VO. Hangover effects on aircraft pilots 14 hours after alcohol ingestion: a preliminary report. *Am J Psychiatry* 1986;143:1546–1550.

74. Miller NS, Gold MS, Cocores JA, Pottash AC. Alcohol dependence and its medical consequences. *NY State J Med* Sept 1988;88:476–481.

75. Cosquitt M, Fielding LP, Cronan JF. Drunk drivers and medical and social injury. *N Engl J Med* 1987; 317:1262–1266.

76. Rashbass C. Russell G. Action of barbiturate drug (amylbarbitone sodium) on the vestibulo-ocular reflex. *Brain* 1961;84:329–335.

77. American Medical Association Department of Drugs, Division of Drugs and Technology. Drugs used for anxiety and sleep disorders. In: *AMA drug evaluations*, 6th ed. Philadelphia: WB Saunders, 1986:81–110.

78. Rall TW. Hypnotics and sedatives; ethanol. In: Gilman AG, et al. (eds). *The pharmacological basis of therapeutics*, 8th ed. New York: Macmillan, 1985:345–382.

79. Schroeder D, Collins W. Effects of secobarbital and D-amphetamine on tracking performance during angular acceleration. *Ergonomics* 1974;17:613–621.

80. Talland G, Quarton G. Methamphetamine and pentobarbital effects on human motor performance. *Psychopharmacology* 1965;8:241–250.

81. Truijens C, Trumbo D, Wagenaar W. Amphetamine and barbiturate effects on human motor performance. *Psychopharmacology* 1965;8:241–250.

82. Smith GM, Beecher HK. Amphetamine, secobarbital and athletic performance: Part II: Subjective evaluations of performance, mood states and physical stress. *JAMA* 1960;172:1502–1514.

83. Findlay LJ, Koller WC. Essential tremor: a review. *Neurology* 1987;37:1194–1197.

84. Shader RI, Greenblatt DJ. Use of benzodiazepines in anxiety disorders. *N Engl J Med* 1993;328:1398–1405.

85. Huber SJ, Paulson GW. Efficacy of alprazolam for essential tremor. *Neurology* 1988;38:241–243.

86. Collomp KR. Effects of benzodiazepine during a Wingate test: interaction with caffeine. *Med Sci Sports Exerc* 1993;25:1375–1380.

87. Payne R. Anatomy and physiology of cancer pain. In: *Management of cancer pain (syllabus of postgraduate course)*. New York: Memorial Sloan Kettering Cancer Center; 1985:1–14.

88. Inturrisi CE. Role of opioid analgesics. *Am J Med* 1984;77:27–37.

89. Inturrisi CE. Narcotic drugs. *Med Clin North Am* 1982;66:1061–1071.

90. Rounsaville B, Jones C, Novelly RA, Kleber H. Neurophysiological functioning in opiate addicts. *J Nerv Ment Dis* 1982;170:209–216.

91. Brown R, Partington J. A psychometric comparison of narcotic addicts with hospital attendants. *J Gen Psychol* 1942;27:71–79.

92. Bruhn P, Maage N. Intellectual and neuropsychological functions in young men with heavy and long-term patterns of drug abuse. *Am J Pychol* 1975;132:397–401.

93. Stein C, Comisel K, Haimerl E, et al. Analgesic effect of intraarticular morphine after arthroscopic knee surgery. *N Engl J Med* 1991;325:1123–1126.

94. Indelicato P. Comparison of diflunisal and acetaminophen with codeine in the treatment of mild to moderate pain due to strains and sprains. *Clin Ther* 1986;8:269–274.

95. Aghababian RV. Comparison of diflunisal and acetaminophen with codeine in the management of grade 2 ankle sprain. *Clin Ther* 1986;8:520–526.

96. Eichner ER: Blood doping: implications of recent research. *Sports Med Dig* 1987;9(11):4–6.

97. Williams MH, Goodwin AR, Perkins R, Bocrie J. Effect of blood reinjection upon endurance capacity and heart rate. *Med Sci Sports* 1973;5:181–185.

98. Brien AJ, Simon TL. The effects of red blood cell infusion on 10-km race time. *JAMA* 1987;257:2761–2765.

99. Robertson RJ, Gilcher R, Metz KF, et al. Hemoglobin concentration and aerobic work capacity in women following induced erythrocythemia. *J Appl Physiol* 1984;57:568–575.

100. Eschbach JW, Egrie JC, Downing MR, Browne JK, Adamson JW. Correction of the anemia of endstage renal disease with recombinant human erythropoietin. Results of a combined phase I and II clinical trial. *N Engl J Med* 1987;316:73–78.

101. Erslev AJ. Erythropoietin. *N Engl J Med* 1991; 324:1339–1344.

102. Higden H. Blood doping among endurance athletes: rationalizations, results and ramifications. *Am Med News* 1985 Sept 27:37.

103. Walker R. Brown A. Test drug surpassed doping. *Calgary Herald* 1988 17 Feb 17:3 OAI.

104. Berglund EB. Effect of erythropoietin administration on maximal aerobic power. *Scand J Med Sci Sports* 1991;1:88–93.

105. Abuse of erythropoietin to enhance athletic performance. *Sports Med Dig* 1991;13:6.

106. Melmed S. Acromegaly. *N Engl J Med* 1990; 322:966–977.

107. Rogol AD. Growth hormone: physiology, therapeutic use, and potential for abuse. *Exerc Sport Sci Rev* 1989;17:352–377.

108. Rudman D, Kutner MH, Blackston RD, Cushman RA, Bain RP, Patterson JH. Children with normal-variant short stature: treatment with human growth hormone for six months. *N Engl J Med* 1981;305:123–131.

109. Van Vliet G. Growth hormone treatment for short stature. *N Engl J Med* 1983;309:1016–1022.

110. Linder B, Cassoria F. Short stature: etiology, diagnosis, and treatment. *JAMA* 1988;260:3171–3175.

111. Wilmore DW. Catabolic illness: strategies for enhancing recovery. *N Engl J Med* 1991;325:695–702.

112. Yarasheski KE, Zachweija JJ, Angelopoulos TJ, Bier DM. Short-term growth hormone treatment does not increase muscle protein synthesis in experienced weight lifters. *J Appl Physiol* 1993;74:3073–3076.

113. Yarasheski KE, Campbell JA, Smith K, Rennie MJ, Holloszy JO, Bier DM. Effect of growth hormone and resistance exercise on muscle growth in young men. *Am J Physiol* 1992;25:E261–267.

114. Kaiser P. Physical performance and muscle metabolism during β-adrenergic blockade in man. *Acta Physiol Scand* 1984;536:1–53.

115. Committee on Substance Abuse Research and Education. *USOC/IOC banned drugs*. United States Olympic Committee, Oct 1986.

116. Stewart KJ, Effron MB, Valenti SA, Kelemen MH. Effects of diltiazem or propranolol during exercise training of hypertensive men. *Med Sci Sports Exerc* 1990;22:171–177.

117. Clonidine vs atenolol for hypertensive aerobic exercisers. *Sports Med Dig* 1989;11:10.

118. Gordon NF, Duncan JJ. Effect of beta-blockers on exercise physiology: implications for exercise training. *Med Sci Sports Exerc* 1991;23:668–676.

119. Choice of a beta-blocker. *Med Lett* 1986;28:20–22.

120. Jacobson BH. Effect of amino acids on growth hormone release. *Phys Sportsmed* 1990;18:63–70.

121. McCarthy P. How much protein do athletes really need? *Phys Sportsmed* 1989;17:170–175.

122. Protein requirements for athletes. *Sports Med Dig* 1990;12:1–3.

123. Slavin JL, Lanners G, Engstrom MA. Amino acid supplements: beneficial or risky? *Phys Sportsmed* 1988;16:221–224.

124. Teman AJ, Hainline B. Eosinophilia-myalgia syndrome: athletes should discard dietary L-tryptophan. *Phys Sportsmed* 1991;19:81–86.

125. *Position stand: weight loss in wrestlers*. Indianapolis: American College of Sports Medicine, 1976.

126. Rosen LW, Hough DO. Pathogenic weight-control behaviors of female college gymnasts. *Phys Sportsmed* 1988;16:140–146.

127. Caldwell JE, Ahonen E, Nousianen U. Differential effects of sauna-, diuretic-, and exercise-induced hypohydration. *J Appl Physiol* 1984;57:1018–1022.

128. Webster S, Rutt R, Weltman A. Physiological effects of a weight loss regimen practiced by college wrestlers. *Med Sci Sports Exerc* 1990;22:229–234.

129. Calabrese LH, Rooney TW. The use of nonsteroidal anti-inflammatory drugs in sports. *Phys Sportsmed* 1986;14:89–98.

130. Hasson SM, Daniels JC, Divine JG, et al. Effect of ibuprofen use on muscle soreness, damage, and performance: a preliminary investigation. *Med Sci Sports Exerc* 1993;25:9–17.

131. Wilkes K, Gledhill N, Smyth R. Effect of acute induced metabolic alkalosis on 800-m racing time. *Med Sci Sports Exerc* 1983;15:277–280.

132. Kozak-Collins K, Burke ER, Schoene RB. Sodium bicarbonate ingestion does not improve performance in women cyclists. *Med Sci Sports Exerc* 1994;26:1510–1515.

133. Jain SC, Singh MV, Rawal SB, et al. Effect of phosphate supplementation on oxygen delivery at high altitude. *Int J Biometeorol* 1987;31:249–257.

134. Kreider RB, Miller GW, Williams MH, Somma CT, Nasser TA. Effects of phosphate loading on oxygen uptake, ventilatory anaerobic threshold, and run performance. *Med Sci Sports Exerc* 1990;22:250–256.

135. Rock CL. Vitamin and mineral needs of older athletes. *Sports Med Dig* 1993;15:7–8.

136. Toxic effects of vitamin overdose. *Med Lett* 1984; 26:73–74.

137. Parry GJ, Bredesen DE. Sensory neuropathy with low-dose pyridoxine. *Neurology* 1985;35:1466–1468.

138. Rebouche CJ, Engel AG. Carnitine metabolism and deficiency syndromes. *Mayo Clin Proc* 1983;58:533–540.

139. Vukovich MD, Costill DL, Fink W. Carnitine supplementation: effect on muscle carnitine and glycogen content during exercise. *Med Sci Sports Exerc* 1994; 26:1122–1129.

140. Decombaz J, Deriaz O, Acheson K, Gmuender B, Jequier E. Effect of L-carnitine on submaximal exercise metabolism after depletion of muscle glycogen. *Med Sci Sports Exerc* 1993;25:733–740.

141. Keith R. Symptoms of carnitine like deficiency in a trained runner taking D,L-carnitine. *JAMA* 1986; 255:1137.

142. Lombardo J. Stimulants and athletic performance: cocaine and nicotine. *Phys Sportsmed* 1986;14:85–90.

143. Van Duser BL, Raven PB. The effects of oral smokeless tobacco on the cardiorespiratory response to exercise. *Med Sci Sports Exerc* 1992;24:389–395.

144. Perkins KA, Sexton JE, Solberg-Kassel RD, Epstein LH. Effects of nicotine on perceived exertion during low-intensity activity. *Med Sci Sports Exerc* 1991; 23:1283–1288.

145. Landers DM, Crews DJ, Boutcher SH, Skinner JS, Gustafsen S. The effects of smokeless tobacco on performance and psychophysiological response. *Med Sci Sports Exerc* 1992;24:895–903.

146. Jaffe J, Jarvik M. Tobacco use and tobacco. In: Lipton M, DeMascio A, Killam K, eds. *Psychopharmacology: a generation of progress*. New York: Raven Press, 1978:1665–1676.

147. Henningfield J, Miyasto K, Jasinki D. Cigarette smokers self administer intravenous nicotine. *Pharmacol Biochem Behav* 1983;19:887–890.

148. Bovet D, Bovet-Nitti F, Oliverio A. Action of nicotine on spontaneous and acquired behavior in rats and mice. *Ann N Y Acad Sci* 1967;142:261–267.

149. Kessler DA. Nicotine addiction in young people. *N Engl J Med* 1995; 333:186–189.

150. Warren KE. Health and economic implications of a tobacco-free society. *JAMA* 1987;258:2080–2086.

151. Eskow RN. Hazards of smokeless tobacco. *N Engl J Med* 1987;317:1229.

152. Dewey W. Cannabinoid pharmacology. *Pharmacol Rev* 1986;38:151–178,

153. Yesavage JA, Leirer VO, Denari M, Hollister LE. Carry-over effects of marijuana intoxication on aircraft pilot performance. *Am J Psychiatry* 1985;142:1325–1329.

154. Hollister L. Health aspects of cannabis. *Pharmacol Rev* 1986;38:1–20.

155. Haynes RC. Adrenocorticotropic hormone; adrenocortical steroids and their synthetic analogs; inhibitors of the synthesis and actions of adrenocortical hormones. In: Gilman AG. *The pharmacological basis of therapeutics*, 8th ed. New York: McGraw-Hill, 1993: 1431–1462.

156. Kerlan RK, Glousman RE. Injections and techniques in athletic medicine. *Clin Sports Med* 1989;8:541–560.

157. Hanley DF. Drug and sex testing: regulations for international competition. *Clin Sports Med* 1986;2:13–17.

158. Fields L, Lange WR, Kreiter NA, Fudala PJ. A national survey of drug testing policies for college athletes. *Med Sci Sports Exerc* 1994;26:682–686.

Sports Neurology, Second Edition,
edited by Barry D. Jordan.
Lippincott–Raven Publishers, Philadelphia © 1998.

4

Functional Anatomy and Biomechanics of the Spine in Sports

Stuart M. Weinstein

*Puget Sound Sports and Spine Physicians, P.S., 1600 East Jefferson Street,
Seattle, Washington 98122*

Within the demands of athletic activity, the spine is subject to acute dynamic overload as well as chronic repetitive exertions. Especially in the athlete, abnormal structure occurring through previous injury or chronic postural adaptations places the spine at risk for further injury. The tolerance of the spinal mechanism to these loads, which is in a general sense determined by the equilibrium between mobility and stability, varies throughout the spinal axis. Understanding the functional anatomy and biomechanics of the spine requires a knowledge of gross and segmental regional kinematics and neurovascular anatomy. This chapter will review relevant aspects of this topic as it relates to athletic injury, with emphasis on the neurologic implications of normal and abnormal anatomy and function.

SPINAL MOBILITY

Although clinically, in the office or on the field, the sports medicine practitioner typically assesses gross spinal motion, it is important to recognize that this does not adequately reflect the complete spinal mechanism. This observed range of motion is actually a summation of segmental motion. Except for the unique anatomic arrangement of the upper cervical spine (from the occiput to C-2), each segment is defined by the three-joint complex: the single discovertebral joint anteriorly and the paired zygapophyseal joints posteriorly (Fig. 1). The cardinal

planes of segmental motion are flexion and extension, torsion and lateral flexion and are all a combination of rotation in a specific plane (i.e., sagittal, axial, and coronal, respectively) plus translation in the same plane (Fig. 2). Gross range of motion may be perceived as "normal" despite the presence of underlying segmental motion abnormalities (i.e., hypo- and hypermobilities) (Fig. 3). Furthermore, segmental motion usually occurs as so-called coupled motion; that is, movement that occurs in one axis is consistently associated with motion that occurs about a second axis (Fig. 4).

The assessment of spinal range of motion may be made clinically or radiographically, in cadavers or living subjects. The cadaveric studies are often performed with the musculature removed, and slightly greater absolute values result. Clinically, total range of motion is relatively easy to determine but not necessarily reflective of a specific pathologic disease or location and therefore may have limited clinical relevance. Segmental motion is more difficult to assess by physical examination, although advanced manual examination techniques (1) do assist in localizing segmental dysfunction to a specific level(s) and may be more predictive of relevant pathomechanics. Both total range of motion and segmental motion are inversely proportional to age, which needs to be considered when evaluating spinal injury in the athlete, especially with increasing numbers of "senior" athletes. Conversely, the cervical

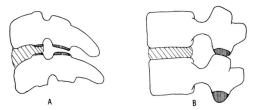

FIG. 1. Diagrammatic representation of the three-joint complex of a typical cervical (**A**) and lumbar (**B**) segment indicating the anterior discovertebral joint and the posterior zygapophyseal joint. In the cervical spine, below the C-3 vertebral body, uncovertebral joints are also present in the posterior aspect of the anterior column. (From ref. 22, with permission.)

spines of younger athletes may in fact exhibit "excessive" range of motion, typically in the upper cervical spine, which is not indicative of a pathologic state (2).

The cervical spine is the most mobile part of the spinal axis, and the potential for sports-induced neurologic injury is proportional to this high degree of mobility. The upper cervical segments [i.e., occiput (C0)-1, C1-2] are unique to the rest of the spinal axis in that there does not exist an intervertebral disc. All planes of range of

motion are available in the cervical spine and coupled motion patterns are well developed. During cervical flexion and extension, sagittal rotation and translation (or shear) occur, the normal upper limit of translation in the middle to lower cervical spine in one direction being approximately 3 mm (3). Another strong coupling pattern occurs between axial rotation and lateral bending, probably because of the oblique orientation of the cervical zygapophyseal joints (Fig. 5). The following are generally accepted levels of maximal segmental range of motion: flexion and extension at the C5-6 level, although head nodding occurs primarily at the C0-1 level owing to the cup-shaped articulation of the occipital condyles and the C-1 facets and rotation of the C1-2 level due to the relationship between the dens and the posterior arch of C-1 (Fig. 6). Approximately 50% of the total available rotation in the cervical spine occurs at the C1-2 level, but because of coupled motion patterns, pure rotation does not take place at any segment. The proportion of rotation to lateral bending increases more rostrally in the cervical spine. Minimal segmental range-of-motion values are also important to recognize as these serve to protect vital neurovascular structures. Rotation and lateral bending are least present at the C0-1 articulation, presumably protecting the vertebral artery from excessive force as it enters the cranium.

Although normal spinal kinematics reveal physiologic coupling patterns, exaggeration of this association (i.e., axial rotation and lateral bending), as can occur with forceful trauma, can directly lead to injury. In particular, the 45° orientation of the middle to lower cervical zygapophyseal joints places the facets at the correct angle for dislocation. For example, lateral bending of the neck to the right is physiologically coupled with rotation of the head to the right as well. The vertebral body rotates right with the spinous process, moving toward the convexity of the curve (Fig. 7). Excessive bending forces the left facet to move too far cephalad, resulting in a facet dislocation on the left.

The thoracic spine with the rib cage is the stiffest and least mobile part of the spine and is vital for erect support. The two main directions

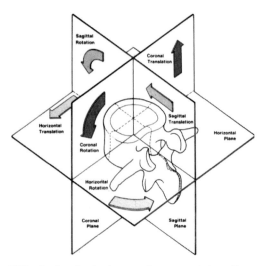

FIG. 2. Cardinal planes of segmental motion. (From ref. 6, with permission.)

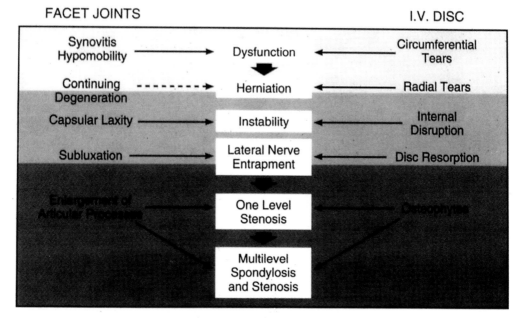

FIG. 3. Segmental motion abnormalities as determined by the interaction between the anterior and posterior elements. The upper box is representative of segmental dysfunction (primarily hypomobility), the middle box is representative of segmental hypermobility, and the lower box is representative of segmental stability. (From ref. 23, with permission.)

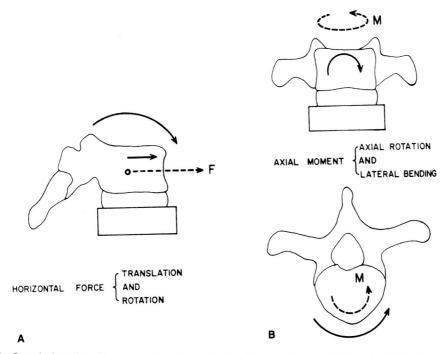

FIG. 4. Coupled motion. Two examples of coupled motion are shown. **A:** An anterior horizontal force, F, produces translation (main motion) and rotation (coupled motion). **B:** Axial torque or moment, M, produces axial rotation (main motion) and lateral rotation (coupled motion). (From ref. 4, with permission.)

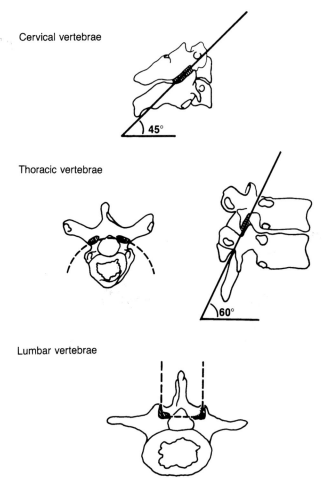

Cervical vertebrae

45°

Thoracic vertebrae

60°

Lumbar vertebrae

FIG. 5. Characteristic zygapophyseal joint orientation in the cervical, thoracic, and lumbar regions. (From ref. 4, with permission.)

of segmental motion within the thoracic spine are sagittal flexion and extension and axial rotation, the latter more evident in the upper thoracic spine from approximately T-1 through T-6 and the former more typical of the lower thoracic segments. An abrupt change in thoracic spine stiffness occurs at approximately the T-9 level. Above this level the thoracic spine acts more like the cervical spine, and below this level it demonstrates motion more typical of the lumbar spine. A strong coupling pattern between sagittal rotation and anterior–posterior translation exists, but other coupling characteristics such as between axial rotation and lateral bending are much weaker than in the cervical spine.

Observed lumbar spine motion is the additive effect of each motion segment from the thoracolumbar junction through the lumbosacral segment, plus lumbopelvic rhythm of the hip joint. The optimal lumbar mechanism provides risk-limited mobility, with the lower lumbar spine generally being the most mobile but also subject to the greatest loads. All cardinal planes of motion occur in lumbar spine with associated coupling characteristics. As in the cervical spine, there is a strong coupling pattern between axial rotation and lateral flexion (Fig. 8). The maximal available segmental range of motion in the lumbar spine occurs at the L4-5 and L5-S1 segments with approximately 20° of flexion and ex-

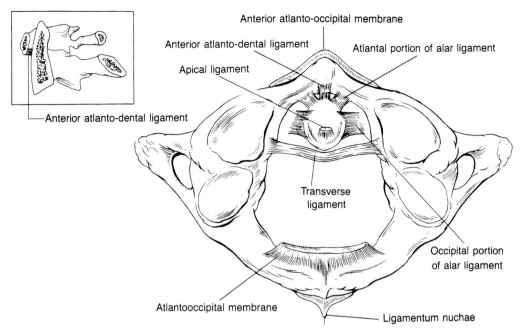

FIG. 6. Cross-sectional depiction of the relationship between the dens and the C-1 vertebral body including the major supporting ligaments. (From ref. 4, with permission.)

tension and 1 to 3 mm of translation at each level. Lateral flexion occurs maximally in the upper lumbar spine, although the absolute range of motion is substantially less (i.e., 5 to 6°) than flexion–extension in the anterior–posterior direction. Little to no lateral flexion occurs at the L5-S1 segment. Axial rotation is variably available at all lumbar segments, but no more than 3°, which provides a protective mechanism for the intervertebral disc.

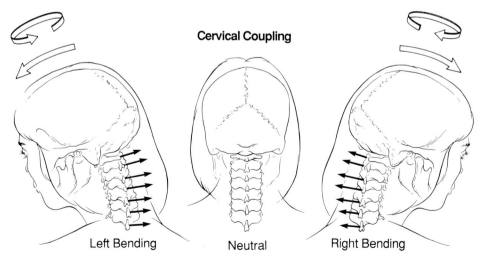

FIG. 7. Cervical spine coupling pattern—lateral bending and rotation. When the head and neck are bent to the right or left, the spinous processes rotate in the opposite direction. (From ref. 4, with permission.)

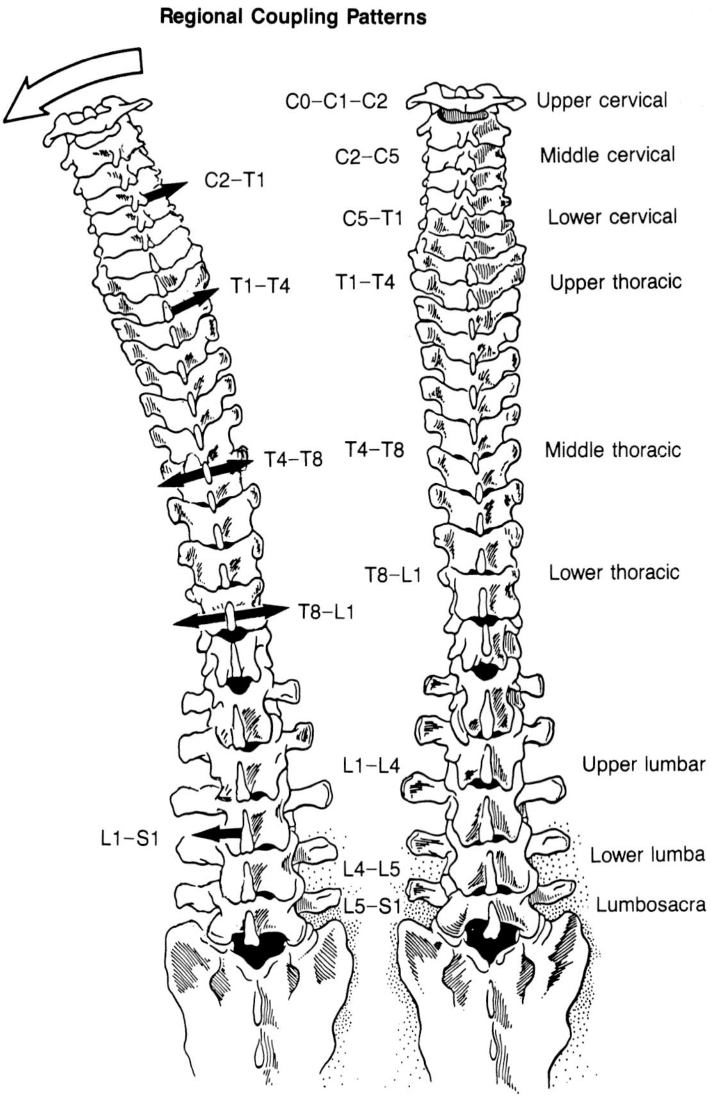

Regional Coupling Patterns

FIG. 8. Composite of the various coupling patterns throughout the spinal axis. In the lumbar spine, side bending to one side results in spinous process rotation to the same side, the opposite of what occurs in the cervical spine. (From ref. 4, with permission.)

SPINAL STABILITY

Throughout the spinal axis, various anatomic components variably contribute to spinal segmental stability, including the intervertebral disc, joints, ligaments, and muscles. Similar to the glenohumeral joint, the instantaneous center of rotation (ICR) principle applies to the three-joint complex as well. The ICR can be defined as a single pivot point around which movement occurs, the location of which can vary through the entire range of motion but is consistent from time to time and at each instant. Maintenance of this ICR provides the most efficient motion with no symptom production and limits shear stresses across the three-joint complex, which in turn limits the tendency for acute injury or chronic degenerative changes to develop. However, the natural aging process, habitual postural alterations, and spinal injury can all lead to alterations in the ICR at any segmental level and often at a combination of levels simultaneously, which can include segmental hypomobility as well as hypermobility.

In the cervical spine, the ligamentous contribution to stability is probably greater than in the thoracic or lumbar spine. These ligaments provide the main restraint in the upper cervical spine complex (4), where neurovascular protection is vital, fixing the occiput to C-2 [via the apical and alar ligaments (5) and tectorial membrane, a rostral continuation of the posterior longitudinal ligament], C-1 to C-2 (via the transverse ligament, maintaining the dens against the posterior arch of C-1, tectorial membrane, and posterior atlantooccipital membrane, which replaces the ligamentum flavum), and the occiput to C-1 (via the anterior and posterior atlantooccipital membranes and possibly the nuchal ligament) (Fig. 6). In addition, in the middle to lower cervical spine, the posterior longitudinal ligament is very well developed, serving to reinforce the posterior disc margin, thus protecting the spinal cord. The ligamentum flavum reinforces the zygapophyseal joint capsule, and a combination of the interspinous, supraspinous, and nuchal ligaments provides posterior segmental stability, limiting excessive anterior translation (Fig. 9).

The bony anatomy of the upper cervical spine is unique. There is no disc above the C-2 vertebral body, and there exists an intimate relationship of the anterior and lateral mass of C-1 with the odontoid process of C-2. Furthermore, the superior facets of C-1 are cup shaped to accommodate the occipital condyles. This unique orientation minimizes rotation and lateral bending at the C0-1 level and, as previously mentioned, protects the vertebral arteries. The zygapophyseal joints of the cervical spine contribute little to stability and, in fact, are oriented to maximize mobility. Conversely, the uncovertebral joints provide stability, particularly to the posterolateral aspects of the intervertebral disc, and also guide motion in the flexion–extension plane (Fig. 10). These are synovial joints, present from C-3 to C-7, and develop postnatally. Uncovertebral joint arthropathy may potentially contribute to abnormal (i.e., painful and/or restricted) motion as well as nerve root impingement resulting from neuroforaminal narrowing or vertebral artery compromise resulting from transverse foramina compromise.

Multiple muscles act on the head and neck to provide stability and generate motion (Table 1). The main action of any muscle is proportional to the length of its lever arm, with shorter muscles acting mainly as segmental stabilizers and longer muscles as prime movers. In general, there is a balance between anterior and posterior muscular activity, with muscle strength and flexibility imbalances contributing to postural alterations. In the cervical spine, a "normal" lordosis places the C5-6 segment anterior to and farthest from the center of gravity. One common dysfunctional posture is the forward head posture as described by hyperextension of the C0-1 and C1-2 segments; hyperflexion of the lower cervical and upper thoracic segments; slackening of the nuchal ligament, which allows shear through the midcervical spine, promoting hypermobility; decrease in the size of the intervertebral foramen potentially leading to radicular symptoms and/or signs; increase in the weight-bearing load of the zygapophyseal joints; shortening of the anterior neck and chest wall myofascial structures and elevation of the first rib leading to thoracic outlet symptoms; and weakness of the cervical flexors, upper thoracic extensors, and scapular stabilizer musculature. As the head is positioned more anteriorly, the distance from the C5-6 segment to the center of gravity increases with concomitant increases in the demand on the posterior cervical musculature by as much as 200%, which in turn abnormally loads both the disc and the posterior elements.

Thoracic spine stability is afforded primarily through the rib cage, which stiffens and strengthens the spine via the costovertebral joints and ligaments, and by effectively increasing the transverse diameter of the spine, thus increasing its resistance to motion in any plane. At most of the costovertebral joints, the head of the rib articulates with the vertebral body at the same level and one rostral, and the rib tubercle articulates with the transverse process at the same level. Both are synovial joints with ligamentous

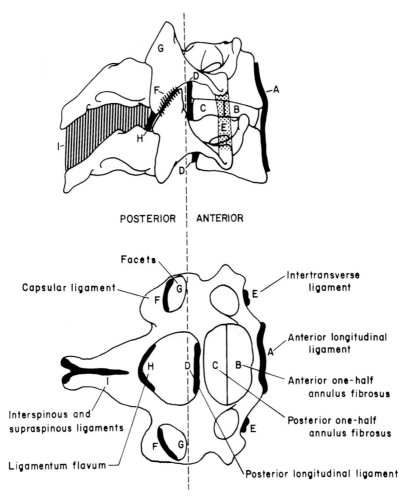

POSTERIOR | ANTERIOR

Facets

Capsular ligament

Intertransverse ligament

Anterior longitudinal ligament

Anterior one-half annulus fibrosus

Posterior one-half annulus fibrosus

Interspinous and supraspinous ligaments

Ligamentum flavum

Posterior longitudinal ligament

FIG. 9. Illustration of the ligamentous structures that participate in stabilizing the middle to lower cervical spine. (From ref. 4, with permission.)

support from the radiate and costotransverse ligaments, respectively (Fig. 11). The zygapophyseal joint and capsule also add to segmental stability. The upper joints protect primarily against anterior translation as the physiologic thoracic kyphosis, which is present because of the slight wedge configuration of the vertebral body and discs, causes the upper thoracic spine to be more prone to instability in flexion. The lower joints protect against axial rotation. The thoracolumbar junction has the highest torsional stiffness. Because of the strong intrinsic stability of these joints, the muscular contribution of most thoracic muscles is as prime movers for movement of the trunk on the pelvis as opposed to segmental stabilizers.

In the lumbar spine, there are multiple factors providing segmental stability, including muscles, ligaments, intervertebral disc, and zygapophyseal joint, with the muscular contribution proportionally the most important in protecting the three-joint complex against excessive shear. The ligamentous structures include the midline ligaments—comprising the supraspinous ligament, interspinous ligament, posterior longitudinal ligament, ligamentum flavum, and zygapophyseal joint capsule—and the anterior longitudinal ligament. The midline ligamentous

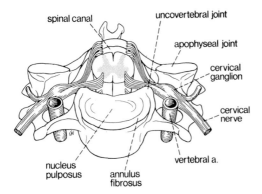

spinal canal

uncovertebral joint

apophyseal joint

cervical ganglion

cervical nerve

vertebral a.

nucleus pulposus

annulus fibrosus

FIG. 10. Diagrammatic representation of a transverse section through the midcervical spine indicating the uncovertebral joint in the postero-lateral position in relationship to the intervertebral disc. The close proximity of the uncovertebral joint to the neuroforamen is also demonstrated. (From ref. 24, with permission.)

structures form a passive restraint system that is engaged with forward bending (Fig. 12). The anterior longitudinal ligament acts to maintain the lumbar lordosis. The lumbar lordosis is an example of the balance between flexibility and stiffness. The advantage of the lumbar lordosis is that it is an ideal posture for axial load bearing. The

TABLE 1. *Muscles affecting head and neck motion*

Flexors	Extensors
Head	
Rectus capitis anterior[a]	Rectus capitis posterior[a]
Rectus capitis lateralis	Obliquus capitis[a,b]
Longus capitis[a]	Splenius capitis[a,b]
Longus colli[a,b]	Longissimus capitis[a,b]
	Semispinalis capitis
Neck	
Sternocleidomastoid[a,b]	Upper trapezius[a,b]
Scalenes (anterior)[a,b]	Splenius cervicis[a,b]
Longus colli[a,b]	"Erector spinae" group
	Iliocostalis cervicis[b]
	Longissimus cervicis
	Spinalis cervicis
	Semispinalis cervicis[a]
	Multifidi[a]
	Rotatores[a]
	Interspinales[a]
	Intertransversarii[a]

[a] Also contributes to axial rotation.
[b] Also contributes to lateral flexion.

load is borne passively by the zygapophyseal joint and ligaments (including the anterior longitudinal ligament, anterior annulus fibrosis, and iliolumbar ligament) and actively by the multifidi. This protects the intervertebral disc and vertebral endplates. The disadvantage is that the lordotic curve is an at risk posture in flexion. The sacrum is tilted forward 40 to 50°, the L-5 vertebral body and L5-S1 disc are wedge shaped, and the lumbosacral angle averages approximately 16° (Fig. 13). The anterior longitudinal ligament resists excessive lumbar extension via tensile force generation and also absorbs energy with axial load.

The ability of the zygapophyseal joint to contribute to lumbar stability is proportional to its geometry (Fig. 14). Articulatory facets that are oriented perpendicular to the sagittal plane restrict forward displacement and shear as the superior facet comes in contact with the inferior facet. The shape of the facet (i.e., flat or curved) further determines how much surface area of contact between facets will occur. Resistance to segmental rotation is afforded by facets that are oriented parallel to the sagittal plane. It is this facet orientation that restricts axial rotation in the lumbar spine to typically no more than 3° per segment, greater than which may result in annular tears.

An intact lumbar intervertebral disc functions in weight bearing (i.e., axial load), bending, and rotation to maintain lumbar stability. With brief axial loads, the mass of the annular fibers resists the external force, whereas with sustained axial loads, the nucleus pulposus acts by transmitting radial pressure to the annulus. Depending on the intactness of the annulus, radial expansion is minimized with equal counterpressure. Also, the nucleus pulposus transmits pressure to the end plate, thus bypassing the annulus altogether. The annulus is the primary structure resisting rotational force. It is arranged in 10 to 20 concentric collagenous lamellae with successive lamellae oriented 65° to the vertical, but in opposite directions (Fig. 15). The 65° angle is optimal to resist both horizontal and vertical forces, with half of the lamellae resisting twisting to the right and half resisting twisting to the left. Last, the resistance to forward bending is derived from the relatively greater thickness of the posterior lamellae and the

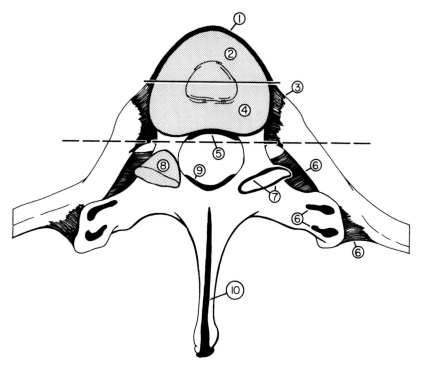

FIG. 11. The major ligaments involved in the thoracic spine: *1,* anterior longitudinal ligament; *2,* anterior half of the annulus fibrosis; *3,* radiate and costovertebral ligaments; *4,* posterior half of the annulus fibrosis; *5,* posterior longitudinal ligament; *6,* costotransverse and intertransverse ligaments; *7,* capsular ligaments; *8,* facet articulation; *9,* ligamentum flavum; *10,* supraspinous and interspinous ligaments. (From ref. 4, with permission.)

greater cross-sectional surface area of the annulus fibrosis posteriorly because of its concave configuration (Fig. 16).

The increase in intradiscal pressure with bending and lifting is due primarily to muscular compressive force and is proportional to the distance of the load being lifted from the body. With forward bending, the posterior annulus stretches and the nucleus pulposus is displaced posteriorly, which is an at-risk posture. The most disc-compromised posture is forward bending, rotation, and lifting a load away from the body. Given the great load demands on the lumbar three-joint complex, which can exceed the intrinsic capacity of these joints, ligaments, and discs, a large muscle contribution is necessary to provide dynamic stability (6).

The muscular components can be divided into posterior muscles—intrinsic and extrinsic—and prevertebral muscles (Table 2). Some muscle groups do provide passive stability as well, such as the erector spinae and hip extensors, generating five times the passive tension of the midline ligaments with forward bending (6). At approximately 90% of maximal lumbar flexion and 60% of hip flexion, the passive force generated in these muscles is fivefold greater than the ligamentous tension generated in the midline ligamentous structures. Dynamically, the contribution of these various muscles changes depending on the activity [i.e., standing posture, extension, lateral flexion, forward flexion, recovery phase (with or without load) and torsion]. With upright posture, little muscle activity occurs, as the lumbar spine is stabilized primarily by ligaments and the zygapophyseal joints. In approximately 75% of people, the line of gravity passes in front of the L-4 vertebral

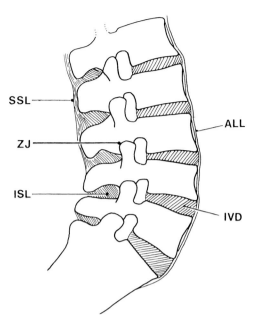

FIG. 12. Lumbar lordosis. Diagrammatic lateral representation of the intact lumbar spine showing its curved shape. *ALL,* anterior longitudinal ligament; *IVD,* intervertebral disc; *ZJ,* zygapophyseal joint; *SSL,* supraspinous ligament; *ISL,* interspinous ligament. (From ref. 6, with permission.)

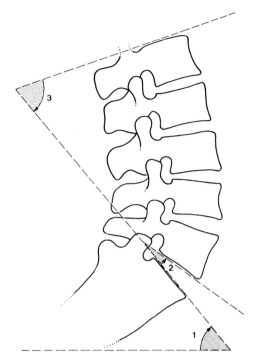

FIG. 13. Lumbar lordosis—some of the angles used to describe the lumbar spine. 1, The angle formed by the top of the sacrum in the horizontal plane. Mean value approximately 50°. 2, The angle between the bottom of L-5 and the top of the sacrum. Mean value approximately 16°. 3, The angle between the top of L-1 and the sacrum, used to measure the lumbar lordosis. Mean value approximately 70°. (From ref. 6, with permission.)

body; thus the multifidi, owing to their force vectors, provide an extension moment. Extension of the lumbar spine from an upright posture is initiated by the shorter segmental lumbar muscles, but with increasing load the longer lever arm erector spinae group is recruited. With lateral flexion, ipsilateral muscular activity initiates the motion, but gravity and bilateral lumbar and trunk muscle activity guide and control motion. During trunk flexion, both lumbar segmental and hip joint motions occur (Fig. 17). With the first 60° of forward bending, the lumbar segments flex with the hip extensors (i.e., gluteus maximus and hamstrings) acting eccentrically to "lock" the pelvis in extension, which maintains tension in the thoracolumbar fascia (see the following), and the erector spinae and multifidi act eccentrically, proportional to the angle of flexion. The next 25° is accomplished primarily by hip joint flexion. The

recovery phase from a forward bent position is essentially a reversal in sequence of forward bending, with the hip extensors, erector spinae, and multifidi all acting concentrically. The act of lifting a weight is basically the recovery phase with a load. To accomplish this with minimal shear across the lumbar segments, the abdominal mechanism (7) via the thoracolumbar fascia is one mechanism that is recruited. The thoracolumbar fascia is a broad soft tissue structure with superficial and deep layers attaching to the spinous processes in the midline, the rib cage superiorly, the pelvis (including the fascia of the gluteus maximus) inferiorly, and the free edge to the internal oblique, transversus

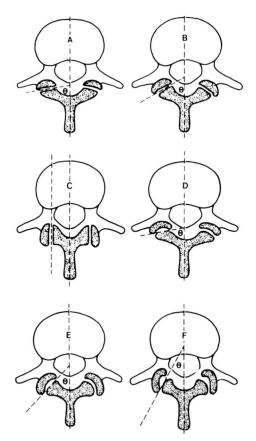

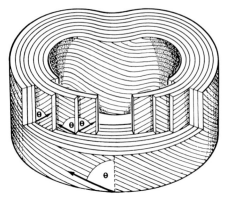

FIG. 15. The detailed structure of the annulus fibrosis. The collagen fibers are arranged in 10 to 20 concentric, circumferential lamellae. The orientation of the fibers alternates in successive lamellae, but their orientation with respect to the vertical is always the same and measures approximately 65°. (From ref. 6, with permission.)

FIG. 14. The varieties of orientation and curvature of the lumbar zygapophyseal joints. **A:** Flat joints oriented close to 90° to the sagittal plane. **B:** Flat joints oriented at 60° to the sagittal plane. **C:** Flat joints oriented parallel (0°) to the sagittal plane. **D:** Slightly curved joints with an average orientation close to 90° to the sagittal plane. **E:** C-shaped joints oriented at 45° to the sagittal plane. **F:** J-shaped joints oriented at 30° to the sagittal plane. (From ref. 6, with permission.)

and throwing on an intact lumbar spine mechanism. In addition, with lifting, tension generated within the thoracolumbar fascia is transmitted directly to the erector spinae muscles via the hydraulic amplifier mechanism. Finally, torsion results from the synergistic effect between the multifidi and the internal oblique as there is no pure trunk or spine rotator. The internal oblique flexes and rotates the trunk but, as previously noted, the multifidi provide an extension moment only, thereby counterbalancing the flexion moment of the internal oblique, resulting in "pure" trunk rotation.

abdominis, and latissimus dorsi laterally (Fig. 18). The fibers of the thoracolumbar facia are organized so that tension that is generated within this structure provides an extension moment to the spine with little shear. The attachment of the thoracolumbar fascia to the latissimus dorsi, which is a strong shoulder internal rotator, provides kinematic evidence of the dependence of proper shoulder mechanics

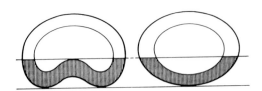

FIG. 16. Intervertebral discs that are concave posteriorly have a greater portion of the annulus fibrosis located posteriorly. Therefore, concave discs have more annulus available to resist the posterior stretch that occurs in flexion and are better protected against annular disruption. (From ref. 6, with permission.)

TABLE 2. *Muscles affecting trunk motion*

Flexors	Extensors	
	Intrinsic	Extrinsic
External oblique[a]	Deep (unisegmental)	Latissimus dorsi
Internal oblique[a]	Interspinalis	Quadratus lumborum
Transversus abdominis	Intertransversarii[a]	Hip extensors
Iliopsoas[b]	Rotatores[a]	Gluteus maximus
	Intermediate (multisegmental)	Hamstrings
	Semispinalis[a]	
	Multifidi[a]	
	Superficial (polysegmental) "erector spinae"	
	Iliocostalis[a,b]	
	Longissimus[a,b]	
	Spinalis[a,b]	

[a] Also contributes to axial rotation.
[b] Also contributes to lateral flexion.

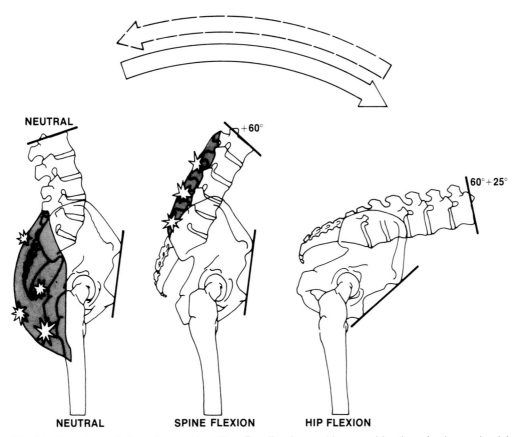

FIG. 17. Muscular activity in forward bending. Bending forward is a combination of spine and pelvic motion. During the spinal flexion phase, hip extensor musculature is active to maintain the pelvis in an extended posture, which maintains tension in a thoracolumbar fascia, and the spinal musculature (erector spinae and multifidi) act to counteract the anterior shear forces that are developed. (From ref. 4, with permission.)

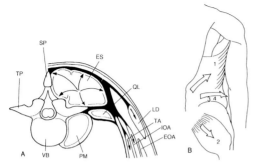

FIG. 18. The thoracolumbar fascia with its attachments. **A:** Cross-sectional diagrammatic representation of the lumbar spine depicting the forces imparted to the thoracolumbar fascia (black) by contraction of the muscles that are attached to it and are contained within it. *SP,* spinous process; *TP,* transverse process; *VB,* vertebral body; *ES,* erector spinae; *LD,* latissimus dorsi; *QL,* quadratus lumborum; *IO,* internal oblique; *TA,* transversus abdominis. **B:** Posterior view of the musculature that attaches to the thoracolumbar fascia. The forces that are generated to the fascia come from the latissimus dorsi from above *(1),* the gluteus maximus from below *(2),* and the internal oblique *(3)* and transversus abdominis *(4)* from the front. (From ref. 25, with permission.)

NEUROVASCULAR ANATOMY

The spinal cord is a component of the central nervous system and extends from the foramen magnum to approximately the L-1 vertebral level, ending in the conus medullaris, below which is the cauda equina (composed of the lumbar nerve roots); therefore, myelopathy can result only from a cervical or thoracic spine injury but radiculopathy can occur anywhere in the spinal axis. The cervical spinal cord is the most susceptible to injury, but intrinsic properties of the spinal neural tissue accommodate the extreme range of motion available in the cervical spine, protecting it from the extreme loads of contact and collision sports. The spinal cord is deformable, with the length changing between 5 and 7 cm from full flexion to full extension of the cervical spine. The spinal cord and dura accommodate this change primarily by simple folding and unfolding of neural tissue, but the final 25% of this dynamic process is accomplished by reversible elastic deformation of neural tissue (Fig. 19).

The size of the spinal cord varies between individuals and within the various regions of the spine itself. The cervical spinal cord ranges from 5 to 12 mm in diameter, usually largest at the upper cervical segments and cervicothoracic segment, whereas the absolute diameter of the bony canal (from C-3 through C-7) is considered stenotic below 12 mm and normal above 15 mm. Cervical extension can also narrow the central spinal canal further, by up to 2 mm (8). The relationship between the size of the spinal cord and the size and shape of the bony canal determines the relative risk of spinal cord injury. The term functional reserve of the spinal canal indicates the "safety margin" of the spinal cord and is qualitatively assessed by the presence of a cerebrospinal fluid (CSF) buffer around the spinal cord and also the shape of the spinal cord (9).

Direct measurement of the bony canal, even by computed tomographic imaging, in and of itself does not accurately determine the relative risk of spinal cord injury from a traumatic event. Further, an indirect measure of bony spinal stenosis using the so-called Torg ratio (10) leads to certain pitfalls. Although the Torg ratio can be used even if the magnification of the x-ray is unknown and it is demonstrated to have high sensitivity, its specificity and positive predictive value for determining spinal stenosis are extremely low (11). The two main pitfalls in the use of this method are (a) that the size of spinal cord relative to the spinal canal is not appreciated, so that even in the presence of a small bony canal, if the spinal cord is relatively small and there is adequate CSF around the cord, then true spinal stenosis probably does not exist, and (b) the ratio may not be applicable to the athletic population for which it was originally designed. Specifically, the numerator of the ratio is the sagittal diameter of the spinal canal measured from the back of a vertebral body to the corresponding spinolaminar line and the denominator is the diameter of the vertebral body (Fig. 20). Because athletes have very large vertebral bodies, the denominator is large and the ratio is smaller and skewed toward the diagnosis of spinal stenosis.

The motor and sensory nerve roots and the spinal nerves are components of the peripheral

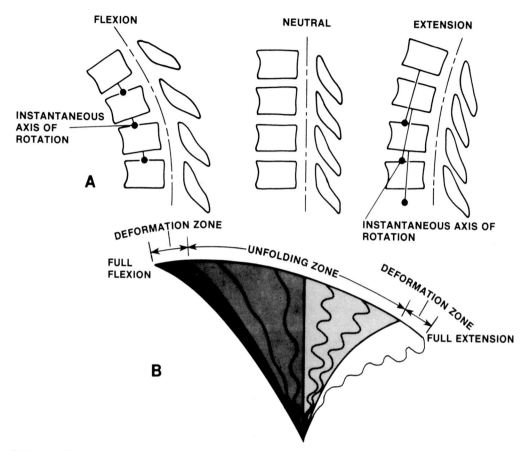

FIG. 19. Diagrammatic representation of the two mechanisms by which the spinal cord accommodates changes in the length of the spinal canal with physiologic flexion and extension. This occurs through unfolding of neural tissue and also elastic deformation. (From ref. 4, with permission.)

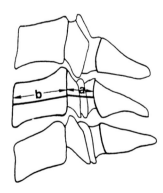

FIG. 20. The Torg ratio. The numerator (*a*) is the distance from the midpoint of the posterior aspect of the vertebral body to the nearest point on the corresponding spinolaminar line, and the denominator (*b*) is the anteroposterior width of the vertebral body. (From ref. 10, with permission.)

nervous system. As there are eight cervical spinal nerves and only seven cervical vertebral bodies, the cervical spinal nerves exit above their correspondingly numbered vertebrae, except that the C-8 spinal nerve exits below the T-1 vertebra. The remaining thoracic and lumbar spinal nerves exit below their correspondingly numbered vertebrae. Each spinal nerve is composed of a ventral (motor) root and a dorsal (sensory) root and then splits into a ventral ramus, providing the myotomes and dermatomes of the extremities and trunk and the dorsal ramus posteriorly innervating the posterior spinal musculature and the zygapophyseal joints, each receiving multilevel innervation (Fig. 21). In evaluating the cross-sectional area of the neuroforamen regionally, in a neutral

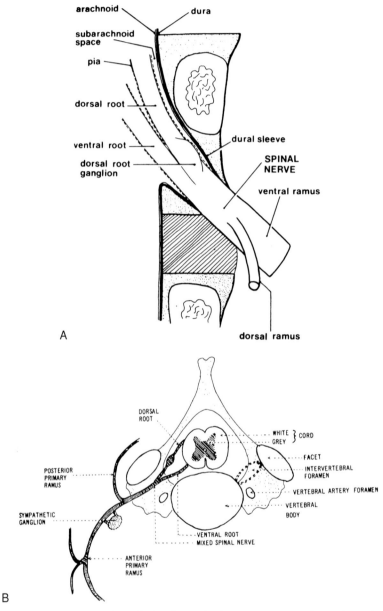

FIG. 21. A: Coronal representation of a lumbar spinal nerve, nerve roots, and meningeal coverings. The nerve roots are invested by pia mater and covered by arachnoid and dura as far as the spinal nerve. The dura of the dural sac is prolonged around the roots as their dural sleeve, which blends with the perineural tissue of the spinal nerve. (From ref. 6, with permission.) **B:** Cross-sectional diagrammatic representation of a cervical spinal nerve and its relationship to the nerve roots and spinal cord. (From ref. 22, with permission.)

posture, the cervical spinal nerve occupies approximately 30% to 35% of the neuroforamen, whereas the lumbar spinal nerves occupy approximately 10% of the intervertebral canal (except at the L-5–S-1 level, in which the L-5 nerve fills approximately 25% of the canal). The relatively "tighter" fit of the cervical nerve root superimposed on the relatively greater range of motion in the cervical spine places the nerve root at risk for compression injury.

The neuroanatomic features of the cervical nerve root–spinal nerve complex provide a foundation for understanding the mechanism of the peripheral nerve injury known as the stinger. Both compression and traction have been implicated as mechanisms of the stinger, although the precise localization of this injury (i.e., cervical versus brachial plexus) has been controversial (12). In general, neural tissue resistance to tensile load is proportional to the number of funiculi (i.e., one nerve bundle, the aggregate of which constitutes the nerve trunk) and the amount of perineurial tissue, whereas the resistance to compressive load is proportional to the size of the intervertebral foramen and the amount of epineurial tissue. In comparing the nerve root–spinal nerve complex to the brachial plexus, it is apparent that the former is more susceptible to both compressive and tensile load for the following reasons: The motor and sensory nerve roots lack perineurial tissue, which develops as an extension of the dura around the spinal nerve; the spinal nerve exits as a single funiculus of a motor and sensory nerve root; the neuroforamen is narrowed with movement of the head and neck into the posterior quadrants; and epineurial tissue is lacking about the spinal nerve (Fig. 22). Furthermore, the anterior nerve root is more vulnerable than the posterior nerve root to traction injury as it lacks the dampening affect of the dorsal root ganglion, it has a thinner dural sheath, and it aligns directly with the spinal cord. This may explain why motor symptoms are more typical than sensory findings in athletes who have residual symptoms after a stinger. Conversely, the brachial plexus resists tensile load because of its plexiform nature and the presence of perineurial tissue and multiple funiculi, but it also resists compressive load because of epineurial

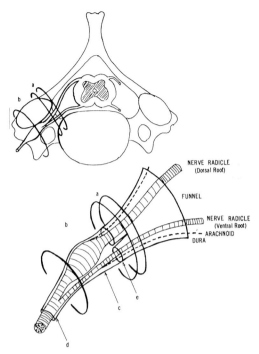

FIG. 22. The nerve root–spinal nerve complex. *(a)* Intervertebral foramen; *(b)* gutter of the transverse process; *(c)* the distal extent of the arachnoid where the arachnoid and dura blend; *(d)* the spinal nerve distal to this point is covered by dural tissue only which forms the perineurium; *(e)* the spinal nerve is formed by a single funiculus of the motor (ventral) and sensory (dorsal) nerve root. (From ref. 22, with permission.)

tissue, which is an extension of the loosely organized epidural sheath of the spinal nerve. Therefore, if the mechanism of the stinger is a traction or a compression event, it is most likely that the nerve root–spinal nerve complex is at greater risk than the brachial plexus for injury.

The spinal components that are considered to be innervated and therefore potential sources of spinal pain include the periosteum of the vertebral body, spinal nerve root including the dorsal root ganglion, dura, radicular arteries and veins, musculotendinous structures, ligaments, zygapophyseal joint capsule and subchondral bone, uncovertebral joints, and the outer one-third of the annulus fibrosis of the intervertebral disc. In particular, the sinuvertebral nerve, which is composed of a recurrent branch of the ventral ramus (i.e., somatic component) and gray rami communicans (i.e., autonomic component), supplies the posterior aspect of the annulus fibrosis in addition to the posterior longitudinal ligament, blood vessels, and dura (Fig. 23). The lateral and anterior aspects of the outer annulus are supplied by gray rami communicans only.

The sympathetic nervous system has an important role in the cervical spine. Postganglionic fibers from the cervical sympathetic chain travel in three distinct pathways: to the peripheral extremity; to the dura, disc, and ligaments via the recurrent meningeal branch; and to the brainstem and carotid plexus. Clinically, the peripheral

branches may have a role in reflex sympathetic dystrophy and the brainstem projections may play a role in the generation of so-called post-traumatic cervical vertigo.

Finally, the vertebral artery is intimately associated with the bony vertebral column. Compression of the vertebral artery can occur within the transverse foramina of the upper six vertebrae by uncovertebral joint osteophytes and by dislocation of the C0-1 and C1-2 joints. Further, the relatively high degree of rotation between C-1 and C-2 subjects the vertebral artery to risk of compression without associated dislocation. Cadaveric studies reveal that 30 and 45° of rotation can occlude the contralateral and ipsilateral vertebral artery, respectively (13, 14). This potential risk is dampened by the presence of a redundant loop of artery between C-1 and C-2 and the limited rotation available at the C0-1 segment.

THE BIOMECHANICAL CONTRIBUTION OF THE SPINE AND TRUNK IN THE OVERHEAD-THROWING ATHLETE

The spine and trunk are key to proper throwing mechanics, including force generation, force transfer, and force attenuation and the prevention of potential neurologic injury (15). The physical principles of force and kinetic energy reveal that the shoulder mechanism alone is inadequate in generating the force (i.e., 60 Nm of internal rotation torque) needed to accelerate the shoulder through an angular velocity of over 7000° per second and to generate a velocity of throwing that is typical of elite athletes. In fact, it is the mass of the trunk that allows it to contribute most of the force (mass × acceleration) and kinetic energy ($\frac{1}{2}$ × mass × velocity^2) to the throwing motion (16). As an example, if the lower body and trunk are removed from the throwing motion, such as in the water polo player, the peak throwing velocity is reduced to approximately half that of a professional baseball pitcher (17). In addition, the spine and trunk allow transfer of force from the lower quadrants to the throwing arm. Creating a rigid cylinder via muscular tension, the ground reactive force that is generated in an anterior–posterior plane is transformed into rotational force.

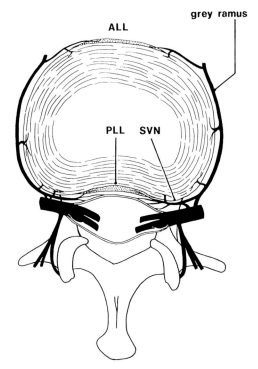

FIG. 23. Cross-sectional diagrammatic representation of the nerve supply of an intervertebral disc. Branches of the gray rami communicans and the sinuvertebral nerves (*SVN*) are shown entering the disc and the anterior and posterior longitudinal ligaments (*ALL, PLL*). Branches from the sinuvertebral nerve also supply the anterior aspect of the dural sac and dural sleeve. (From ref. 6, with permission.)

The different stages of throwing each play a unique role in the transfer of force from the ground to the throwing extremity (18). The wind-up phase is one in which potential energy is stored in the trunk. A very tightly packed wind-up position early in the throwing phase maximizes trunk velocity later. The late cocking and acceleration phase transfers this potential energy into kinetic energy. If the trunk "opens up" too early, energy is lost and less arm velocity and control result. Furthermore, the anterior glenohumeral joint is subject to tensile load and the resultant potential instability may lead to neurovascular injury about the thoracic outlet. The trunk also acts as a force attenuator, protecting the shoulder from the extreme tensile loads in the follow-through phase. As the trunk rotates forward and bends laterally, it reacquires energy, thus dissipating the distraction forces on the shoulder and associated nerves such as the suprascapular nerve.

Each region of the spinal axis contributes to efficient throwing. The lumbar spine provides a level foundation that remains stable throughout the throwing motion. The vertical orientation of the lumbar zygapophyseal joints favors flexion–extension and the ability to maintain lumbar lordosis, which has an important role in throwing. Lumbar lordosis is universal in baseball pitchers in the cocking phase. A "controlled" lordosis allows adequate preloading of the abdominal musculature such that with initiation of the acceleration phase, contralateral trunk flexion and rotation are most efficient (15). Excessive or passive lordosis, which may result from muscle fatigue, results in less preload of the abdominal musculature, which results in less efficient throwing with loss of control and velocity. The ability of the trunk to flex laterally is also critical in that it is trunk flexion that creates the abduction moment for the humerus (19,20). Despite the various throwing styles (i.e., overhead, three-quarters position, or sidearm), the humerus and trunk have a relatively fixed relationship of between 90 and 110° and thus it is trunk motion that initiates arm abduction. This is accomplished in part by efficient preloading of the trunk and abdominal musculature. As mentioned earlier, the thoracolumbar fascia also plays a significant role in the throwing motion. In addition to its ability to stabilize the lumbar spine, it has a direct attachment to the latissimus dorsi, which is a strong shoulder internal rotator and a prime mover of the shoulder in the acceleration phase of throwing.

The thoracic spine also contributes to proper throwing. The degree of thoracic kyphosis influences the position of the scapula and thus the glenohumeral joint. Proper scapular rotation is critical for maintaining the instantaneous center of rotation about the glenohumeral joint (21). In addition, the oblique orientation of the thoracic zygapophyseal joint facilitates transfer of ground reactive force to rotational acceleration in the upper body.

Finally, the cervical spine has a role in throwing. The cervical zygapophyseal joints are oriented more horizontally and the proportionally larger amount of available cervical segmental range of motion allows target acquisition that influences trunk position in all phases of throwing.

REFERENCES

1. Maitland GD. *Vertebral manipulation,* 5th ed. London: Butterworths, 1986:73–87.
2. Swischuk LE. Anterior displacement of C2 in children: physiologic or pathologic? *Radiology* 1977;122:759–763.
3. White AA, Johnson RM, Panjabi MM, Southwick WO. Biomechanical analysis of clinical stability in the cervical spine. *Clin Orthop* 1975;109:85.
4. White AA, Panjabi MM. *Clinical biomechanics of the spine,* 2nd ed. Philadelphia: JB Lippincott Co, 1990: 283–292.
5. Dvorak J, Panjabi MM. Functional anatomy of the alar ligaments. *Spine* 1987;12:183–189.
6. Bogduk N, Twomey LT. *Clinical anatomy of the lumbar spine,* 2nd ed. Melbourne: Churchill Livingstone, 1991: 83–105.
7. Gracovetsky S, Farfan H, Heleur C. The abdominal mechanism. *Spine* 1985;10:317–324.
8. Penning L. Some aspects of plain radiography of the cervical spine in chronic myelopathy. *Neurology* 1962; 12:513–519.
9. Cantu RC. Sports medicine aspects of cervical spinal stenosis. In: Holloszy JD, ed. *Exercise and sports sciences reviews,* vol 23. Baltimore: Williams & Wilkins, 1995:399–409.
10. Torg JS, Pavlov H, Genuario SE, et al. Neurapraxia of the cervical spinal cord with transient quadriplegia. *J Bone Joint Surg Am* 1986;68A:1354–1370.
11. Herzog RJ, Wiens JJ, Dillingham MF, Sontag MJ. Normal cervical spine morphometry and cervical spinal stenosis in asymptomatic professional football players. Plain radiography, multiplanar computed tomography, and magnetic resonance imaging. *Spine* 1991;16:S178–S186.
12. Herring SA, Weinstein SM. Electrodiagnosis in sports medicine. *Phys Med Rehabil State of the Art Reviews* 1989;3:809–822.

13. Fielding JW. Cineroentgenography of the normal cervical spine. *J Bone Joint Surg Am* 1957;39A:1280.
14. Selecki BR. The effects of rotation of the atlas on the axis: experimental work. *Med J Aust* 1969;1:1012.
15. Young JL, Herring SA, Press JM, Casazza BA. The influence of the spine on the shoulder in the throwing athlete. *J Back Musculoskeletal Rehabil* 1996;7:5–17.
16. Toyoshima S, Hoshikawa T, Miyashita M, Aguri T. Contribution of the body parts to throwing performance. In: *Biomechanics IV*. Baltimore: University Park Press, 1974:169–174.
17. Whiting WC, Puffer JC, Finerman G, Gregor RT, Maletis GB. Three-dimensional cinematographic analysis of waterpolo throwing in elite performers. *Am J Sports Med* 1985;13:95–98.
18. Jobe FW, Tibone JE, Jobe CM, Kvitne RS. The shoulder in sports. In: Rockwood CA Jr, Matsen FA III, eds. *The Shoulder*. Philadelphia: WB Saunders, 1990: 961–990.
19. Atwater AE. Biomechanics of overarm throwing movements and of throwing injuries. *Exerc Sport Sci Rev* 1979;7:43–85.
20. Feltner ME. Three dimensional interactions in a two segment kinetic chain. Part II: Application to the throwing arm in baseball pitching. *Int J Sports Biomech* 1989;5:420–450.
21. Kibler WB. Role of the scapula in the overhead throwing motion. *Contemp Orthop* 1991;22:525–532.
22. Calliet R. Neck and arm pain, 2nd ed. Philadelphia: FA Davis Co, 1981.
23. Kirkaldy-Willis WH, Burton CV. Managing back pain, 3rd ed. Edinburgh: Churchill Livingstone, 1992.
24. Bland JH. Disorders of the cervical spine: diagnosis and medical management, 2nd ed. Philadelphia: WB Saunders, 1994.
25. Porterfield JA, DeRosa C. Mechanical low back pain: prospectives and functional anatomy. Philadelphia: WB Saunders, 1991.

Sports Neurology, Second Edition,
edited by Barry D. Jordan.
Lippincott–Raven Publishers, Philadelphia © 1998.

5

Electromyography: Clinical Applications

Peter Tsairis

Hospital for Special Surgery, 535 East 70th Street, New York, New York 10021

Clinical electrophysiologic studies are an extension of the neurologic examination and should not provide a clinical diagnosis of the patient's illness. In the assessment of function of the peripheral nervous system or of motor unit disorders, the electromyographic (EMG) study consists of two parts. The standard procedures involve either observation of an evoked muscle response to galvanic stimulation of peripheral motor or sensory nerves or recording of electrical activity detected by a needle electrode inserted into a skeletal muscle. These studies may indicate abnormalities that characterize the nature of the disease process and its location within the motor unit. Similarly, it can be ascertained whether the disease process involves sensory nerves or motor nerves or both. In addition, electrophysiologic data can help distinguish axonopathies from myelinopathies.

Although most electromyographers feel that there are no specific waveforms that are pathognomonic of specific diseases, abnormalities of neuromuscular junction physiology may be diagnostic of either myasthenia gravis or the myasthenic syndrome. Usually the abnormalities on the electromyogram serve as objective criteria of motor unit dysfunction. These results must be integrated with the results of other studies and the clinical examination in arriving at a clinical diagnosis.

This chapter briefly reviews the common electrophysiologic techniques and their application to dysfunction of the motor unit encountered in sports-related injuries. For reviews of the technical aspects of performing nerve conduction studies

and needle electromyography, the reader is referred to standard sources on this subject (1,2).

MOTOR UNIT ANATOMY AND PHYSIOLOGY

The motor unit is defined as the lower motor neuron (anterior horn cell, axon, and terminal nerve endings) and all muscle fibers innervated by it. The thousands of muscle fibers that compose a mammalian skeletal limb muscle are organized into motor units. In the cat, three physiologic types of motor units have been identified, and each type has a unique and uniform histochemical enzymatic staining reaction, namely a histochemical profile (3). In the major limb muscles there may be 200 to 300 motor units, and each unit may have 400 to 1000 muscle fibers regardless of the physiologic type. Anatomically, muscle fibers of a single motor unit are not grouped together in fascicles. Many studies have shown that the fibers of one motor unit are diffusely distributed throughout many fascicles and interdigitate with fibers of other motor units to produce a mosaic pattern. This evidence supports the physiologist's concept that the motor unit is a functional and anatomic entity and is the basic quantal unit of muscle movement. This concept is the key to understanding the pathophysiology of nerve and muscle disorders.

Table 1 shows a classification of three histochemical fiber types in mammalian muscle, based on correlative physiologic and histochemical studies of single motor units in the cat. Type FF motor units are fast-contracting, fatigue-sensitive

TABLE 1. *Histochemical reactivity of myofibers in single motor units of the cat gastrocnemius muscle*

Histochemical profile	Physiological type		
	FF	FR	S
Myofibrillar ATPase	High	High	Low
ATPase activity—preincubation at pH 4.65	Intermediate	Low	High
Diphosphopyridine nucleotide dehydrogenase, succinate dehydrogenase	Low	Intermediate	High
Periodic acid–Schiff staining (presumed glycogen content)	High	Intermediate to high	Low
Phosphorylase	High	Intermediate to high	Low
Capillary network	Scant	Rich	Rich

From ref. 3, with permission.

units that have muscle fibers with presumably high glycogen content, low oxidative capacity, and sparse capillary supply. Fibers of these units correspond to type II muscle fibers. It is suggested that these units depend on anaerobic glycolysis for energy. Their histochemical profile could explain their rapid fatigue, because their glycogen has been shown to be depleted quickly during repetitive muscle activity. Fibers of SS units have relatively less glycogen, high oxidative activity, and a rich capillary supply and correspond to type I muscle fibers. These units are slow contracting and fatigue resistant and most likely utilize aerobic pathways for energy. FR motor units are in the intermediate class physiologically and histochemically. For example, they have both aerobic and anaerobic capabilities and probably utilize either source of energy, depending on the type of stress imposed on the muscle. These different but interrelated motor unit groups in a single muscle may be utilized by the peripheral nervous system for various types of movement, such as sustained tonic muscle contraction or short-lived phasic muscle movement (3).

Different types of histochemical reactivities are shown to indicate metabolic differences between motor units or even muscle fibers. In any mammalian limb muscle, the percentage of each fiber type may vary depending on the predominant physiologic function of the muscle or on the stress imposed on the muscle. Most limb muscles are histochemically heterogeneous (two or three fiber types) because they may be called on to perform various functions. However, some are histochemically homogeneous; that is, they have a predominance of one fiber type. For example, a tonic slow-contracting muscle such as the soleus muscle of the calf characteristically has a majority of fibers that are uniformly rich in oxidative activity, low in glycogen content, and intermediate in myosin adenosine triphosphatase (ATPase) activity. On the other hand, the flexor digitorum muscles are primarily fast contracting and have fibers that are predominantly rich in glycolytic and myosin ATPase activity. Although the gastrocnemius muscle is considered a "white muscle" and is fast contracting, it has a mixture of fiber types that are rich in both glycolytic and oxidative activities. These histochemical variations are also characteristic of human limb muscles and must be taken into account when interpreting a muscle biopsy in the evaluation of a patient with muscle weakness.

CLINICAL APPLICATIONS

At times it may be difficult for the neurologist to determine whether muscle weakness or wasting or some other type of motor dysfunction is a result of a disease of the motor unit. In some instances the muscle dysfunction may be attributable to pain, a psychiatric disorder (conversion reaction), muscle disuse, or even central nervous system disease. In these instances the clinical electrophysiologic analysis is of the utmost importance in determining whether there is or is not a disease of the motor unit. Furthermore, in early stages of neuromuscular disease the EMG findings may be the only objective evidence of dysfunction of the motor unit.

Peripheral Nerve Injury

Damage to peripheral nerves, whether in sports injuries or not, is likely to result from either direct trauma, stretch or traction on the nerve, or severe compression with or without associated ischemia. Nerve conduction studies are the key to assessment of these injuries. Stimulation of a peripheral motor or sensory nerve is synchronized with recording equipment to permit accurate measurement of the time required for the nerve impulse to pass from a point of stimulation to a pickup electrode placed over the muscle belly innervated by the nerve in question. Techniques have been developed for the study of both motor and sensory nerve conduction, and normal values have been established for each peripheral nerve and for variations from children to the elderly. When muscle weakness or numbness or paresthesias suggest peripheral nerve injury, a normal response of the muscle to stimulation of the involved nerve indicates that the injury is proximal to the site of the stimulus or that it is not severe enough to produce demyelination or axonal damage (wallerian degeneration). The earliest sign of degeneration of a nerve is failure of the nerve to respond to electrical stimulation below the site of injury; this usually occurs 3 days after injury. Injury to a peripheral nerve may not be severe enough to have caused degeneration and may produce only a conduction block or neurapraxia.

In addition, one may find a delayed conduction velocity between two stimulation sites on the nerve or an increase in the F-wave latency. The F-wave latency represents an action potential traveling antidromically along motor nerves to the anterior horn cell and then back to the muscle. Lastly, one may see only temporal dispersion of the compound muscle action potential on stimulation of the nerve; this is when the conduction time is not uniformly decreased in all nerve fibers, which results in an increase in the duration of the action potential (polyphasia).

In general, slow conduction velocities, delayed distal latencies and F-waves, normal compound motor action potentials (CMAPs), temporal dispersion, and absence of fibrillations characterize a pure demyelinating neuropathy. Conversely, relatively preserved motor conduction velocities, distal latencies, and F-waves; decreased CMAPs; and fibrillations on electromyography constitute the findings of axonal degeneration (neuronopathy) (Table 2).

In cubital tunnel syndromes (ulnar nerve injury), stimulation of the ulnar nerve several centimeters above the elbow shows delayed conduction across the elbow, and/or fibrillations of the interossei, if axonal damage is significant. The same applies to carpal tunnel syndrome. Neurapraxias may occur in acute inflammatory polyradiculoneuropathy, in pressure palsies associated with diabetes mellitus, or as a result of mechanical compression. For the most part, nerve conduction studies are easy to perform at common sites of pressure, for example, at the carpal tunnel (median nerve), cubital tunnel (ulnar nerve), head of the fibula (peroneal nerve), or ankle (posterior tibial nerve at the tarsal tunnel). With surface stimulation of a deep peripheral nerve, errors may occur as a result of spread of a strong current through deep subcutaneous tissues and along nerves distal to the desired point of stimulation. In these cases, this can be avoided by using a monopolar needle electrode as a stimulus, placing it adjacent to the nerve in order to localize the point of stimulation.

Regeneration activity or reinnervation begins almost immediately after nerve injury. As mentioned, motor or sensory conduction may remain normal for several days distal to the site of injury. Low conduction velocities observed during reinnervation are felt to be related directly to the small diameter of the regenerating nerve fibers. Significant slowing of motor conduction occurs in a variety of demyelinating polyneuropathies and indicates selective dropping out of the larger diameter fast-conducting motor or sensory (proprioceptive) fibers. The temperature of the limb and age of the patient affect conduction times (4). Therefore, measure the temperature of the limb before beginning a nerve conduction study, and warm a cold extremity for at least 10 minutes before beginning the study.

TABLE 2. *Electrophysiology: segmental demyelination (myelinopathy) and axonal degeneration (axonopathy)*

Features	Myelinopathy	Axonopathy
Motor conduction		
MCV	Slow	Normal[a]
DL	Delayed	Normal[a]
Neurapraxia	Present	Not present
CMAP amplitude	Normal	Decreased
Temporal dispersion	Present	Not present
F-wave response	Absent or delayed	Normal[a]
Sensory conduction		
SCV	Slow	Normal
DL	Delayed	Normal
SNAP amplitude	Normal	Decreased
Needle electromyography		
Fibrillations	None	Present
Fasciculations	None	Present
MUAPs		
Recruitment	Decreased	Decreased
Configuration	Polyphasic	Irregular or normal

MCV, Motor conduction velocity; SCV, sensory conduction velocity; DL, distal latency; CMAP, compound motor action potential; SNAP, sensory nerve action potential; MUAP, motor unit action potential.

[a] Abnormally slow in neuronopathies (anterior horn cell diseases, severe demylinating neuropathy).

Needle electromyography may not show any abnormalities for 2 to 3 weeks after a nerve injury. Early on, there may be a reduction in the number of motor unit action potentials generated from the muscle during voluntary effort. Spontaneous fibrillation potentials after insertion or movement of the needle electrode (abnormal insertional activity) may appear 10 to 14 days after an injury. Denervation activity in the form of fibrillations does not occur until 2.5 to 3 weeks after the nerve has been injured. The shorter the length of nerve between the site of injury and the muscle, the earlier the appearance of fibrillations. Fibrillations are present until reinnervation occurs or until the muscle becomes atrophic. In completely or nearly completely denervated muscle, fibrillation potentials gradually decrease in number and in some instances may be difficult to detect after 1 year.

Brachial Plexus Injury and Thoracic Outlet Syndrome

Lesions in the brachial plexus or of nerves around the shoulder girdle can usually be differentiated from root compression either by stimulating the respective nerves in question (axillary or suprascapular) or by observing the pattern of needle EMG abnormalities in the muscle innervated by either one of those nerves. For example, if a patient presents with pain and/or weakness around the shoulder and one finds evidence of denervation limited to the spinatii with or without slowing of suprascapular motor conduction, this should indicate a suprascapular neuropathy rather than partial compression of the fifth or sixth cervical root. In root compression one may find denervation activity in the cervical paraspinal muscles. This can sometimes be a difficult EMG examination because of incomplete relaxation or because of the overlapping muscles in that area. This again emphasizes the importance of the clinical examination in the overall assessment of the patient. Injury to the dorsal scapular nerve may be distinguished from C-5 root lesions by denervation signs found only in the rhomboid muscles. Injuries to the axillary nerve may be distinguished from either C-5 or C-6 root lesions by denervation signs found only in the deltoid muscle or teres minor. The same applies for the musculocutaneous nerve that innervates the biceps brachii and the radial nerve that innervates the brachioradialis and/or supinator or forearm extensors.

Nerve conduction studies are usually normal in most thoracic outlet syndromes. They are usually abnormal when there is an unequivocal neurologic deficit. For example, in thoracic outlet syndromes caused by a cervical rib with associated hand weakness, one usually finds delayed distal sensory conduction along the ulnar and sometimes the median nerve and fibrillations of intrinsic hand muscles.

Cervical Root Compression and/or Avulsion

Peripheral motor conduction is usually normal in these lesions. Evoked muscle action potentials are usually small, particularly if there is a significant amount of muscle atrophy. In most cases sensory nerve conduction abnormalities and/or needle EMG abnormalities are present. The sensory action potential recorded from mixed nerves such as the ulnar or peroneal nerves is composed predominantly of impulses originating from large afferent fibers that conduct at a velocity higher than that of motor fibers. When one sees an abnormality of sensory nerve conduction, it is usually an indication of involvement of the large myelinated fibers (those subserving touch and vibration) rather than involvement of motor fiber conduction. In general, the sensory nerve action potential or evoked response is normal in neuromuscular junction disorders and myopathies.

In cervical root compression syndromes, there is normal motor conduction, sensory conduction may be absent or the sensory action potential may be small or delayed. This abnormality coupled with needle EMG abnormalities usually implies spinal root compression or an intrinsic radiculopathy. The sensory action potential is preserved in the presence of lesions proximal to the dorsal root ganglion; for example, it may be preserved despite loss of sensation after a root avulsion. In this situation the F-wave latency, which is a type of motor conduction study, may be delayed or absent. Not all electrophysiologic studies of suspected nerve root compression syndromes are of diagnostic value. In these situations, the clinical examination coupled with cervical myelography

and/or neuroimaging scans is equally important. In some cases of nerve root compromise, one may detect chronic denervation activity in several cervical myotomes, but this in effect does not necessarily indicate the vertebral level of root damage. For example, a laterally extruded herniated disc between C-5 and C-6 will compress the C-6 root, whereas a more centrally extruded disc at the same level may affect the C-7 root. If the root compression is exerted long enough to produce degeneration of axons, one may see fibrillation potentials earlier in paraspinal muscles than in limb muscles. Fibrillations may persist until reinnervation occurs or until the muscle atrophies or degenerates. When reinnervation takes place, there may be a reduction in the amount of fibrillation. The earliest sign of reinnervation is the appearance of small-amplitude, highly polyphasic potentials of short duration ("nascent potentials"). These may be present several weeks before there is clinical or other evidence of functional recovery. The appearance of nascent polyphasic potentials should be a source of encouragement to the patient and is justification for continued conservative management. As reinnervation takes hold, motor unit potential activity increases and the form of the action potential normalizes.

Lumbar Root Lesions

Injury to a single nerve root resulting from compression by a herniated disc causes denervation only in the muscles that receive innervation from the affected root. Routine nerve conduction studies are usually normal in the analysis of lumbar root lesions. F-wave latencies and/or H-reflexes are of some value. Localization of a nerve root lesion depends on the finding of fibrillation potentials either in the muscles of the extremity that receive innervation from the anterior primary ramus of the spinal nerve or in lumbar paraspinal muscles that receive innervation from the posterior primary ramus of the spinal nerve or both. Therefore, both lumbar paraspinal and limb muscles should be evaluated in these cases. Trauma to the spinal cord may damage anterior horn cells and thus cause fibrillations in muscles innervated by the segments involved. When anterior horn cells are involved, the fibrillations may be minimal, fasciculations may be more prominent, and voluntary motor unit action potentials may be quite large and irregular or polyphasic in configuration.

In summary, electrophysiologic studies assess the degree of neurologic injury; in doing so they provide (a) an indication of a level or segment of involvement, (b) an estimate of the degree of damage, and (c) a baseline for serial follow-up studies as deemed clinically useful.

Electrophysiologic Analysis of Selective Nerve Injuries in Athletes

Severe injuries to the shoulder may result in selective damage to the suprascapular nerve, axillary nerve, musculocutaneous nerve, or long thoracic nerve. Anterior or posterior shoulder dislocations may injure the suprascapular nerve and inferior dislocations may injure the axillary nerve. In both cases there may be a motor conduction delay. By stimulating the suprascapular nerve at Erb's point and recording from the appropriate innervated muscle (5,6) one can localize the level of the lesion. Long thoracic nerve palsy may occur with overuse injuries. For example, it may occur in weight lifters, tennis players, swimmers, and gymnasts. It may also occur spontaneously without any known provocation. This nerve may be examined in a similar fashion by measuring conduction to the serratus anterior muscle with stimulation at Erb's point (7,8). Injuries to the musculocutaneous nerve are much less common an association with shoulder injury. The musculocutaneous nerve can be examined in a similar fashion by stimulating the nerve at Erb's point and examining conduction to the biceps muscle (9).

Cubital Tunnel Syndrome

Trauma to the elbow may produce an ulnar neuropathy related either to direct injury to the elbow or to a stretch–dislocation injury to the nerve at the level of the cubital fossa. This nerve injury can be documented by a nerve conduction study and needle EMG analysis. The ulnar nerve is a mixed nerve and therefore both motor and sensory functions can be assessed. There may be a motor conduction block at the elbow, an absent or delayed distal ulnar sensory evoked response, or both. Sometimes the level of entrapment may be significantly proximal to the elbow. The level of injury can be determined by an "inching technique" in the nerve conduction study (10). Needle electromyography may reveal hyperirritability of ulnar innervated muscles, in the form of positive waves, or partial denervation activity, in the form of fibrillations.

CONCLUSIONS

Clinical electrophysiology of the peripheral and central nervous system requires a great deal of technical skill and clinical sophistication. None of these studies should be done routinely without a clear understanding of the basic clinical problem. It would not be feasible to examine in a set order all muscles that might be involved in the various types of motor unit disorders. The peripheral nerves and muscles for needle electromyography must be selected according to the problem presented by the individual patient. All electromyographers must understand the diverse clinical problems that may be encountered in order to justify the plan of examination. The examination may be modified in order to obtain the necessary information with the least amount of discomfort to the patient.

Electrical activity of muscle is greatly affected by the interaction between the patient and the electromyographer. For example, if the patient is tense and not relaxed, it may alter baseline activity in the muscle, which may be interpreted as abnormal. It is essential that an electromyographer is thoroughly familiar with (a) the anatomy and innervation of skeletal muscle, (b) the clinical aspects of various neuromuscular disorders, and (c) the significance of various forms of abnormal electrical activity, which he or she should be able to distinguish from artifact.

REFERENCES

1. Ahlskog JE. *Clinical examinations in neurology*, 6th ed. St. Louis: Mosby–Year Book, 1991.
2. Oh SJ. *Clinical electromyography: nerve conduction studies*, 2nd ed. Baltimore: Williams & Wilkins, 1993.

3. Burke RE, Tsairis P. Anatomy and innervation ratios in motor units of cat gastrocnemius. *J Physiol* (Lond) 1973; 234:749.

4. Howard JE, McGill KC, Dorfman LJ. Age effects on properties of motor unit action potentials: ADEMG analysis. *Ann Neurol* 1988;24:207.

5. Aiello I, Serra G, Traina GC, Tugnoli V. Entrapment of the suprascapular nerve at the spinoglenoid notch. *Ann Neurol* 1982;12:314.

6. Kraft GH. Axillary, musculocutaneous and suprascapular nerve latencies. *Arch Phys Med Rehabil* 1972;53:382.

7. Kaplan PE. Electrodiagnostic conformation of long thoracic nerve palsy. *J Neurol Neurosurg Psychiatry* 1980;43:50.

8. Petura JE, Trojaberg W. Conduction studies of the long toracic nerve in serratus anterior palsy of different etiologies. *Neurology* 1984;34:1033.

9. Trojaberg W. Motor and sensory conduction in the musculocutaneous nerve. *J Neurol Neurosurg Psychiatry* 1976;39:890.

10. Miller RG. The cubital tunnel syndrome. *Ann Neurol* 1979;6:56.

Sports Neurology, Second Edition,
edited by Barry D. Jordan.
Lippincott–Raven Publishers, Philadelphia © 1998.

6

Electromyography and the Study of Muscle Kinesiology and Fatigue

Joseph H. Feinberg

*Department of Sports Medicine, Kessler Institute for Rehabilitation, 1199 Pleasant Valley Way,
West Orange, New Jersey 07052*

Electromyography (EMG) is a technique with broad and powerful applications. It is most commonly used to diagnose neurologic and muscle disorders. More recently, EMG has also been used to study muscle kinesiology and muscle fatigue. This has helped us better understand the biomechanics of sports, the pathomechanics of injuries, and more appropriate rehabilitation programs. This chapter reviews the neurophysiology and technical factors relevant to the study of muscle kinesiology and fatigue. Work that has been done studying muscle kinesiology and muscle fatigue is reviewed and its clinical relevance discussed.

NEUROPHYSIOLOGY OF THE MOTOR UNIT

EMG is the study of the myoelectric signal, the electrical signal generated when a muscle's motor units contract. A motor unit consists of the muscle fibers innervated by an axon. The more muscle fibers per axon or the larger the muscle fiber diameter, the greater the size of the motor unit and the amplitude of the myoelectric signal. Muscles with motor units that have a low ratio of axon to muscle innervation such as a hand intrinsic (a ratio of 1:110) are designed for skilled activities; muscles with a larger ratio such as the medial gastrocnemius muscle (a ratio of 1:1770) are designed for a quicker burst of power (1).

Motor units are catergorized according to the twitch time of their muscle fibers. The faster the twitch, the higher the muscle fiber conduction velocity. The muscle fibers are broken down into slow-twitch fibers, also known as type I, and fast-twitch fibers, also known as type II (2). Type 2 fibers are further subdivided into IIA, IIB, and IIC (3). The predominance of type I or type II fibers determines whether a muscle is designed for longer endurance activities, such as the soleus, which is rich in type I, or activities that require short, quick bursts of power, such as the quadriceps, which is rich in type II (4–6).

ANALYSIS OF THE MYOELECTRIC SIGNAL

Motor units have a diphasic or triphasic configuration, an amplitude, and firing rates that depend on many factors (7). As a muscle attempts to generate a greater force, the motor unit firing rate increases, and with a further increase in force additional motor units are recruited.

When studying muscle kinesiology or fatigue, many motor units are recruited and overlap each other. Instead of individual motor unit analysis, amplitude, frequency analysis, and muscle fiber conduction velocity of the entire myoelectric signal are studied.

Amplitude can be measured as the height of the signal from the baseline to the peak, from peak to trough, or by taking the root mean square (8). Amplitude can be used for studying muscle firing patterns (9–18) but because the EMG/force relationship is not always linear (19–25), it can not be used to reliably predict force. Muscle length, the type of contraction, muscle fatigue, motor unit size, strength of the individual muscle fibers, and the amount and rate of motor units contracting are all variables that affect this.

A motor unit can be analyzed by determining the frequencies of its action potential. This is based on the rate of rise and fall of the action potential or the speed with which there is a change in polarity of the action potential phases. This should not be confused with the frequency that represents the firing rate of a motor unit. After a myoelectric signal is recorded, a fast Fourier transformation is performed (26,27) and a power spectrum is obtained. The mean or median frequency is then determined.

The median frequency will be dependent on the fiber type distribution of the muscle being studied (fast twitch versus slow twitch) (28,29) and muscle fiber diameter (30). It will vary with muscle fatigue (21,22,31) and muscle force (32–37). Fast twitch muscle fibers conduct and depolarize electrically faster (approximately four times) than slow twitch (38–43). They therefore have inherently higher frequencies than slow twitch motor units (28,29). Larger diameter fibers, which are usually type II, also conduct at a faster rate and have higher frequencies than smaller diameter fibers (25).

Slowing of muscle fiber conduction velocity occurs during a sustained contraction (44,45). This slowing causes a decrease in the median frequency (33,44,46,47,48). Therefore, analysis of the power spectrum can be done to determine muscle fatigue.

TECHNICAL ASPECTS OF EMG

EMG Electrodes

An EMG signal must be recorded with a recording and reference electrode. Electrodes can be skin surface or intramuscular and can be used to study muscle firing patterns (9–16) and follow muscle fatigue (21,22,49–55) (Fig. 1). Intramuscular electrodes record a broader range of frequencies than surface electrodes (8).

Electrode Placement

Electrode placement can affect both the amplitude and frequency of the myoelectric signal (4,32,56). Amplitude will be dependent on muscle fiber orientation and location of the motor point (8). The median frequency will depend both on the distance from the motor point and the distribution of type I and type II fibers within the muscle (1). Motor point identification with electrical stimulation is a more precise method for reproducing electrode placement than using gross anatomic landmarks (57,58). Depth of penetration should also be accurately reproduced when inserting intramuscular electrodes (28,29).

Filtering of the Myoelectric Signal

Filtering of the myoelectric signal reduces the range of frequencies that an electrode records. The farther the electrode is from the signal's source and the greater the amount of tissue there is between them, the more the signal is filtered (30,59). Frequencies greater than approximately 500 Hz are filtered out when using surface electrodes. Therefore, intramuscular electrodes record a broader range of frequencies than surface electrodes (8). Because it is a drop in the higher frequencies that occurs in early muscle fatigue (21,22,31,51,52,60), intramuscular electrodes are probably more sensitive indicators of muscle fatigue than surface electrodes; however, their intersession reliability has not yet been well demonstrated (61).

Electrode Surface Area and Interelectrode Distance

Electrode surface area and interelectrode distance both affect amplitude and frequency (8,62). This is especially true for fine wire electrodes, with which the amount of exposed wire (recording area) can vary. Motion of the electrodes after insertion can change the interelectrode distance and is difficult to detect. Separate insertion of the two electrodes with a set interelectrode distance may help minimize this (63) (Fig. 1). Several isometric contractions prior to recording are felt to help anchor the wires (8).

ELECTROMYOGRAPHY AND MUSCLE KINESIOLOGY

EMG has played a vital role in relating muscle function to the biomechanics of sports. It is one

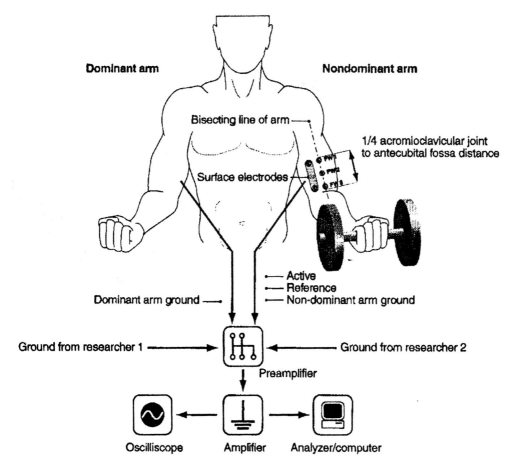

FIG. 1. Electrode placement on and in the biceps brachii of the nondominant arm. Each fine wire (FW) electrode is placed as shown. A surface bar electrode is placed just medial to the fine wire electrodes. Any of the five electrodes could be used as an active or reference electrode for a given configuration. A total of eight preamplifiers accept the eight different signals from the biceps. Ground electrodes are placed as above. Preamplifier, amplifier, and oscilloscope connections are also shown.

of the most accurate objective methods of determining when a muscle is contracting. This is particularly important for complex activities in which many muscles may act in a synergistic manner. This has led to a greater understanding of muscle firing patterns and muscle contraction patterns.

EMG can determine whether a muscle is active or at rest, but there are limitations that are often overlooked. One cannot differentiate on the basis of the myoelectric signal alone whether a muscle is contracting concentrically, isometrically, or eccentrically (20). The EMG amplitude for an eccentric contraction is lower than the amplitude recorded for a concentric contraction that produces the same force (20). This is because of

the role noncontractile elements play in generating force during an eccentric contraction. An agonist cannot be differentiated from an antagonist. The EMG signal is not a reliable indicator of force because the relationship between the EMG amplitude and muscle force is often not linear.

Although necessary for joint stability and motor coordination, cocontraction patterns may lead to early muscle fatigue and overuse injuries and impair muscle coordination. As motor skills improve, cocontractions should be reduced and motor skills can be accomplished more efficiently. EMG can be used as a biofeedback technique to help accomplish this.

Shoulder Function

The use of EMG in studying shoulder function has given us a clearer understanding of the biomechanics of overhead sports. Prime movers of the arm are the deltoid, pectoralis major, and latissimus dorsi. The four rotator cuff muscles, the supraspinatus, infraspinatus, teres minor, and subscapularis, are responsible for maintaining glenohumeral joint congruity and stability. The most common shoulder injuries in sports are to the rotator cuff or glenohumeral ligament–labral complex; however, motion of the entire upper extremity is dependent on the stability and motion of the scapula. This is controlled by the scapulothoracic movers and stabilizers, the trapezius, rhomboids, serratus anterior, levator scapulae, and pectoralis minor. The scapula's only static link to the body is the acromioclavicular joint. This underscores the importance of the scapulothoracic muscles in the biomechanics of shoulder motion.

One of the earliest EMG studies of shoulder function demonstrated a synergistic action between the supraspinatus and deltoid during abduction and flexion of the arm (64). The three remaining muscles of the rotator cuff functioned as glenohumeral stabilizers by depressing the humeral head during arm elevation. This is necessary to maintain glenohumeral compression for adequate cartilagenous nutrition. It also helps to prevent excessive glenohumeral motion, which may damage the static stabilizers, the glenohumeral ligaments, and labrum.

Muscle activity during shoulder elevation and depression was studied in three different planes (65). This study suggested that the supraspinatus and subscapularis are important dynamic stabilizers primarily during glenohumeral elevation and served as a foundation for later studies of shoulder biomechanics.

Work has been done to develop better rehabilitation programs by determining which exercises best activate muscles of the shoulder (66–68). The findings have been used to structure more appropriate rehabilitation programs and better isolate muscle groups; however, because the isolation of muscles is not activity or sport specific, the functional carryover of these exercises should be more thoroughly explored. Furthermore, the fact that EMG activity does not have a linear relationship with force is often overlooked.

The Shoulder in the Throwing Athlete

The throwing of a baseball has been studied extensively. High-speed photography has broken the motion of throwing into five phases: the windup, early cocking, late cocking, acceleration, and follow-through or the deceleration phase (Fig. 2). Muscle firing patterns have also been studied during these five phases with both surface and intramuscular electrodes (9,11). In

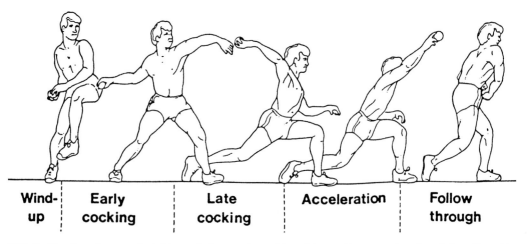

| Wind-up | Early cocking | Late cocking | Acceleration | Follow through |

FIG. 2. The five phases of pitching: windup, early cocking, late cocking, acceleration, follow-through.

one study, fine wire intramuscular electrodes were used to study shoulder muscles during pitching (9). This report included the deltoid and rotator cuff. It demonstrated the greatest EMG activity of all four rotator cuff muscles in late cocking and follow-through, the two extremes of motion. This supports the concept that the entire cuff functions to maintain joint stability and protect the static elements of the glenohumeral joint.

A second study (10) evaluated the biceps, triceps, pectoralis major, latissimus dorsi, and serratus anterior. In this study, the triceps, latissimus dorsi, and pectoralis major appear to be contracting eccentrically to decelerate the forearm and arm in late cocking prior to contracting concentrically as accelerators during the acceleration phase. The contraction patterns of the serratus anterior were not consistant and therefore difficult to interpret.

The Elbow in the Throwing Athlete

Valgus overload to the elbow can occur during the late cocking to acceleration phase of throwing. It can lead to medial (ulnar) collateral ligament injuries, ulnar neuritis, and osteochondritis of the capitellum. The pronator teres, flexor carpi radialis, and ulnaris act as dynamic stabilizers of the anteromedial elbow joint and give support to the medial collateral ligament (MCL). Muscle contraction patterns have been studied in the elbow to determine whether there were differences between pitchers with MCL insufficiency and those without injury to the MCL (14). The extensor carpi radialis brevis and longus had greater activity in the injured pitchers than in the uninjured pitchers when throwing both a fastball and a curveball. Injured pitchers had less activity in the extensor carpi radialis and pronator teres when throwing a fastball. These differences were seen in the late cocking and acceleration phases when the MCL undergoes the greatest stress from valgus overload. Decreased activity in the pronator teres may have made the MCL, and potentially the ulnar nerve and radiocapitellar joint, more susceptible to injury. Cocontraction of the wrist extensors in injured pitchers may lead to early fatigue of the wrist flexors, making the MCL more susceptible to injury.

The Elbow in Racquet Sports

Tennis elbow or lateral epicondylitis is one of the most common injuries to tennis players at all levels of competition. Elbow mechanics have been studied in all three major tennis strokes, the forehand, backhand, and serve, using high-speed photography and EMG analyses to better understand the pathophysiology of this condition (15).

The serve has been broken down into five phases, which are similar to those in overhead throwing: windup, early cocking, late cocking, acceleration, and follow-through (Fig. 3). There was low activity in all muscle groups in the windup. Activity in the extensor carpi radialis brevis (ECRB) and extensor digitorum communis (EDC) increased in early cocking and continued to increase in late cocking. The flexor carpi radialis (FCR), pronator teres (PT), and ECRB were all very active during acceleration, with some increase in activity in the EDC and extensor carpi radialis longus (ECRL). All muscles then dropped off to low activity during early follow-through, with only the biceps increasing in activity in late follow-through. The wrist extensors appear to be undergoing an eccentric cocontraction during the acceleration phase. This may be necessary to help stabilize the wrist and better control motion, but an eccentric overload of the wrist extensors could lead to lateral epicondylitis.

The forehand is broken down into preparation, acceleration, and early and late follow-through (Fig. 4). Only the ECRL was moderately active during preparation. Three extensors, the ECRB, ECRL, and EDC, had high activity during acceleration. The FCR had moderate activity. Only the ECRB and biceps remained highly active during early follow-through, while the EDC and FCR had moderate activity. In late follow-through the ECRL and ECRB remained moderately active while all other muscles had low activity. The isometric or eccentric cocontraction of the wrist extensors probably helps to stabilize the wrist during acceleration but with eccentric overload could lead to lateral epicondylitis.

The backhand was also broken down into preparation, acceleration, and early and late follow-through (Fig. 5). All muscles had low activity in preparation. During acceleration, the ECRB, ECRL, and EDC had high activity while the PT had moderate activity. The ECRB had

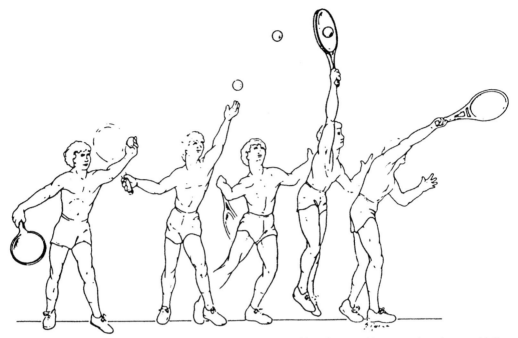

FIG. 3. Five phases of the tennis serve: windup, early cocking, late cocking, acceleration, and follow-through.

high activity in early follow-through. The EDC, ECRL, FCR, and PT had moderate activity. All muscles then dropped to low activity in late follow-through. These muscle firing patterns do not demonstrate any clear risk factors for developing lateral epicondylitis.

The Shoulder in Swimmers

Shoulder pain is a common complaint in swimmers. These patients often present with signs of supraspinatus impingement that may be secondary to underlying glenohumeral hypermobility or impaired scapula rotation and elevation. To better understand the pathophysiology of their condition, electromyographic analysis has been performed during the free-style stroke (12). The stroke was broken down into pull-through and recovery phases (Fig. 6). The deltoids, supraspinatus, upper trapezius, and rhomboids were very active from late pull-through through early

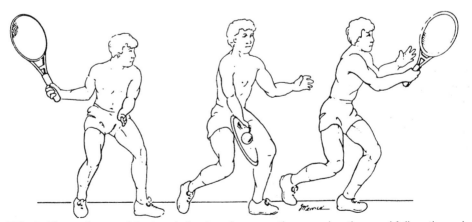

FIG. 4. Three phases of the tennis forehand: preparation, acceleration, and follow-through.

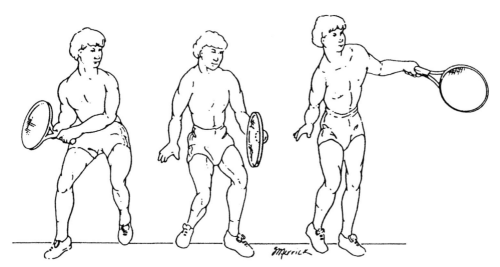

FIG. 5. Three phases of the tennis backhand: preparation, acceleration, and follow-through.

recovery. As the deltoids elevate the humerus, the supraspinatus helps to maintain glenohumeral congruity preventing superior migration of the humeral head. The rhomboids and upper trapezius stabilize and elevate the scapula head. The subscapularis was very active during late pull-through and continued to increase in activity into early recovery. Activity declined but was still very significant in late recovery. The infraspinatus was minimally active during early and late recovery, and the teres minor was moderately active between early and late pull-through. The serratus anterior was moderately active throughout the entire stroke, playing a key role in scapula stabilization and rotation. The pectoralis major was highly active in middle pull-through, and the latissimus dorsi was very active in late pull-through. Both are major propulsors of the swimmer during pull-through of the freestyle stroke.

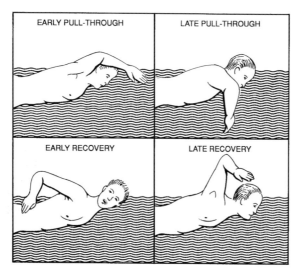

FIG. 6. Four phases of the freestyle stroke: early recovery, late recovery, early pull-through, and late pull-through.

The Painful Shoulder in Swimmers

Swimmers with painful shoulders were studied by the same methodology used for those with normal shoulders (13). There were more similarities than differences. The functional significance of the muscle firing patterns is unclear, but a decrease seen in serratus anterior activity could potentially lead to impingement. A decrease that was seen in subscapularis activity could lead to less glenohumeral stabilization. The increase in rhomboid activity may lead to limitions in scapula motion.

Quadriceps Function in Patellofemoral Syndrome

Patellofemoral syndrome is one of the most common causes of knee pain. Although it is considered to be primarily an overuse injury, many biomechanical factors, including the Q angle, hyperpronation, femoral anteversion, tibial torsion, geometry of trochlea groove, patella baja or alta, quadriceps muscle imbalances, weakness in the gluteal muscles, tight lateral capsular retinaculum, and lax medial capsular retinaculum, are felt to play a role in the etiology of this condition (69–72). The quadriceps consists of four major subdivisions all innervated by the femoral nerve: vastus medialis (VM), vastus intermedius (VI), vastus lateralis (VL), and rectus femoris (RF). The VM is then further divided into the vastus medialis oblique (VMO) and vastus medialis longus (VML). Anatomic studies have demonstrated that the oblique fibers of the VMO come from the adductor magnus or longus, which are primarily obturator nerve innervated but may have a small tibial nerve component as well (73). The subdivisions of the quadriceps act synergistically to maintain a balance of force vectors as the patella is pulled through the trochlear groove. Many believe that an imbalance in function between the VM and VL may lead to or be contributory to anterior knee pain or patellofemoral syndrome (70,74–80).

EMG has been used to study quadriceps function and determine whether there are muscle imbalances, primarily between the VMO and VL, that could cause abnormal patella tracking (81–85). Most studies performed are limited because the relationship between EMG activity and muscle force is not consistently linear. Comparing muscle balance solely on the basis of EMG activity is probably not valid. There was also no attempt to identify the muscle motor points and standarize electrode placement.

In one study (81) using a surface EMG analysis, a group of patients with patellofemoral pain syndrome (PFPS) was compared with an asymptomatic control group. There were no significant differences between the two groups in the ratio of VMO to VL electromyographic activity with the knee at several angles. There was a decrease in the VMO-to-VL ratio of EMG activity in a subset of the PFPS group who had Q angles greater than 22°. This occurred at 15° of knee extension. Others have demonstrated similiar findings (70, 71).

The EMG activities of the VMO and VL were compared during both concentric and eccentric isokinetic exercises at 60 and 120° per second (82). VMO activity was greater than VL activity throughout the entire range tested (10 to 85°) and the VMO/VL ratio increased with an increase of the knee flexion angle. The VMO/VL ratio was similar for eccentric and concentric contraction at 60° per second. Eccentric contractions at both 60 and 120° per second were also similar, but the VMO/VL ratio was greater for concentric contractions at 120° per second.

Surface EMG was used to compare the reflex response times of the VMO and VL following a patella tendon tap (83). There was an increase in the VL response time in patients with PFPS compared with asymptomatic controls, but there were no differences in VMO response time. These findings demonstrated a reversal of the muscular firing order between the VMO and VL in patients diagnosed with PFPS compared with asymptomatic individuals.

Another study looked at the relationship between the VMO and VL in a group of asymptomatic females (84). Using fine wire intramuscular electrodes, they found no difference in the EMG activity of the VMO or VL throughout full range of knee motion.

Many of these studies suggest that a VMO–VL imbalance exists at specific angles of knee flexion and is dependent on the type of muscular contraction (eccentric vs. concentric), the speed of contraction, and the Q angle. The relationship between muscle imbalance and patellofemoral symptoms can be proved significant only when clinical trials show that symptoms are reduced when they are corrected.

Knee Rehabilitation

Electromyography has been used to help develop more effective exercise programs for knee rehabilitation (86–97). Studies have been performed to determine whether there are exercises that preferentially strengthen the vastus medialis.

One study compared EMG activities in the rectus femoris and the vastus medialis during straight-leg raises and quadriceps sets in asymptomatic patients and patients with a history of knee surgery or knee pathology (92). In both groups there was greater activity in the the vastus medialis during quadriceps sets and greater activity in the rectus femoris during a straight-leg raise. There was also greater activity in the both the rectus femoris and vastus medialis in patients with a history of knee surgery or knee pain during straight-leg raises and quadriceps sets. Quadriceps sets are an isometric contraction for both the rectus femoris and vastus medialis. A straight-leg raise is an isometric contraction for the vastus medialis but a concentric contraction for the rectus femoris. Comparison of the electrical activities (and the related forces) of the VM and RF undergoing different types of contractions (concentric vs. isometric) may not be valid. The RF is a two-joint muscle and also acts as a hip flexor, whereas the VM is a one-joint muscle. A more valid comparison may have been between the VM and VL, both one-joint muscles.

Another EMG study was done to determine which exercises led to better activation and isolation of the VMO (93). Utilizing fine wire electrodes, the researchers compared the myoelectric signals of the VMO and VL with hip adduction (knee fully extended) and with medial tibial rotation (knee flexed 30°). The VMO had greater activity with adduction. Similar results were found in a study that used surface EMG electrodes. There were no significant differences, however, with medial tibial (internal) rotation.

These studies may give a more scientific basis for structuring a rehabilitation program for patients with patellofemoral syndrome and enhance our understanding of its pathophysiology. The effect of these exercises has largely been anecdotal, and few if any outcome studies have been done to support their efficacy.

Muscle Function in the Anterior Cruciate Ligament–Deficient Knee

Patients with a torn anterior cruciate ligament (ACL) have increased anteromedial rotation of the tibia. Dynamic stabilizers of the knee, the hamstrings can compensate for a torn ACL by pulling the proximal tibia posteriorly. EMG activity in the quadriceps and hamstrings has been studied to determine whether an ACL disruption changes the normal muscle firing patterns (101, 98,99). No consistent differences in EMG firing patterns of the knee muscles were found when patients with intact and torn ACLs were compared. One study demonstrated an increase in biceps femoris (lateral hamstring) activity and simultaneous decrease in quadriceps activity in ACL-deficient patients during the swing-to-stance transition at normal walking speeds (100). During this phase the leg was accelerating forward with the entire lower extremity. Just prior to heel strike, the lower extremity decelerated. The hamstrings probably fired to prevent the tibia from subluxing anteriorly. The hamstrings were less active than in normal individuals during mid-stance and terminal stance. The tibial–femoral compression forces with weight bearing may have been enough to prevent any tibial translation. This does not explain why hamstring activity was reduced compared with control subjects.

EMG activity in the quadriceps and hamstrings of ACL-deficient patients both braced and unbraced was compared with that in subjects with an intact ACL (101). They also found an increase in lateral hamstring activity during swing in the unbraced ACL-deficient knee. There was an increase in medial hamstring activity during the stance phase that was confirmed in another study (99), as well as a decrease in quadriceps activity. The hamstrings appear to be compensating for the absent ACL. Bracing of the ACL-deficient knee does not appear to alter firing patterns.

Another study looked at the relationship between the ACL, hamstrings, and quadriceps (95) by stressing an intact ACL. The hamstrings were excited and the quadriceps inhibited. This suggested that with anteromedial stress on the tibia, sensory feedback via the ACL may cause the hamstrings to pull the tibia back posteriorly.

Coactivation patterns of quadriceps and hamstring muscle have been studied in athletes (96). Hypertrophy of the quadriceps impaired hamstring coactivation. Strengthening the hamstrings reduced this.

Quadriceps and hamstring contraction patterns have been studied using surface EMG in ACL-intact individuals comparing open and closed kinetic chain exercises (102). A cocontraction of the hamstring and quadriceps occurred only during the closed-chain exercises.

Popliteus function in ACL-deficient patients has been studied to determine whether the popliteus plays a role in anterolateral instability (103). No significant difference between those with an intact ACL and those with complete tears was found.

Additional Kinesiologic Research

The studies just reviewed reflect only a representation of the extensive amount of kinesiologic research that has been done using EMG as an indication of muscle function. The golf swing has been studied in both men and women (16–18); the butterfly and breaststroke have been studied in swimmers (12); the back muscles have been studied in wrestlers and tennis players (104); and lower extremity muscle mechanics have been studied in ballet dancers (105), cyclists (106,107), and runners (108,109). The role of muscles as dynamic stabilizers has been studied in patients with ankle (110) and shoulder (111–114) instability. Neuromuscular control of squat lifting has also been studied (115).

ELECTROMYOGRAPHY AND MUSCLE FATIGUE

One of the most exciting applications of EMG has been in the study of fatigue in muscle at the level of the muscle fiber. Although fatigue can occur at the neuromuscular junction in conditions such as myasthenia gravis or myasthenic syndrome, it normally occurs at the muscle fiber level in healthy individuals. Understanding fatigue patterns may help design exercise programs that will prevent injuries, improve athletic performance, and better rehabilitate the injured. Mentioned earlier were the advantages and disadvantages of intramuscular versus surface electrodes. Many technical obstacles still exist, but the potential use both as a research tool and in the clinical setting make this a method deserving of further study.

Changes in three components of the myoelectric signal are indicative of early muscle fatigue. These are (a) slowing of the muscle fiber conduction velocity, (b) a decrease in the dominant frequency of the power density spectrum, and (c) an increase in the amplitude prior to mechanical failure (60). A drop in the median frequency occurs during a sustained muscle contraction with muscle fatigue. The drop is believed to be secondary to muscle fiber conduction velocity slowing (44,116,117). This is probably due to a change in the concentration of metabolic by-products (117). A dropout of type II fibers and increase in recruitment of type I fibers during fatigue may also play a role. This decline is linear. As a muscle sustains a contraction while maintaining a constant force, there is a linear decline in the median frequency. A more precipitous drop in the median frequency occurs with mechanical failure (21).

In addition to monitoring changes in median frequency, the root-mean-square (RMS) and rectified signals, both representative of the myoelectric amplitude, have been used as indicators of muscle fatigue. During a sustained contraction, the amplitude actually increases but then drops precipitously at the point of mechanical failure. Increased motor unit recruitment during fatigue has been one explanation for the initial increase in signal amplitude (31,118).

Twitch properties (fast twitch vs. slow twitch) of the muscle fibers of a motor unit determine the rate of fatigability. Slow-twitch fibers utilizing aerobic metabolic pathways have greater endurance than fast-twitch fibers. This has been demonstrated electromyographically in fatigue studies by following both the increase in an integrated EMG signal and the decrease in the power density spectrum. One study showed that the biceps, which has a higher fast-twitch fiber concentration, fatigued at a much greater rate than the soleus, which has a higher slow-twitch fiber concentration, during similar sustained isometric contractions (31). Others have revealed similar findings (36).

One of the earlier studies on fatigue of shoulder muscles used both surface and fine wire EMG (119). The supraspinatus, not accessible with a surface electrode, was studied with fine wire electrodes. Surface electrodes were used for the trapezius, infraspinatus, deltoid, and biceps. Both an increase in RMS and drop in mean power frequency were used as indicators of fatigue. The supraspinatus and upper trapezius were the first muscles to fatigue. Because intramuscular electrodes are more sensitive in detecting fatigue than surface electrodes, a comparison between the supraspinatus and all other muscles is not valid.

EMG studies of quadriceps function during knee extension were done to determine whether fatigue caused an imbalance of the VMO and VL (120). No significant differences were found in the drop in median frequency during short-arc quadriceps sets.

The median frequencies of paraspinal muscles in patients with low back pain (LBP) were compared with those in individuals with no history of LBP (121). A drop in the initial median frequency (IMF) was found in association with an increase in the force level of muscle contraction in both groups. This is contrary to the usual increase in IMF seen during an increase in contraction of limb muscles. This was felt to occur secondary to an increase in recruitment of smaller diameter type II muscle fibers. Patients with LBP were found to have a 10% to 15% lower IMF in the longissimus muscle at the L-1 level. A decline in the median frequency was greater in LBP patients in the multifidus (L-5) and iliocostalis (L-2). These results are consistent with those from several other studies (122–125).

SUMMARY

EMG is a powerful technique for studying muscle kinesiology and fatigue in sports medicine. Electrode placement, filtering characteristics, signal processing, the type of electrodes used, fiber type distribution, and the type of muscle contraction are all variables that affect the quality of the myoelectric signal. Both surface and intramuscular electrodes have been used in the study of muscle kinesiology. This has led to a greater understanding of stroke (golf, swimming, and tennis) and throwing mechanics, gait patterns, and muscle firing patterns in pathologic conditions such as patellofemoral syndrome, ACL tears, and shoulder and ankle instability. More effective rehabilitation and training programs have been developed. EMG is one of the few objective methods for determining muscle fatigue. Surface EMG electrodes have been the most reliable and commonly used method. Intramuscular electrodes appear to be more sensitive for detecting myoelectric indicators of fatigue and are necessary when studying deep muscles; however, significant technical limitations still exist and reproducibility has not been well demonstrated. A greater understanding of muscle fatigue patterns may further clarify the pathophysiology of many overuse injuries and help in their prevention.

Acknowledgments

I would like to thank Neil Spielholz, Ph.D., Steven Kirshblum, M.D., and Kevin O'Connor for their critical comments regarding the manuscript. I would also like to thank Kathy Pugliese for her assistance in preparation.

REFERENCES

1. Feinstein B, Lindegard B, Nyman E, et al. Morphological studies of motor units in normal human muscles. *Acta Anat* 1955;23:124–142.
2. Engel WK. Fiber-type nomenclature of human skeletal muscle or histochemical purposes. *Neurology* 1974; 24:344–348.
3. Brooke MH, Kaiser KK. Muscle fibre types: how many and what kind? *Arch Neurol* 1970;23:369–379.
4. Johnson MA, Polgar J, Weightman D, Appleton D. Data on the distribution of fiber types in thirty six human muscles: an autopsy study. *J Neurol Sci* 1973; 18:111–129.
5. Gollnick PD, Sjodin B, Karlsson J, Jansson E, Saltin B. Human soleus muscle: a comparison of fiber composition and enzyme activities with other leg muscles. *Pflugers Arch* 1974;348:247–255.

6. Edgerton VR, Smith JL, Simpson DR. Muscle fibre type populations of human leg muscles. *Histochem J* 1975;7:259–266.

7. Johnson EW. The EMG examination. In: Johnson EW, ed. *Practical electromyography.* Baltimore: Williams & Wilkins, 1988:1–21.

8. Basmajian JV, DeLuca CJ. *Muscles alive: their functions revealed by electromyography,* 5th ed. Baltimore: Williams & Wilkins, 1958.

9. Jobe FW, Tibone JE, Perry J, Moynes D. An EMG analysis of the shoulder in throwing and pitching. *Am J Sports Med* 1983;11(1):3–5.

10. Jobe FW, Moynes D, Tibone JE, Perry J. An EMG analysis of the shoulder in pitching. *Am J Sports Med* 1984;12(3):218–220.

11. Pappas AM, Zawacki RM, McCarthy CF. Rehabilitation of the pitching shoulder. *Am J Sports Med* 1958; 13:223–235.

12. Nuber GW, Jobe FW, Perry J, Moynes DR, Antonelli D. Fine wire electromyography analysis of muscles of the shoulder during swimming. *Am J Sports Med* 1986; 14(1):7–11.

13. Scovazzo ML, Browne A, Pink M, Jobe FW, Kerrigan J. The painful shoulder during freestyle swimming: an electromyographic cinematographic analysis of twelve muscles. *Am J Sports Med* 1991;19(6):577–582.

14. Glousman RE, Barron J, Jobe FW, Perry J, Pink M. An electromyographic analysis of the elbow in normal and injured pitchers with medial collateral ligament insufficiency. *Am J Sports Med* 1992;20(3):311–317.

15. Morris M, Jobe FW, Perry J, Pink M, Healy BS. Electromyographic analysis of elbow function in tennis players. *Am J Sports Med* 1989;17(2):241–247.

16. Jobe FW, Perry J, Pink M. Electromyographic shoulder activity in men and women professional golfers. *Am J Sports Med* 1989;17(6):782–787.

17. Pink M, Perry J, Jobe FW. Electromyographic analysis of the trunk in golfers. *Am J Sports Med* 1993; 21(3): 385–388.

18. Bechler JR, Jobe FW, Pink M, et al. Electromyographic analysis of the hip and knee during the golf swing. *Clin J Sport Med* 1995;5(3):162–166.

19. VanderHelm FC. Analysis of the kinematic and dynamic behavior of the shoulder mechanism. *J Biomed* 1994;27:527–550.

20. Moritani T, Muramatsu S, Muro M. Activity of motor units during concentric and eccentric contractions. *Am J Phys Med* 1988;66:338–351.

21. DeLuca CJ, Sabbahi MA, Stulen FB, Bilotto G. Some properties of the median frequency of the myoelectric signal during localized muscular fatigue. *Proceedings of the 5th International Symposium on Biochemistry of Exercise* 1983:175–186.

22. DeLuca CJ. Myoelectrical manifestations of local muscular fatigue in humans. *CRC Crit Rev Biomed Eng* 11:251–279.

23. Woods JJ, Bigland–Ritchie B. Linear and non-linear surface EMG/force relationships in human muscles: an anatomical/functional argument for the existence of both. *Am J Phys Med* 1983;62:6:287–299.

24. Lawrence JH, DeLuca CJ. Myoelectric signal vs force relationship in different human muscles. *J Appl Physiol* 1983;54:1653–1659.

25. Solomonow M, Baratta R, Zhou BH, Shoji EH, D'Ambrosia R. The EMG force model of electrically stimulated muscles: dependence on control strategy and predominant fiber composition. *IEEE Trans Biomed Eng* 1987;34:692–703.

26. Hannaford L, Lehman S. Short time Fourier analysis of the electromyogram: fast movements and constant contraction. *IEEE Trans Biomed Eng* 1986;BME-33:1173–1181.

27. LeFever RS, DeLuca CJ. The contribution of individual motor units to the EMG power spectrum. *Proceedings 29th Ann Conf Eng Med Biol* 1976:56.

28. Gerdle B, Wretling ML, Henricksson-Larsen K. Do the fibre-type proportion and the angular velocity influence the mean power frequency of the electromyogram? *Acta Physiol Scand* 1988;134:341–346.

29. Moritani T, Gaffney FD, Charmichael T, Hargis J. Interrelationships among muscle fiber types, electromyogram and blood pressure during fatiguing isometric contraction. In: Winter DA, Norman RW, Wells RP, Hayesk C, Patla AE (eds). *Biomechanic IX-A.* Champaign, IL: Human Kinetics, 287–292.

30. Bilodeau M, Goulet C, Nadeau S, Arsenault AB, Gravel D. Comparison of the EMG power spectrum of the human soleus and gastrocnemius muscles. *Eur J Appl Physiol* 1994;68:395–401.

31. Moritani T, Nagata A, Muro M. Electromyographic manifestations of muscular fatigue. *Med Sci Sports Exerc* 1982;14:198–202.

32. Roy SH, DeLuca CJ, Schneider J. Effects of electrode location on myoelectric conduction velocity and median frequency estimates. *J Appl Physiol* 1986; 61:1510–1517.

33. Broman H, Bilott G, DeLuca CJ. Myoelectric signal conduction velocity and spectral parameters: influence of force and time. *J Appl Physiol* 1985;58:1428–1437.

34. Kranz HK, Williams AM, Cassell J, Caddy DJ, Silberstein RB. Factors determining the frequency content of the electromyogram. *J Appl Phsiol* 1983;55:392–399.

35. Bilodeau M, Arsenault AB, Gravel D, Bourbonnais D. EMG power spectra of elbow extensors during ramp and step isometric contractions. *Eur J Appl Physiol* 1991;63:24–28.

36. Komi PV, Tesch P. EMG frequency spectrum, muscle structure and fatigue during dynamic contractions in man. *Eur J Appl Physiol* 1979;42:41–50.

37. Moritani T, Muro M. Motor unit activity and surface electromyogram power spectrum during increasing force of contraction. *Eur J Appl Physiol* 1987;56:260–265.

38. Buchtal F, Schmalbruch H. Contraction times and fibre types in intact human muscle. *Acta Physiol Scand* 1970;79:435–452.

39. Brust M, Cosla HW. Contractility of isolated human skeletal muscle. *Arch Phys Med* 1967;48:543–555.

40. Eberstein A, Goodgold J. Slow and fast twitch fibers in human skeletal muscle. *Am J Physiol* 1968; 215:535–541.

41. Barnard RJ, Edgerton VR, Peter JB. Effect of exercise on skeletal muscle. II. Contractile properties. *J Appl Physiol* 1970;28:767–770.

42. Close R. The relation between intrinsic speed of shortening and duration of the active state of muscle. *J Physiol (Lond)* 1965;180:542–559.

43. Barany M. ATPase activity of myosin correlated with speed of muscle shortening. *J Gen Physiol* 1967; 50:197–218.

44. Lindstrom LH, Magnusson RI. Interpretation of myoelectric power spectra: a role and its application. *Proc IEEE* 1977;65:653–662.

45. Mortimer T, Magnusson R, Petersen I. Conduction velocity in ischemic muscle: effect on EMG power spectrum. *Am J Physiol* 1970;131:1324–1329.

46. Brody LR, Pollock MT, Roy SH, DeLuca CJ, Celli B. pH-induced effects on median frequency and conduction velocity of the myoelectric signal. *J Appl Physiol* 1991;71:1878–1885.

47. Beliveau L, Helal JN, Gaillard E, Van Hoecke J, Atlan G, Bouissou P. EMG spectral shift and P-NMR–determined intracellular pH in fatigued human biceps brachii muscle. *Neurology* 1991;41:1998–2001.

48. Stashuk D, DeLuca C. Median frequencies of cannula and surface detected myoelectric signals. *Proc Ninth Annual IEEE EMBS Conference Boston* 1987:661.

49. Broman H, Bilotto G, DeLuca CJ. Myoelectric signal conduction velocity and spectral parameters: influence of force and time. *J Appl Physiol* 1985;58:1428–1437.

50. Horita T, Ishiko T. Relationships between muscle lactate accumulation and surface EMG activities during isokinetic contractions in man. *Eur J Appl Physiol* 1987;56:18–23.

51. Merletti R, Knaflitz M, DeLuca CJ. Myoelectric manifestations of fatigue in voluntary and electrically elicited contraction. *J Appl Physiol* 1990;69;1810–1820.

52. Merletti R, Sabbahi MA, DeLuca CJ. Median frequency of the myoelectric signal: effects of muscle ischemia and cooling. *Eur J Appl Physiol Occup Physiol* 1984;52:258–265.

53. Richie DH, DeVries HA, Endo CK. Shin muscle activity and sports surfaces: an electromyographic study. *J Am Podiatr Med Assoc* 1993;83:181–190.

54. Petrofsky SJ, Lind AR. The influence of temperature on the amplitude and frequency components of the EMG during brief and sustained isometric contractions. *Eur J Appl Physiol* 1980;44:189–200.

55. Viitasalo JT, Komi PV. Effects of fatigue on isometric force- and relaxation-time characteristics in human muscle. *Acta Physiol Scand* 1981;111:87–95.

56. Rosenfalck P. *Intra- and extracellular potential fields of active nerve and muscle fibers.* Copenhagen: Academisk Forlag, 1969.

57. Gath I, Stalberg E. The calculated radial decline of the extracellular action potential compound with in situ measurements in the human brachial biceps. *Electroencephalogr Clin Neurophysiol* 1978;44:547–552.

58. Delagi EF, Perotta A. *Anatomic guide for the electromyographer,* 2nd ed. Springfield, IL: Thomas, 1980.

59. Bilodeau M, Bertrand-Arsenault A, Gravel D, Bourbonnais D, Kemp F. The influence of gender on the EMG power spectrum statistics of elbow flexors and extensors. *IEEE Eng Med Biol Soc* 1991;13:841–842.

60. Arendt-Nielsen L, Mills KR. Muscle fibre conduction velocity, mean power frequency, mean EMG voltage and force during submaximal fatiguing contractions of human quadriceps. *Eur J Appl Physiol* 1988;58:20–25.

61. Krivickas LS, Nadler SF, Davies MR, Petroski GF, Feinberg JH. Spectral analysis during fatigue. *Am J Phys Med Rehabil* 1996;75:1139–1143.

62. Sable AW, Haig AJ, Alba HM, et al. Effect of wire electrode surface area on power spectrum during fatigue. *Muscle Nerve* 1991;14:885.

63. Davis BA, Krivickas LS, Maniar R, Newandee DA, Feinberg JH. The reliability of monopolar and bipolar fine-wire electromyographic measuirement of muscle fatigue. *Med Sci Sports Exerc* (*in press*).

64. Inman VT, Saunders JB, Abbot LC. Observations on the function of the shoulder joint. *J Bone Joint Surg* 1944;26:1–30.

65. Shevlin MG, Lehmann JF, Lucci JA. Electromyographic study of the function of some muscles crossing the glenohumeral joint. *Arch Phys Med Rehabil* 1969;50:264– 270.

66. Rowlands LK, Wertsch JJ, Primack SJ, Spreitzer AM, Roberts MM. Kinesiology of the empty can test. *Am J Phys Med Rehabil* 1995;74:302–304.

67. McCann PD, Wootten ME, Kadaba MP, Bigliani LU. A kinematic and electromyographic study of shoulder rehabilitation exercises. *Clin Orthop* 1993;288:179–188.

68. Townsend H, Jobe FW, Pink M, Perry J. Electromyographic analysis of the glenohumeral muscles during a baseball rehabilitation program. *Am J Sports Med* 1991;19:264–272.

69. Hunter HC. Patellofemoral arthralgia. *J Am Osteopath Assoc* 1985;85:580–585.

70. Mariani PP, Caruso I. An electromyographic investigation of subluxation of the patella. *J Bone Joint Surg Br* 1979;61B:169–171.

71. Souza DR, Gross MT. Comparison of vastus medialis obliquus: vastus lateralis muscle integrated electromyographic ratios between healthy subjects and patients with patellofemoral pain. *Phys Ther* 1991;71:310–320.

72. Huberti HH, Hayes WC. Patellofemoral contact pressures. *J Bone Joint Surg Am* 1984;66A:715–724.

73. Bose K, Kanagasuntheram R, Osman MBH. An anatomic and physiologic study. *Orthopedics* 1980;3:880–883.

74. Hughston JC. Subluxation of the patella. *J Bone Joint Surg Am* 1968;50A:1003–1026.

75. Fox TA. Dysplasia of the quadriceps mechanism. *Sug Clin North Am* 1975;55:199–226.

76. Outerbridge RE, Dunlop JAY. The problem of chondromalacia patellae. *Clin Orthop* 1975;110:177–196.

77. Trillat A, Dejour R, Puddu GC. La sublussazione recidivante della rotula. *G Ital Ortop Traumatol* 1975;1:209–219.

78. Mansat C, Duboureau L, Cha P, Dorbes R. Desequilibre rotulien et instabilite rotatoire externe du genou. *Rev Rhum Mal Osteo-Articulaires* 1977;44:115–123.

79. Perugia L. La patologia del meccanismo estensore. Read at the International Meeting of the Society of Knee Surgery, Rome, 1977.

80. McConnell J. The management of chondromalacia patellae: A long term solution. *Aust J Physiother* 1986;32(4):216–223.

81. Boucher JP, King MA, Lefebvre R, Pepin A. Quadriceps femoris muscle activity in patellofemoral pain syndrome. *Am J Sports Med* 1992;20:527–532.

82. Sczepanski TL, Gross MT, Duncan PW, Chandler JM. Effect of contraction type, angular velocity, and arc of motion on VMO:VL EMG ratio. *J Orthop Sports Phys Ther* 1991;14:256–262.

83. Voight ML, Wieder DL. Comparative reflex response times of vastus medialis obliquus and vastus lateralis in normal subjects and subjects with extensor mechanism dysfunction. *Am J Sports Med* 1991;19:131–137.

84. Reynolds L, Levin TA, Medeiros JM, Adler NS, Hallum A. EMG activity of the vastus medialis oblique and the vastus lateralis in their role in patellar alignment. *Am J Phys Med* 1983;62:61–69.

85. Basmajian JV, Harden TP, Regenos EM. Integrated actions of the four heads of quadriceps femoris: an electromyographic study. *Anat Rec* 1971;172:15–20.

86. Pocock GS. Electromyographic study of the quadriceps during resistive exercise. *J Am Phys Ther Assoc* 1963; 43:427–434.

87. Allington R, Baxter, ML, Koepke GH, Christopher RP. Strengthening techniques of the quadriceps muscles: an electromyographic evaluation. *J Am Phys Ther Assoc* 1966;46:1173–1176.

88. Gough JV, Ladley G. An investigation into the effectiveness of various forms of quadriceps extension. *Phys Ther* 1971;57:356–361.

89. Skurja M, Perry J, Gronley J, Hislop HJ. Quadriceps action in straight leg raise versus isolated knee extension (EMG and tension study). *Phys Ther* 1980;60:582.

90. Antich TJ, Brewster CE. Modification of quadriceps femoris muscle exercises during knee rehabilitation. *Phys Ther* 1985;66:1246–1251.

91. Lieb FJ, Perry J. Quadriceps function. *J Bone Joint Surg Am* 1971;53A:749–758.

92. Soderberg GL, Minor SD, Arnold K, et al. Electromyographic analysis of knee exercises in healthy subjects and in patients with knee pathologies. *Phys Ther* 1987;67:1691–1696.

93. Hanten WP, Schulthies SS. Exercise effect on electromyographic activity of the vastus medialis oblique and vastus lateralis muscles. *Phys Ther* 1990; 70: 561–565.

94. Wheatley MD, Jahnke WD. Electromyographic study of the superficial thigh and hip muscles in normal individuals. *Arch Phys Med* 1951;32:508–515.

95. Solomonow M, Baratta R, Zhou BH, Shoji H, D'Ambrosia R. The EMG-force model of electrically stimulated muscles: dependence on control strategy and predominant fiber composition. *IEEE Trans Biomed Eng* 1987;BME-34:692–702.

96. Baratta R, Solomonow M, Zhou BH, Letson ED, Chuinard R, D'Ambrosia R. Muscular coactivation: the role of the antagonist musculature in maintaining knee stability. *Am J Sports Med* 1988;16:113–122.

97. Gryzlo SM, Patek RM, Pink M, Perry J. Electromyographic analysis of knee rehabilitation exercises. *J Orthop Sports Phys Ther* 1994;20:36–43.

98. Carlson S. Nordstrand A. The coordination of the knee muscles in some voluntary movements and in the gait in cases with and without knee injuries. *Acta Chir Scand* 1968;134:423.

99. Tibone JE, Antich MS, Fanton GS, Moynes DR, Perry J. Functional analysis of anterior cruciate ligament instability. *Am J Sports Med* 1986;14:276–284.

100. Limbird TJ, Shiavi R, Frazer M, Borra H. EMG profiles of knee joint musculature during walking: changes induced by anterior cruciate ligament deficiency. *J Orthop Res* 1988;6:630–638.

101. Branch TP, Hunter R, Donath M. Dynamic EMG analysis of anterior cruciate deficient legs with and without bracing during cutting. *Am J Sports Med* 1989;17:35–41.

102. Lutz GE, Palmitier RA, An KN, Chao EY. Comparison of tibiofemoral joint forces during open-kinetic-chain and close-kinetic-chain exercises. *J Bone Joint Surg Am* 1993;75A:732–739.

103. Weresh MJ, Gabel RH, Brand RA, Tearse DS. Popliteus function in ACL-deficient patients. *Iowa Orthop J* 1994;14:85–93.

104. Sward L, Svensson M, Zetterberg C. Isometric muscle strength and quantitative electromyography of back muscles in wrestlers and tennis players. *Am J Sports Med* 1990;18:382–386.

105. Trepman E, Gellman RE, Solomon R, Murthy K, Micheli LJ, DeLuca CJ. Electromyographic analysis of standing posture and demi-plié in ballet and modern dancers. *Med Sci Sports Exerc* 1994;26:771–782.

106. Jorge M, Hull ML. Analysis of EMG measurements during bicycle pedaling. *J Biomech* 1986;19:683–694.

107. deGroot G, Welbergen E, Clijsen L, Clarijs J, Cabri J, Antonis J. Power, muscular work, and external forces in cycling. *Ergonomics* 1994;37(1):31–42.

108. Montgomery WH, Pink M, Perry J. Electromyographic analysis of hip and knee musculature during running. *Am J Sports Med* 1994;22:272–278.

109. Reber L, Perry J, Pink M. Muscular control of the ankle in running. *Am J Sports Med* 1993;21:805–810.

110. Karlsson J, Andreasson GO. The effect of external ankle support in chronic lateral ankle joint instability: an electromyographic study. *Am J Sports Med* 1992; 20:257–261.

111. Pande P, Hawkins R, Peat M. Electromyography in voluntary posterior instability of the shoulder. *Am J Sports Med* 1989;17:644–648.

112. Suzuki R, Ito N, Kuwahara K. An electromyographical study on loose shoulder. *Fourth Congress of Int Soc Electrophysiol Kinesiol* 1979:114–115.

113. Kronberg M, Brostrom L, Nemeth G. Differences in shoulder muscle activity between patients with generalized joint laxity and normal controls. *Clin Orthop* 1991;269:181–192.

114. Glousman R, Jobe F, Tibone J, Moynes D, Antonelli D, Perry J. Dynamic electromyographic analysis of the throwing shoulder with glenohumeral instability. *J Bone Joint Surg Am* 1988;70:220–226.

115. Scholz JP, McMillan AG. Neuromuscular coordination of squat lifting. II: Individual differences. *Phys Ther* 1995;75:133–144.

116. Stalberg E. Propagation velocity in human muscle fibers in situ. *Acta Physiol Scand* 1967;70(Suppl):287.

117. Stulen FB, DeLuca CJ. Frequency parameters of the myoelectric signal as a measure of muscle conduction velocity. *IEEE Trans Biomed Eng* 1981;BME-28:515–523.

118. Blank A, Gonen B, Magora A. The size of active motor units in the initiation and maintenance of an isometric contraction carried out to fatigue. *Electromyogr Clin Neurophysiol* 1979;19:535–539.

119. Hagberg, M. Electromyographic signs of shoulder muscular fatigue in two elevated arm positions. *Am J Phys Med* 1981;60:111–121.

120. Grabiner MD, Koh TJ, Miller GF. Fatigue rates of vastus medialis oblique and vastus lateralis during static and dynamic knee extension. *J Orthop Res* 1991; 9:391–397.

121. Roy SH, DeLuca CJ, Casavant DA. Lumbar muscle fatigue and chronic lower back pain. *Spine* 1989; 14:992–1001.

122. DeVries HA. EMG fatigue curves in postural muscles: a possible etiology for idiopathic low back pain. *Am J Phys Med* 1968;47:175–181.

123. Jayasinghe WJ, Harding RH, Anderson JAD, Sweetman BJ. An electromyographic investigation of postural fatigue in low back pain—a preliminary study. *Electroencephalogr Clin Neurophysiol* 1978;18:191–198.

124. Kraus H, Raab W. *Hypokinetic disease,* Springfield, IL: Charles C Thomas Publisher, 1961.

125. Nicolaisen T, Jorgensen K. Trunk strength, back muscle endurance and low back trouble. *Scand J Rehabil Med* 1985;17:121–127.

Sports Neurology, Second Edition,
edited by Barry D. Jordan.
Lippincott–Raven Publishers, Philadelphia © 1998.

7

Neuroradiology of Sports-Related Injuries

Robert D. Zimmerman

Department of Radiology, New York Hospital/Cornell Medical Center,
525 East 68th Street, New York, New York 10021

It is the purpose of this chapter to review the role of neuroradiologic studies in the evaluation of patients with sports-related injuries. The imaging features of sports-related injuries do not differ from the imaging features of neurotrauma in general, although the nature of the sport may produce a preponderance of one or more types of traumatic lesions. Therefore this chapter provides a general review of the imaging features of neurotrauma, followed by a discussion of injuries likely to occur with individual activities (e.g., boxing).

The mainstay of structural neuroimaging (the detection of normal and pathologic anatomic states) in head trauma is computed tomography (CT) (1–4), but magnetic resonance imaging (MRI) has been utilized with increasing frequency because of improved detection and characterization of the sequelae of trauma (5–11) (Figs. 1 and 2). Subject to availability, MRI will probably replace CT in the assessment of patients with head trauma. CT will continue to play a significant role in cases in which MRI cannot be performed and in cases in which skull fracture is likely (e.g., in-line skating accidents) (Fig. 2). The ability to detect subtle traumatic lesions and to identify and characterize incidental pathologic foci is particularly important for boxers, who are at much greater risk for repeated head trauma than the general population. In one series of 21 boxers, MRI proved superior to CT in detecting focal and diffuse intracranial injuries (12).

The evaluation of spinal injuries is also undergoing rapid evolution. Traditionally, plain radiographs and CT have been used to assess the osseous spine. To evaluate the contents of the spinal canal, myelography has been required. The introduction of high-speed helical CT has made it possible to assess the osseous structures rapidly and accurately (13–17). MRI can be used to demonstrate noninvasively intra- and extraspinal soft tissue injuries, including lesions that previously could not be detected by any imaging technique (17–19).

A variety of new imaging techniques for the assessment of central nervous system function are now being used or are under investigation. Fast spin echo (FSE) techniques have produced a 4- to 20-fold reduction in scan time. This has made it possible to perform studies that were impractical in the past because of scan time. One such technique is fluid-attenuated inversion recovery (FLAIR) (Fig. 3). This is a sequence that is heavily T2 weighted for brain but uses an inversion pulse to null the signal from cerebrospinal fluid (CSF), eliminating the difficulty of differentiating the normal high intensity of CSF from the hyperintensity of a pathologic process.

The introduction of more powerful high-speed gradients (e.g. >20 millitesla) makes it possible to perform even faster examinations such as single-shot FSE (SSFSE) and echo-planar imaging (EPI), which can be used to obtain a single slice in as little as 20 msec. Increased scan speed also makes it possible to perform an ever-expanding variety of structural and "functional" (fMRI) sequences in patients in a reasonable amount of time (e.g., 30 minutes) (20–29).

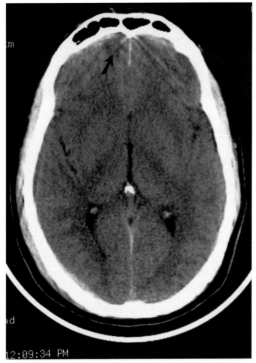

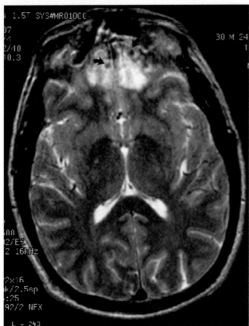

A. *MR spectroscopy (MRS):* Alterations in energy metabolites, neuronal markers, and lactic acid can be detected with this technique.

B. *Diffusion-weighted imaging (DWI):* Motion of water molecules can be detected using flow-sensitive sequences similar to those employed for phase-contrast MR angiography. The amount of freely diffusing water (DWI) increases with vasogenic (extracellular) edema and decreases with cytotoxic edema (cell swelling with shrinkage of the extracellular space). DWI can demonstrate abnormalities when routine T2-weighted (T2W) and FLAIR images are normal (20,21).

C. *Perfusion-weighted imaging (PWI):* The use of contrast agents to detect alterations in blood flow, blood volume, and mean transit time was developed with CT and has been adapted to MRI using paramagnetic contrast agents. As the contrast agent passes through the cerebral vessels, it causes signal loss that is proportional to the amount of contrast present (20,21).

D. *Magnetization transfer (MT):* The amount and proportion of free and macromolecular bound water can be assessed by using a radiofrequency (RF) pulse that suppresses the protons that are exchanging between the two water pools. The size of these proton pools varies in a number of disease processes, in particular those affecting white matter such as diffuse axonal injury (DAI).

E. *Activation studies:* Using sequences that are sensitive to blood oxygen levels, it is possible to map the location of brain activity during various cognitive tasks [blood oxygenation level dependent (BOLD) imaging], thus potentially identifying abnormal patterns of brain activity.

Functional data can also be obtained with other imaging techniques. Positron emission tomography (PET) (23,24) and the more readily available single-photon emission computed tomography (SPECT) (25–27) can assess brain function and activation using labeled energy compounds (glucose) or oxygen. It is now possible to measure and map the electromagnetic activity of the brain using magnetoencephalography (MEG) (28,29).

FIG. 1. Frontal contusions in a boxer. Computed tomography (**A**) is grossly normal, although there is some subtle heterogeneous density in the right frontal lobe (*arrow*). T2-weighted magnetic resonance (**B**) reveals bifrontal hyperintense edema with small hypointense foci of acute hemorrhage.

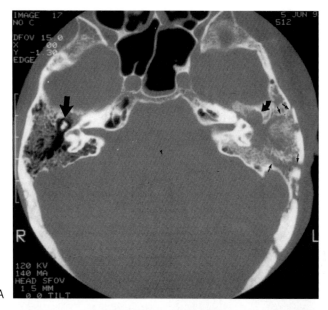

A

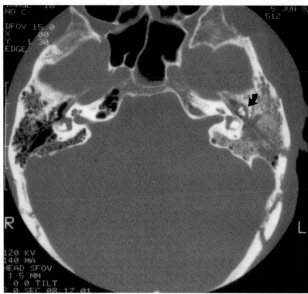

B

FIG. 2. In-line skating injury. The patient, without protective headgear, fell backward. Thin-section computed tomographic (CT) scans (**A** and **B**) through petrous bones reveal opacification of mastoid air cells and the epitympanic space. Fractures extend through petrous bone (*small arrows*). Note absence of ossicles (**A**) in their normal position in the epitympanic space [compare with the position of contralateral ossicles (*arrow*)]. Ossicles were dislocated and displaced inferiorly (*curved arrow* in **B**). CT scan at level of frontal lobes (**C**) is normal. T2-weighted magnetic resonance scan (**D**) at the same level reveals bifrontal hemorrhagic contusions.

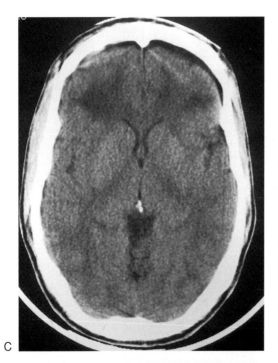

C

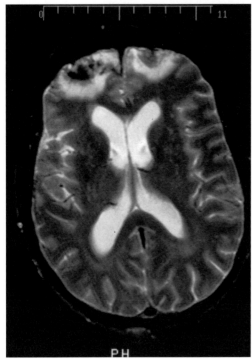

D   P H

FIG. 2. *Continued*

Data from fMRI, PET, SPECT, and MEG can be electronically superimposed on high-resolution MRI images, further improving the spatial resolution of these modalities (28). These new techniques, used singly or in combination, may make it possible to identify, characterize, and treat acute and chronic lesions of the brain and spinal cord earlier than with previously available techniques including routine "structural" MRI. This, in turn, may prevent or limit permanent impairment.

IMAGING STRATEGIES

CT revolutionized the evaluation of traumatized patients because of its great sensitivity and specificity. It replaced all previous modalities (including plain radiographs) as the chief and usually sole diagnostic tool in the evaluation of patients with head trauma (1,2). Nevertheless, it is recognized that CT is relatively insensitive to a few important lesions, especially those occurring near the surface and deep within the brain. CT also fails to detect the underlying causes of posttraumatic syndrome (concussions) (7,12,27,28,30,31).

MRI is more sensitive than CT in detecting most intracranial lesions (7–11) (Figs. 1 and 2). MRI is particularly valuable in the identification of superficial lesions such as small subdural hematomas and nonhemorrhagic contusions that cannot be seen with CT. These lesions occur adjacent to the calvarium and can be obscured on CT by artifact from the bone (in particular above the irregular orbital roof, where most contusions occur) (7). The absence of artifact from bone and the ability to perform multiplanar imaging have made it possible to identify and characterize these superficial intracranial lesions in a manner that is impossible with CT (Fig. 3). MRI has also proved superior to CT in detecting deep brain lesions including shear injuries (DAI) because of its greater sensitivity to changes in white matter (33) (see Figs. 7 and 9).

In the past, the feasibility of using MRI in acute head trauma has been limited by long scan times, difficulty of monitoring patients and life support, and scanner availability. These problems have diminished as scan time has decreased dramatically

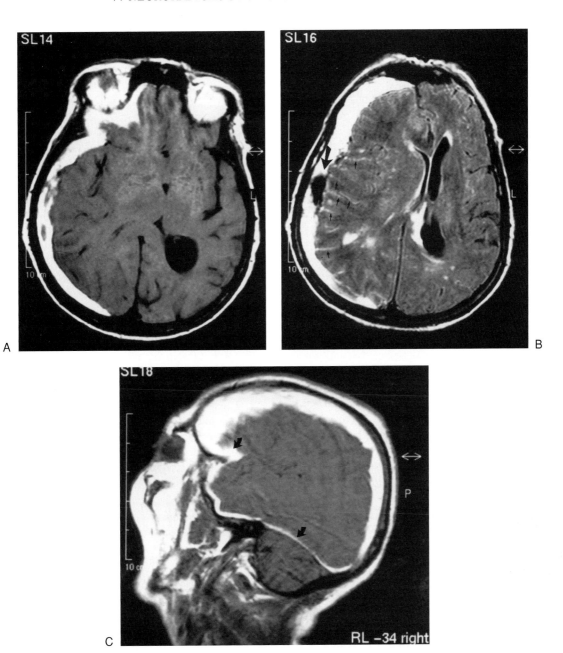

FIG. 3. Acute subdural hematoma in a football player. Axial T1-weighted (T1W) scan (**A**), fluid-attenuated inversion recovery (FLAIR) (**B**), and sagittal T1W scan reveal a large subacute subdural hematoma with a focus of recurrent acute hemorrhage (*arrow,* **B**). Note the extension over the orbital roof and superior tentorial surface seen on a sagittal image (*arrows,* **C**), which cannot be appreciated on axial images. Subarachnoid hemorrhage is well seen with FLAIR (*small arrows*).

and equipment for monitoring and maintaining acutely ill patients in the MRI environment has been manufactured (32). The proliferation of MRI scanners has been viewed with alarm, but this increased capacity makes it possible to utilize MRI as a screening test in head trauma.

Routine ("anatomic") MRI does have limitations. Patients with postconcussive syndromes typically have normal MRI scans even when they have severe functional impairment (7,12). The correlation between extent of dysfunction and MRI findings in patients with DAI is better than with CT, but MRI is not sufficiently accurate to allow confident prediction of the patient's outcome. New functionally based MRI sequences such as DWI (20), MT (22), and MRS promise to solve some of these problems by allowing more accurate demonstration of derangement of brain anatomy and function in both the acute and chronic phase of disease.

IMAGING OF INTRACRANIAL HEMORRHAGE

One additional potential limitation of MRI is the ability to detect hemorrhage, in particular acute subarachnoid hemorrhage (SAH) and hyperacute (<24 hours) intracerebral hemorrhage. On CT scans, the appearance of hemorrhage is straightforward and well known (34). Acute hematomas are hyperdense relative to brain because of the globin fraction of the hemoglobin molecule. This hyperdensity is readily apparent on scans obtained between 1 and 10 days after trauma and is specific enough to allow accurate diagnosis. As the globin is destroyed and removed, the density of blood diminishes and the ability to characterize a lesion as hemorrhagic is lost.

On MRI, the appearance of hemorrhage is much more complex (35–37). Intensity varies dramatically over time and with each pulse sequence. It is dependent on multiple factors, including the water content of the clot, the integrity of the red cells, and the presence of various paramagnetic hemoglobin breakdown products (e.g., deoxyhemoglobin and methemoglobin) that dramatically alter the intensity of blood.

During the first postictal week, hematoma intensity changes rapidly. On T1-weighted [short relaxation time (TR), short echo time (TE)] images, hematomas are initially mildly hyperintense relative to white matter. The intensity diminishes to mild hypointensity during days 2 and 3, and the hematomas become markedly hyperintense on approximately postictal day 4 because of the T1-shortening effect of methemoglobin. On T2-weighted (long TR, long TE) images, hematomas are initially hyperintense (Fig. 4). After 12 to 24 hours, they become markedly hypointense because of the presence of intracellular deoxyhemoglobin, and after approximately 5 days intensity increases and the hematomas again become hyperintense because of red cell lysis (Fig. 3).

Because of the complex findings of acute hemorrhage on MRI, radiologists were initially reluctant to advocate its use in the assessment of hemorrhagic lesions. With experience it has become clear that the ability to detect acute hemorrhage with MR is equal to that with CT. The addition of pulse sequences such as gradient echo (standard and EPI) and FLAIR has improved our ability to detect hyperacute and acute hemorrhage within the brain and subarachnoid spaces to the point where it is conceivable that in the near future it will be possible (given scanner availability) to use MRI as the primary tool for the assessment of patients with acute head trauma (38).

Magnetic resonance imaging is more sensitive than CT in detecting subacute hemorrhage (36). Hemorrhage is characteristically hyperintense relative to brain on all pulse sequences from 1 week to 1 month after the ictus. On CT, hematoma density diminishes gradually, becoming isodense relative to brain at approximately 10 to 20 days and hypodense thereafter. Isodensity and hypodensity are nonspecific findings that may be seen with various lesions; thus MRI is superior to CT in specifically identifying zones of subacute hemorrhage.

ACUTE TRAUMA

Extracerebral Hematomas

The size, shape, and location of an extracerebral hematoma depend on the relationship of the lesion to the dura and on the mechanism of trauma (4,10,39). MRI is superior to CT in detecting all

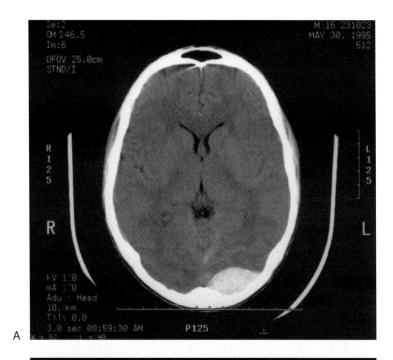

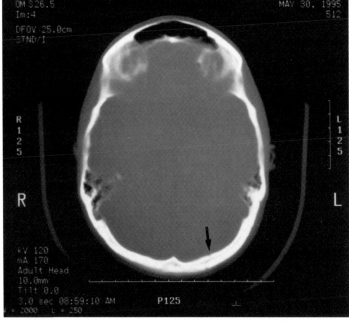

FIG. 4. Epidural hematoma (EDH) secondary to a bicycle accident. The rider was not wearing a helmet. Computed tomography (**A** and **B**) reveals a lentiform hyperdense EDH adjacent to the torcular and transverse sinus. A fracture (*arrow,* **B**) was identified at the level of the transverse sinus. Axial T2-weighted magnetic resonance imaging (T2W MRI)(**C**) and sagittal T1W MRI (**D**) reveal a lentiform hematoma of mixed intensity (hyperacute) with a hypointense rim representing displaced dura (*small arrows,* **C** and **D**). Note that the hematoma is contiguous with the transverse sinus, which is occluded (*large arrow,* **D**). Findings are indicative of venous EDH.

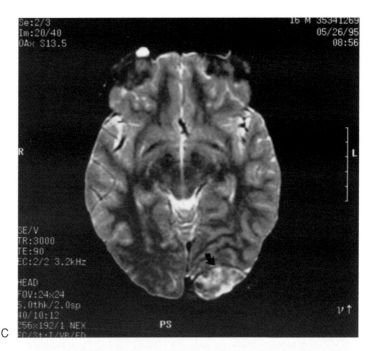

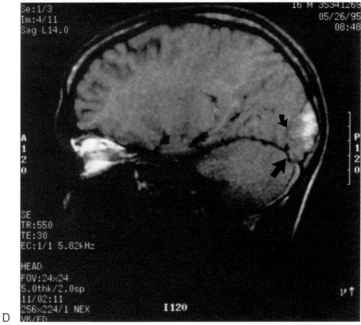

FIG. 4. *Continued*

extraaxial hematomas (7–11), even when the hemorrhage is isointense to adjacent brain. The absence of bone artifact, multiplanar scanning capacity, and high contrast between brain and spinal fluid make it possible to visualize the displaced brain surface directly on MRI in a manner that is impossible with CT, thus allowing excellent visualization of all extracerebral hematomas.

Epidural hematomas (EDHs) (Fig. 4) are secondary to fracture and result from falls or direct blows to the head (10,36). Although all fractures result in some bleeding, large EDHs occur when the fracture produces rupture of a major calvarial vessel such as the middle meningeal artery. This leads to extravasation of blood under arterial pressure. The dura is tightly adherent to the inner table of the skull and therefore the hematomas are focal and bulge into the adjacent compliant brain. EDHs occur most commonly along the course of the middle meningeal artery. Occasionally, severe trauma results in laceration of a major dural venous sinus (e.g., the superior sagittal sinus). The hematoma is centered on the sinus and straddles multiple intracranial compartments (4). In contrast, arterial EDHs tend to stop at venous sinuses because the dura is most tightly adherent at these locations.

On CT and MRI, EDHs present as focal lentiform (medially convex) masses adjacent to major arterial or venous structures (1,3,4,10). Fractures and associated extracranial soft tissue masses are detected in over 90% of cases.

Subdural hematomas (SDHs) (Fig. 3) result from acceleration–deceleration or torsion injury and are commonly encountered in falls. SDHs result from hemorrhage into the tissue plane between the dura and the arachnoid, usually as a result of rupture of bridging cortical veins as they extend to the dural venous sinuses (1,3,4,10,39). The venous hemorrhage is under low pressure and there is slow bleeding that dissects freely through the extensive, continuous-convexity subdural space (39), producing a thin but extensive crescentic collection on imaging studies. Occasionally, SDHs result from laceration of a superficial cortical artery. These hematomas expand rapidly and are virtually always associated with parenchymal damage. They therefore have an extremely poor prognosis.

Large-convexity SDHs are easily detected with CT, but narrow lesions may be missed because of an artifact from the adjacent hyperdense bone. These lesions are more apparent on MRI because of its superior identification of superficial brain anatomy. The size and extent of a subdural hematoma are always better assessed by MRI than by CT, and 30% of SDHs are detected by MRI alone (7). Because the lesions detected with MRI alone are small, surgical management is not affected. In athletic injuries, the identification of an SDH certainly affects decisions about when and whether the patient may return to his or her sport.

Parenchymal Injury

The most common parenchymal injury is the contusion (Figs. 1 and 2). In a closed-head injury the brain is damaged by a direct (coup) impact transmitted through the skull and indirectly by the rapid deceleration of the contralateral portion of the brain as it strikes the inner table of the skull (contracoup) (1–3,10,11,39). Contusions are usually cortical or subcortical, and they most commonly involve the frontal, temporal, and occipital poles. The inferior frontal lobes are particularly prone to contusion because the floor of the anterior fossa is rough and irregular. As the frontal lobes slide along these irregular surfaces, the brain is abraded. Pathologically there is an admixture of various amounts of hemorrhage, edema, and brain tissue within the injury. Mild injuries may be nonhemorrhagic, but in severe cases a frank hematoma may form.

On CT, contusions are identified as irregular, ill-defined, moderately hyperdense superficial masses. Surrounding hypodensity is present as a result of edema and bland contusion (1–3). Small and/or nonhemorrhagic contusions are difficult to identify with CT (Figs. 1 and 2). Inferior frontal and temporal contusions may be obscured by hyperdense artifacts from adjacent frontal and temporal bones. Serial studies often demonstrate increasing edema and a mass effect and progressive hemorrhage. Occasionally, the initial CT scan is completely normal, but follow-up studies 1 or 2 days later demonstrate large areas of hemorrhage. Round or oval, homogeneous hyperdense masses represent frank hematomas. Complete disruption of brain tissue results in a "contusion tear," a large, irregular, hyperdense triangular lesion that extends from a broad base on the cortex to a narrow apex at the ventricular margin (3,10,11,39).

The presence and extent of parenchymal damage are more accurately assessed by MRI, which is more sensitive to increased tissue water (edema and nonhemorrhagic contusion) and because artifacts from the frontal and temporal bones are not present (5–11). Hypointensity on T2W, FLAIR, and in particular gradient echo or EPI scans indicates the presence of hemorrhage with a sensitivity that equals or surpasses that of CT.

Injury to deep portions of the brain occurs when acceleration–deceleration produces shear forces leading to diffuse axonal injury (Figs. 5 and 6). Shearing injuries are usually diffuse and distributed throughout the supratentorial white matter. In severe cases, areas of hemorrhage may develop in the corpus collosum, basal ganglia lateral corticomedullary junction, and posterior brainstem (10,11,39,40). Nonhemorrhagic lesions cannot be detected with CT; therefore deep hemorrhages, even when small, are often associated with a poor prognosis because they tend to occur in association with extensive (but undetectable by CT) shearing injuries. Follow-up examinations often show rapid development of severe atrophy.

MRI is superior to CT in the detection of DAI (Fig. 5) (7–11, 33). Foci of white matter edema (of any cause) are much more easily visualized with MRI than are petecheal hemorrhages. Gradient echo and EPI sequences are particularly efficacious in demonstrating these small hemorrhages. Despite these improvements, the correlation between MRI findings and clinical outcome is not perfect. When there are extensive posttraumatic white matter edema and petecheal hemorrhage and/or there is involvement of the basal ganglia or brainstem, the prognosis is poor. Less extensive or focal changes (e.g., isolated hemorrhage in the corpus collosum) are less predictive of outcome (Fig. 6). A focal deep hemorrhage may be an indicator of more extensive injury but it may also

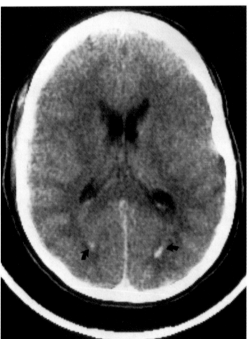
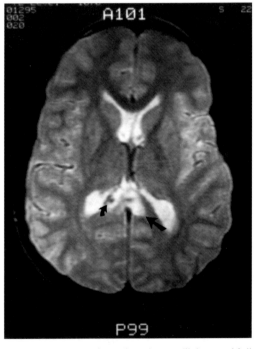

A   B

FIG. 5. Diffuse axonal injury (DAI) in a teenager rendered comatose after a head-on collision and fall during a soccer match. Computed tomography (**A**) reveals only intraventricular hemorrhage layering in the occipital horns of the lateral ventricles. On a T2-weighted scan (**B**), there is edema of the splenium of the corpus callosum (*large arrow*) with central hypointensity (*small arrow*) reflecting the presence of acute hemorrhage.

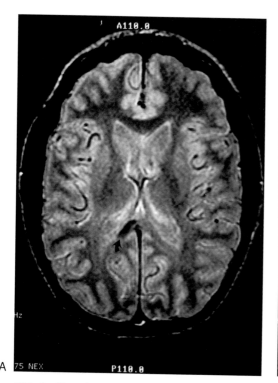 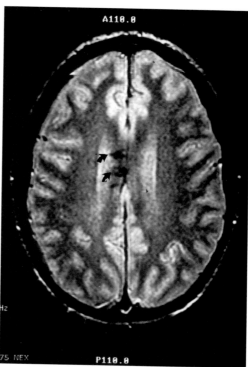

FIG. 6. Chronic diffuse axonal injury with recovery. The patient was in coma for 1 month after a biking accident. Magnetic resonance imaging was done 6 months after full recovery. The patient was wearing a helmet. Axial proton density images reveal areas of hypointensity indicative of chronic hemorrhage in the splenium (**A**) and body (**B**) of the corpus callosum (*arrows*).

represent an isolated axonal injury. Studies have demonstrated alterations in the magnetization transfer ratio of the white matter in the absence of abnormalities on routine MRI that seem to correlate better with outcome (22).

Both CT and routine MRI are usually normal in patients with posttraumatic syndrome (concussions) (7,10,11). Evaluations of MRI scans of amateur boxers after blows to the head have not demonstrated significant abnormalities (31). MRI does have value in this setting, however, because it allows the demonstration of subtle focal lesions such as small subdural hematomas, bland contusions, and incidental lesions (e.g., arachnoid cysts) that may produce findings that mimic postconcussive states (12).

Imaging techniques that are based on physiologic rather than structural changes have shown promise in detecting changes in patients with posttraumatic syndrome. PET and SPECT may be used to assess metabolic changes in the brain such as al-

terations in glucose metabolism (23–27). MEG has shown transient alterations in the distribution of brain magnetic activity in patients with posttraumatic symptoms (29). Subtle changes in tissue water and macromolecular composition may be detected with DWI (20) and MT MR sequences (22). These studies may prove particularly useful in assessing the extent of damage (transient or permanent) in athletes such as boxers and football players who are subject to recurrent head injury.

CHRONIC INJURY

The sequelae of prior trauma may be demonstrated by both CT and MRI. In most patients with significant injuries, focal atrophy or encephalomalacia develops at the site of injury. In severe or recurrent trauma, diffuse atrophy can be seen. Posttraumatic atrophy is commonly encountered in veteran boxers, especially those with dementia. A cavum septum pellucidum has also been reported as a common finding in these patients (Fig. 7) (41,42).

Magnetic resonance imaging is superior to CT in detecting the sequelae of trauma (7,10). The multiplanar capacity and absence of bone artifact make it possible to define the extent of focal lesions more accurately. Focal atrophy, encephalomalacia, and old hemorrhage all appear hypodense on CT scans but each has distinctive intensities on MR images. Diffuse atrophy is detected by both modalities, but MRI is superior in determining the extent of posterior fossa atrophy. The extent of diffuse atrophy is a better prognostic indicator of outcome than is the presence or extent of white matter injury.

VASCULAR INJURY

Damage to the cervical carotid or vertebral arteries with secondary cerebral infarction may result from various sports-related activities (43,44). With rapid, violent turning or twisting of the head or occasionally with a direct blow to the neck, the arteries are crushed against adjacent bony vertebral structures and the vessel intima is damaged, producing a subintimal hematoma, which can dissect along the vessel over the next several hours. Infarction is generally embolic rather than occlusive because most patients are young and have sufficient collateral flow to maintain circulation to the affected vascular distribution. This lesion occurs in diving or surfing injuries but may also be seen with any rapid head movement.

Symptoms of acute infarction are typically delayed until about 8 to 12 hours after the injury. Diagnosis may be complicated by the latency. In some patients with severe trauma, the onset of symptoms is relatively rapid, and clinical and CT findings may be interpreted as the result of direct cerebral injury rather than infarction caused by cervical vascular trauma. In cases in which trauma is mild and the onset of deficit is delayed, the patient may not report the history of neck injury, thinking it inconsequential or unrelated to

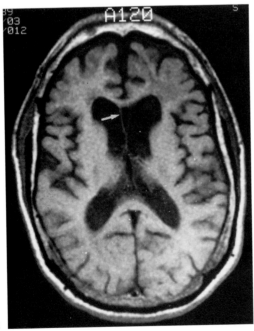 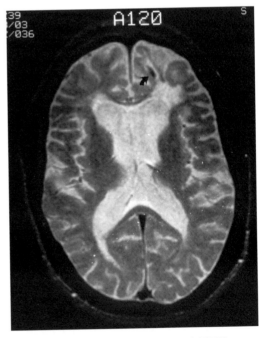

A   B

FIG. 7. A retired boxer with chronic traumatic encephalopathy (CTE). A T1-weighted (T1W) scan (**A**) reveals generalized atrophy and focal encephalomalacia (mild hypointensity) in the left frontal lobe. A small CSP (*arrow*) is present. On a T2W scan (**B**), atrophy is also visible. Left frontal gliosis or encephalomalacia is hyperintense with a small central focus of hypointensity representing old hemorrhage (*arrow*).

the subsequent neurologic deterioration. Because the intracranial vessels are intrinsically healthy, there is often good recovery.

On CT scans a focal area of hypodensity in the peripheral middle cerebral artery distribution is typically encountered. Although characteristic of infarction, it may be difficult to distinguish from a large bland contusion. Posterior fossa infarcts related to vertebral damage may be difficult to detect with CT. Infarcts are more easily appreciated with MRI, especially in the posterior fossa. Arterial occlusion may be directly demonstrated as absence of the normal arterial flow void. The intramural clot (dissection) can be directly visualized as a peripheral area of hyperintensity surrounding a central focus of hypointensity that represents the residual lumen ("target" sign) (44) (Fig. 8). Magnetic resonance angiography (MRA) can confirm the presence of dissection by showing the occluded vessel or the narrowed lumen and the adjacent intramural clot. The combination of MRI and MRA is superior to conventional angiography, which can demonstrate only nonspecific occlusion or stenosis. Serial MRI and MRA often demonstrate recanalization and resolution of the intramural clot.

SPINAL TRAUMA

The workup of spinal injuries is more complicated than that of head trauma because it is not possible to define the nature and extent of spinal injuries with any single modality (13–17). Plain-film radiography remains the most commonly employed screening test (14). Plain films allow assessment of spinal alignment and identification of many fractures, but stability, especially after flexion injury, cannot always be determined.

The initial evaluation is performed to determine the stability of the spinal column (14). If an unstable injury is present, damage to the spinal cord may ensue unless care is taken in moving the patient. Films are first obtained with a cross-table lateral technique to minimize the patient's motion. Localizing signs such as a fracture or soft tissue injury are identified, and the alignment of the vertebral bodies is assessed. The signs of instability range from obvious phenomena such as multiple fractures and severe dislocation to subtle changes such as flaring of the spinous processes. Stability is dependent on the integrity of the posterior vertebral elements and their ligamentous attachments. Some fractures are stable, whereas soft tissue injury of the posterior ligaments can produce instability without fracture (14). Knowledge of the mechanism of injury is an important aid in the assessment of stability. Direct trauma to the spine usually results in focal bone disruption. More commonly, trauma is the result of flexion, extension, rotation, or compression. Instability usually results from the flexion component of the injury. Rupture of the interspinous ligament leads to flaring of the spinous processes on plain films. With more severe injury, the zygapophyseal joint capsule is disrupted, and the inferior articulating facet of the superior vertebral body may slip forward anterior to the superior articulating facet of the more inferior body. Once this occurs, the facets become locked and incapable of returning to their normal position. More severe flexion injuries cause compression and disruption of the intervertebral disc and an anterior compression or teardrop fracture of the vertebral body. Even in severe injuries the cord may not be initially damaged, so the radiographic detection of instability is key in preventing subsequent development of spinal pathology.

Extension injuries less often produce spinal instability but are more likely, when severe, to cause damage to the spinal cord as bony spinal elements are displaced posteriorly into the spinal canal. Axial loading injuries such as may occur in cranial crown injuries in football produce upper cervical extension injuries and commonly result in severe damage to the cord (45–47).

The anterior–posterior dimension of the spinal canal is also assessed on plain radiographs. The canal should be at least 70% of the adjacent vertebral body. Patients with small canals (congenital stenosis) are prone to develop acute transient cord dysfunction with cervical trauma (45).

CT scanning has been used with increasing frequency to evaluate patients with cervical spine injuries (13–16). The advent of helical scanners has dramatically improved the efficacy of CT by making it possible to obtain thin-section scans of the entire cervical spine in a short period of time. These images can be reformatted in sagittal and

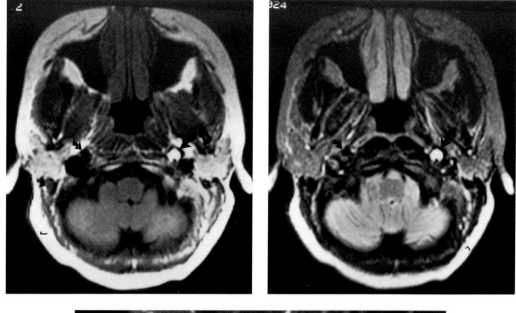

A   B

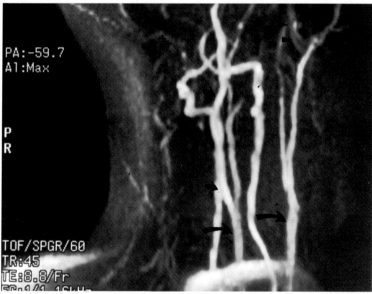

C

FIG. 8. Carotid dissection in a skier. Axial T1-weighted (T1W) and T2W images (**A** and **B**) reveal a round focus of hyperintensity in the wall of the left internal carotid artery (*arrows*). Note the small eccentric focus of hypointensity at the posterior margin representing residual lumen. Normal right carotid artery (*small arrows*) is seen as a large hypointense focus (normal flow void). Oblique reconstruction of magnetic resonance angiogram (**C**) reveals normal flow in both common carotid arteries (*large arrows*) and the right internal carotid artery (*small arrows*). There is absence of flow in the left internal carotid artery. An intramural clot produces subtle hyperintensity along the course of the upper cervical left internal carotid artery (*arrowheads*).

coronal planes to provide critical information about alignment, joint pathology, and complex fractures. Studies have demonstrated that helical CT is superior to plain radiography in the detection of fractures in the cervical spine (16) and several authors have advocated routine cervical CT in conjunction with cranial CT in patients with severe head injures (17).

As good as CT has become, it is still not possible to assess the contents of the spinal canal with this modality. Myelography in combination with CT has been used to detect cord compression by bone fragments, swelling or epidural hemorrhage, and cord swelling, but this invasive technique cannot provide information about the nature of cord injuries. MRI has been utilized with increasing frequency to assess the contents of the canal. Direct visualization of the cord is routinely obtained and therefore cord compression, EDH, cord edema, and cord hematomas can be directly and noninvasively identified (17–19). Fractures are not as well seen as with CT, but with MRI it is possible to identify ligamentous injuries that can produce instability. In order to use MRI for patients with cervical trauma, MRI-compatible stabilization devices have been devised.

A much more common sequela of athletic activity is chronic spinal injury. One of the by-products of the general increase in exercise has been an increase in the number of patients presenting with sequelae of chronic recurrent spinal trauma. Disc herniation, spinal stenosis, and neural canal stenosis are commonly encountered (45). In the lumbar region, plain radiographs are often normal or demonstrate nonspecific degenerative changes, even in the presence of stenosis or herniated nucleus pulposus (HNP). Spinal stenosis is diagnosed when the canal is narrowed, usually by a combination of degenerative disc disease, hypertrophic degenerative arthritis of the zygapophyseal joints, and hypertrophy of the ligamentum flavum. In many patients this is superimposed on a congenitally narrow spinal canal. Alterations in the normal angulation and contour of the zygapophyseal joints (facet tropism) may produce congenital narrowing and predispose to the development of severe degenerative arthritis, which leads to spinal stenosis. L4-5 is the most commonly and severely involved level of stenosis.

L3-4 is the next most commonly involved level. Spinal stenosis is difficult to quantify. When the spinal canal is narrower than 1 cm in any dimension, clinically significant stenosis is often present. It must be remembered, however, that both the spinal canal and the thecal sac vary in size, so direct measurement of the spinal canal is an unreliable indicator of stenosis. The most reliable finding of stenosis is relative narrowing of the canal and distortion of the thecal sac. When the sac narrows at L3-4 and/or L4-5 relative to L1-2 and then widens again at L5-S1, spinal stenosis is present. Distortion of the thecal sac and obliteration of epidural fat are usually present with symptomatic stenosis.

HNP results from rupture of the annulus fibrosis with extension of disc material into the spinal canal (45,46). This produces a focal ventral soft tissue mass that obliterates epidural fat, displaces or obscures the nerve root, and compresses the anterior–lateral aspect of the thecal sac.

MRI of the lumbar spine has a sensitivity that equals or surpasses that of CT (46,48,49). The use of both axial and sagittal images makes it possible to identify free fragments of disc material that have migrated superiorly or inferiorly away from the parent disc. Disruption of the annulus fibrosis may be visualized in many cases, a direct sign of herniation. In addition, sagittal MRI allows routine demonstration of the conus medullaris, thus eliminating the possibility (always present with CT) of missing an intrinsic tumor that is mimicking an HNP. MRI is also more sensitive than all other modalities (plain films, CT, or RN scans) in demonstrating degenerative discs, infection, and spinal metastases.

The chronic sequelae of cervical and thoracic trauma are best imaged by MRI. Stenosis, HNP, cord compression, and chronic cord injuries (e.g., posttraumatic cysts) are directly visualized. The introduction of phase array coils and fast spin-echo techniques has made it possible to perform high-resolution imaging of the entire spine in a reasonable amount of time.

BOXING AND MARTIAL ARTS

In boxing and martial arts, head injuries are common and inevitable because victory is directly achieved by rendering the opponent unconscious (50). Neuroimaging studies may be performed for two distinct purposes. First, they are used to evaluate fighters who suffer from acute neurologic disturbances during a match. Second, they may be used to detect evidence of brain damage resulting from the chronic and cumulative effects of multiple matches, in particular chronic traumatic enecephalopathy (CTE) (50–53).

Acute Injury

Minor head injuries without permanent neurologic sequelae are common. CT and MRI scans of boxers who have been knocked out without residual focal neurologic deficits are normal (12), as are studies of patients who suffer from concussions induced by other types of head injury (7,10,11). This is not surprising, given that the events producing the alteration in consciousness occur at the level of the cell membrane without sufficient amounts of hemorrhage or edema to be detected by CT and MRI. Abnormalities have been detected in patients with minor head trauma using functional techniques such as SPECT and MEG (23–29). If these techniques prove reliable, it should be possible to assess objectively the extent of brain injury and monitor the return to normal function. With this information, decisions about when and whether to allow a boxer to resume his career could be made in a manner that prevents or limits subsequent brain damage (54).

Severe acute head injuries, especially those that produce fixed neurologic dysfunction, are fortunately rare in boxers. In the same 2-year study already described there were only four hospital admissions for neurologic dysfunction in a 2-year period (involving over 400 fighters per year), one of which resulted in death (55). This low rate of serious neurologic injury is probably a result of stringent medical supervision.

The types of lesions encountered depend on the mechanism of injury. Fractures and associated adjacent epidural hematomas or parenchymal contusions are not commonly encountered as a direct result of blows to the head because of the use of gloves and padding of the ring (56).

A severe blow to the head can produce sufficient acceleration and rotation to cause SDHs, contrecoup contusions, and shear injuries to the brain. Severe injuries may also result from a fall after the boxer has been rendered unconscious with rapid deceleration as the head strikes the canvas. This in turn may lead to the development of acute subdural hematomas and contusions in a classic coup–contrecoup distribution. Subdural hematomas are the most commonly encountered lesions and they account for most of the deaths associated with boxing (41,52,56). Severe DAI leads to death or a vegetative state, but minimal shear injuries are associated with recovery (33). The cumulative effect of multiple subclinical shear injuries might account for the later development of dementia and atrophy.

Occasionally, CT or MRI performed to evaluate a boxer for acute neurologic abnormality provides evidence of prior trauma. Chronic subdural hematomas, zones of encephalomalacia, porencephaly, and focal atrophy may be encountered. Imaging studies may also reveal incidental lesions that are causatively unrelated to boxing. These findings are, nevertheless, important because they may render the boxer more susceptible to injury during subsequent matches (12).

Chronic Injury

Chronic, often progressive, neurologic dysfunction is more common than severe acute injury. This syndrome, variously termed, punch-drunk syndrome, dementia pugilistica, or, more recently and generally, chronic traumatic encephalopathy, typically begins near or after the end of the fighter's career. Its onset may be delayed for several decades. Pathologic studies of boxers suffering from CTE demonstrate cerebral and cerebellar atrophy, a high incidence of cavum septum pellucidum (Fig. 7), and stretching and atrophy of deep structures such as the hypothalamus and fornix (39,51,56,57).

These findings are well demonstrated by CT or MRI in retired boxers. It would, of course, be much more important if these changes (or their precursors) could be detected in active boxers at a time when intervention could prevent or at least limit the severity of CTE.

Studies have demonstrated a correlation between the number of knockouts and/or number of bouts and the presence of atrophy (30,51,52). Amateur fighters have the lowest incidence of atrophy, presumably reflecting the use of headgear and diminished severity and number of blows to the head (31). These studies were limited because of the small number of subjects, mixed populations (professional and amateur, active and retired fighters), and possibility of selection bias. A major methodologic limitation is the difficulty in documenting objective evidence of mild atrophy on CT scans. There is significant normal variation in ventricular and sulcal size in normal young adults, and the appearance of these structures is influenced by technical factors such as slice thickness and scan quality.

These problems were addressed in a study of 338 consecutive CT scans of active professional boxers (42). In order to avoid the difficulties inherent in assessing the degree of atrophy, only three grades of ventricular–sulcal size were assigned and the studies were reviewed by two neuroradiologists who were blinded to all clinical data concerning the boxers. The incidence of pathologic findings was quite low. Only 25 (7.4%) examinations were clearly abnormal, demonstrating moderate to severe brain atrophy and/or focal hypodense lesions. Of the studies, 238 (70%) were normal and 75 (22%) showed borderline ventricular and/or sulcal prominence (more than expected for age) but were not unequivocally abnormal. The presence of borderline or dilated ventricles correlated with a prior history of knockout or technical knockout (TKO) but not with number of bouts or won–lost record (42).

Cavum septum pellucidum (CSP) was identified in 13% of the fighters. This is a normal developmental anatomic structure, which usually regresses by early childhood. The CSP may persist in a few patients into adulthood as a large rectangular spinal fluid space between the frontal horns of the lateral ventricles. In boxers, it is postulated that rotational forces cause the two layers of ependyma that make up the septum to tear apart (Figs. 7 and 9). The CSPs encountered in active boxers are smaller than those seen in the general population and are difficult to detect with CT and MR scanners of poor quality (42). This finding may be useful as an objective indicator of early atrophy in boxers who otherwise demon-strate normal or borderline dilated spinal fluid spaces (Fig. 9).

Serial neuroimaging studies can detect progressive neurologic injury. Serial CT scans of 45 active professional boxers (21) obtained over an average duration of 31 months revealed evidence of progressive brain injury in six fighters (13%). Three boxers had progressive atrophy and three developed a CSP. Progressive changes on serial CT scans were associated with having more than ten losses ($p<0.05$) (58).

These studies do offer some hope that we will be able to identify evidence of chronic injury earlier and more accurately. The use of functional imaging studies should add to our ability to identify fighters at risk for the future development of CTE (23–29).

CONTACT SPORTS

Head injuries are common in football and hockey (59). The use of protective headgear has dramatically reduced the frequency and severity of head injuries in these sports, but concussions still occur. A single event is usually not significant, but recurrent episodes can lead to permanent damage just as they can in boxers (59).

The use of headgear has had a paradoxical effect on the incidence of severe cervical trauma. "Spearing," a tackling technique in which the defensive player drives the crown of his helmet into the opposing player, can lead to axial loading and cervical fracture with cord damage (45–47). The same injury occurs in hockey when a player is checked into the "boards" from behind at high speed (60). Changes in the rules governing these sports have reduced the incidence of these injuries, but education of coaches, players, and the public is necessary to eliminate these catastrophic events.

Collisions between players can lead to head trauma in sports such as soccer and basketball, which are not traditionally considered contact sports (Fig. 5). Because headgear is not utilized, fractures with or without associated epidural hematomas and contusions are more common than in football and hockey. CTE has been reported in soccer players. It has been postulated that this may result from striking the ball with the

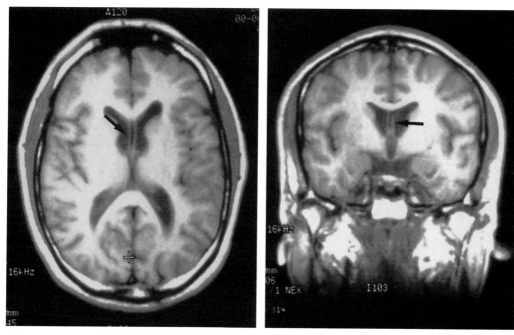

FIG. 9. Cavum septum pellucidum in an active veteran boxer. Axial and coronal T1-weighted images reveal a small CSP (*arrows*) in an active veteran fighter. No other abnormalities were noted in this study of a boxer without dementia.

head, but studies indicate that CTE is the result of multiple collisions (61).

HIGH-SPEED SPORTS

Horseback riding (62), biking (63,64), skiing, ice skating, roller skating, skateboarding, and in-line skating (roller blades) (65,66) are sports in which head and spine injuries occur as a result of collisions and falls. The incidence of head injuries in these sports is directly related to the use of protective headgear. In horseback riding and biking, the widespread use of helmets has led to a dramatic decrease in the incidence of severe head trauma. In sports in which helmets are not routinely used, the frequency and severity of head injury are much greater (Fig. 4).

This is most apparent with the dramatic increase in the rate of occurrence of severe head injuries in in-line skaters. As this relatively new sport has become extremely popular over the past few years, the number of severe head injuries has grown at an alarming rate. Few skaters wear protective headgear. (Ironically, most skaters do wear wrist and knee guards, perhaps reflecting the

relative importance they place on the functions their brains, wrists, and knees, respectively.)

When helmets are not used, fractures with associated EDHs and contusions are the most common injuries (Fig. 2). In-line skaters tend to fall backward at high speeds and therefore have a predilection for petrous fractures. SDHs and DAI may occur as well if there is a significant decelerational or rotational component.

EXTREME SPORTS

Massive injuries and death are the usual consequence of human error, equipment failure, or just bad luck in extreme sports such as skydiving, hang gliding, extreme skiing, and mountain climbing. Bungee jumping (67) is a new addition to the spectrum of highly dangerous activities that some individuals seem to crave. It has the advantage (?) over more rigorous sports that it requires no training or preparation. For the most part, these patients rarely live long enough to be evaluated by imaging studies. The few that do survive have multicompartment massive injury.

REFERENCES

1. French BN, Dublin AB. The value of computerized tomography in 1000 consecutive head injuries. *Surg Neurol* 1977;7:171–183.
2. Snoek J, Jennett B, Adams JH, et al. Computerized tomography after recent severe head injury in patients without acute intracranial hematoma. *J Neurol Neurosurg Psychiatry* 1979;42:215–225.
3. Brant-Zawadzki M, Pitts LH. The role of CT in the evaluation of head trauma. In: Federle NP, Brant-Zawadzki M, eds. *Computed tomography in the evaluation of trauma.* Baltimore: Williams & Wilkins, 1982:1–59.
4. Zimmerman RD, Danziger A. Extracerebral trauma. *Radiol Clin North Am* 1982;20:105–121.
5. Hans JS, Kaufman B, Alfidi RJ, et al. Head trauma evaluated by magnetic resonance and computed tomography: a comparison. *Radiology* 1984;150:71–77.
6. Snow RB, Zimmerman RD, Gandy SE, et al. Comparison of magnetic resonance imaging and computed tomography in the evaluation of head trauma. *Neurosurgery* 1986;18:45–52.
7. Kelly AB, Zimmerman RD, Snow RB, et al. Head trauma: comparison of MRI and CT—experience in 100 patients. *AJNR* 1988;9:699–703.
8. Gentry LR, Godersky JC, Thompson B, Bunn VD. Prospective comparative study of intermediate field MR and CT in the evaluation of closed head injury. *AJNR* 1988;9:91–100.
9. Gentry LR, Godersky JC, Thompson B. MR imaging of head trauma: review of the distribution and radiopathologic features of traumatic lesions. *AJNR* 1988;9:101–110.
10. Gentry LR. Head trauma. In: Atlas SW, ed. *Magnetic resonance of the brain and spine.* Philadelphia: Lippincott–Raven Publishers, 1996:611–648.
11. Gentry LR. Imaging of closed head injury. *Radiology* 1994;191:1–17.
12. Jordan BD, Zimmerman RD. Computed tomography and magnetic resonance imaging: comparisons in boxers. *JAMA* 1990;263:1670–1674.
13. Brant-Zawadzki M, Minagi H. CT in the evaluation of spine trauma. In: Federle MP, Brant-Zawadzki M, eds. *Computed tomography in the evaluation of trauma.* Baltimore: Williams & Wilkins, 1982:106–152.
14. Gehweiler JAQ, Osborne RL, Becker RF. *The radiology of vertebral trauma.* Philadelphia: WB Saunders, 1980.
15. Borock EC, Gabram SG, Jacobs LM, Murphy MA. A prospective analysis of a two-year experience using computed tomography as an adjunct for cervical spine clearance. *J Trauma* 1991;31:1001–1005.
16. Nunez DB, Zuluaga A, Fuentes-Bernardo DA, Rivas LA, Becerra JL. Cervical spine trauma: how much do we learn by routinely using helical CT? *Radiographics* 1996;16:1307–1318.
17. Cornelius RS, Leach JL. Imaging evaluation of cervical spine. *Neuroimaging Clin North Am* 1995;5:451–463.
18. Davis SJ, Teresi LM, Bradley WG, Ziemba MA, Bloze AE. Cervical spine hyperextension injuries: MR findings. *Radiology* 1991;180:245–251.
19. Flanders AE, Croul SE. Spinal trauma. In: Atlas SW, ed. *Magnetic resonance of the brain and spine.* Philadelphia: Lippincott–Raven Publishers, 1996:1161–1206.
20. Moseley ME, Wendkand ME, Kucharczyk J. Magnetic resonance imaging of diffusion and perfusion. *Top Magn Reson Imaging* 1991;3:50–67.
21. Fisher M, Prichard JW, Warach S. New magnetic resonance techniques in acute ischemic stroke. *JAMA* 1995;274:908–911.
22. Smith DH, Meaney DF, Lenkinski RE, et al. New magnetic resonance imaging techniques for the evaluation of traumatic brain injury. *J Neurotrauma* 1995;12:573–577.
23. Roberts MA, Manshadi FF, Bushnell DL, Hines ME. Neurobehavioural dysfunction following mild traumatic brain injury in childhood: a case report with positive findings on positron emission tomography (PET). *Brain Inj* 1995;9:427–436.
24. Worley G, Hoffman JM, Paine SS, et al. 18-Fluorodeoxyglucose positron emission tomography in children and adolescents with traumatic brain injury. *Dev Med Child Neurol* 1995;37:213–220.
25. Prayer L, Wimberger D, Oder W, et al. Cranial MR imaging and cerebral ^{99m}Tc HM-PAO-SPECT in patients with subacute or chronic closed head injuries and normal CT examinations. *Acta Radiol* 1993;34:593–599.
26. Bavetta S, Nimmon CC, McCabe J, et al. A prospective study comparing SPECT with MRI and CT as prognostic indicators following severe closed head injury. *Nucl Med Commun* 1994;15:961–968.
27. Masdeu JC, Van Heertum RL, Kleiman A, et al. Early single-photon emission tomography im mild head trauma. A controlled study. *J Neuroimaging* 1994;4:177–181.
28. Walter H, Kristeva R, Knorr U, et al. Individual somatotopy of primary sensorimotor cortex revealed by internodal matching of MEG, PET, and MRI. *Brain Topogr* 1992;5:183–187.
29. Gallen CC, Sobel DF, Lewine JD, et al. Neuromagnetic mapping of brain function. *Radiology* 1993;187:863–867.
30. Casson IR, Sham R, Campbell EA, et al. Neurologic and CT evaluation of knock-out boxers. *J Neurol Neurosurg Psychiatry* 1982;45:170–174.
31. Holzgraefe M, Lemme W, Funke W, Felix R, Felten R. The significance of diagnostic imaging in acute and chronic brain damage in boxing. A prospective study in amateur boxing using magnetic resonance imaging (MRI). *Int J Sports Med* 1992;13:616–620.
32. Kanal E. Shellock FG. Patient monitoring during clinical MR imaging. *Radiology* 1992;185:623–629.
33. Mittl RL, Grossman RI, Hiehle JF, et al. Prevalence of MR evidence of diffuse axonal injury in patients with mild head injury and normal head CT findings. *AJNR* 1994; 15:1583–1589.
34. New PF, Arnow S. Attenuation measurements of whole blood and blood fractions in computed tomography. *Radiology* 1976;121:645–649.
35. Gomori JM, Grossman RI, Goldberg HI, et al. Intracranial hematomas: imaging by high field MR. *Radiology* 1985;157:87–93.
36. Zimmerman RD, Heier LA, Snow RB, et al. Acute intracranial hemorrhage: intensity changes on sequential MR scans at 0.5 T. *AJNR* 1988;9:47–57, and *AJR* 1988;150:651–661.
37. Hayman LA, Taber KH, Ford JJ, Bryan RN. Mechanisms of MR signal alternation by acute intracerebral blood: old concepts and new theories. *AJNR* 1991;12:899–907.

38. Noguchi K, Ogawa T, Inugami A, et al. Acute subarachnoid hemorrhage: MR imaging with fluid-attenuated inversion recovery pulse sequences. *Radiology* 1995; 196:773–777.

39. Lindberg R. Pathology of cranio-cerebral injuries. In: Newton TH, Potts DE, eds. *Radiology of skull and brain.* St Louis: Mosby, 1977;3:3049–3087.

40. Zimmerman RA, Bilaniuk LT, Gennerelli T. Computed tomography of shearing injuries of the cerebral white matter. *Radiology* 1978;127:393–396.

41. Unterharnscheidt F. About boxing: review of historical and medical aspects. *Tex Rep Biol Med* 1970;28: 421–495.

42. Jordan BD, Jahre C, Hauser WA, et al. CT of 388 active professional boxers. *Radiology* 1992;185:509–512.

43. Batzdorf U, Benson JR, Maclederhi JH. Blunt trauma of the high cervical carotid artery. *Neurosurgery* 1979; 5:195–201.

44. Goldberg HI, Grossman RI, Gomori JM, Asbury AK, Bilaniuk LT, Zimmerman RA. Cervical internal carotid artery dissecting hemorrhage: diagnosis using MR. *Radiology* 1986;158:157–161.

45. Torg JS, Sennett B, Pavlov H, Leventhal MR, Glasgow SG. Spear tackler's spine. An entity precluding participation in tackle football and collision activities that expose the cervical spine to axial energy inputs. *Am J Sports Med* 1993;21:640–649.

46. Tall RL, De Vault W. Spinal injury in sport: epidemiologic considerations. *Clin Sports Med* 1993;12:441–448.

47. Bishop PJ. Factors related to quadriplegia in football and the implications for intervention strategies. *Am J Sports Med* 1996;24:235–239.

48. Haughton VM, Williams AL. *Computed tomography of the spine.* St. Louis: Mosby, 1982.

49. Czervionke LF, Haughton VM. Degenerative disease of the spine. In: Atlas SW, ed. *Magnetic resonance of the brain and spine.* Philadelphia: Lippincott–Raven Publishers, 1996;1093–1160.

50. Morrison RG. Medical and public health aspects of boxing. *JAMA* 1986;255:2475–2480.

51. Sironi VA, Scotti G, Ravgnati L, et al. Scans and EEG findings in professional pugilists: early detection of cerebral atrophy in young boxers. *J Neurosurg Sci* 1982;26:165–168.

52. Ross RJ, Cole M, Thompson JS, et al. Boxers: computed tomography, EEG, and neurosurgical evaluation. *JAMA* 1983;249:211–213.

53. McLatchie G, Brooks N, Galbraith S, et al. Clincal neurological examination, neuropsychology, electroencephalography, and computed tomographic head scanning in active boxers. *J Neurol Neurosurg Psychiatry* 1987; 50:96–99.

54. Kelly JP, Nichols JS, Fillet CM, Lillehei KO, Rubinstein D, Kleinschmidt-DeMasters K. Concussion in sports: guidelines for the prevention of catastrophic outcome. *JAMA* 1991;266:2867–2899.

55. Jordan BD, Campbell EA. Acute injuries among professional boxers in New York State: a two year survey. *Physician Sports Med* 1988;16:87–91.

56. Jordon BD. Neurologic aspects of boxing. *Arch Neurol* 1987;44:453–459.

57. Lampert PW, Hardman JM. Morphologic changes in the brains of boxers. *JAMA* 1984;251:2676–2679.

58. Jordan BD, Jahre C, Hauser WA, Zimmerman RD, Peterson M. Serial computed tomography in professional boxers. *J Neuroimaging* 1992;2:181–185.

59. Wilberger JE. Minor head injuries in American football. Prevention of long term sequelae. *Sports Med* 1993;15: 338–343.

60. Reynen PD, Cancy WG. Cervical spine injury, helmets, and face masks. *Am J Sports Med* 1994;22:167–170.

61. Jordan SE, Green GA, Galanty HL, Mandelbaum BR, Jabour BA. Acute and chronic brain injury in United States National Team soccer players. *Am J Sports Med* 1996;24:205–210.

62. Hamilton MG, Trammer BI. Nervous system injuries in horseback-riding accidents. *J Trauma* 1993;34:227–232.

63. Frank E, Frankel P, Mullins RJ, Taylor N. Injuries resulting from bicycle collisions. *Acad Emerg Med* 1995;2:200–203.

64. Mellion MB. Common cycling injuries. Management and prevention. *Sports Med* 1991;11:52–70.

65. Calle SC, Eaton RG. Wheels-in-line skating injuries. *J Trauma* 1993;35:946–951.

66. Schieber RA, Branche-Dorsey CM, Ryann GW. Comparison of in-line skating injuries with rollerskating and skateboard injuries: *JAMA* 1994;271:1856–1858.

67. Vanderford L, Meyers M. Injuries and bungee jumping. *Sports Med* 1995;20:369–374.

Sports Neurology, Second Edition,
edited by Barry D. Jordan.
Lippincott–Raven Publishers, Philadelphia © 1998.

8

Neurologic Problems in the Special Olympics

Richard D. Birrer

Catholic Medical Center of Brooklyn and Queens, Inc.,
88-25 153rd Street, Jamaica, New York 11432

Let me win,
but if I cannot win,
let me be brave in the attempt.

Special Olympics Motto

BACKGROUND

Founded in 1968 as a summer day camp, held at the home of Eunice and Sargent Shriver, the Special Olympics opened the door to competitive sports for persons with disabilities. Since then, the program has expanded to all 50 states and 140 countries. Approximately 1 million athletes compete worldwide, and the program is a member of the International Olympic Committee and U.S. Olympic Committee on sports for the disabled (1). There are 22 Olympic-style organized sport programs, divided into winter and summer, individual and team events (Table 1). All official sports follow internationally accepted sports rules that are adapted to the needs of athletes. Grouping of athletes is by ability and age in order to equalize competition. Training, fitness, and sport skill development are part of the program, although they are emphasized to different degrees at the local level. For motivated athletes, "graduation" from Special Olympics to regular sports programs (i.e., Special Olympics Unified Sports) may be the ultimate goal.

ELIGIBILITY AND SELECTION

Although the local, regional, and national organizations have some flexibility for determining who may compete, the standard participation criteria are (a) age 8 and older and (b) intellectual functioning significantly below average (e.g., mental handicap), cognitive delay, or significant learning or vocational problem (2, sect L, pp 7–8).

Participation in Special Olympics events requires a preparticipation physical examination. The examination can be performed individually or by the station method using a sports health team. The former is more cost effective. In one study, 70% to 75% of sports-significant abnormalities were reported by questionnaire (3). Whereas 1% to 3% of nondisabled, nonretarded athletes had sports-significant abnormalities on screening history and physical examination, the incidence approached 40% in the Special Olympics population. Neurologic (16%) and ophthalmologic (15%) problems made up over 75% of the abnormalities, with musculoskeletal (6%) and medical (5%) constituting the remaining (3). A history of seizures constituted 75% to 80% of the neurologic problems and was the most common diagnosis. The remaining neurologic conditions included spina bifida, cerebral palsy, hemiparesis, aphasia, and autism. The predominant eye abnormality was the presence of monocular vision (60%), although cataracts, myopia, blindness, and amblyopia commonly occurred. Musculoskeletal problems include amputation, previous orthopedic procedure (e.g., fusion, plates, screws, rods), arthritis, and subluxation or dislocation, particularly of the cervical spine (i.e., Down syndrome). Arrhythmias, congenital heart abnormalities, undescended testis, skin infection, deafness, and endocrinopathies were common medical abnormalities.

TABLE 1. *Summer and Winter Special Olympics sports*

Alpine skiing	Aquatic athletics
Badminton	Basketball
Bocce	Bowling
Cross-country skiing	Cycling
Ice hockey	Equestrian
Floor hockey	Football (soccer)
Figure skating	Golf
Gymnastics	Power lifting
Roller skating	Sailing
Softball	Speed skating
Snowshoeing	Table tennis
Team handball	Tennis
Volleyball	

An area of particular concern is the cervical spine in the athlete with Down syndrome. Certain sports are often medically contraindicated for such individuals because of the suspected risk of spinal trauma associated with atlantoaxial instability. The instability is present in 13% (10% to 40%) of children with Down syndrome (2,4–6). The instability can be assessed accurately only by radiography and not by clinical criteria including general laxity assessment (7). Therefore, the practice standard has been the requirement of not only a medical examination but also lateral cervical spine radiographs in flexion and extension for all individuals with Down syndrome intending to compete in the Special Olympic Games (2,8–10). Repeated x-ray studies may or may not be recommended for individuals with normal findings if done at an early age. Follow-up is necessary for asymptomatic individuals with increased distance. Where indicated, operative stabilization is recommended.

The normal atlantoaxial distance (anterior surface of the odontoid process to the posterior aspect of the anterior atlas arch) is 2.5 mm or less in adults and 5 mm or less in children. It should be noted that many other cervical spine anomalies are identified, some more common than an increased atlanto-dens interval (e.g., occiput–C-1 instability, odontoid dysplasia, precocious arthritis, C-1 hypoplasia, spondylolysis, and spondylolisthesis). Approximately 85% of those with Down syndrome have no radiographic evidence of instability (11), 13% to 14% show radiographic evidence of instability but are asymptomatic, and 1% to 2% have symptoms that may require treatment. Symptoms include weakness, neck tilt, neck pain, gait disturbance, hypertonicity or sensory abnormalities in the upper or lower extremities, or loss of bowel or bladder control.

Because the natural history of cervical spine instability is unknown and controlled long-term longitudinal studies are lacking, guidelines have been subjected to closer scrutiny. Most observers agree that the majority of individuals with cervical spine instability remain entirely asymptomatic (12,13). Work involving 400 children and young adults with Down syndrome (6) suggested that there is no clinical reason to bar these individuals from playing certain sports and no need to screen them by radiography for participation clearance. A computed tomographic scan or magnetic resonance image should be obtained for more definite assessment if there are clinical and radiographic signs of cord compression.

INJURY PROFILE

There have been only two published studies on injuries sustained by contestants in the Special Olympics (14,15). Of the injuries, 45% to 60% were musculoskeletal (e.g., sprains, strains, contusions, abrasions) and 40% to 50% were medical. No neurologic injuries were noted, although there were two (1%) seizures in the study by Wekesa and Onsongo (14). The latter occurred several hours after the sport activity and did not affect further training or participation. There were 11 (5%) headaches, but none prevented continued participation or training.

RECOMMENDATIONS (2,8)

1. Seizure precautions in all sports and recreational activities in which there might be a risk of severe injury if a convulsion were to occur: swimming, diving, gymnastics (apparatus use), skiing, speed skating, and equestrian events.

2. Eye protection (polycarbonate lenses) in missile-type sports for monocular athletes. Eye protection is recommended for Alpine and cross-country skiing, floor and poly hockey, softball, basketball, soccer, and volleyball.

3. Restriction of Down syndrome athletes with cervical subluxation from Special Olympic training or competition in certain sports: diving, gymnastics, pentathlon, squat lift in power lifting, high jump, soccer, Alpine skiing, swimming utilizing flip turns, butterfly stroke, diving starts, or any competitive event or warm-up exercise that places undue stress on the head and neck.[1]

4. Until the Department of Health and Human Services (DHHS) and the Special Olympic guidelines are modified, radiographic clearance of the cervical spine is necessary for all Down syndrome athletes participating in high-risk recreational or sports activities.

CONCLUSION

The Special Olympics program is highly beneficial, particularly in terms of social adjustment and life satisfaction (15). This risk for neurologic injury is probably negligible for athletes participating in the Special Olympic Games. Although all health care practitioners need to be aware of the current screening guidelines for the Down syndrome athlete, more recent research suggests that participation of such individuals can be optimized without radiographic assessment of the cervical spine.

Every effort should be made to maximize the involvement of handicapped athletes in sports and recreational activities. For the handicapped, given satisfactory physical health, it is probably a greater source of happiness and pride than for the able-bodied.

---

[1]The restriction can be waived by an acknowledgment of risks signed by the adult athlete or his or her parent or guardian if the athlete is a minor *and* written certifications from two physicians excluding the examining physician of record.

REFERENCES

1. Songster T. The Special Olympics sports program: an international sport program for mentally retarded athletes. In: Sherrill C, ed. *Sport and disabled athletes.* Champaign, IL: Human Kinetics, 1984:73–79.
2. *Official Special Olympics summer sports rules 1992–1995,* rev ed, Washington, DC: Special Olympics International, 1992.
3. McCormick DP, Ivey FM, Gold DM, et al. The preparticipation sports examination in Special Olympics athlete. *Tex Med* 1988;84(4):39–43.
4. Davidson RG. Atlantoaxial instability in individuals with Down syndrome: a fresh look at the evidence. *Pediatrics* 1988;81:857–865.
5. Cope R, Olson S. Abnormalities of the cervical spine in Down syndrome: diagnosis, risks, and review of the literature with particular reference to the Special Olympics. *South Med J* 1987;80(1):33–36.
6. Cremers MJG, Bol E, de Roos F, et al. Risk of sports activities in children with Down syndrome and atlantoaxial instability. *Lancet* 1993;342:511–514.
7. Cremers MJG, Beyer JHM. No relation between general laxity and atlantoaxial instability in children with Down syndrome. *J Pediatr Orthop* 1993;13:318–321.
8. *Official Special Olympics winter sports rules 1994–1998.* Washington, DC: Special Olympics International, 1994.
9. Committee on Sports Medicine: Atlantoaxial instability in Down syndrome. *Pediatrics* 1984;74:152–154.
10. *Guidelines for cervical spine screening in Down syndrome.* Standing Medical Advisory Committee, Department of Health and Human Services, 1986.
11. Alvarez N, Rubin L. Atlantoaxial instability in adults with Down syndrome: a clinical and radiological survey. *Appl Res Ment Retard* 1986;7:67–78.
12. Pueschel SM, Scola FH. Atlantoaxial instability in individuals with Down syndrome: epidemiologic, radiographic, and clinical studies. *Pediatrics* 1987;80:555–560.
13. Goldberg MJ. Spine instability and the Special Olympics. *Clin Sports Med* 1993;12:507–515.
14. Wekesa M, Onsongo J. Kenyan team care at the Special Olympics—1991. *Br J Sports Med* 1992;26:128–133.
15. Birrer RB. The special Olympics: an injury overview. *Physician Sports Med* 1984;12(4):95–97.
16. Klein T, Gilman E, Zigler E. Special Olympics: an evaluation by professionals and parents. *Ment Retard* 1993;31(1):15–23.

Sports Neurology, Second Edition,
edited by Barry D. Jordan.
Lippincott–Raven Publishers, Philadelphia © 1998.

9

Paralympics and the Physically Disabled Athlete

Arnold M. Illman

4180 Sunrise Highway, Massapequa, New York 11758

The purpose of this chapter is to present an overview of athletics for the physically disabled. This serves as an introduction to familiarize the reader with the differences and similarities of sport between this group of athletes and their able-bodied counterparts. It attempts to give an overview of the problems encountered, the gains made, and the goals that should be attained over the immediate future.

Athletes who are physically disabled compete in many of the same sports as their able-bodied counterparts, but because of their handicaps, they must often utilize modified implements. Subdivision of the athletes is a prime concern so that competition among them is fair. For the physician who becomes involved in this form of athleticism, merely clearing an individual for sports by performing a physical examination is not sufficient. The physician must understand not only the kinesiology of the sport concerned but also the problems specific to each type of disability. The doctor must be able to understand each athlete's potential in order to allow people with dissimilar disabilities to compete against one another in both modified and unmodified sporting events.

In order to appreciate the complexity of this sports movement, it is important to understand how it came into being, to what degree it has evolved, and into what it might eventually develop.

In the 1940s, Dr. Guttman, a German physician who relocated during World War II from Germany to England, felt that many people who had sustained spinal cord injuries were not achieving their full potential with conventional rehabilitative methods. He felt that both the mind and the body would be better served if sports could to be utilized in therapy. The patients and hospital staff at Stoke Manderville in England were quite enthusiastic over this idea, and thus sports for the physically handicapped were born.

At first the games, although competitive, were essentially therapeutic in value. As time passed and the potential of these people was better appreciated, competition became more intense. Teams were formed and competitions between countries, rudimentary at first, were developed. Standards had to be developed in order to make these games meaningful. Athletes from different countries got to know one another, so the competitions had a strong social overtone. Physicians essentially controlled the sports in those days. Strict limitations were invoked in order to protect the athletes from being injured. The athletes started to train for these competitions and sent out a message that the old restrictions, laid down by the physicians, prevented them from competing at as high a level as they thought they could.

At about this time, because of the large number of countries involved and the intense interest that was developing in these games, specific disabilities became divided into specific organizations: for example, the Cerebral Palsy Organization; the International Sports Organization for the Disabled (ISOD), which included all amputees; and Les Autres (people with disabilities that do not necessarily fall into specific categories).

ISOD promotes sports development for all amputees and other athletes who have locomotor disabilities that are not attributed to people with cerebral palsy, spinal cord injuries, or amputations (e.g., those with dwarfism, multiple sclerosis, or severe scoliosis). Each of these international organizations became expert in the development of sports for those with the disability it represented. They organized their own competitions, local, regional, national, and international. They helped the potential athletes with specific disabilities to become better trained. They fostered the development of specific equipment for specific injuries, e.g., special prosthesis for running, sleds for ice hockey, etc.

It became apparent that within each disability, there were significant differences in physical potential (e.g., there were below-knee amputees and above-knee amputees). As a result, a classification system became necessary to allow athletes with the same types of disabilities to compete with one another in an equitable manner. Physical examinations were performed on the athletes in order to determine their level of disability. Athletes with similar amounts of disability were placed in the same classes. Each class was a separate entity as far as each sporting event was concerned. These classes were developed by a group of physicians and technical sports experts.

As the years passed and training and the level of competition exceeded even the most optimistic projections of the earlier proponents of this sports movement, it became more apparent that experts in kinesiology were needed. Experimentation was carried out to develop wheelchairs that were light and had less wind resistance and less friction, in order to help the sport keep up with the intense fervor of the athletes. Every 4 years, conferences were held to pool information and incorporate changes in classification.

World games and paralympic competition became more popular. These competitions were set up as international games with those with each disability competing individually, often at the same venue as those with other disabilities. All sports were represented. During these games it became obvious that there was redundancy in the competitions and that individuals with different disabilities might be able to compete with one another in the same class if an adequate classification system could be developed. Athletes with different disabilities could ultimately be integrated as long as their potential level of competition was known. Some athletes and countries felt that there would be unfairness because of the seemingly impossible task of joining these people together in competition. However, after a few years it became clear that this mode of competition could be fair.

Data from scientific studies were collected and the more sophisticated knowledge that was obtained from these studies resulted in frequent changes in classification rules. Athletes and officials then felt that because the sports were so different, the sport should have a greater role than the disability in the development of this movement. At this point, experts in each sport, including technical experts, kinesiology experts, and physicians, formed their own international sports organizations in order to keep in step with the added training and enthusiasm of the athletes. The individual sports, with the help of the international disability organizations, further refined their rules. Subsequently, it was felt that anatomic classifications of the athletes' disabilities was not sufficient and that a method of functional evaluation for athletes in particular sports was needed. Athletes were first examined to determine their anatomic level of disability and then watched while they were put through certain functional tests closely related to the sport in which they were to compete.

Although this method appears to be fair and realistic, it has significant drawbacks. Some athletes tend to "hold back" when they are being tested functionally, either because they do not wish to burn themselves out before an event or possibly to be placed in a less competitive group in order to win. In addition, sometimes a highly trained athlete is placed in a higher class than he or she probably belongs in, so a person with severe disability who trains hard and is essentially an overachiever may be placed in a more difficult class. Thus, it becomes apparent that this method of functional classification requires mature classifiers in order to make the system work. This cuts down the number of classifiers who could be utilized and also implies that the methodology might be too subjective.

The International Paralympic Committee (IPC) was formed to parallel the International Olympic Committee (IOC) in able-bodied sports. This organization is made up of individual national paralympic committees and international sports federations. It supervises the multidisability games known as paralympic competitions and world competitions that occur every 4 years.

The philosophy of the IPC is to organize games in which the highest caliber athletes in each sport, from every country, can compete at a level that most closely emulates the level of able-bodied athletes. These sporting competitions have shown how versatile people with physical disabilities can be. Competition is as intense as in able-bodied events. Most countries have realized the positive public relation advantages of this type of event and have become quite active in sponsoring these athletes.

For the purposes of IPC competitions, all athletes are physically examined by classifying teams made up of physicians, physical therapists, and officials. Each sport has developed an outline of classes into which each athlete is placed. This outline has been developed and modified over many years. In some sports, the athlete is then observed in simulated competition in order to confirm or change the class in which he or she would be placed to make for a more meaningful competition. The overall classification system is adapted from each international federation for the disabled sports and modified in order to allow competition among people with different disabilities.

Because of the intensity of these competitions, overzealous athletes are occasionally misled and found to be guilty of substance abuse. As a result, drug testing has become mandatory. The IPC utilizes the same standards in methodology for drug testing as the IOC. The sanctions that are administered to these athletes and countries are the same as in able-bodied sports.

Another difficulty with this method of classification is the determination of minimal disability or the criteria used to determine whether a person is disabled in order to compete. The true disabled athlete must be protected from individuals who have a problem that, although it might prevent them from competing as able-bodied Olympians (e.g., a rotator cuff or arthritis of the knee), nonetheless is not allowed in these games.

Thus, games for the physically handicapped have evolved from a rehabilitation exercise program in the mid-1940s to sophisticated competitions that differ from sports for the able-bodied in allowing people with dissimilar physical problems to compete against one another. The methodology of classification has changed considerably since its inception and is still imperfect. Without classification, athletic events among the disabled could not exist. This is considerably different from the situation in able-bodied sports, in which no such differentiation is made. Recently, there has been greater interest in the types of orthotics and prostheses that are used in disabled sports, for with the evolution of more advanced prostheses, medals can be won. Unfortunately, at this point some of the third world countries do not have the financial support to utilize these devices in order to have their athletes compete at their highest potential.

TYPES OF EVENTS

Usually, the supporting events are adapted for the disabled while utilizing the basic rules for able-bodied sports. What follows is a listing of the more common sporting events utilized in the disabled movement with a small description of the major adaptations that have been designed for disabled athletes over the years.

Wheelchair Tennis

The athletes have a mobility-related disability. The ball is usually taken on the second bounce; the second bounce can be out of the court. The athlete must remain in the wheelchair at all times. This requires stamina, unusual adaptation for the use of the wheelchair as far as mobility is concerned, and coordination on the part of the athlete.

Volleyball

There are two types of volleyball competition.

Standing Volleyball

Essentially, rules for the able-bodied are followed. Most athletes are amputees and each athlete is given a point value from 1 to 8, 1 being the least disabled and 8 being the most disabled. A team is limited to a set number of points on the court at one time. Therefore, coaching strategy is important. The game is played on a wooden floor with a normal net height.

Sitting Volleyball

The net is lowered and the buttocks must touch the court during play. Because of the nature of the game, occasionally both shoulders and back, rather than buttocks, may make contact with the court. The game requires an unusual amount of athleticism because of balance problems and the speed of ball movement. Many able-bodied athletes have attempted to play this game and have failed because of awkwardness and inability to adapt to the sitting position during play.

Nordic and Alpine Sports

Skis have been modified to allow greater participation. Stabilizers have been added to monoskis. Often, spinal cord–injured individuals ski down in a sledge-like apparatus. Amputees usually require one ski, occasionally with stabilizers on the poles. There are limitations to the modifications allowed that are based on the degree of disability. Blind skiers go down with a partner holding a guideline between them. Speeds reaching 45 miles per hour are not the exception in the downhill skiing competition.

Speed Racing

Speed racing is usually carried out on sledges. The athletes use two sticks to propel themselves forward; there is no steering device on the unit.

Ice Sledge Hockey (Fig. 1)

The usual rules of ice hockey are followed but the game is played with athletes in sledges. The hockey stick is short and has small teeth for traction on the ice in order to propel the sledge. Sledge hockey team is based on a point system similar to that utilized in standing volleyball. Slightly modified hockey pads and helmets are worn.

Archery

The degree and type of disability determine whether the athlete competes from the standing or sitting position, the length (and thus power) of the bow, and the distance of the target. Individuals with poor spinal balance may use straps to prevent forward movement in the wheelchair during release of the bow.

Field Events, Including High Jump, Long Jump, Javelin, and Discus (Figs. 2 and 3)

People are placed in classes that are determined by their ability to stand or sit. All amputees, except for those with bilateral above-knee amputations, are required to throw from a standing position. This requires tremendous strength and balance on the part of the athlete in order to discharge the implement in throwing events. Close observation of the functional classification of spinal cord–injured individuals is extremely important because of the large numbers of athletes with mixed spinal cord lesions and the importance of trunk balance in the ability of the athlete to compete. Racing groups are determined by level of spinal cord lesion when athletes use a wheelchair as an implement to race. Recently, amputees have been joined with some ambulatory individuals with cerebral palsy and spinal lesions. Wheelchairs are adapted for racing (Fig. 4). They are made of lightweight material with good aerodynamic features. Blind athletes run tethered to a companion by a lead line. Some athletes run in the direction of sound. The length of races varies from 100 m to a full marathon.

Cycling

Blind individuals, amputees, and athletes with cerebral palsy can compete in this sport. Adaptations

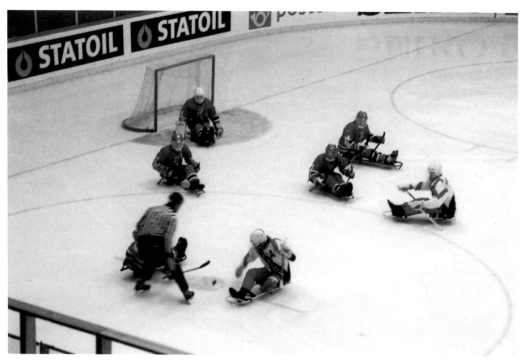

FIG. 1. Sledge hockey, Lillehammer, 1994.

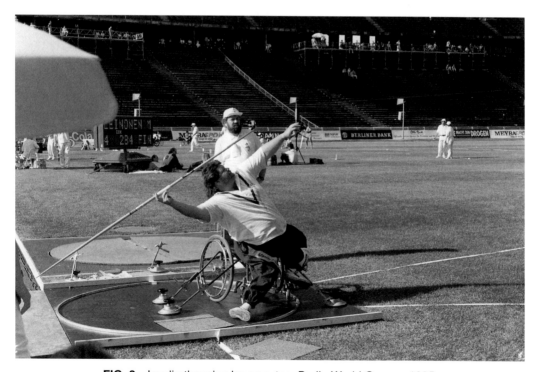

FIG. 2. Javelin throwing by amputee, Berlin World Games, 1995.

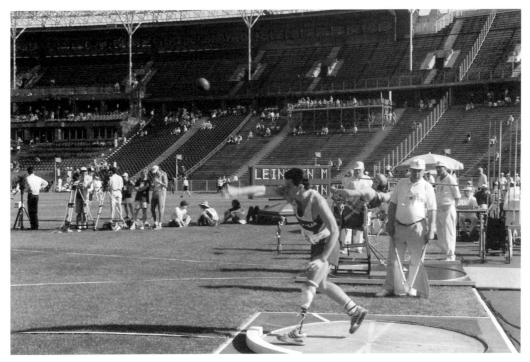

FIG. 3. Amputee, Berlin World Games, 1995.

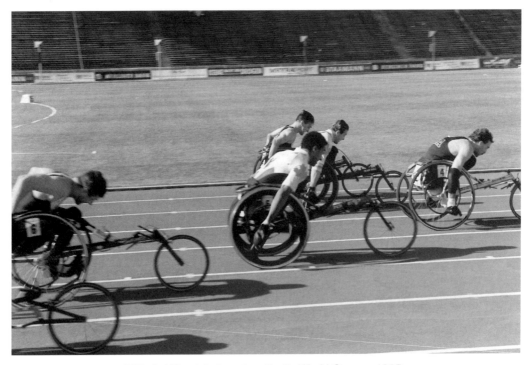

FIG. 4. Wheelchair racing, Berlin World Games, 1995.

for the steering device and pedals can be used. Races vary from 1500 to 20,000 m.

Equestrian

All disability groups participate in dressage competition. Adaptations of the saddle are used to keep the athlete in control and upright.

Long Bowling

Long bowling is usually performed from the wheelchair or standing position; normal rules are followed.

Power Lifting

This is an open competition. The only qualification that must be met is that of the minimal disability described by various disability groups. Only the bench press is contested. Amputees have a formula by which weight is added to their bodies to compensate for the loss of weight caused by amputation. The only significant variation from that of able-bodied bench press competitions is that both legs must be on the bench and no greater than a 20° flexion contracture of the elbow is allowed.

Shooting

In principle, this is similar to archery.

Swimming

All of the disabilities compete with one another. Classification is determined by a combination of anatomic and functional evaluations. No flotation devices are allowed.

Table Tennis

All types of motor disabilities compete; regular table tennis rules are utilized with minimal modifications.

Amputee Soccer

Amputee soccer is played mostly in the South American and Eastern European countries. Regular soccer rules are utilized. Amputees may not use a prosthesis but can use one crutch. The crutch can be used as a leg in moving the ball.

Wheelchair Basketball

Play is on a point system depending on the degree of functional disability of the athletes. The movement of the ball down the court is the same as in able-bodied basketball; double dribbling is not allowed. The athlete must compete from the wheelchair.

Other Events

In addition to the preceding sports, other, somewhat less popular sports that are played are water polo, sailboat racing, fencing, badminton, snooker, and bocce.

It is quite apparent that sports for the disabled, in modified form, parallel all sporting events for the able-bodied. Today, paraplegics are even doing scuba diving, and golf among blind and wheelchair-bound athlete has been gaining in popularity on a local basis. Some amputees and blind athletes have competed with the able-bodied in wrestling. Amputee groups are requesting the inclusion of boxing as a demonstration sport. In today's world, there is essentially no barrier to any individual competing in most accepted sports.

SPORTS INJURIES PECULIAR TO DISABLED ATHLETES

Almost every injury that can occur in the able-bodied athlete can occur in the disabled groups. Some of these injuries, however, have a greater impact on the disabled individual because loss of function in these athletes, theoretically, can result in permanent loss of independence. However, this situation is quite rare. Often, disabled athletes have limited access to top-level coaches and trainers in their local area. Disabled athletes may not be as mobile in getting to their instructers as their able-bodied counterparts, and the funding to do so is often limited.

Many coaches who work with able-bodied athletes have limited understanding of the problems facing disabled athletes while training. As a result, poor training techniques are often developed. Weight training can be used incorrectly, resulting in body abuse. Stretching is often neglected. Distance often isolates the disabled athlete from others with the same problems, so communication and exchange of ideas often do not take place except during competitions. Many of these athletes have become acclimated to a certain level of discomfort and consequently tend not to heed their bodies' warning signs.

Regional training sessions have been developing in each country in order to help the athletes come closer to their potential. It is important to note that personality factors strongly influence these athletes. Often, after a severe accident or when an individual is born with physical problems, rehabilitation is mandatory. Less than 1% of these people become so motivated during their rehabilitation that they exceed their expectations and achieve what is to their friends an unbelievable level of physical independence. Some of these athletes tend to overuse their bodies and to develop tunnel vision to the extent of ignoring everything else in order to overcome their problems. This group of individuals often become top athletes, but they tend to overtrain and become injured. Their psychologic outlook is so demanding that they often do not consider themselves disabled and feel that their results in competition should come close to those of able-bodied Olympians. This positive thinking is important for the athletes, but they sometimes devote their lives to perfecting their bodies in sport to the exclusion of everything else.

The shoulder is the most commonly injured joint in these athletes. Wheelchair athletes use their shoulders to propel themselves and lift themselves in and out of chairs. In order to do this, at the earliest phase of their rehabilitation, weight training becomes necessary. Some of these individuals go on to power lifting or become field event specialists. For some individuals, the training and competition become counterproductive, because overuse of the shoulders causes injury to their rotator cuffs, which sometimes cannot be repaired. These athletes are in a constant training mode because of the specific requirements of normal daily activities. As

the athlete ages, circulation to the rotator cuff decreases, so repair to control ensuing shoulder pain, rotator-cuff tears, and so forth is not always efficacious. Often, athletes are not well informed and essentially self-destruct and lose their independence in activities of normal living. Their credo of mind over matter that brought them to the point of being athletes can cause significant damage if their trainers and coaches are not cognizant of these problems. Extremely close supervision is required to control the athlete's training program.

Amputees have different problems because of their stumps. Skin breakdown can occur, especially in people engaged in field and track events. Sometimes this is due to poor fitting of the prosthesis and sometimes to overuse in training for an athletic event. Amputees are quite susceptible to neck and back disorders. Arm amputees use shoulders to control their prosthesis, and often their balance is disturbed when they are involved in moving sports. Neck spasm with radiation occurs, and this can be difficult to resolve if an individual has to compete in more than one event during one competition. Also, herniation of lumbar discs occurs, especially among above-knee amputees who must hyperextend their back in order to ambulate and control their prosthesis. This becomes a difficult problem to treat in the running athletes.

Many of these athletes do not accept treatment readily because they may need to use crutches to allow their stumps to heal properly. The amputees, having worked so hard to become ambulatory, tend not to want to "regress," so they often compete less efficiently with stump problems. Stump problems in athletes become more severe than in the normal amputee population and can lead to secondary body strain. Stress fractures through the stump have been noted. Athletes often apply local anesthetic material to the stump in order to run the race, and this compounds their problems when the race is over. Prosthetic breakdown occurs during workout and races, which leads to extra strain on the athlete's stump. Amputees are always problematic. Sometimes surgical procedures are carried out in order to remove neuromas. Prostheses have to be modified in the running athlete in order to give relief to areas where neuromas are suspected. Sometimes, because of the nature of the phantom pain, it is difficult to discern between that and radiculitis resulting from herniated discs.

Another problem that decreases the top performances of good athletes is the fact that some amputees may be receiving chemotherapy for cancer. Their stamina is diminished because of changes in their blood composition and the toxicity of the chemotherapeutic materials, and this can lead to secondary injuries. In addition, the possibility of metastatic spread, although unknown at the time of competition and training, is real. These people are required to have frequent general medical evaluations.

Athletes with cerebral palsy are susceptible to seizure disorders. Occasionally, a poorly regulated athlete, can have a seizure during training and/or competition, leading to falls and secondary injuries.

Occasionally, a seizure occurs during a movement in sport and an athlete falls. Fractures, however, are rare. Concussions are even rarer, but sometimes a diagnostic problem arises and one tries to discern between a poorly communicative individual with cerebral palsy and a person who has sustained brain trauma. Motion fractures and muscle tears may result from the trauma of running. If simple muscle massage does not alleviate the situation, the physician must be attuned to the fact that more significant problems exist. Diagnostic testing is indicated. Discomfort from muscle spasm, which is present in the able-bodied athlete, can be intensified in the individual with cerebral palsy because of contraction of the joints and extensor spasm of the lower back. Again, the problem of discerning between radiculitis and intensified spasm of the back in the running athlete must be solved.

Because of their spasticity, which is evident, much time and an increased number of personnel are required to maintain athletes of this type. The high level of athleticism required usually results in exclusion of the individuals with athetoid cerebral palsy. If a significant component of this is present, balance problems may lead to injuries.

Athletes must be monitored closely because of their abnormal lower lumbar bone configuration, as pedicle malformation can lead to severe spinal stenosis. Athletes who are involved in field events and power lifting must be queried constantly about whether they have leg symptoms in order to rule out the possibility of herniation of discs or herniation of lumbar discs.

Spinal cord–disabled athletes must be carefully monitored for fluid loss because of their change of autonomic nervous system function. Fluid loss in competition must be especially controlled in this group of athletes. Also, they are susceptible to hyperthermia related to their inability to lose heat from self-absorption.

Fracture through a paralyzed limb can occur as a result of falls, because this area is anesthetic. Often simple splinting may be all that is indicated, although it is not encouraged. Occasionally, athletes hide the fact that they have fractures and continue to compete and train. Clonus is regularly encountered, but static positioning of the limb is all that is needed and this does not usually lead to any injuries.

Loss of sensation can result in skin breakdown. Because the patient does not perceive discomfort, the first symptom of skin breakdown can be sepsis. Therefore, skin care is mandatory, especially among spinal cord–injured athletes who twist in chairs, resulting in friction trauma to the skin and skin breakdown. Athletes tend to hide this problem; therefore the coach and responsible officials must inspect these athletes for decubitus that may be hidden from view.

BIBLIOGRAPHY

Cerebral Palsy—International Sports and Recreation Association (CP-ISRA). *Classification and sports rules manual,* 6th ed. Edwalton Nottingham, UK: CP-ISRA, 1993.
International Paralympic Committee handbook. Brugge, Belgium: IPC, 1994.
International Sports Organization of the Disabled handbook. Toronto: ISOD, 1994.
International Stoke-Mandival Wheelchair Sports Federation official rules. Aylesbury Bucks, England: Guttmann Sports Center, 1992.

Sports Neurology, Second Edition,
edited by Barry D. Jordan.
Lippincott–Raven Publishers, Philadelphia © 1998.

10

Rehabilitation of the Neurologically Impaired Athlete

Yasoma B. Challenor

Department of Physical Medicine and Rehabilitation, Columbia University College of Physicians and Surgeons, New York, New York 10032

For the able-bodied person it is difficult to separate the effects of physical exercise and training from those related to the experience of recreation in normal growth and development. Early in childhood, the physically able child learns the concepts of individual and team sports and exercise activities, of winning and losing, and of competition. Recreation may or may not involve exercise accompanying the experience of these activities.

With the onset of central nervous system lesions or peripheral nerve injury, however, the common misconception may be that recreation must become a non–exercise-related, sedentary activity. In American society, participation in individual and team sports or the continuation of sports participation enhances a person's perception of self-worth as well as respect for the abilities of others; these aspects are still available to the handicapped person. The social interaction and enjoyment of training and participation in team and individual sports need not be lost for the person with a nervous system injury. The need is to establish a reasonable match between the performance allowed by the disabling condition and the residual physical ability, with preparation for and selection of safe sports activities.

Sports profiling is one way to address this need. Sports profiling involves gathering information about the physiologic, neuromuscular, psychologic, and sports-preference status of an individual to match the individual to the attributes necessary for participation in sports activities. A typical profile includes measurements of neuromuscular coordination, sensory integration, muscle strength, joint flexibility, and cardiorespiratory status. These are then matched with the performance characteristics required for a given sport as well as with the level of sports performance (strenuous contact sports or strenuous noncontact sports with low levels of exertion) (1).

Sports profiling for the neurologically impaired athlete should be viewed as a guide and not as a limitation. Quite often we marvel at the compensations and adaptations that individual athletes have discovered for themselves. Our role in rehabilitating the neurologically impaired athlete is to facilitate this process of adaptation to sports or to use the profiling to aid in the selection of a sport for an athlete who requires redirection to a different sport outlet or to an altered exertional level.

Warming up is as necessary a process for the impaired athlete as for any other athlete. The prescribed warm-up activities are not only sport specific but also tailored to the nature of the injury and the requirements of the disability (2,3). For example, an athlete with some degree of spasticity would work on extremely slow, sustained stretch without a ballistic component, because ballistic stretch would elicit the hyperactive stretch reflex characteristic of spasticity and would resist the muscle elongation that is the goal of the stretch. Slow or fast repetitive, non-resistive exercise of large muscle groups or tailored calisthenics would then follow.

Conditioning exercises would be sport specific as well as individual specific. For instance, a freestyle swimmer would have exercises to strengthen back extensors, pectoral muscles, latissimus dorsi, hip flexors and extensors, and quadriceps. This would be in contrast to the 100-yard dash runner, for whom exercises would be chosen to strengthen hip and knee extensors for driving and push-off power; anterior deltoids and pectorals for reciprocal arm motion; and gastrocnemius, soleus, and hip and knee extensor exercises for the explosive initial acceleration at the start of the activity (4).

Consideration of this differential from one sport to another introduces the concept of exercise prescription. In general, this exercise prescription is most knowledgeably developed by the physiatrist (specialist in physical medicine and rehabilitation) or the orthopedist. Because there is a tendency to focus on energy conservation for the injured athlete, warm-up activities may be short-changed or skipped, to the detriment of the athlete. Just as with the able-bodied athlete, the preexercise warm-up enhances flexibility and performance and decreases the risk of muscle strain resulting from sudden exertion (5,6).

REHABILITATION OF THE BRAIN-INJURED ATHLETE

Intracranial disorders that result in impairment of neuromuscular function and control may have a wide variety of causes, manifestations, and prognoses. The following considers the specific neuromuscular control problems that must be dealt with for the return of the athlete to or preparation for sports participation.

Spasticity

Corticospinal tract lesions are generally signaled by increased muscle tone, exaggerated stretch reflexes, and pathologic reflexes. These physical signs contribute minimal information to understanding the functional distortions imposed by the spasticity, however. Spasticity implies a total disorder of the initiation, sequencing, grading, isolation, and timing of motor control, often with impaired sensation as well. Different components of this sequence of control may be more involved than others. There may be a significant latency from the moment of ideation or formulation of the plan to begin movement to the actual start of the movement. The tension required for the specific act formulated may be either a great deal more than needed or significantly less than needed. If sufficient tension for the task is developed, it may be difficult to maintain (motor impersistence). Once the required tension is obtained it may be difficult to release, involving yet another latency period from formulation of the idea to release and the accomplishment of the start of that motion.

The requisite activity may call for activation of selected muscles, but the spasticity may cause significant overflow into antagonist muscles or proximal muscles not required for the task. This overflow of spasticity may delay, hinder, distort, or prevent the required activity. Generally, the faster the individual tries to perform, the more the distortion is imposed by the spasticity (7).

The specific components involved in distorting this entire sequence of coordination must be analyzed and dealt with not only from a remedial point of view but also in terms of matching and profiling (8). For example, a patient with a latency in initiating movement would not be encouraged to participate in a sport that required a fast reaction time for performance or safety. Preferred activities would be those that do not make great demands on refinement of movement (9,10).

Classification of injury according to functional level becomes quite important in selecting sports as well as in making competition fair and appropriate. Athletes with spasticity can benefit from the type of classification used by the National Association of Sports for Cerebral Palsy. According to this functional classification, class I refers to a quadriplegic or triplegic person using a wheelchair and experiencing moderate to severe spasticity in the limbs involved. There may be severe control problems in the upper extremities and torso, with partial or no ability to propel a wheelchair. This individual might be profiled for a swimming event if he or she had 25% available range of motion in the upper extremities. In contrast, a class II individual has moderate to severe involvement of four limbs without ambulatory skills but retains the ability to propel the wheelchair with the legs and has better upper extremity range of motion than class I individuals. There is at least 40% range of motion in the upper extremities, which would allow participation in a wide range of field activities.

The class III individual has moderate involvement of three or four limbs, with fair functional strength and only moderate control problems, and has 60% available range of motion in the upper extremities. A class IV individual is essentially paraparetic with good functional strength in the arms and torso. A class V individual is moderately paretic, hemiparetic, or paraparetic and manages regular daily activities without a wheelchair. There is 80% normal range of motion in the upper extremities. A class VI quadriparetic or triparetic individual is able to ambulate with some supportive devices other than orthotics, which allows participation in foot races and a wide range of field events. A class VII individual is moderately paretic, hemiparetic, or minimally quadriparetic. Although moderate, this deficit is apparent to the lay observer. A class VIII individual has a minimal handicap, such as minimal hemiparesis or monoparesis, that is detectable only on neurologic examination; such an individual has free ability to run and jump (11), and the lay observer may be unaware of a deficit.

When rehabilitation functional goals are set after brain injury, the injured individual may be powerfully motivated by having realistic sports participation as one of the goals toward which to aim. Some of the more strenuous or repetitive aspects of the rehabilitation process may be enhanced by incorporating selected movements or patterns that will later be used in sports participation. In general, improvement after intracranial lesions may be expected to continue for at least 1 year after injury, with the fastest improvement being in the first 6 months. For children, this recovery process may last as long as 30 to 36 months.

Ataxia

Ataxia of cerebellar origin may involve dysmetria, nystagmus, scanning speech, intention tremor, and varying degrees of trunk and head titubation. In the course of rehabilitation, manual joint approximation or resisted activities tend to enhance sensory awareness of moment-to-moment joint position. Enhancements of sensory feedback may then be utilized to improve limb control. Kinesthetic cues supplement visual control of motion. Enhancement of kinesthetic cueing also lessens the random nature of movements attempted, so that the oscillations imposed by the ataxia may be smoothed; timing and amount of corrective effort to be applied are better assessed using these kinesthetic cues (12).

For the individual with a significant head and trunk titubation, sports activities involving the sitting position or adapted to allow sitting may be introduced. In general, sports that involve targeting (archery and dart throwing) may be less rewarding than activities such as calisthenics, swimming, or bicycling.

Disorders of Sensation

Disordered or impaired sensory acuity or disorders of interpretation of sensation may accompany neuromuscular deficits of central origin. The patient may also have difficulty integrating sensory information with functional activities to be performed (13,14). Although it is not possible to change or restore sensation, it is possible to direct attention to the type of sensory information available to prevent habits of disuse. An early association between the sensory information that is available and improved functional performance needs to become habitual.

Loss of special senses such as hearing or sight does not preclude active sports participation. Blind athletes can run races holding onto a guide wire, can play sports using balls with a bell incorporated in the sphere, or may be involved in field sports with verbal cueing from a coach. The hearing-impaired athlete who wishes to participate in track and field may use a light start signal rather than the traditional starting gun. The hearing-impaired athlete would probably have little difficulty participating in most of the sports on the activities checklist given in Table 1.

Central nervous system lesions that restrict one part of the visual field necessitate compensatory retraining for awareness of objects or

TABLE 1. *Sample activity checklist*

Activity[a-d]	Energy expenditure level[e]
Archery	3
Badminton	3–6
Baseball, softball	4–5
Basketball	7–9
Bicycling	2
Bowling	2
Calisthenics	3–4
Canoeing	2–4
Dancing	2–5
Dart throwing	2
Fencing	8
Football	6–8
Golf	2–3
Group games, relays	6–9
Gymnastics	5–9
Hockey (floor and field)	2–6
Horseback riding	
Walk	2
Trot	3
Posted trot	4
Jogging	7–8
Karate, judo	6–9
Kayaking	2–4
Martial arts	6–9
Ping-Pong	4
Sailing	3
Shuffleboard	2
Skating (ice and roller)	6
Soccer	5–6
Swimming	4–7
Tennis	4–6
Volleyball	4–6
Walking	2–5
Weight training	5–9
Wrestling	6–9

  [a] Nonparticipatory (spectator, scorekeeper, or referee).
  [b] Limited participation (tabletop versions of games, assisted and nonresisted movement, graded endurance).
  [c] Moderate participation (active movement, gravity-resisted movements, minimal resisted movements, graded endurance, as tolerated).
  [d] Full participation (total participation with regard to endurance and resisted movement).
  [e] Energy expenditure levels: 1, 1.5 to 2.0 metabolic equivalents (METS or 2 to 2.5 kcal/min); 2, 2 to 3 METS (2.5 to 4 kcal/min); 3, 3 to 4 METS (4 to 5 kcal/min); 4, 4 to 5 METS (5 to 6 kcal/min); 5, 5 to 6 METS (6 to 7 kcal/min); 6, 6 to 7 METS (7 to 8 kcal/min); 7, 7 to 8 METS (8 to 10 kcal/min); 8, 8 to 9 METS (10 to 11 kcal/min); 9, 10+ METS (11+ kcal/min).

activities in that visual field. There may be a restriction on contact sports or sports in which an incoming missile (ball, javelin, and the like) may not be perceived. There are many medical specialties that can assess sensory and motor dysfunctions. Disorders of sensory interpretation and sensory motor integration that result from intracranial lesions are often numerous, subtle, and difficult to delineate. These deficits should be addressed by a knowledgeable physician–therapist team. Once deficits are documented, it may subsequently be difficult to pinpoint a causal relationship between signs of dysfunction on standardized testing and the actual performance observed in functional situations. Therapists should not face this challenge unaided or unsupervised.

REHABILITATION OF THE SPINAL CORD–INJURED ATHLETE

For the athlete, regardless of the level of skill, loss of function secondary to spinal cord injury is a devastation beyond the ability of a verbal description to encompass. For some athletes with a permanent disability, the suggestion that wheelchair competition is a possibility may appear to be a cruel distortion. The lower the anatomic level of the spinal lesion, however, the greater the expected independence of function and the more expansive the options for sports participation (7) (Table 2).

The official medical classification developed by the National Wheelchair Athletic Association has been well established for years and works well in achieving a reasonable match for spinal cord–injured athletic competitors (15). Class IA includes all cervical lesions with incomplete or complete quadriplegia, with both hands involved and weakness of the triceps as well as severe weakness of the trunk and lower extremities, interfering with trunk balance and control and producing inability to walk. Class IB is also a cervical level, complete or incomplete, but with preservation of normal or good triceps (4 or 5 on manual muscle testing). Class IC is also a cervical level but with normal or good finger flexion and extension for grasp and release; there is no intrinsic hand muscle function, however. Trunk

TABLE 2. *Spinal cord functional levels*

	Quadriplegia				Paraplegia			
Function	C-4	C-5	C-6	C-7 and C-8	T-1 to T-10	T-10 to L-2	L-3 and L-4	L-5 and S-1
Intact muscle groups	Diaphragm, neck muscles	Deltoid, biceps, rotator cuff	Pectorals, extensor carpi radialis, serratus	Triceps, latissimus dorsi, extensor and flexor digitorum	Thenar, digital intrinsic, intercostals, paraspinals	Abdominals, lower paraspinals, intercostals	Quadriceps, hip adductors	Hamstrings, gluteus medius and maximus
Muscle actions	Respiration: abdominal and accessory	Shoulder flexion, abduction and external rotation, forearm flexion and supination	Shoulder internal rotation, wrist extension	Elbow extension, full wrist and finger control	Fairly good thoracic expansion, weak hip hiking	Spinal erect support, full thoracic expansion, weak hip flexion	Knee extension	Hip extension and abduction
Functional goals								
Eating	+/–	+/–	+/–	+	+	+	+	+
Dressing	–	+/–	+/–	+/–	+	+	+	+
Toilet	–	–	+/–	+/–	+	+	+	+
Bed mobility	–	May use biceps and sling to turn	+/–	+	+	+	+	+
Wheelchair adaptations	Electric: head or mouth control	Electric: arm control	Wheel rim extensions	–				–
Independence	–	+/–	+/–	Nearly complete	Complete	Complete with curbs	Long distance use only	–
Employment								
Homebound	–	–	–	+/–	+	+	+	+
Outside job	–	–	–	–	+	+	+	+
Automobile driving	–	–	–	+/–	+/–	+	+	+
Public transportation	–	–	–	–	–	+/–	+	+
Functional ambulation	–	–	–	–	Rare	+/–	+	+
Brace components	Environmental controls	Ball-bearing arm supports, hand and wrist splints	Universal cuff, tenodesis splint	Hand splints (occasionally)	Leg, hip, and back control and crutches	Leg and hip control and crutches	Ankle control only and crutches	Partial ankle control only

Adapted from *Practice of pediatrics*, vol 4, Kelley VC, ed., with permission of JB Lippincott Company, © 1979.

imbalance and impaired ambulation are equivalent in all the class I categories.

In class II the lesion becomes defined as producing paraplegia below T-1 and including T-5 levels, so there is total loss of or poor abdominal muscle strength (0 to 2 on manual muscle testing) and no useful trunk balance for sitting. Class III refers to complete or incomplete paraplegia with disability below T-5 and including T-10, so that upper abdominal muscles and spinal extensor musculature are sufficient to provide some degree of trunk balance for sitting. Sitting balance is impaired to some extent. Class IV is again a complete or incomplete paraplegic level with a disability below T-10 and extending down to and including L-2. There is no quadriceps or very weak quadriceps function (0 to 2 on manual muscle testing) as well as gluteal muscle paralysis. Class V refers to complete or incomplete paraplegia below L-2 with quadriceps graded between 3 and 5 on manual muscle testing. In wheelchair sports activities, force is required to make the wheels turn for a given distance; thus work is performed. The shorter the time in which a given amount of work is performed, the greater the amount of power required. Most wheelchair athletic activities (other than weight lifting) require repetitive contractions against submaximal resistance. The wheelchair user must propel the wheelchair with the muscles of the upper body and upper extremities, which are less efficient than the muscles of the lower extremities. Arm cranking and wheelchair ergometry can be used to assess physiologic responses to exercise in spinal cord–injured athletes (16).

Wheelchair sports include tennis, bowling, basketball, field events such as wheelchair sprints and distance races, slalom activities for maneuvering a wheelchair around or over various obstacles with the greatest possible speed, table tennis, putting the shot, javelin, archery, weight lifting, and even martial arts (17,18). The challenging nature of some of the track events is illustrated by the slalom, in which the wheelchair is required to jump onto and off a platform and maneuver through ramp activities and turns in tiny distances. Agility in maneuvering between flagged gates and strength and endurance for performance of these maneuvers in the shortest possible time are required. These activities call for considerable balance, coordination, control, and judgment.

Efforts have been made to keep standard national rules for each sport as close to normal guidelines as possible, with some adaptations to allow safe wheelchair use by participants with different degrees of disability. For international competition, the classification according to disability level becomes extensive, and the five classifications already listed for spinal cord injury are expanded to ten competitive categories. Technologic advances have led to lightweight, maneuverable wheelchairs with low-slung seats to lower the center of gravity for stability as well as canted wheels for stability and maneuverability. Pneumatic racing tires, adjustable bracket frames for rapid modification, and steering knobs near the coaster rims for high-speed racing are all options. Overall reduction in wheelchair weight lessens energy expenditure.

Wheelchair-associated injuries may vary from ulnar nerve compression in the tunnel of Guyon, caused by pressure against the wheel rim, to minor blisters and callus formation secondary to skin friction and pressure. Cuts, abrasions, and lacerations may occur from contact with metal components of the wheelchair or from trapping of fingers between wheelchair parts or within the spokes. Protection of insensitive buttock areas is required to prevent damage from sheer forces caused by movement of the buttocks across the wheelchair seat. Many athletes prefer not to use seat belts so that, if they fall, they can fall freely away from the wheelchair. Fractures associated with falls are not common but can occur. Preparation of the upper extremities for wheelchair sports participation includes stretches similar to those used by swimmers for shoulder joints and for the back. Specific activities aimed at strength (progressive resistive exercises), endurance (repetitive submaximal exercises), or power (maximal energy expenditure in the least amount of time) may be tailored for the specific sport in which the athlete will participate.

Osteoporosis caused by paralytic muscle disuse remains a significant problem for spinal cord–injured athletes. In general, there are two major factors for counteracting osteoporosis: weight bearing is the minimal contributor, and muscle activity is the major contributor (19).

Electrical muscle stimulation for exercise of nondenervated muscles has been proposed as a means of increasing blood supply to muscles, improving cardiorespiratory conditioning, and lessening the degree of paralytic osteoporosis. In the spinal cord–injured patient, spasticity may to some extent lessen, but not remove, the problem of osteoporosis. Although the etiology of heterotopic ossification has not been clarified, microtrauma on a repetitive basis has been implicated. This microtrauma may be totally unperceived because of anesthesia or impaired sensation below the level of the spinal lesion. With this factor in mind, athletes must be cautious about repetitive incidental trauma around major joints. Heterotopic ossification tends to be periarticular, with the joint surfaces themselves remaining unaffected. Nevertheless, the extent of the ossification may be great enough to immobilize joints; this is particularly seen as extraarticular ankylosis around the hip.

Not only must microtrauma from direct sports participation be guarded against, but also overzealous exercise must be avoided (20,21). Prevention of heterotopic ossification relies on control of subcutaneous or deeper infection; regular, gentle, passive mobility of joints; and in selected patients the use of etidronate disodium, which blocks the formation of crystalline hydroxyapatite.

Signs and symptoms of heterotopic ossification may begin as early as 2 months and as late as 6 to 8 months after spinal cord injury; symptoms include swelling, restricted motion, and occasional pain if some sensation is preserved. The bone isoenzyme alkaline phosphatase level is elevated. Even before roentgenographic signs appear, bone scans may be positive. The bone scan becomes normal once the ossification turns into mature bone, however. The roentgenographic picture then shows mature bone with distinct margins and trabeculations.

REHABILITATION OF THE ATHLETE WITH PERIPHERAL NERVE DISORDER

Polyneuropathy

Acute or postinfectious polyneuropathies usually involve only temporary loss of ambulation because of their distally predominant involvement (22). The greatest challenge to the athlete with polyneuropathy, as well as to the therapeutic team, is the application of graded strengthening activities without overfatigue. The concept of overwork or overfatigue retarding recovery of reinnervating muscle remains controversial (23). Nevertheless, the patient with peripheral nerve involvement is the neurologically injured person most likely to experience this phenomenon. This is particularly true of the athlete. Normal peripheral nerve innervation to the motor unit in a functioning muscle group involves a considerable amount of reserve strength, which is not used during ordinary daily activity. Repeated or sustained contractions of muscles during activity recruit different populations of muscle fibers so that there is a smooth maintenance of the performance level without overfatigue of any one population.

Peripheral neuropathy diminishes the reserve and distorts the recruitment of motor units as well as limiting the number of recruitable motor units available. In addition, the peripheral neuropathy may involve impaired sensation, so that subjective perceptions of fatigue or overuse are diminished. When this feature of decrease in available motor units is combined with impaired sensory feedback and the excessively high motivation of the athlete to regain normal performance, susceptibility to overfatigue is definitely present.

Overwork weakness may be difficult to diagnose and has been described as having two characteristics: a decrease in strength or endurance related to a specific task or activity and failure to regain strength that was demonstrable during a specific exercise (23,24). If one relies on overall loss of strength to establish the presence of overwork weakness, the diagnosis may be delayed to a point where recovery is decelerated or impaired.

Early in the diagnostic assessment of polyneuropathy, electrodiagnostic studies begin to give clues to the possibility of overfatigue. During electromyography of muscles involved by peripheral neuropathy, it is sometimes possible to see dropping out of recruited motor units during sustained or repeated contraction. This often corresponds clinically to manual muscle testing, with repeated contractions against the same resistance resulting in a diminished excursion of joint motion with each contraction. Single-fiber electromyography may also aid in establishing the presence of fatigue phenomena.

It is also important in history taking to elicit signs of fatigue with the awareness that in the well-motivated athlete there may be reluctance to admit to these signs. Single-resistance testing of muscles during manual muscle testing does not reveal this, so several repetitions on manual muscle testing become mandatory.

The physician managing the patient as well as the therapist or athletic trainer working toward restoration of strength and function must be familiar with the signs of fatigue in the area being exercised. These signs include, but may not be limited to, the appearance of fatigue tremors and fasciculations during exercise, the appearance of substitution patterns to compensate for a fatiguing muscle (often accompanied by greater use of proximal muscles that are usually not required in performing the task at hand, diminished excursion of joint motion with repeated contractions of muscles, decreased resistance tolerated during successive contractions, and subjective feelings of muscle fatigue on the part of the athlete. The athlete as well as the therapist, trainer, and physician must understand the possibility of overwork fatigue in order to cooperate in monitoring to prevent its appearance during rehabilitation.

Mononeuropathy

Injury to isolated peripheral nerves may occur during the course of sports performance (e.g., cyclists' palsy) or may be due to trauma unrelated to sports events. As recovery from weakness progresses, serial electromyography may be helpful in revealing the degree of fatigability of muscles. Electromyographic kinesiology may be used to supplement visual observation of proximal compensations. Injury to mixed nerves may cause not only lack of cutaneous sensation but also impairment or distortion of kinesthetic awareness of moment-to-moment muscle tension and joint position (25). Thus muscle strengthening alone may not be sufficient to restore well-coordinated movement.

Biofeedback may be useful in this situation, not only to provide an external cue to impaired internal awareness of muscle activation but also to provide cues for discouraging use of undesirable compensatory muscle contractions. Generally, the biofeedback is of use early in the course of reinnervation but may not be useful after reliable voluntary activation of desirable muscle tension levels has been reached. Reeducation of sensory awareness should also be part of the retraining after peripheral nerve injury (26,27). This includes reeducation of diminished sensory cues to identify shapes, weight, textures, and sensory figure–ground experiences as well as reeducation for perception of position in space.

As soon as it is feasible, the reeducation and rehabilitation process should be transferred to the specific sports activity that is the athlete's goal. As recovery continues, part of the physician's ongoing monitoring must include direct observation of the sport being performed. In general, this is more likely to be part of the assessment done by the athletic trainer or therapist, but the physician must be aware of the specific activities and biomechanics involved in the sport being performed to assess whether the challenge of the sport adequately matches the available neuromuscular control that the injured athlete has achieved.

Recovery from Neuropathy

In both generalized and isolated peripheral neuropathy, one of the goals of the rehabilitation program is to protect distally reinnervating muscles and intrinsic muscles during the process of strengthening and recovery. Supplementary splinting may be needed to accomplish this goal. As each step in recovery and adjustment of the rehabilitation programming occurs, the athlete must be fully aware of the reasons for changes and restrictions for protection so that cooperation with the sequenced application of rehabilitation modalities is optimal.

During the early stages of recovery from peripheral nerve injury or polyneuropathy, attention must be given to trying to maintain general cardiorespiratory training levels despite the basic pathology. Pool therapy is often beneficial for this goal. In severe, acute polyneuropathies the buoyant effect of the water may also be useful for initiating the process of ambulation until inherent muscle control can support the body weight against the pull of gravity on dry land. Swimming may be a useful means of maintaining general conditioning, even for isolated peripheral nerve injuries, during the early stages of recovery when the specific sports performed by the athlete may not be possible. Conditioning activities can also be tailored according to the part of the body injured. Bicycling or stationary skiing activities can be used while awaiting recovery from upper extremity injury, and stationary rowing or upper extremity bicycle ergometry may be used while awaiting lower extremity recovery.

CONCLUSION

In 1984, the games of the twenty-third Olympiad in Los Angeles included wheelchair track and field events for the first time as demonstration sports. This had the beneficial effect of introducing to the sports-minded public the awareness of events tailored for the injured athlete, which had been taking place as international wheelchair games for many years. The popular press and news media have made the public aware of the Special Olympics program created by the Joseph P. Kennedy, Jr. Foundation. Fewer people may be aware that the U.S. Olympic program has created a Committee for the Handicapped in Sports, which comprises representatives of major organizations promoting both international and national competitions for the handicapped athlete. The number of organizations devoted to promoting sports activities for the injured athlete grows from year to year. More and more rehabilitation centers are incorporating sports activities in their recreation and therapeutic programs. Injured athletes appear in television commercials and are popular motivational speakers (28). The medical profession is becoming aware of the need for physical activity for the injured or disabled person as well as for the "well" person (29).

It is to be hoped that this trend continues. In a society that is oriented toward fitness and sports participation, physically handicapped individuals need the challenges of sports participation as well as the opportunities for recreational and competitive sports performance. An additional sign of growth in this area will be the continued emergence of these sports activities from the medical realm into the social sports world.

REFERENCES

1. Birrer RB, Daller IA. The exercise prescription. *NY State J Med* 1987;318:106–112.
2. Curtis KA. Wheelchair sports medicine: Part 3: Stretching routines. *Sports Spokes* 1981 Oct:16–18.
3. Jackson RW, Fredrickson A. Sports for the physically disabled. *Am J Sports Med* 1979;7:293–296.
4. Challenor YB: Exercise and the handicapped child. *Semin Neurol* 1981;1:358–364.
5. Anderson B, Burke ER. Scientific, medical and practical aspects of stretching in the exercise prescription. *Clin Sports Med* 1991;10(1):63–86.
6. BenKibler W, Chandler J. Sport-specific conditioning. *Am J Sports Med* 1994;22:424–432.
7. Challenor YB, Gonzales EG, Turner N. Rehabilitation in neuromuscular disorders. In: Kelley VC, ed. *Practice of pediatrics,* Chap 100. Hagerstown, MD: Harper & Row, 1979:1–23.
8. Kottke FJ. Halpern D, Easton JLM. The training of coordination: Part 1. *Arch Phys Med Rehabil* 1978; 59:567–568.
9. Halpern D. Therapeutic exercises for cerebral palsy. In: Basmajian JV, ed. *Therapeutic exercises,* 3rd ed. Baltimore: Williams & Wilkins, 1978:281–306.
10. Challenor YB, Gold AP. Cerebrovascular disease in children and remediation of neuromuscular residua. In: Downey IA, Low NL, eds. *The child with disabling illness: principles of rehabilitation.* New York: Raven Press, 1982:105–120.
11. National Association of Sports for Cerebral Palsy. *Rules, classification, and national records. Sports manual.* New Haven, CT: National Association of Sports for Cerebral Palsy, 1978:1–10.
12. Kottke FJ. Halpern D, Easton JLM. The training of coordination: Part 2. *Arch Phys Med Rehabil* 1978; 59:569–570.
13. Kinaesthesia. *Lancet* 1973;473–474. Editorial.
14. Dellon AL, Kallman CH. Evaluation of functional sensation in the hand. *J Hand Surg* 1983;8:161–164.
15. Corcoran PJ, Goldman RF, Hoerner EF, et al. Sports medicine and the physiology of wheelchair marathon racing. *Orthop Clin North Am* 1980;11:697–716.
16. Wicks JR, Oldridge NB, Cameron BJ, et al. Arm cranking and wheelchair ergometry in elite spinal cord–injured athletes. *Med Sci Sports Exerc* 1983;15:224–231.
17. Linden P. Aikido. The gentle martial art. *Sports Spokes* 1978 Jan/Feb:8–10.
18. Pandavela J, Gordon S, Geodon G, et al. Martial arts for the quadriplegic. *Am J Phys Med* 1986;65:17–29.
19. Abramson AS, Delagi EF. Influence of weight-bearing and muscle contraction on disuse osteoporosis. *Arch Phys Med Rehabil* 1961;42:147–151.
20. Rossier AB, Bussat P, Infante F. Current facts on paraosteoarthropathy (POA). *Paraplegia* 1973;2:36.

21. Guttmann L. Soft tissue calcifications and ossifications. In Guttmann L, ed. *Spinal cord injuries.* London: Blackwell Scientific, 1973:207.

22. Cavanagh JB. The problems of neurons with long axons. *Lancet* 1984;1284–1287.

23. Bennett RL, Knowlton GC. Overwork weakness in partially denervated skeletal muscle. *Clin Orthop Relat Res* 1958;12:22–29.

24. Lieberman JS, Taylor RG, Fowler WM Jr. Fatiguing muscle weakness: an overlooked phenomenon in patients with neurogenic dysfunction. *Arch Phys Med Rehabil* 1981;62:515.

25. Moberg E. The role of cutaneous afferents in position sense, kinaesthesia, and motor function of the hand. *Brain* 1983;106:1–19.

26. Dellon AL, Jabaley ME. Reeducation of sensation in the hand following nerve suture. *Clin Orthop Relat Res* 1982;163:75–79.

27. Dellon AL, Curtis RM, Edgerton MT. Reeducation of sensation in the hand after nerve injury and repair. *Plast Reconstr Surg* 1974;54:297–305.

28. Stein J. Physical activity from rehabilitation to independent community function: the role of physical activity in handicapping conditions. *Clin Sports Med* 1991;10(1): 211–221.

29. Pate RR, Pratt M, Blair SN, et al. Physical activity and public health—a recommendation from the Centers for Disease Contol and Prevention and the American College of Sports Medicine. *JAMA* 1995; 273:402–407.

PART II

Neurologic Disorders in the Athlete

Sports Neurology, Second Edition,
edited by Barry D. Jordan.
Lippincott–Raven Publishers, Philadelphia © 1998.

11

Emergency Management of Cervical Spine Injuries

Thomas T. Lee, Glen R. Manzano, and Barth A. Green

University of Miami School of Medicine,
P.O. Box 016960, Department of Neurological Surgery, Miami, Florida 33101

Recreational, amateur, and professional sports occupy a high level of importance in present-day American society. Beyond being a source of exercise and entertainment to the average American, competitive professional sports is a multimillion dollar industry that employs a number of talented and physically gifted athletes. The motivation to participate in competitive, aggressive sports has led to bigger, faster, and stronger athletes and has subsequently increased the velocity of collisions and severity of injuries. This is especially significant when one considers acute cervical spine injuries.

The management of a suspected spinal cord injury begins at the moment of injury and involves a multidisciplinary team of health care professionals (1). Because of the serious implications of a neck injury, strict guidelines have been developed for the treatment of these patients.

CLASSIFICATION OF CERVICAL INJURIES

The principal forces responsible for a cervical spinal column injury include axial compression, flexion, extension, rotation, shear, distraction, and a combination of these forces (2,3). The spinal column is divided into three columns, as classified by Denis. This is defined by the advent of computed tomography, which visualizes the vertebral body in axial views and is also capable of reconstructing images in sagittal and coronal orientations. The three columns are anterior, middle, and posterior. The anterior column consists of the anterior half of the vertebral body, anterior half of the annulus fibrosus, and the anterior longitudinal ligament. The middle column consists of the posterior half of the vertebral body, the posterior half of the annulus fibrosus, and the posterior longitudinal ligament. The posterior column consists of the posterior arch, interspinous ligament, supraspinous ligament, and ligamentum flavum. Several categories exist for classifying the types of fractures that commonly result from these forces.

Compression Fracture

This is a fracture of the anterior column with middle column intact. This fracture is generally stable. Neurologic deficit is rare. When the anterior body collapses, the intact middle column acts as a hinge, imposing tensile force on the posterior ligamentous structures. In general, only expectant treatment and orthotic bracing are necessary, especially in the cervical region. For thoracolumbar compressions, if the anterior vertebral column height reduction is 50% or greater, the likelihood of posterior column failure is significant (4). For a kyphotic angle of greater than 30°, a vertebral body height decrease of more than 50%, or if a patient who undergoes subsequent laminectomies, there has been a report of increased long-term deformity (5). A stabilization is recommended for these circumstances.

Burst Fracture

In such a fracture, the predominant mechanism is axial loading. Combination with flexion or rotation causes the characteristic patterns seen with burst fractures. A characteristic feature of this type of injury is failure of the middle column, which is not present in a compression fracture (Fig. 1A and B). Posterior column fractures may also be associated and make this type of fracture even more unstable. A unique burst fracture of the C-1 ring has been termed a Jefferson fracture.

Denis (6) proposed several key features of burst fractures: (a) comminution of the vertebral body, (b) loss of posterior vertebral body height, (c) retropulsion of bony and ligamentous or disc material into the spinal canal, (d) fracture of the lamina, and (e) increase in interpediculate space. The initial degree of canal compromise was reported by Lemons et al. (7) to correlate directly with the degree of neurologic deficit, although other reports disputed this claim. Forty-seven percent of the patients with a burst fracture sustained neurologic deficits. These injuries are generally stable unless posterior injuries (especially facets, pars interarticularis, or ligaments) are present, in which case the fracture should be stabilized. If there is associated neurologic deficit or radiographic signs of cord or nerve decompression, the authors generally advocate decompressive surgery followed by internal fixation.

Fracture-Dislocation

Such fractures are characterized by the failure of all three columns. The forces involved may be compression, rotation, tension, extension, and shear. Such an injury is most frequently associated with a spinal cord pathology and neurologic deficit (6). By definition, a fracture dislocation is an unstable three-column injury and requires internal fixation with arthrodesis. Three subtypes of fracture-dislocations have been described.

Type A injury is the result of combined flexion–rotational forces. Although initially described in mining accident victims (8), this may also occur as a result of a fall or an ejection from a motor vehicle in an accident. The characteristic computed tomographic scan shows the superior

and inferior vertebral bodies to be rotated on axial images. Facet disruption, canal compromise, and articular surface fracture are frequently observed. In the cervical region, unilaterally perched facet is generally associated with incomplete injury or even a relatively normal neurologic examination (9).

Type B fracture-dislocation is caused by the force of shear across the horizontal plane. Both anterolisthesis and retrolisthesis of the superior vertebral body are possible, depending on the direction of the impact.

Type C injury is a bilateral facet dislocation (Fig. 2) caused by the flexion–distraction mechanism. It resembles a seat belt type of injury, but associated anterior column failure is also present. The anterior column failure most frequently involves the intervertebral disc or the anterior vertebral body. The anterior longitudinal ligament is stripped but not torn (6), as significant superior vertebral subluxation can occur. For a bilaterally locked facet in the cervical region, in contrast to a unilaterally locked facet, significant neurologic deficits are generally present.

Hangman's Fracture

This unique fracture occurs at the axis (C-2) level, with the predominant vector of force being hyperextension. Classically, bilateral posterior ring fractures at the pedicles are observed. The patients are frequently neurologically intact, owing to the relatively large cervical canal at this level. Although it was named for cervical fractures associated with hanging, this injury is now most often caused by a motor vehicle accident. An uncomplicated hangman's fracture can be treated with a rigid external orthosis such as a rigid cervical collar or halo fixation (10,11).

Odontoid Fracture

Three types of odontoid fractures have been identified (12–14). Type I fracture goes through the tip of the dens, and type II fracture (Fig. 3) goes through the junction between the base of the dens and the anterior arch of C-2. Type III fracture extends into the cancellous bone of the C-2 body. These fractures were divided into subtypes A and B to describe the osseous and transverse

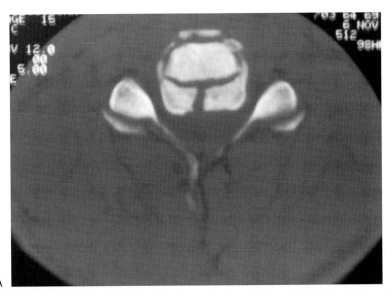

A

FIG. 1. A: Computed tomographic scan through the body of C-5, demonstrating a burst fracture with involvement of both the anterior and middle columns.

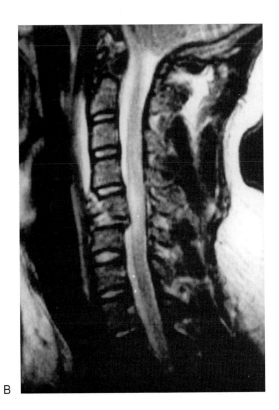

B

FIG. 1. B: Cervical magnetic resonance T2-weighted sagittal view demonstrated the "burst" component impinging on the cord anteriorly. Moderate cord signal change is noted.

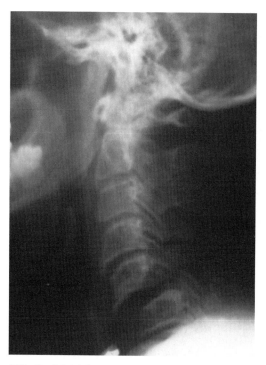

FIG. 2. C5-6 bilateral locked facet resulted in a 50% anterolisthesis of C-5 on C-6. The patient was completely quadriplegic below C-5.

ligament involvement by Dickman et al. (15). In general, type I and III fractures heal spontaneously with external fixation devices. Owing to a poorer vascular supply, type II odontoid fractures frequently do not fuse with only external fixation (12). Neurologic deficits are not usually associated with these injuries.

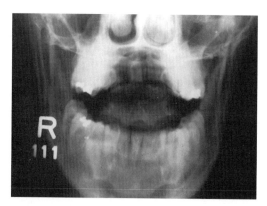

FIG. 3. Open-mouth view of the odontoid showed a linear lucency through the base of the dens consistent with a type II odontoid fracture.

Miscellaneous Injuries

Other common injuries of the upper cervical spine include atlantooccipital dislocation (distraction), C1-2 rotatory subluxation, Jefferson fracture (C-1 ring burst fracture caused by axial loading), and atlantoaxal dislocation. Isolated spinous process, unilateral articular process, transverse process, or laminar fractures are frequently observed but do not require surgical intervention. A traumatic herniated disc should also be included in the differential diagnosis and ruled by magnetic resonance imaging (MRI). Any neurologic worsening or increasing pain should prompt a follow-up evaluation, including plain films and MRI.

INITIAL MANAGEMENT OF ATHLETIC ACUTE CERVICAL INJURIES

On-the-Field Assessment

All patients sustaining major trauma must be deemed by medical personnel to have a spinal cord injury until proved otherwise. The first step in treating a "downed" athlete with a suspected cervical injury is an assessment of breathing and circulation (16). If an athlete with a cervical spine injury is not breathing, cardiopulmonary resuscitation should be initiated. If the athlete is wearing a helmet with a face mask, the face mask should be removed without taking off the helmet (Fig. 4A–C). Labored breathing may be an indicator of a high cervical injury. In all cases of spinal injury, oxygen should be administered as soon as it is available, and ventilation should be carefully monitored.

A preliminary neurologic examination should also be administered on the field (16). Once mental status has been established, the athlete should be questioned about neck or back pain and extremity numbness or weakness. A diagnosis of spinal cord injury should dictate subsequent handling and transport of the player.

Transport

In transporting an individual with a suspected spinal cord injury, it should be remembered that continuous movement of an injured spinal cord

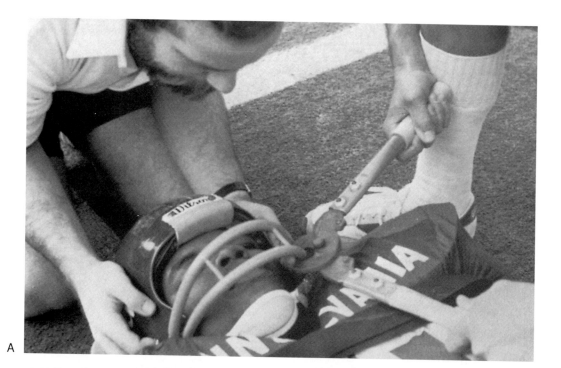

A

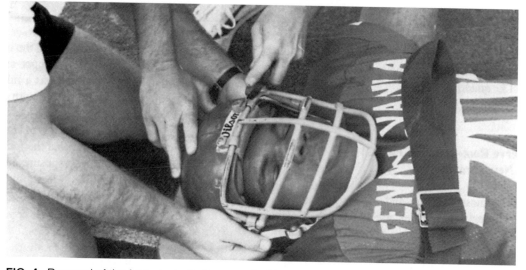

B

FIG. 4. Removal of the face mask. **A:** Remove double and single masks with bolt cutters. Head and helmet must be securely immobilized. **B:** Remove cage-type masks by cutting the plastic loops with a utility knife. Make the cut on the side of the loop away from the face. **C:** Remove the entire mask from the helmet so that it does not interfere with further resuscitation efforts. (From Torg JS, ed. *Athletic injuries to the head, neck, and face.* Philadelphia: Lea & Febiger, 1982. Copyright JS Torg.)

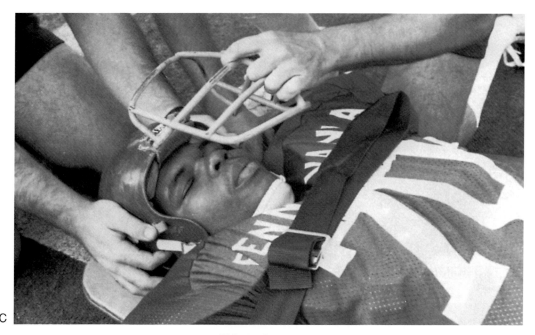

C

FIG. 4. *Continued.*

could inflict further damage, causing further neurologic deterioration. (17,18). When the transport team arrives, the patient must be placed in the supine position on a spine board (Fig. 5) to facilitate transport (Fig. 6). This often involves turning or lifting the athlete. A popular and effective method of doing this is one described by Watkins, which involves using a team of five people headed by a physician (16,19). The physician should control the head and ensure proper alignment with the shoulders and torso. A cervical collar, if applicable, can aid in immobilizing the patient. However, if a helmet is being worn, it should not be removed until the athlete reaches the hospital (Fig. 7A and B). Immobilization of the head can be achieved by securing it on either side with rolled blankets and taping or by strapping it to the board. The rest of the body can also be secured with straps, making sure that they do not interfere with proper breathing.

EMERGENCY ROOM PROTOCOL

The initial emergency room evaluation of spinal cord injury should proceed in a multidisciplinary fashion. Significant head injuries, as well as sys-

temic trauma, can be associated with a spinal cord injuries (20–22). Spinal shock and respiratory muscle failure should be considered in patients with cervical injuries, which can cause a "sympathectomy" syndrome consisting of hypotension and bradycardia, because of unopposed vagal tone. This must be distinguished from hemorrhagic shock of other etiologies. Fluid support, appropriate hemodynamic monitoring, including a pulmonary artery catheter and arterial line, and pressors may be necessary.

Upon arrival at the emergency room, a baseline full neurologic examination should be performed. When the patient is hemodynamically and respiratorily stabilized and the neurologic status has been assessed, plain radiographs of cervical, thoracic, and lumbosacral spine should be obtained.

If the patient shows any sign of a spinal cord injury, the high-dose methylprednisolone protocol outlined by the National Spinal Cord Injury Study II is recommended (22). The loading dose can be given within 8 hours of the injury; 30 mg/kg of methylprednisolone is given as slow bolus in the first hour, followed by an infusion of 5.4 mg/kg/h for 23 hours. Appropriate gastritis

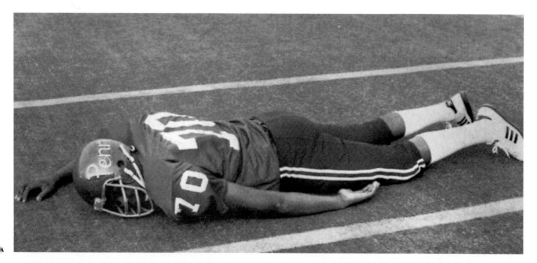

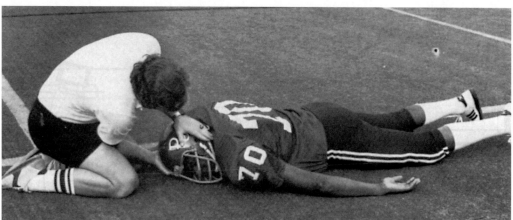

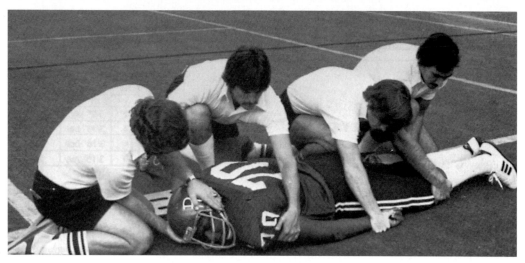

FIG. 5. A: Athlete with suspected cervical spine injury who may or may not be unconscious. Any unconscious athletes should be managed as though they had significant neck injury. **B:** After checking the airway, the leader immediately immobilized the head and neck unit. **C–E:** The athlete is logrolled onto the spine board. (From Torg JS, ed. *Athletic injuries to the head, neck, and face.* Philadelphia: Lea & Febiger, 1982. Copyright JS Torg.)

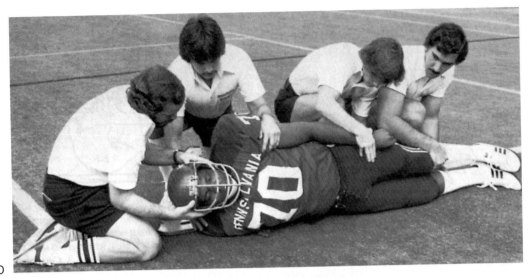

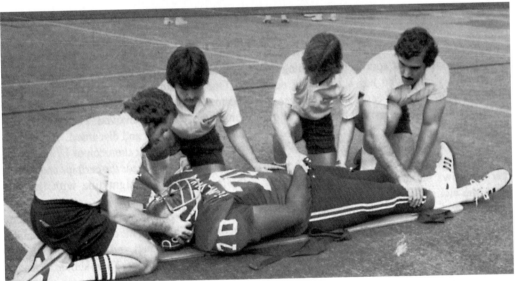

FIG. 5. *Continued.*

or ulcer prophylaxis should be given. In the study conducted by Bracken et al. (22), a benefit of high-dose steroid was observed in incomplete spinal cord injury, as complete motor injury with or without sensory sparing did not show major improvement. This study, however, excluded patients who subsequently underwent decompression and stabilization. The benefit of the steroid should be weighed against the possible complication of infection and gastrointestinal hemorrhage. No steroid is infused in cases of

penetrating injuries because of possible visceral involvement.

The authors generally do not place patients under cervical traction until appropriate radiographic studies are obtained in the emergency department. Significant risks of increasing neurologic deficits exist, especially in young patients with distraction-type injury and ligamentous laxity and patients with ankylosing spondylitis (1). Overdistraction and increased spinal deformity are definite considerations in these patients. When

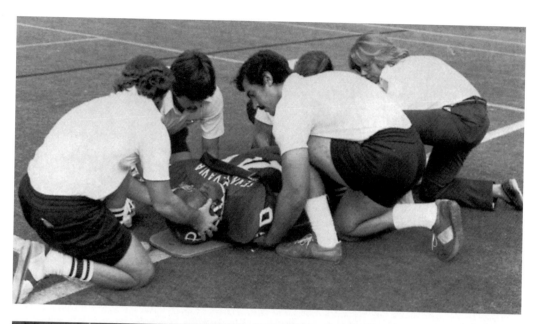

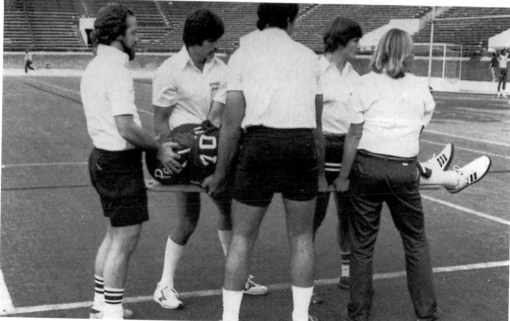

FIG. 6. Lifting and carrying the athlete. Four members of the medical support team lift the athlete on the command of the leader. The leader maintains the manual immobilization of the head. The spine board is not recommended as a stretcher. An additional stretcher should be used for transporting the patient over long distances. (From Torg JS, ed. *Athletic injuries to the head, neck, and face.* Philadelphia: Lea & Febiger, 1982. Copyright JS Torg.)

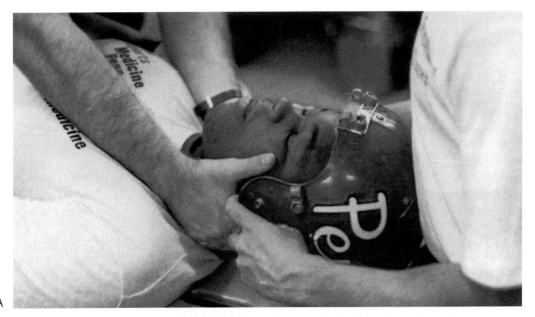

A

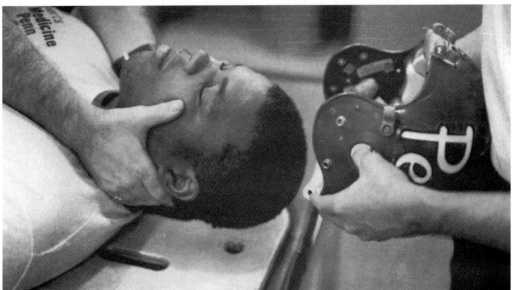

B

FIG. 7. Removal of the helmet. **A:** The helmet should be removed only when permanent immobilization can be instituted. The helmet may be removed by detaching the chin strap, spreading the earflaps, and gently pulling the helmet off in a straight line with the cervical spine. **B:** The head must be supported under the occiput during and after removal of the helmet. (From Torg JS, ed. *Athletic injuries to the head, neck, and face.* Philadelphia: Lea & Febiger, 1982. Copyright JS Torg.)

there is obvious cervical fracture or dislocation on plain cervical radiographs, traction with an MRI-compatible Gardner-Wells tong is applied and 5 pounds per interspace of total traction is initiated. The same amount of traction is applied for

patients without clear fracture or malalignment who present with a definite cervical level of injury. Posttraction plain radiographs are obtained to ascertain the realignment and to check for overdistraction. If reduction cannot be achieved, the patient is then fiberoptically intubated with minimal neck manipulation. After benzodiazepine and muscle relaxants are administered, manual reduction and realignment under fluoroscopy are attempted. In the authors' experience, the majority of the patients could be reduced by these means and generaly no acute surgical realignment and stabilization are needed. The patient is maintained in a cervical collar under traction on a Rotorest treatment table to avoid undue motion. If the manual reduction under fluoroscopy and muscle relaxant fails, the patient needs to be reduced under general anesthesia intraoperatively. A simultaneous fusion, after operative reduction of the fracture or subluxation, is necessary to provide immediate stability in these cases.

After cervical fracture reduction and other plain films of the spine, computed tomography (CT) can be utilized to image areas poorly visualized by the plain films and areas of suspected injury on the plain film. These images provide detailed bone anatomy near the site of injury and may be invaluable in preoperative planning. CT scanning, however, is not the diagnostic tool of choice for detecting soft tissue or ligamentous injuries, herniated discs, or an epidural hematoma. Its sensitivity for an intramedullary lesion is similarly low. MRI or CT with myelography may be needed to assess soft tissue or cord injury. The authors prefer MRI because of greater anatomic detail, the ability to evaluate soft tissue injury, and capability of multiplanar imaging. CT myelography is reserved for patients with incompatible metal implants or medical conditions.

EVALUATION OF NECK PAIN IN ATHLETES

Because of the degree of physical impact and exertion, athletes are prone to develop neck pain of various etiologies. Common causes of neck pain are hyperflexion and hyperextension injuries, which have a muscular or tendinous component and generally do not require an extensive workup (23). The history should identify the possible mode and mechanism of injury. Any exacerbating factor or movement should be ascertained. The presence of a "trigger point" may also aid

in the diagnosis. A full neurologic examination testing all sensory, motor, reflex, and long-tract signs and sphincter function should be performed. A set of adequate plain cervical radiographs visualizing down to the cervical–thoracic junction (top of T-1) is a relatively inexpensive screening test (24). In addition to detecting a usual fracture, it can detect a unilateral locked facet, a subtle rotatory subluxation, or odontoid fractures. If no neurologic deficit or radiographic abnormality is detected, a trial of conservative treatments, including rest, soft cervical collar, massages, compress application, and nonsteroidal antiinflammatory drugs, generally leads to symptomatic relief. Occasionally, a trial of trigger point injection may be necessary to alleviate the symptoms.

If the symptoms are persistent despite conservative treatments or any abnormality is detected on the neurologic examination or screening radiographs, the patient is placed in a rigid cervical collar and appropriate imaging studies are done. All patients would undergo MRI and a CT scan for the reasons mentioned in the previous section. Any neurologic deterioration in a previously neurologically intact patient would prompt the same investigation.

CRITERIA FOR RETURN TO PLAY

The guidelines for return to contact sports after a cervical spine injury focus on the status of signs and symptoms and on radiographic findings (25). Radiographic studies normally try to rule out spinal cord compression or injury from fracture or stenosis.

Defining stenosis from radiographic measurements had, for years, been complicated by magnification error. A ratio method developed by Torg et al. (26) and Pavlov et al. (27), which corrects for this magnification error, and advances in modem imaging techniques such as MRI have made diagnosing radiographic stenosis an easier task.

Basically, three scenarios exist with injured athletes after treatment. The first of these is the athlete with persistent neurologic deficit. This is an absolute contraindication for return to contact sports, as further neurologic deterioration is likely. There

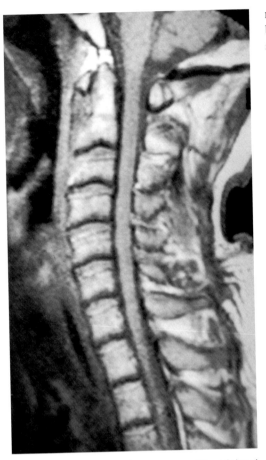

FIG. 8. Sagittal magnetic resonance T1-weighted image demonstrated a narrow cervical canal with decreased canal/vertebral body ratio. No focal traumatic injury was seen.

are numerous examples in the literature of athletes who returned to play without resolution of symptoms and suffered subsequent neurologic complications (28). Another possibility is an athlete with resolution of signs and symptoms but radiographic evidence of stenosis (Fig. 8) or instability. This is a relative contraindication for return to play, as subsequent injury is likely to aggravate or result in cord compression and result in neurologic deficit. Literature in sports medicine, neurology, and radiology supports the notion that spinal stenosis predisposes a patient to spinal cord injury (28). Finally, an athlete with resolution of symptoms and unremarkable radiographic studies is normally cleared for return to play. With an unremarkable radiographic evaluation, the athlete with minimal

residual neck pain may return to practice while being closely observed for any progression of symptoms of spinal cord or nerve root injury.

REFERENCES

1. Green BA, David C, Falcone S, Razack N, Klose KJ. Spinal cord injuries in adults. In: Youmans JR, et al., eds. *Neurological surgery,* 4th ed. Philadelphia: WB Saunders, 1996:1969–1990.
2. Eismont FJ, Garfin SR, Abitol J. Thoracic and upper lumbar spine injuries. In: Browner BD, Jupiter JB, Levine AM, et al., eds. *Skeletal trauma.* Philadelphia: WB Saunders, 1993:729–803.
3. Lebwohl NH, Starr JK. Surgical management of thoracolumbar fractures. In: Greenberg I, ed. *Handbook of head and spine trauma.* New York: Marcel Dekker, 1993:593–646.
4. Maiman DJ, Pintar FA. Anatomy and clinical biomechanics of the thoracic spine. *Clin Neurosurg* 1990; 38:296.
5. Bohlman HH. Treatment of fractures and dislocations of the thoracic and lumbar spine. *J Bone Joint Surg Am* 1985;76A:165–169.
6. Denis F. The three column spine and its significance in the classification of acute thoracolumbar spinal injuries. *Spine* 1983;8:817–831.
7. Lemons VR, Wagner FC Jr, Montesano PX. Management of thoracolumbar fractures with accompanying neurological injury. *Neurosurgery* 1992;30: 667–671.
8. Holdsworth FW. Fractures, dislocations and fracture-dislocation of the spine. *J Bone Joint Surg Br* 1963; 45B:6.
9. Sim E. Vertical facet splitting: a special variant of rotary dislocations of the cervical spine. *J Neurosurg* 1995; 82:239–243.
10. Hartman JT, Palumbo F, Hill BJ. Cineradiography of the braced normal cervical spine: a comparative study of five commonly used cervical orthoses. *Clin Orthop* 1975; 109:97–102.
11. Wolf JW, Johnson RM. Cervical orthoses. In: The Cervical Spine Society, ed. *The cervical spine.* Philadelphia: JB Lippincott Co, 1983:54–61.
12. Hadley MN, Browner CM, Liu SS, et al. New subtype of acute odontoid fractures (type IIA). *Neurosurgery* 1988;22:67–71.
13. Hadley MN, Diclanan CA, Browner CM. Acute traumatic atlas fractures: management and long term outcome. *Neurosurgery* 1988;23:31–35.
14. Hadley MN, Dickman CA, Browner CM. Acute axis fractures: a review of 229 cases. *J Neurosurg* 1989;71: 642–647.
15. Dickman CA, Greene KA, Sonntag VK. Injuries involving the transverse atlantal ligament: classification and treatment guidelines based upon experience with 39 injuries. *Neurosurgery* 1996;38(1):44–50.
16. Feuer H. History, examination and acute management of spinal injury. In: Nicholas JA, Hershman EB, eds. *The lower extremity and spine in sports medicine.* St. Louis: Mosby, 1995.
17. Green BA, Eismont FJ. Acute spinal cord injury: a systems approach. *Cent Nerv Syst Trauma* 1984;1(2): 173–195.

18. Green BA, Eismont FJ, O'Heir JT. Pre-hospital management of spinal cord injuries. *Paraplegia* 1987;25: 229–238.

19. Watkins RG. Neck injuries in football players. *Clin Sports Med* 1986;5:223.

20. Eisenburg HM, Cayard C, Papancolaua FF. The effects of three potentially preventable complications on outcome after severe closed head injury. In: Ishar S, Nagai H, Brock M, eds. *Intracranial pressure*, 5th ed. Tokyo: Springer-Verlag, 1983:549–553.

21. Klauber MR, Toutant SM, Marshall LF. A model for predicting delayed intracranial hypertension following severe head injury. *J Neurosurg* 1984;61:695–699.

22. Bracken MB, Shepard MJ, Collins WF, et al. A randomized, controlled trial of methylprednisolone or naloxone in the treatment of acute spinal-cord injury. Result of the second National Acute Spinal Cord Injury Study. *N Engl J Med* 1990;322:1405–1411.

23. Travis RL. Hyperextension and hyperflexion injuries of the cervical spine. In: *Youman's* ed. *Neurological surgery*, 4th ed. Philadelphia: WB Saunders, 1996: 2037–2042.

24. Rahim KA, Stambough X. Radiographic evaluation of the degenerative cervical spine. *Orthop Clin North Am* 1992;23:395–403.

25. Cantu RV, Cantu RC. Guidelines for return to contact sports after transient quadriplegia. *J Neurosurg* 1994; 80:592–594.

26. Torg IS, Pavlov H, Genuario SE, et al. Neurapraxia of the cervical spinal cord with transient quadriplegia. *J Bone Joint Surg Am* 1986;68:1354–1370.

27. Pavlov H, Torg IS, Robie B, et al. Cervical spinal stenosis: determination with vertebral body ratio method. *Radiology* 1987;164:771–775.

28. Cantu RC. Cervical spinal stenosis: challenging an established detection method. *Physician Sports Med* 1993;21(9):57–63.

Sports Neurology, Second Edition,
edited by Barry D. Jordan.
Lippincott–Raven Publishers, Philadelphia © 1998.

12

Soft Tissue Injuries and Disc Disease of the Cervical Spine

Barry D. Jordan

*Reed Neurological Research Center, University of California
at Los Angeles School of Medicine, 710 Westwood Plaza, Los Angeles, California 90095-1769*

A variety of cervical spine disorders can be encountered in sports (Table 1). Although the majority of cervical spine disorders or injuries experienced by the athlete tend to be benign and self-limited, more serious and life-threatening injuries can also occur. The current chapter reviews some of the more common injuries to the cervical spine (i.e., soft tissue injuries and disc disease) seen in sports.

SOFT TISSUE INJURIES

Soft tissue injuries of the neck and cervical spine include contusions, muscle strain, and ligamentous sprain. Although these injuries are more frequently encountered in the contact and collision sports, they can occur in almost any sport.

Neck Contusion

The athlete presenting with a neck contusion often reports a history of direct trauma to the neck, from either an object (e.g., lacrosse stick, tennis racquet) or the body part of another athlete (e.g., elbow, knee). Typically, these injuries tend to be benign and self-limited, unless associated with more severe injury to the anterior neck (e.g., fracture of the trachea, carotid artery trauma, or cervical spine fracture). Traumatic injury to the vascular structures of the neck may be associated with stroke (see Chapter 23). The physical examination of the athlete with a neck contusion may demonstrate visual evidence of trauma (e.g.,

ecchymosis or hematoma). The athlete may exhibit a limited range of motion secondary to pain. The pain tends to be localized to the primary area of trauma. Pain radiating down an upper extremity or paresthesias of an upper extremity should alert the clinician to a more serious injury. In addition, any upper extremity weakness should alert the examiner to possible neurologic injury. The results of neurologic examination in a neck contusion should be within normal limits. Any athlete who has an abnormal neurologic examination after direct trauma to the neck should be immobilized and plain radiographs obtained to rule out fracture and/or instability of the cervical spine. In neck contusion, plain radiographs are negative for fractures, dislocations, and instability. The standard treatment should include rest, ice, and/or analgesics as indicated. Because these injuries tend to be benign and self-limited, return to competition is seldom a major concern.

Cervical Strain or Sprain

The cervical strain or sprain syndrome is one of the most commonly encountered injuries of the cervical spine in sports. The athlete presenting with a cervical muscle strain or ligamentous sprain typically complains of a "jamming" or "twisting" injury to the neck followed by pain that is exacerbated by motion. Potential mechanisms of injury may include hyperextension, hyperflexion, lateral flexion, flexion–rotation, extension–rotation, and axial loading. The neck

TABLE 1. *Disorders of the cervical spine in sports*

Neck contusion
Cervical strain or sprain
Nerve root neuropraxia
Spinal cord neuropraxia
Disc disease
Spondylosis
Fracture or dislocation
Epidural hematoma
Neurovascular injury
Spinal deformities

pain tends to be localized without radiation down the upper extremities. The athlete should not experience any weakness or sensory changes (e.g., numbness, tingling, pins and needles) in the upper or lower extremities. Weakness or sensory changes of the upper or lower extremities after injury to the cervical spine should alert the clinician to the possibility of a more serious injury (e.g., cervical fracture, disc herniation).

On examination, the athlete experiencing a cervical strain or sprain may exhibit a painful restricted range of motion of the neck. This may be accompanied by muscle spasms involving the cervical musculature. The athlete should have a negative Spurling sign. A positive Spurling sign is suggestive of cervical nerve root irritation and indicative of a more serious injury to the cervical spine. The neurologic examination should be within normal limits. The athlete should exhibit normal strength and sensation in the upper extremities. Deep tendon reflexes should be physiologic and symmetric. Asymmetric reflexes in the upper extremities are suggestive of a cervical radiculopathy. Hyperactive reflexes in the lower extremities with a positive Babinski sign may be indicative of a myelopathy.

In a cervical strain or sprain, radiologic investigations are within normal limits. Plain radiographs are negative for fracture, dislocation, or cervical instability but may demonstrate straightening of the cervical spine or loss of the normal cervical lordosis. Computed tomography (CT) or magnetic resonance imaging (MRI) is seldom indicated unless a more serious cervical spine injury is suspected.

The management of cervical strain or sprain syndrome is conservative. When a more serious cervical spine injury has been ruled out, the standard treatment should include rest or restriction of activity, cryotherapy for the initial 24 to 48 hours, analgesics or antiinflammatories, and heat. Immobilization with a soft cervical collar may provide temporary relief, but it should not be utilized for long periods of time. Immobilization for longer than 2 weeks may result in atrophy and weakness of the cervical musculature. Once a pain-free full range of motion is achieved, the athlete should participate in a neck strengthening and exercise program. The athlete can return to competition after achieving a painless, spasm-free, full range of motion of the cervical spine.

CERVICAL DISC DISEASE

Both cervical disc degeneration and cervical disc herniation can be encountered in the athlete. Disc degeneration can occur as an isolated entity or be a component of a generalized degenerative process of the cervical spine (i.e., cervical spondylosis). Disc degeneration and subsequent spondylosis occur with minor repetitive trauma to the cervical spine. With prolonged trauma and/or aging the intervertebral disc loses its water content, elasticity, and cushioning ability with resultant disc space narrowing. The mechanics of the spine are then altered, with decreased motion at the involved levels and compensating increased motion and even instability at the adjacent levels (1). As disc degeneration increases, cervical spondylosis develops. Cervical spondylosis represents a spectrum of degenerative and soft tissue (e.g., disc ligaments) changes of the cervical spine (Table 2). Cervical disc herniation can also occur as isolated phenomenon or be associated with cervical spondylosis. In addition, cervical disc herniation may be

TABLE 2. *Cervical spondylosis*

Degenerated disc with or without herniation
Disc space narrowing
Osteophytes (bone spurs or bone ridges)
Vertebral body fusion
Spinal stenosis
Neuroforaminal stenosis
Instability with slight subluxation
Thickening of the ligaments

associated with other forms of neurotrauma to the cervical spine (e.g., fracture, dislocation).

The athlete who presents with an acute disc herniation develops sudden onset of sharp neck pain with or without radiation down the upper extremities. Cervical disc herniation can result from direct trauma to the cervical spine or from a hypertension–hyperflexion (whiplash) type of injury. Cervical disc herniation has also been described in weight lifting after forceful exertion during a lift (2) and in amateur scuba divers secondary to gas microbubbles causing cervical disc degeneration (3). If a cervical disc herniation compresses an exiting nerve root, the athlete may experience a cervical radiculopathy characterized by radicular pain, paresthesias, and/or weakness in an upper extremity. The differential diagnosis of cervical radiculopathy includes focal entrapment neuropathies in the upper extremity, brachial plexopathy, and shoulder disease (Table 3). Symptoms involving both upper extremities and/or the lower extremities after trauma to the cervical spine should alert the clinician to the possibility of a cervical myelopathy. Transient quadriparesis secondary to cervical disc herniation causing a decreased anterior–posterior diameter can also occur (see Chapter 14).

The evaluation of an athlete with cervical disc disease should include a detailed physical and neurologic examination along with the appropriate radiologic and electrophysiologic investigations when indicated. On the general physical examination, the athlete may experience painful

and restricted range of motion of the cervical spine possibly associated with paracervical muscle spasm. Unlike the case of cervical strain or sprain, the athlete may exhibit radicular findings if an exiting cervical nerve root is compromised. The associated motor, sensory, and reflex changes are dependent on the nerve root involved. Neurologic findings associated with selected cervical nerve root injuries are presented in Table 4. The detailed neurologic examination should also determine whether the athlete is experiencing a cervical myelopathy. Neurologic signs of a cervical myelopathy include spasticity, weakness, sensory loss, and/or hyperflexia of the lower extremities (Table 5). Bowel and bladder symptoms may also be a clinical indicator of cervical myelopathy. The acute onset of a cervical myelopathy in an athlete experiencing neck trauma constitutes a medical emergency (see Chapter 11). Any athlete experiencing neck pain with radicular and/or myelopathic symptoms should have plain radiographs obtained to rule out fracture, dislocation, or instability. Cervical disc degeneration with or without herniation may be evidenced as disc space narrowing on plain radiographs. Radiologic confirmation of cervical disc disease is best accomplished by MRI. Although CT scanning can identify disc herniation, it is less sensitive than MRI unless it is performed along with myelography. However, CT scanning does afford the advantage of detecting osseous degenerative changes that may often accompany degenerated or herniated discs. Electrophysiologic testing may provide additional diagnostic information for those suspected of having a radiculopathy and/or myelopathy. Electromyography and nerve conduction studies can confirm the presence of a cervical radiculopathy and rule out peripheral neuropathies of the upper extremities. Somatosensory evoked potential may be useful in supporting the diagnosis of cervical myelopathy (see Chapter 5).

The management of cervical disc disease in the athlete is dependent on the severity of the injury and the extent of neurologic involvement. In the athlete without a fracture, dislocation, or significant neurologic deficit (i.e., progressive radiculopathy and/or myelopathy), conservative therapy should be instituted. The initial manage-

TABLE 3. *Differential diagnosis of cervical radiculopathy*

Focal entrapment neuropathies
  Median nerve
    Pronator syndrome
    Anterior interosseous syndrome
    Carpal tunnel syndrome
  Ulnar nerve
    Cubital tunnel syndrome
    Guyon's canal
  Radial nerve
    Supinator syndrome
  Thoracic outlet syndrome
Brachial plexopathy (e.g., "stinger" or "burner")
Shoulder disease

TABLE 4. *Neurologic examination of cervical nerve roots*

Nerve root	Disc level	Motor	Sensory	Reflex	Comments
C-3	C2-3	Neck muscle weakness	Back of neck	None	Phrenic nerve paralysis if severely involved
C-4	C3-4	Neck muscle weakness	Back of neck	None	Phrenic nerve paralysis if severely involved
C-5	C4-5	Deltoid	Lateral arm	Biceps	Can also test biceps muscle, supraspinatus muscle
C-6	C5-6	Wrist extension	Lateral forearm	Brachioradialis	Wrist extension is not pure C-6
C-7	C6-7	Triceps	Middle finger	Triceps	May also test strength of wrist flexors and finger extensors
C-8	C7-T1	Finger flexors	Medial forearm and little finger	Finger flexor	Painless weakness and atrophy may be the only signs
T-1	T1-2	Interossei	Medial arm	Finger flexor	Incomplete Horner's sign may be present (i.e., miosis and/or ptosis)

ment should include rest and removal from the offending activity, supplemented with anti-inflammatories, analgesics, and/or muscle relaxants. In addition, immobilization utilizing a soft cervical collar may provide rest for the paracervical musculature and limit motion that may exacerbate neck pain. Other modalities such as moist heat, ultrasonography, and transcutaneous nerve stimulation may also provide symptomatic relief. The role of traction in the treatment of cervical disc disease is controversial, and traction is contraindicated in malignancy, cord compression, infection, osteoporosis, and rheumatoid arthritis (4). Most athletes improve with conservative therapy within 6 weeks. For a patient who fails to respond to the treatment approach outlined, trigger point injections with lidocaine or corticosteroid may be helpful in decreasing paravertebral muscle spasm and tenderness.

Indications for surgical intervention in cervical disc disease include intractable pain that fails to resolve with conservative therapy, a significant and/or progressive neurologic deficit, or bowel or bladder symptoms associated with a myelopathy.

Whether an athlete who exhibits a cervical disc herniation should participate in contact or collision sports needs to be addressed on an individual and clinical basis. In general, an athlete who has a disc herniation that is associated with a residual neurologic deficit should not be allowed to compete in a contact or collision sport. Furthermore, a disc herniation that significantly

compromises the anteroposterior diameter of the spinal canal (i.e., abutting or compressing the spinal cord) and is associated with a transient quadriparesis that resolves should also be considered a relative contraindication to participation. In sports in which falls are likely (e.g., equestrian, cycling) athletes with disc herniations associated with a neurologic deficit should be advised concerning potential risks if they were to fall. However, determination concerning participation should be approached on an individual basis and should consider the radiologic,

TABLE 5. *Neurologic signs in cervical myelopathy*

Motor
1. Increased tone or spasticity in the lower extremities
2. Weakness of the lower extremities
3. Ataxia or difficulty controlling lower extremities while walking

Sensory
1. Impaired sensation to pain, light touch, or temperature that may correspond to a level
2. Impaired position and/or vibration in the lower extremities with dorsal column involvement

Reflexes
1. Hyperactive deep tendon reflexes in the lower extremities
2. Hypoactive deep tendon reflexes in the upper extremities if nerve roots are involved (i.e., associated with cervical radiculopathy)
3. Positive Babinski's reflex

Autonomic
1. Bowel or bladder symptoms

neurologic, and sport-specific aspects. Although athletes who undergo a cervical discectomy and single-level fusion are often allowed to return to contact or collision sports, clinical and/or epidemiologic evidence supporting this decision is limited.

CONCLUSION

Soft tissue injuries and cervical disc disease represent the more commonly encountered cervical spine injuries in sports. In the athlete who presents with neck pain, a careful neurologic examination along with the appropriate radiologic investigations must be undertaken to rule out more serious and potentially life-threatening injuries to the cervical spine.

REFERENCES

1. Clark CR. Indications and surgical management of cervical myelopathy. *Semin Spine Surg* 1989;1:254–261.
2. Jordan BD, Istrico R, Zimmerman RD, et al. Acute cervical radiculopathy associated with weightlifting. *Physician Sports Med* 1990;18(1):73–76.
3. Reul J, Weis J, Jung A, et al. Central nervous system lesions and cervical disc herniations in amateur divers. *Lancet* 1995;345:1403–1405.
4. Boden SD, Wiesel SW. Conservative treatment of cervical disc disease. *Semin Spine Surg* 1989;1:229–232.

Sports Neurology, Second Edition,
edited by Barry D. Jordan.
Lippincott–Raven Publishers, Philadelphia © 1998.

13

Fractures and Dislocations of the Cervical Spine

Louis H. Rappoport, *Frank P. Cammisa, Jr., *Patrick F. O'Leary

Arizona Spine Consultants, Ltd., 6036 North 19th Avenue,
Suite 306, Phoenix, Arizona 85015;
*The Hospital For Special Surgery, 535 East 70th Street, New York, New York 10021

Although cervical spine fractures and dislocations are relatively uncommon in athletes, they represent a significant proportion of athletic injuries producing permanent disability. Consequently, the sports medicine physician must acquire a comprehensive understanding of potential athletic cervical spine injuries. A thorough comprehension of cervical spine anatomy and biomechanical considerations that govern these injuries provides the key components of the knowledge base. This core information can then be used for mastering the principles and guidelines for diagnostic evaluation and treatment of specific injury patterns. In addition, as athletic participation continues to increase, additional objective data concerning the epidemiology and biomechanics of cervical spine injuries are available for analysis. The availability of this information has made it possible to establish principles and guidelines for the prevention of athletic cervical spine injuries.

EPIDEMIOLOGY

Epidemiologic analysis of athletic cervical spine injuries can be useful in detecting specific injury trends and may identify associated risk factors. The data can be used to institute proper training and educational programs for athletes and team personnel. In addition, sports-specific rules and equipment modifications can be implemented after analysis of this information in order to limit the incidence of serious cervical spine injuries. For example, after the implementation of rules changes in football, the National Football Head and Neck Injury Registry reported a dramatic reduction in cervical spine injuries resulting in permanent quadriplegia [1].

Cervical spine injuries have been reported in many sporting activities, including football, gymnastics, rugby, trampoline jumping, ice hockey, racquet sports, water sports, skiing, snowmobiling, automobile racing, motorcycle racing, mountain climbing, horseback riding, skydiving, hang gliding, parachuting, and track and field events [1–19]. Contact sports, high-speed sports, and sports associated with unpredictable variables (i.e., skydiving) have been correlated with the greatest risk for cervical spine injury.

A review of retrospective studies yields an incidence of spinal injuries in sports of 5% to 15%. However, the limitations of these studies tend to decrease the reported incidence. There is a tendency to underreport athletic cervical spine injuries for three reasons. First, the overwhelming majority of spinal injuries are self-limited and do not come to the attention of health care personnel. Second, most athletes are reluctant to report minor injuries to team personnel. Third, many athletic injuries occur in the practice setting, when health care personnel may not be present [20]. In a prospective study evaluating head and neck injuries in college football players between 1975 and 1982, 18% of players reported sustaining a neck injury (2). Although the majority of these injuries were reported as minor (55%), the remaining 45% experienced at least transient neurologic symptoms or deficits. In a prospective investigation of permanent cervical cord injuries in football between 1977 and 1989, Cantu and Mueller (5) reported an injury incidence of 0.62 per 100,000 in junior high and high school players and 1.64 per 100,000 in college players.

DIAGNOSIS AND TREATMENT OF ACUTE CERVICAL SPINE FRACTURES AND DISLOCATIONS

In the treatment of cervical spine injuries, the key principles are prevention of further neurologic injury and rapid relief of any spinal cord compression. In cases in which spinal deformity is present, early controlled realignment may result in satisfactory neural element decompression. Skeletal traction (i.e., Gardner-Wells tong or halo traction) is commonly used for realignment of the cervical spine. After realignment, specific surgical methods can be utilized for decompression of persistent mechanical compression of the spinal cord. Surgical treatment may require an anterior, posterior, or combined approach, depending on the nature and location of the pathology. In cases in which satisfactory realignment has been achieved and there is no radiographic evidence of persistent significant neural element compression, the patient can be temporarily immobilized in traction or a halo vest. In these situations, further specific treatment (operative versus nonoperative) depends on the pathologic diagnosis. If spinal realignment is not successful, urgent open reduction and stabilization may be required to achieve neural element decompression.

The majority of athletic cervical spine injuries are relatively minor and respond favorably to nonoperative treatment. However, the physician must be cognizant of injuries that require more aggressive management. In general, the indications for surgical treatment are (a) neurologic deficit secondary to neural element compres-

sion, (b) instability, and/or (c) significant spinal deformity.

UPPER CERVICAL SPINE INJURIES

Atlantooccipital Dislocation

Injuries at the atlantooccipital junction are rare in athletes, but may occur in situations of high-speed trauma (Fig. 1). The majority of these injuries are fatal because of neurologic compromise and resultant respiratory arrest. If the patient should survive, urgent controlled realignment and halo vest immobilization should initially be performed. The use of cervical traction is contraindicated in the management of these highly unstable injuries, because of the significant risk of distraction of neural tissues. When the patient is stabilized, posterior occipitocervical fusion (occiput to C-1 or C-2) is recommended as the definitive treatment for these pure ligamentous injuries.

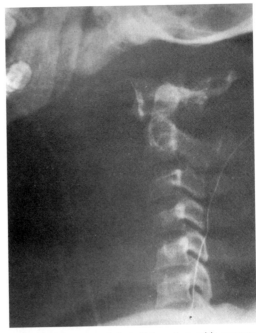

FIG. 1. Atlantooccipital dislocation with severe displacement. (From *OKU sports medicine.* Rosemont, IL: American Academy of Orthopaedic Surgeons, 1994, Fig. 6, p. 279.)

C-1 Fractures

Fractures of the atlas (C-1) can be divided into four types: (a) anterior arch fracture or avulsion, (b) posterior arch fracture, (c) lateral mass fracture, and (d) burst (Jefferson's) fracture. The predominant mechanism of injury resulting in these fractures is axial compressive loading, which forces the occipital condyles into the lateral masses of C-1. Symptoms associated with C-1 fractures include neck pain and headaches. Resultant neurologic injuries are rare, as these are decompressive injuries. Visualization of these fractures can be difficult with conventional radiographs. Plain tomography and/or computed tomography (CT) may be necessary for complete diagnostic evaluation of the fracture pattern. An open-mouth odontoid view should be utilized for the evaluation of potential C-1 lateral mass displacement.

Secondary forces (shear, flexion, extension, and/or rotation) contribute to the specific injury pattern. Because of the presence of these secondary forces, the radiographic evaluation should be carefully scrutinized to rule out associated contiguous or noncontiguous cervical spine injuries. In patients with posterior arch fractures, approximately 50% have an associated cervical spine injury (21). The most common associated injuries are posteriorly displaced odontoid fractures and traumatic spondylolisthesis of the axis (C-2).

Fractures of the anterior arch of C-1 generally result from avulsion of the longus colli muscle(s). These injuries are stable and can be managed with a rigid cervical orthosis. Isolated posterior arch fractures are also considered to be stable injuries and can be treated with a rigid orthosis or halo vest, generally for 3 months. As noted previously, associated cervical spine injuries are relatively common with posterior arch fractures and may take priority in the treatment of these patients.

Unilateral fractures of the lateral mass of C-1 are usually limited to one side of the neural arch. However, an additional posterior arch fracture on the contralateral side has been reported (21). Asymmetric displacement of the affected lateral mass can be visualized on the open-mouth radiograph.

A burst (Jefferson's) fracture of C-1 represents combined anterior and posterior arch fractures on both sides of the neural arch. This fracture pattern usually occurs as a result of a pure axial loading force on the cervical spine. Most commonly, the open-mouth radiograph reveals symmetric displacement of the lateral masses. Spence et al. (22) have shown that a total lateral mass displacement greater that 6.9 mm indicates concomitant rupture of the transverse ligament. The clinical significance of associated transverse ligament insufficiency with regard to the development of C1-2 instability is debatable. In a clinical evaluation of atlas fractures, Levine and Edwards (21) reported that late C1-2 instability did not seem to occur in patients with associated transverse ligament insufficiency, regardless of whether lateral mass reduction was achieved. In their investigation, no patient was noted to have an atlantodens interval (ADI) greater than 5 mm on flexion–extension radiographs after fracture healing. The authors hypothesized that the secondary soft tissue stabilizing structures (i.e., the alar ligaments) remain intact in patients with this injury pattern, precluding the development of gross C1-2 instability.

The need for reduction of lateral mass displacement remains uncertain. The development of posttraumatic C1-2 facet arthrosis has not been definitively correlated with the presence or absence of residual lateral mass displacement (23). Thus, painful nonunions and malunions of atlas fractures appear to occur, but specific risk factors have yet to be established.

The majority of lateral mass and Jefferson's fractures can be effectively treated with halo vest immobilization until fracture healing, generally within 3 months. Fracture healing can be assessed using CT or plain tomography. After fracture healing, dynamic flexion–extension lateral radiographs should be obtained to rule out significant C1-2 instability. In patients with significant lateral mass displacement (>7 mm), skeletal traction can be utilized to achieve lateral mass reduction, if desired. Continuous axial traction for a minimum of 6 weeks is necessary to maintain reduction, as a halo vest cannot provide satisfactory cervical spine distraction. When early fracture healing has been documented, these patients can be immobilized in a halo vest until definitive fracture union. Alternatively, surgical reconstruction of fractures with significant lateral mass displacement can be performed. This technique employs anterior reduction and plate fixation via a transoral approach and allows preservation of rotation at the C1-2 motion segment (24).

The management of patients who develop chronic C1-2 instability requires careful assessment of the status of the posterior arch fracture(s). If a solid union of the posterior arch fracture(s) has been achieved with halo vest immobilization, a posterior C1-2 arthrodesis is recommended. If the posterior arch fracture(s) has not healed, the options for surgical management include (a) posterior occiput-C2 arthrodesis, (b) posterior C1-2 transarticular screw fixation (Magerl technique) (25), and (c) transoral anterior C1-2 reduction and plate fixation (24). The latter two techniques preserve motion at the occipitocervical motion segment. They can be used as the initial treatment for the rare patient who presents with C1-2 instabil-

ity at acute fracture presentation. It should be emphasized that these latter procedures are technically demanding and require proper training before their clinical use.

Atlantoaxial Instability Without Fracture

The atlantoaxial ligamentous complex (transverse, apical, and alar ligaments) can rupture without concomitant fracture, resulting in atlantoaxial instability. These pure ligamentous injuries can occur after severe flexion loads to the cervical spine. A significant increase in the ADI on lateral flexion–extension radiographs confirms the diagnosis (Fig. 2). The ADI is normally less than 3 mm in adults or less than 4 mm in children. The transverse ligament has been shown to rupture in the ADI range of 3 to 5 mm. An ADI greater than 5 mm is indicative of insufficiency of the remaining atlantoaxial ligamentous complex (26). Athletes with preexisting rheumatoid arthritis or connective tissue disease

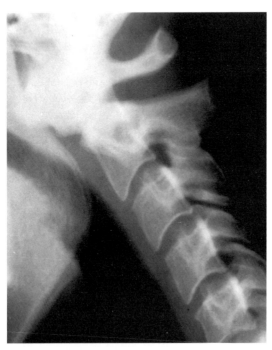 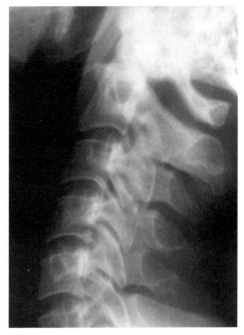

FIG. 2. Atlantoaxial instability. Flexion lateral radiograph (*left*) and extension lateral radiograph (*right*) revealing dynamic C1-2 instability. (From *OKU sports medicine.* Rosemont, IL: American Academy of Orthopaedic Surgeons, 1994, Fig. 7, p. 280.)

may be at increased risk for this injury, as less force may be required to produce injury. Spinal cord injury can result from odontoid process compression of the cord against the posterior arch of C-1. Fortunately, neurologic injury is rare, as there is a large space available for the cord at the C1-2 level. As these are pure ligamentous injuries, surgical stabilization is required. Stabilization can be achieved via a posterior C1-2 fusion, most commonly utilizing a wire construct.

C1-2 Rotatory Subluxation

Atlantoaxial rotatory subluxation is seen most commonly in children; however, it may also occur in adults. Spontaneous occurrence has been reported in children after an upper respiratory infection, or it may result from trauma. This injury is rarely reported in athletes. The mechanism of injury is theorized as being combined distraction and axial rotation, which results in subluxation of the lateral C1-2 facet articulation. These patients generally present with a painful torticollis and have extreme apprehension upon attempted range of motion of the neck. In chronic cases, the facet subluxation can become fixed in a nonanatomic position. Associated neurologic injury rarely occurs.

Atlantoaxial rotatory subluxation has been classified into four types, depending on the severity and direction of C-1 displacement and the presence and severity of associated increase in the ADI (27). Many of these injuries are missed on initial radiographic screening. The open-mouth radiograph usually demonstrates a "wink" sign, defined as overriding of the C1-2 facet articulation on the side of subluxation, with the contralateral joint appearing normal. Flexion–extension lateral radiographs should be obtained for ADI evaluation. The fixed association of the C1-2 articulation can be readily demonstrated utilizing dynamic CT scans in the left and right axial rotation positions.

In children, acute injuries are generally managed successfully with a brief course of cervical traction, followed by collar immobilization. In adults, acute injuries can usually be reduced with skeletal traction. If reduction is successful, halo vest immobilization for 8 to 12 weeks is recommended. If closed reduction is not possible in acute cases, open reduction and posterior C1-2 arthrodesis are required. Posterior C1-2 fusion is also recommended for recurrent deformities, injuries associated with significant C1-2 instability (ADI > 5 mm), and in all cases in which a concomitant neurologic deficit is present. Transoral direct anterior reduction and C1-2 plate fixation have also been proposed for the treatment of irreducible or unstable injuries (24). Closed reduction with traction is frequently unsuccessful in cases of chronic subluxation (>3 months), and fusion is generally required for pain relief.

Odontoid Fractures

Fractures of the odontoid process have been classified by Anderson and D'Alonzo (28) into three types on the basis of fracture location. Type 1 fractures represent a ligamentous avulsion (alar ligaments) of the tip of the odontoid process, type 2 fractures occur through the neck of the odontoid process, and type 3 fractures occur at the base of the odontoid and extend into the body of C-2. In addition, odontoid fractures should be assessed for the severity of displacement and angulation at the fracture site. Diagnosis is often possible on evaluation of plain radiographs, including an open-mouth view. The prevertebral soft tissues at the C-2 level should be carefully evaluated on the lateral radiograph, as abnormal widening represents an indirect sign of injury. In some cases, tomography (plain or CT) may be necessary to confirm the diagnosis and to determine the fracture pattern. Radiographs should also be evaluated for the presence of a concomitant posterior arch fracture of C-1, because if this is present, alteration of the treatment plan may be necessary.

Type 1 fractures are rare injuries and are considered stable, as they occur cephalad to the intact transverse ligament. However, lateral flexion–extension radiographs should always be obtained to rule out definitively significant C1-2 instability. These injuries can be treated symptomatically with a cervical collar.

Type 2 fractures represent the most common fracture of the odontoid process. These fractures can result from hyperextension, flexion, rotation, or lateral forces, in variable combinations. In general, the treatment of these fractures remains controversial, because of the increased risk for nonunion with this fracture pattern. Overall, type 2 fractures have a nonunion rate of 15% to 85%, even in the presence of adequate immobilization. Risk factors for nonunion include age greater than 50 years, displacement greater than 5 mm, posterior (versus anterior) displacement, and improper treatment (i.e., halo vest overdistraction) (29–31). In a multicenter investigation, Clark and White (32) reported a 68% nonunion rate for type 2 fractures treated with halo vest immobilization. In the same study, type 2 fractures with more than 10° of angulation or more than 5 mm of translation managed by surgical stabilization achieved a significantly greater union rate.

In athletes without risk factors for nonunion, initial management can consist of halo vest immobilization in a reduced position for 12 weeks. Fracture healing and stability can then be assessed with tomography and flexion–extension lateral radiographs. Nonunions of type 2 odontoid fractures can be effectively managed with a posterior C1-2 arthrodesis. Athletes with significant risk factors for nonunion can be considered for primary C1-2 fusion in the acute setting.

Wire constructs are most commonly utilized for posterior C1-2 stabilization. Newer techniques have been recommended that preserve axial rotation at the C1-2 motion segment. These include direct anterior odontoid screw fixation (30,33) and transoral reduction and plate fixation (R. Louis, personal communication, 1993). These newer techniques are particularly useful in cases in which a concomitant posterior arch fracture of C-1 is present. In this situation, the use of a standard C1-2 wire construct is precluded, unless the posterior arch fracture achieved solid union during initial halo vest management. The transarticular C1-2 fusion technique of Magerl (25,34) has also been recommended for the treatment of specific injury patterns.

Type 3 fractures generally have a high rate of union, as they extend into the cancellous bone of the C-2 body. They can be managed effectively with halo vest immobilization for 12 weeks. Impacted, nondisplaced type 3 fractures can al-

ternatively be treated in a rigid cervical orthosis. Follow-up radiographic evaluation should be routinely performed to assess for fracture union and stability.

Traumatic Spondylolisthesis of C-2

Traumatic spondylolisthesis of the axis is most commonly known as a hangman's fracture. These injuries may occur in athletes participating in many sports activities, including football, ice hockey, gymnastics, high-speed racing, and aquatic and equestrian sports. These bipedicular fractures are usually diagnosed on a routine lateral radiograph, where significant anterior translation of C-2 on C-3, including complete facet dislocation, can be present in some cases. Tomography can be helpful in the assessment of complex fracture patterns. The severity of instability can be assessed on supervised flexion–extension lateral radiographs in the awake, intact patient. Neurologic injury related to the fracture is uncommon but may be seen in some cases with associated C2-3 facet dislocation. The modification of the Effendi classification by Levine and Edwards (35) classifies these injuries into four fracture types.

Type I fractures are nondisplaced or have less than 3 mm of C2-3 translation present. There is no associated angulation with this fracture type. Combined hyperextension and axial loading is theorized to be the mechanism of injury (35). As there is no significant ligamentous injury, these fractures are considered stable, and most patients achieve successful union after orthotic immobilization for approximately 3 months.

Type II fractures have both significant translation (>3 mm) and angulation. A two-stage mechanism of injury has been hypothesized for this fracture type. An initial hyperextension-loading force results in a longitudinal fracture through the neural arch and is subsequently followed by secondary flexion and compression forces (35). These secondary forces act to disrupt the C2-3 disc space and posterior longitudinal ligament. The anterior longitudinal ligament remains intact. Initial treatment consists of fracture reduction using halo traction (10 to 20 pounds) with the neck in a slightly extended position. The intact anterior longitudinal ligament prevents overdistraction at the C2-3 segment. Further treatment is guided by the severity of initial fracture translational displacement. In patients with moderately displaced fractures (3 to 6 mm of initial translation), halo vest immobilization can be utilized until fracture union, generally in 2 to 3 months. This treatment approach yields successful results in the majority of these cases. Patients with severely displaced fractures (>6 mm of initial translation) should ideally be maintained in traction for 4 to 6 weeks to allow early fracture union in the reduced position, as early mobilization in a halo vest often results in a significant loss of fracture reduction and a resultant higher nonunion rate. Once early fracture union has been documented, halo-vest immobilization can be utilized until complete fracture union (3 months total) (36).

Type IIA fractures have radiographic evidence of significant angulation but minimal translational displacement. The hypothesized mechanism of injury is flexion and distraction (35). These fractures represent a variant of the type II fracture, with the line of fracture being more oblique and posterior, in a position just anterior to the facet joints. The use of traction in the treatment of this injury pattern is contraindicated, as it may result in a significant increase in angulation and widening of the posterior disc space. These fractures should be treated with immediate halo vest immobilization, utilizing gentle axial compression for fracture reduction. Fracture union generally occurs after 3 months of halo vest immobilization.

Type III fractures have radiographic evidence of severe angulation and translation, in association with a unilateral or bilateral C2-3 facet dislocation. These injuries result from flexion-compression forces. As these fractures have the potential for severe deformity and instability, associated neurologic injuries are more commonly present. As the facets are often "free floating," closed reduction may be unsuccessful. However, if closed reduction is achieved, it may be unstable. Therefore, open reduction and stabilization are usually required. Current stabilization alternatives include (a) posterior C2-3 oblique wiring with adjuvant halo vest immobilization and (b) posterior C-2 screw compression osteosyn-

thesis of the bipedicular component (Judet technique) in combination with plate fixation for stabilization of the C2-3 segment (37–39). The latter technique utilizes lateral mass screw fixation in C-3 and generally provides rigid fixation, obviating the need for halo vest immobilization.

MIDDLE CERVICAL SPINE INJURIES

Athletic cervical spine injuries at the C3-4 level are rare. However, they appear to be distinctly different from injuries occurring in other regions of the cervical spine. In evaluating 25 cases of C3-4 injuries in football players, Torg et al. (40) reported the following significant findings: (a) a predominance of ligamentous and intervertebral disc injuries versus bone injuries, (b) a greater association of transient quadriplegia with an acute disc herniation, (c) increased difficulty in achieving successful closed reduction of unilateral or bilateral facet dislocations with skeletal traction, and (d) favorable neurologic recovery after early, aggressive management. Specific treatment of these injuries is otherwise similar to that recommended for other regions of the cervical spine.

LOWER CERVICAL SPINE INJURIES

Injuries of the lower cervical spine segments differ from those occurring in the upper cervical spine, as there is a decreasing ratio of canal diameter to cord diameter, increasing the risk of a concomitant neurologic injury. Injury patterns include (a) avulsion fractures, (b) compression fractures, (c) facet injuries (subluxation/dislocation and/or fracture), (d) vertebral body burst fractures, and (e) teardrop fractures. All patients must be carefully evaluated for the presence of instability, spinal deformity, and/or neural element compression.

Avulsion Injuries

Spinous process ("clay shoveler's") fractures have been reported in power lifters and football players (8,11). These fractures most commonly occur at the C-7 level. Although several mechanisms of injury have been proposed for these fractures, most clinicians feel that spinous process avulsion fractures occur as a result of a sudden contracture of the trapezius and rhomboid muscles. Alternatively, avulsion of a spinous process can result from a sudden, severe flexion force, with resultant force transmission through the supraspinous and interspinous ligaments. Isolated spinous process fractures are stable injuries and are effectively managed with a cervical orthosis for symptomatic treatment.

Another type of avulsion injury is represented by the extension teardrop fracture. In this case, there is an avulsion of the anteroinferior corner of the vertebral body by the anterior longitudinal ligament at its insertion point. The mechanism of injury is a sudden hyperextension force. Although extension teardrop fractures most commonly occur at C-2, they can also occur in the lower cervical spine. Associated disc disruption can occur at the time of initial injury and may lead to late segmental disc degeneration. Treatment consists of brief symptomatic immobilization in a cervical collar.

Compression Fractures

Compression fractures of the lower cervical spine are characterized by loss of anterior vertebral body height to a variable degree. Although the middle spinal column must remain intact, there may be associated posterior column ligamentous insufficiency in more severe fractures. Complete diagnostic radiographic evaluation may include flexion–extension lateral views, CT scan, and/or magnetic resonance imaging (MRI) studies of the cervical spine. These studies also help to rule out associated injuries. The presence and severity of instability can be analyzed using established radiographic parameters (41).

In cases of isolated fractures with less than 25% loss of anterior vertebral body height, treatment can consist of orthotic immobilization, as these are considered stable injuries. In fractures with greater than 50% loss of anterior vertebral body height, there is often an associated tensile failure of the posterior ligamentous complex. As a result, significant segmental instability may be present. MRI is particularly useful in evaluating for the presence of posterior soft tissue disruption in these cases. If significant segmental instability

is present, operative stabilization and fusion are required, because of the unpredictable nature of healing of the posterior injury. In the majority of cases, surgical stabilization can be performed utilizing segmental spinous process wiring. However, in the presence of a concomitant posterior element fracture (spinous process, lamina, and/or facet), spinous process wiring and fusion of an adjacent normal motion segment are usually required. Although alternative wiring techniques (e.g., oblique wire stabilization) can be used in this setting, the procedure of choice appears to be posterior fusion with lateral mass screws and plate fixation. The latter procedure restricts the fusion to the involved segmental level (37,39). In athletes with severe compression, concomitant anterior column reconstruction may be necessary to prevent possible failure of the posterior stabilization construct.

Facet Joint Injuries

Injuries of the articular facets can be divided into subluxations or dislocations, fractures, or combination injuries. Facet injuries can occur either unilaterally or bilaterally. Neurologic deficits can be associated with all facet injury patterns, ranging from single-root deficits to spinal cord injury.

Isolated unilateral and bilateral facet dislocations are pure ligamentous injuries, anatomically representing disruption of the supraspinous ligament, interspinous ligament, ligamentum flavum, and facet capsule(s). The basic diagnosis can generally be made from a routine lateral radiograph of the cervical spine. However, plain tomography, CT scan, and MRI evaluation may be helpful in demonstrating concomitant fractures and the severity of soft tissue injury. MRI is particularly useful in evaluating for the presence of a concomitant disc herniation, which may be seen in association with facet subluxations or dislocations, more commonly in the setting of bilateral injuries (42). The treating physician must be aware of the possibility of associated disc herniation, as spinal reduction maneuvers can result in further disc extrusion and resultant neurologic injury.

Unilateral facet dislocations occur as a result of a combination of flexion–rotation and axial compressive loading. Radiographically, this results in approximately 25% vertebral body subluxation, as visualized on the lateral projection. In addition, the lateral radiograph may reveal a "perched" facet or complete facet dislocation, with the latter having a radiographic appearance resembling a bow tie (43).

The mechanism of injury for bilateral facet dislocations is severe flexion and axial loading. As in unilateral facet dislocations, this may result in perched facets or complete facet dislocations. On the lateral radiograph, there is noted to be approximately 50% vertebral body subluxation at the injured segment. Because of the greater degree of subluxation with these injuries, neurologic deficits are more commonly present than with unilateral dislocations.

The treatment of facet dislocations remains controversial. Because of the significant risk of concomitant disc herniation, many clinicians argue that all of these patients should undergo routine myelographic or MRI evaluation of the cervical spine before attempted closed or open reduction. Although this approach appears to be ideal, there are inherent technical, logistic, and financial issues raised by this plan of treatment. Eismont et al. (42) have outlined a reasonable approach for the management of these patients. All patients should initially be placed in skeletal traction. For patients who are neurologically intact, skeletal traction up to a maximum of 50 pounds can be applied for attempted closed reduction, utilizing careful radiographic and neurologic monitoring. If successful closed reduction is achieved and the neurologic status is unchanged, the patient can be placed in temporary halo vest immobilization, and an MRI can be performed to rule out disc herniation before definitive surgical treatment. If there is no evidence of disc herniation, segmental posterior stabilization and fusion are recommended, as these are ligamentous injuries and sufficient healing is unpredictable. Stabilization with spinous process wiring is sufficient in most cases. In cases in which there is radiographic evidence of a concomitant disc herniation, anterior cervical discectomy and fusion should be performed before posterior stabilization (Fig. 3). Some clinicians have recommended a pure anterior treatment approach for the latter

group of patients, utilizing plate fixation for stabilization (44,45). However, the use of anterior stabilization for the treatment of a posterior injury pattern remains controversial at this time.

In cases in which closed reduction is difficult, an urgent MRI should be obtained to rule out concomitant disc herniation. If there is no evidence of disc herniation, treatment can proceed with posterior open reduction and stabilization. If a disc herniation is found, anterior discectomy and fusion are performed before posterior open reduction and stabilization. In addition, Eismont et al. (42) recommend immediate MRI evaluation of patients who present with a significant neurologic deficit, as well as those who develop worsening symptoms or progressive neurologic deficit during attempted closed reduction.

Facet fractures may present to the clinician as isolated injuries, but they more commonly occur in association with facet dislocations or other cervical spine injuries. Facet fractures may be either unilateral or bilateral in location. These fractures can often be visualized on lateral and oblique cervical spine radiographs, although CT imaging (with sagittal reconstruction) and/or conventional tomography can be obtained for diagnostic evaluation and treatment planning (Fig. 4).

Neurologic deficits can be seen in association with unilateral facet fractures. These can range from isolated nerve root deficits to spinal cord syndromes. Although reduction of unilateral facet fractures can generally be achieved with traction, significant residual rotational instability necessitates posterior surgical stabilization and fusion in most cases. Many clinicians have recommended oblique segmental wiring for stabilization of these injuries, as this provides greater resistance to rotational forces than standard spinous process wiring techniques. Alternatively, posterior stabilization using lateral mass screws and plate fixation provides excellent stability and has been recommended by some investigators (37–39).

As with unilateral facet fractures, bilateral facet fractures are usually diagnosed in association with dislocations or other injury patterns. In these patients, the severity of instability depends on the fracture location. Fractures occurring at the base of the superior facets result in a loss of the posterior bony buttress and consequently allow significant segmental translation and potential neural element compression. Fractures that are restricted to the extreme apical portion of the superior facets generally preserve some stability via the remaining portion of the bony facet buttress. Inferior facet fractures generally occur at the base and less commonly result in a neurologic deficit. The management of bilateral facet fractures is similar to that used for unilateral facet fractures.

Vertebral Body Burst Fractures

Vertebral body burst fractures occur as a result of severe axial compressive loading, usually in combination with secondary hyperflexion forces. Anatomically, these injuries are characterized by a comminuted fracture of the posterior vertebral body, or middle spinal column, which usually results in variable bone retropulsion into the spinal canal. Posterior ligamentous disruption and/or posterior element fractures are often associated with this injury pattern and may result in significant segmental kyphosis. As a result of the canal encroachment and spinal deformity, spinal cord injury is often present in these patients, ranging from complete to incomplete deficits.

The initial diagnosis of a burst fracture can generally be established from evaluation of the plain radiographs. However, additional radiographic techniques are needed to define fully the pathologic anatomy. The CT scan provides detailed analysis of the bone elements and evaluates the extent of spinal canal compromise. MRI is utilized to assess the severity of neural element compression, posterior ligamentous injury, and parenchymal spinal cord injury (Fig. 5).

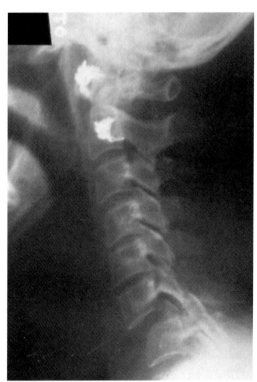
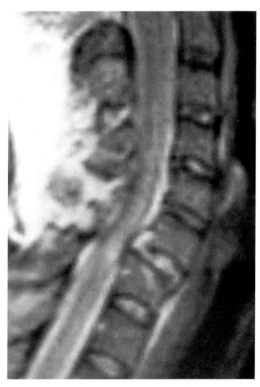

A   B

FIG. 3. Bilateral facet dislocation with concomitant disc herniation. **A:** Lateral radiograph reveals bilateral C6-7 facet dislocation. **B:** Magnetic resonance image showing associated C6-7 disc herniation. The patient underwent an initial anterior cervical decompression and fusion, followed by posterior fusion with wire stabilization.

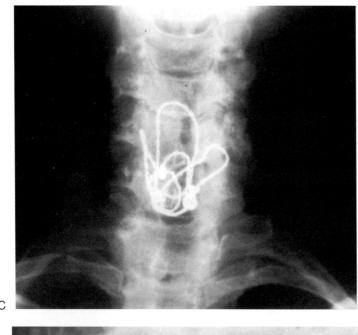

C

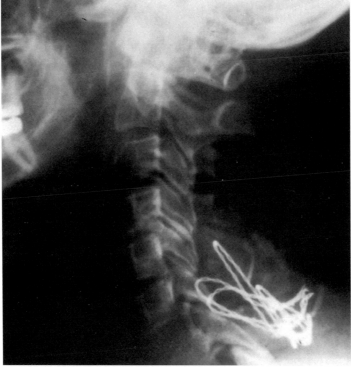

D

FIG. 3. Anteroposterior (**C**) and lateral (**D**) postoperative radiographs illustrating combined anterior and posterior stabilization and fusion. (From *OKU sports medicine.* Rosemont, IL: American Academy of Orthopaedic Surgeons, 1994, Fig. 8, p. 284.)

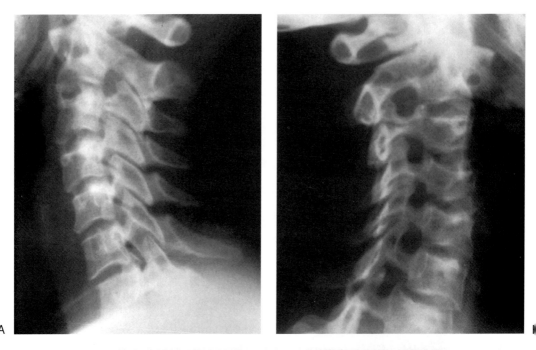

A

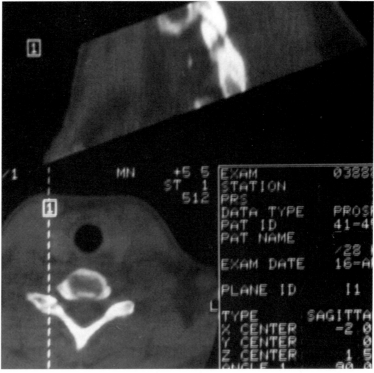

C

FIG. 4. C6-7 unilateral facet fracture. Lateral **(A)** and oblique **(B)** radiographs reveal unilateral facet fracture at C6-7 with foraminal encroachment. **C:** Axial computed tomographic scan with sagittal reconstruction visualize the fractured facet. (From Nicholas JA, Hershman EB, eds. *The lower extremity and spine in sports medicine.* St. Louis, MO: Mosby, 1995: vol 2, Fig. 50-14, p. 1129.)

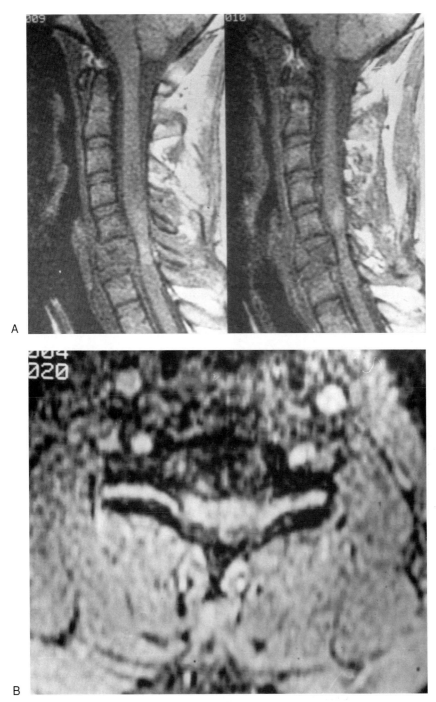

FIG. 5. C-6 burst fracture. Sagittal **(A)** and axial **(B)** magnetic resonance images reveal vertebral body comminution and bony retropulsion into the spinal canal, with resultant spinal cord compression. Increased signal intensity within the spinal cord (sagittal view) is indicative of intrinsic spinal cord injury. (From Nicholas JA, Hershman EB, eds. *The lower extremity and spine in sports medicine.* St. Louis, MO: Mosby, 1995: vol 2, Fig. 50-15, p. 1130.)

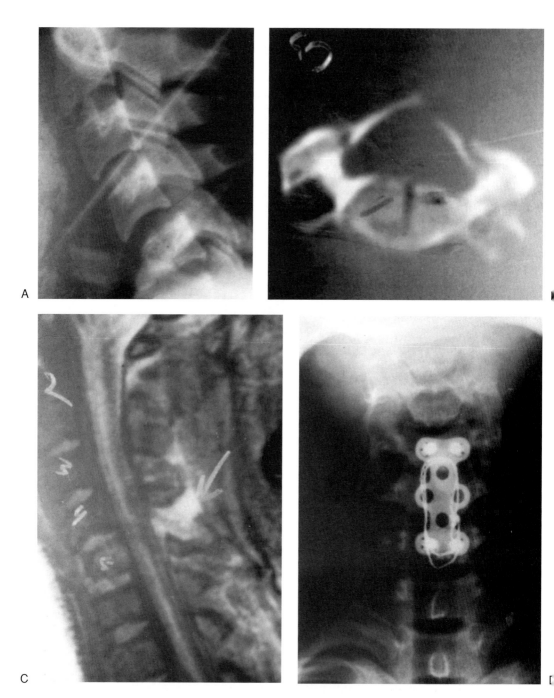

FIG. 6. C-5 teardrop fracture. **A:** Lateral radiograph showing a displaced fracture of the anteroinferior portion of the C-5 vertebral body with mild retrolisthesis of the posteroinferior portion of C-5. Widening of the C4-5 interspinous process distance is apparent. **B:** Axial computed tomographic scan reveals a sagittally oriented fracture of the vertebral body and posterior element fractures. **C:** Sagittal magnetic resonance imaging reveals C4-5 posterior ligamentous disruption. The patient underwent an anterior cervical decompression and fusion with unicortical plate fixation, followed by a posterior fusion with wire stabilization. Anteroposterior **(D)** and lateral **(E)** postoperative radiographs showing the combined anterior and posterior stabilization and fusion. (From Nicholas JA, Hershman EB, eds. *The lower extremity and spine in sports medicine.* St. Louis, MO: Mosby, 1995: vol 2, Fig. 50-16, p. 1131.)

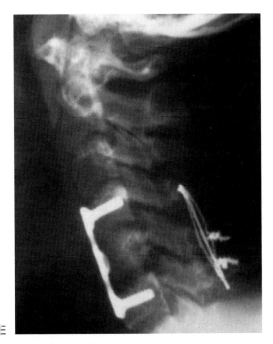

FIG. 6. *Continued.*

As these are severe destabilizing injuries, adjuvant anterior plate fixation is recommended to augment stabilization (44,45). Some investigators have recommended anterior reconstruction and plate stabilization as the sole procedure in patients with associated posterior ligamentous insufficiency, but this treatment approach remains controversial. In a biomechanical analysis of cervical spine internal fixation techniques, anterior plate fixation did not result in adequate stabilization of flexion-type injuries associated with posterior ligamentous disruption (46). Therefore, even with the use of anterior plate fixation, additional posterior stabilization is recommended in most cases. Interspinous process wire fixation achieves secure stabilization in most cases, provided the posterior bone elements are intact. In patients who have associated spinous process or lamina fractures, lateral mass screws and plate fixation provide excellent spinal stability while limiting the fusion to the injured level(s) (37,39,47).

After completion of the clinical assessment, athletes can initially be placed in skeletal traction. This may not only yield significant spinal realignment but may also result in decompression of the spinal canal by way of ligamentotaxis of the retropulsed bone fragments. Once traction is in effect, an MRI can be obtained to evaluate for the presence and severity of residual canal encroachment. If there is no evidence of residual neural element compression and spinal realignment has been successful, patients can be temporarily immobilized in traction or a halo vest, with surgical stabilization performed when feasible. If residual canal compromise is present and there is an associated incomplete neurologic deficit, urgent anterior surgical decompression is required.

Most burst fractures represent unstable three-column injuries, and therefore combined anterior and posterior surgical stabilization and fusion is recommended for the treatment of these injuries. The initial stage consists of anterior corpectomy with spinal canal decompression. This is performed with the patient maintained in skeletal traction. Reconstruction of the anterior and middle spinal columns can be achieved using tricortical iliac crest or fibula strut grafts.

Teardrop Fractures

These fractures represent three-column injuries and are characterized by (a) a displaced fracture of the anteroinferior corner of the superior vertebral body, (b) segmental disc disruption, and (c) posterior ligamentous injury or fracture. Retrolisthesis of the posteroinferior portion of the involved vertebral body generally occurs, and this results in variable degrees of neural element compression. As a result, there is a relatively high incidence of neurologic deficit, ranging from root injuries to complete spinal cord injuries (48). These injuries result from severe flexion–axial loading forces.

The diagnostic evaluation and treatment are similar to those used for burst fractures. Combined anterior and posterior stabilization and fusion is recommended in most cases, as these fractures represent grossly unstable injuries (Fig. 6).

Lamina Fractures

Fractures of the lamina generally occur in association with other major cervical spine injuries (e.g., burst fractures). On a rare basis, fractures of the lamina can occur as isolated injuries, resulting from extension–axial loading forces. In cases in which a lamina fracture is visualized or suspected, a comprehensive radiographic assessment is indicated to rule out concomitant injuries. In patients with isolated lamina fractures without evidence of neural element compression and/or instability, treatment consists of rigid orthotic immobilization until fracture healing (6 to 8 weeks). Flexion–extension lateral radiographs should be obtained after fracture healing to rule out instability.

Lateral Mass Fractures

Fractures of the lateral mass represent a complete separation of the lateral mass from the involved vertebral body and thereby result in disruption of the facet joints directly above and below the involved vertebra (Fig. 7) (49). These fractures also generally occur in association with other cervical spine injuries (e.g., facet dislocation) but on occasion can be present as isolated injuries. An associated vertebral artery injury may rarely be present, as the fracture plane may course through the transverse foramen. As lateral mass fractures result in significant instability, surgical reduction, stabilization, and fusion are mandatory. Utilizing a posterior approach, the involved lateral mass can be reduced under direct vision before stabilization. Traditionally, interspinous process wire stabilization of the adjacent segments has been recommended for the treatment of these injuries. However, lateral mass plate fixation may be the best approach, as the intermediate screw can be used to stabilize the fractured lateral mass (39). Associated injuries may require combined anterior–posterior surgical treatment.

MAJOR LIGAMENTOUS INJURIES

The posterior ligamentous complex can be disrupted as a result of severe axial compression–flexion injuries to the cervical spine. This may result in significant segmental instability. Radiographically, segmental spinous process widening is present, associated with a variable degree of translation and/or angulation at the injured level. In some cases, instability may be detected only on dynamic lateral flexion–extension radographs, thus supporting the need for dynamic radiographs in the trauma setting (Fig. 8). Investigators have established radiographic parameters for the determination of clinical instability (41). Translational instability has been defined as 3.5 mm or more displacement in the sagittal plane, and angular instability has been defined as a minimal difference of 11° between adjacent spinal segments. In some patients, MRI may be useful in analyzing the extent and severity of soft tissue injury.

The clinical entity of subacute instability has also been reported in the trauma setting, although not specifically in athletes (50). It has been defined as the development of radiographic instability within 3 weeks of cervical spine injury, in association with a normal initial radiographic evaluation of the patient. It has been speculated that subacute instability develops as a result of elastic and plastic deformation of the ligamentous structures and intervertebral disc. These patients are also noted to have a normal initial neurologic evaluation. However, at follow-up there is often a neurologic deficit associated with the instability pattern. Given the potential for the development of subacute instability, follow-up radiographs (including flexion–extension views) and neurologic assessment have been recommended for patients who sustain a cervical spine injury, despite a normal initial evaluation. This may be particularly important for the athlete with persistent neck pain, despite a normal neurologic examination and normal initial radiographs.

As sufficient healing is unlikely to occur in patients with isolated soft tissue lesions, segmental posterior stabilization and fusion are recommended for athletes with significant ligamentous instability. In the majority of cases, stabilization can be achieved with spinous process wiring (51).

HYPEREXTENSION INJURIES

Hyperextension injuries occurring in athletes with preexisting cervical spondylosis (Fig. 9) can result in significant neurologic deficits, most commonly the central cord syndrome (52). This

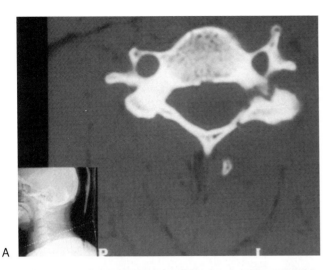

A

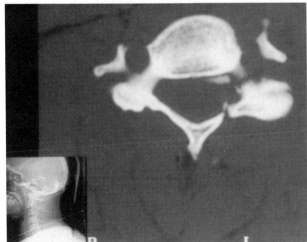

B

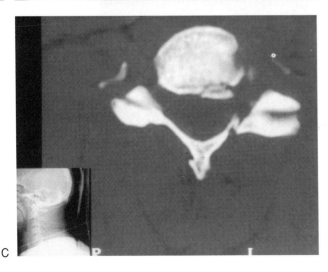

C

FIG. 7. C-5 lateral mass separation fracture with concomitant complete C5-6 transdiscal injury and associated anterior cord syndrome. **A:** Axial computed tomographic (CT) image reveals left lateral mass separation fracture. The pedicle fracture line courses just posterior to the intertransverse foramen. **B** and **C:** Axial CT images showing C-5 inferior endplate fractures, associated with the severe C5-6 transdiscal injury. The injury pattern resulted in severe instability at the C5-6 level and left C4-5 facet disruption secondary to the displaced C-5 lateral mass fracture. Because of the severe instability, the patient underwent a combined anterior–posterior stabilization procedure. The first phase consisted of a C5-6 anterior cervical decompression and fusion, with unicortical plate fixation. The second phase consisted of a C4-6 posterior fusion, with lateral mass plate fixation. The extension of the posterior fusion to include the C4-5 level was required because of the C4-5 facet disruption. Anteroposterior **(D)** and lateral **(E)** postoperative radiographs showing the combined anterior and posterior stabilization and fusion. **F:** Sagittal magnetic resonance image 11 weeks after injury showing persistent increased signal within the spinal cord, despite the patient's improving neurologic status. (From Nicholas JA, Hershman EB, eds. *The lower extremity and spine in sports medicine.* St. Louis, MO: Mosby, 1995: vol 2, Fig. 50-17, p. 1133.)

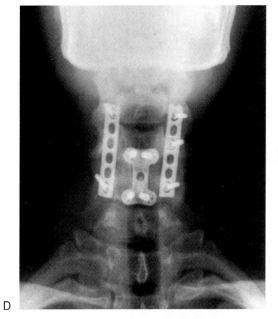

D

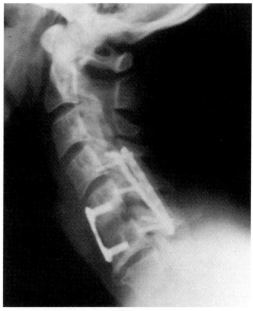

E

F

FIG. 7. *Continued.*

may occur despite the absence of a cervical spine fracture. In these patients, a hyperextension force may result in compression of the spinal cord between the buckled ligamentum flavum posteriorly and the vertebral body osteophytes anteriorly. The lateral radiograph may reveal slight retrolisthesis of the cephalad vertebral body, indicative of disruption of the intervertebral disc and longitudinal ligaments to a variable degree (53). MRI can be utilized to evaluate the presence and severity of soft tissue injury, extradural neural element compression, and intrinsic cord injury (54).

Most cases can be effectively treated nonoperatively with orthotic immobilization and close neurologic monitoring. In athletes with significant soft tissue disruption, instability, and/or extradural neural element compression, surgical decompression and/or stabilization is recommended.

PREVENTION OF CERVICAL SPINE INJURIES

The key to prevention of cervical spine injuries is strict education of athletes and all team personnel. The educational process should be started as early as possible in the career of the athlete. Frequent reinforcement of injury prevention methods is recommended. Each prospective athletic participant must be advised of the nature of the specific sport and the various mechanisms of injury. The proper use of protective equipment should be presented in detail, as this may prevent certain injuries (e.g., "burners" in football players). The technical aspects of the specific sport should be carefully outlined to the athlete (e.g., blocking and tackling in football).

Good physical conditioning of the athlete may not only improve performance but also help to

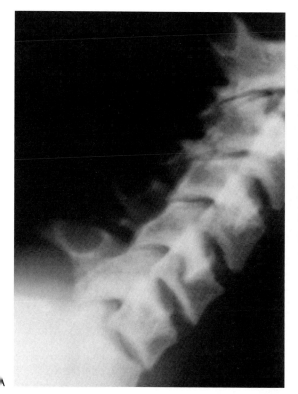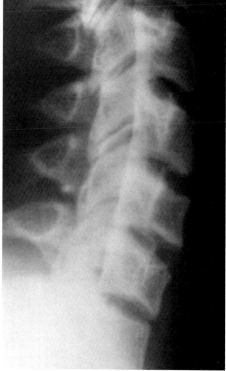

B

FIG. 8. C6-7 traumatic instability secondary to posterior ligamentous complex disruption. Lateral **(A)** flexion and extension **(B)** radiographs showing dynamic segmental instability.

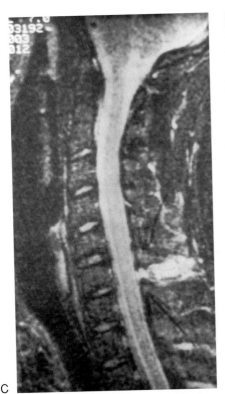

C

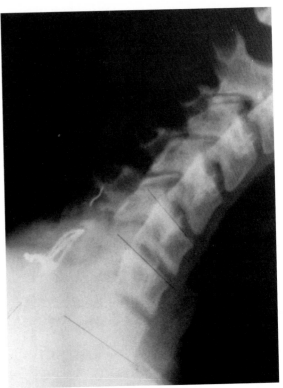

D

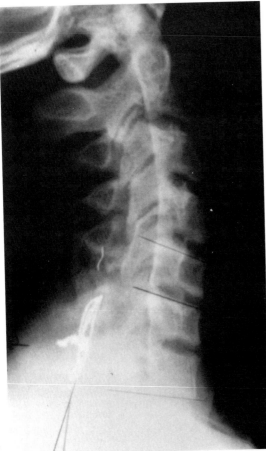

E

FIG. 8. C: T2-weighted sagittal magnetic resonance image illustrates the posterior ligamentous injury. The patient underwent a posterior fusion with spinous process wire stabilization. Flexion **(D)** and extension **(E)** postoperative lateral radiographs reveal a solid fusion. (From *OKU sports medicine.* Rosemont, IL: American Academy of Orthopaedic Surgeons, 1994, Fig. 3, p. 276.)

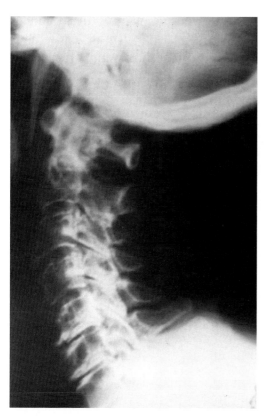

FIG. 9. Cervical spondylosis. (From *OKU sports medicine.* Rosemont, IL: American Academy of Orthopaedic Surgeons, 1994, Fig. 5, p. 278.)

prevent injuries. The selection of a proper physical fitness program begins with the preparticipation physical examination. On the basis of this assessment, an appropriate training program can be designed for the specific sport at issue and the appropriate skill level. For example, in football players, neck-strengthening exercises play a vital role in the prevention of cervical spine injuries. The fitness level of the athletes should be followed throughout their careers. The preparticipation physical examination is also used as a screening process for the detection of significant underlying orthopedic conditions. If a significant condition is found, preclusion of the prospective athlete from specific sports that are known to have a higher risk for cervical spine injury may be necessary.

RETURN TO PLAY

In the management of patients who have sustained a cervical spine injury, investigators have developed classification systems in an attempt to predict the risk for future injury with continued athletic participation. These systems have been based predominantly on clinical experience, as limited objective data are available for use as a foundation for this decision-making process (19,55,56). In general, each specific case must be evaluated with respect to the injury pattern, the sport in question, and the age and activity level of the athlete.

Athletes who have sustained cervical sprains or strains, intervertebral disc injury, or minor fractures and avulsions are permitted to return to contact activities when the clinical evaluation reveals (a) no reported cervical spine symptoms, (b) full, painless cervical spine range of motion, (c) full muscle strength, (d) no evidence of radiographic instability, and (e) a normal neurologic evaluation (57–59). If these criteria are not met, the athlete should be restricted from participation in certain contact activities.

Other criteria have been established for return to contact activities after specific bone or ligamentous injuries (59). Athletes who have undergone single-level anterior cervical decompression and fusion for disc herniation may be permitted to return to contact activities as long as a solid fusion is present and the preceding criteria have been achieved. Athletes who have evidence of a solid single-level posterior fusion may be treated in a similar fashion. Athletes who are status post multilevel cervical fusions should be restricted from participation in certain contact sports, because of the altered biomechanics of the cervical spine. In these cases, loads are distributed over fewer motion segments, resulting in an increased risk for the development of degenerative changes in the facets and intervertebral discs of the remaining motion segments (59).

REFERENCES

1. Torg JS, Vegso JJ, Sennett B. The National Football Head and Neck Injury Registry: 14-year report on cervical quadriplegia (1971–1984). *Clin Sports Med* 1987; 6:61–72.

2. Albright JP, McAuley E, Martin RK, Crowley ET, Foster DT. Head and neck injuries in college football: an eight-year analysis. *Am J Sports Med* 1985;13:147–152.

3. Brady TA, Cahill BR, Bodnar LM. Weight training–related injuries in the high school athlete. *Am J Sports Med* 1982;10:1–4.

4. Bruce DA, Schut I, Sutton LN. Brain and cervical spine injuries occurring during organized sports activities in children and adolescents. *Clin Sports Med* 1982;1: 495–514.

5. Cantu RC, Mueller FO. Catastrophic spine injuries in football (1977–1989). *J Spinal Disord* 1990;3: 227–231.

6. Cheng CL, Wolf AL, Mirvis S, Robinson WL. Bodysurfing accidents resulting in cervical spinal injuries. *Spine* 1991;17:257–260.

7. Frymoyer JW, Pope MH, Kristiansen T. Skiing and spinal trauma. *Clin Sports Med* 1982;1:309–318.

8. Herrick RT. Clay shoveler's fracture in power-lifting. A case report. *Am J Sports Med* 1981;9:29–30.

9. McCoy GF, Piggot J, Macafee AL, Adair JV. Injuries of the cervical spine in schoolboy rugby football. *J Bone Joint Surg Br* 1984;66B:500–503.

10. Mueller FO, Blyth CS. Fatalities from head and cervical spine injuries occurring in tackle football: 40 years' experience. *Clin Sports Med* 1987;6:185–196.

11. Nuber GW, Schafer MF. Clay shoveler's injuries: a report of two injuries sustained from football. *Am J Sports Med* 1987;15:182–183.

12. Paley D, Gillespie R. Chronic repetitive unrecognized flexion injury of the cervical spine (high jumper's neck). *Am J Sports Med* 1986;14:92–95.

13. Scher AT. Diving injuries to the cervical spinal cord. *South Afr Med J* 1981;59:603–605.

14. Scher AT. Rugby injuries of the spine and spinal cord. *Clin Sports Med* 1987;6:87–99.

15. Tator CH. Neck injuries in ice hockey: a recent, unsolved problem with many recent contributing factors. *Clin Sports Med* 1987;6:101–114.

16. Torg JS, Das M. Trampoline-related quadriplegia: review of the literature and reflections on the American Academy of Pediatrics position statement. *Pediatrics* 1984;74:804–812.

17. Torg JS, Pavlov H, Genuario SE, et al. Neuropraxia of the cervical spinal cord with transient quadriplegia. *J Bone Joint Surg Am* 1986;68A:1354–1370.

18. Torg JS. Trampoline-induced quadriplegia. *Clin Sports Med* 1987;6:73–85.

19. Watkins RG. Neck injuries in football players. *Clin Sports Med* 1986;5:215–246.

20. Garrick JG, Requa RK. Injuries in high-school sports. *Pediatrics* 1978;61:465.

21. Levine AM, Edwards CC. Fractures of the atlas. *J Bone Joint Surg Am* 1991;73A:680–691.

22. Spence K, Dedser D, Sell K. Bursting atlantal fracture associated with rupture of the transverse ligament. *J Bone Joint Surg Am* 1970;52A:543–549.

23. Segal LS, Grimm JO, Stauffer ES. Non-union of fractures of the atlas. *J Bone Joint Surg Am* 1987;69A: 1423–1434.

24. Harms J. Orthopaedics-traumatology I, rehabilitationskrankenhaus, Karlsbad-Langensteinbach, Germany. Personal communication, 1993.

25. Grob D, Magerl F. Operative Stabiliserung bei frakturen von C1 und C2. *Orthopade* 1987;16:46.

26. Fielding JW, Cochran GV, Lawsing JF, Hohl M. Tears of the transverse ligament of the atlas. *J Bone Joint Surg Am* 1974;56A:1683–1691.

27. Fielding J, Hawkins R. Atlantoaxial rotatory fixation. *J Bone Joint Surg Am* 1977;59A:37–44.

28. Anderson L, D'Alonzo R. Fractures of the odontoid process of the axis. *J Bone Joint Surg Am* 1974;56A: 1663–1674.

29. Hadley MN, Browner C, Sonntag VKH. Axis fractures: a comprehensive review of management and treatment in 107 cases. *Neurosurgery* 1985;17:281–290.

30. Montesano P, Anderson P, Schlehr F, Thalgott J, Lowery G. Odontoid fractures treated by anterior odontoid screw fixation. *Spine* 1991;3S:33–37.

31. Schatzker J, Rorabeck CH, Waddell JP. Non-union of the odontoid process. *Clin Orthop* 1975;108:127.

32. Clark CR, White AA. Fractures of the dens: a multicenter study. *J Bone Joint Surg Am* 1985;67A: 1340–1348.

33. Etter C, Coscia M, Jaberg H, Aebi M. Fixation of dens fractures with a cannulated screw system. *Spine* 1991; 3S:25–32.

34. Jeanneret B, Magerl F. Primary posterior fusion C1/2 in odontoid fractures: indications, technique, and results of transarticular screw fixation. *J Spinal Disord* 1992;5: 464–475.

35. Levine AM, Edwards CC. The management of traumatic spondylolisthesis of the axis. *J Bone Joint Surg Am* 1985;67A:217–226.

36. Levine AM, Edwards CC. Treatment of injuries in the C1-C2 complex. *Orthop Clin North Am* 1986;17:31–44.

37. Anderson PA, Henley MB, Grady MS, Montesano PX, Winn HR. Posterior cervical arthrodesis with AO reconstruction plates and bone graft. *Spine* 1991;16:S72–S79.

38. Jeanneret B, Magerl F, Ward EH, Ward J. Posterior stabilization of the cervical spine with hook plates. *Spine* 1991;16:S56–S63.

39. Nazarian SM, Louis RP. Posterior internal fixation with screw plates in traumatic lesions of the cervical spine. *Spine* 1991;16:S64–S71.

40. Torg JS, Sennett B, Vegso JJ, Pavlov H. Axial loading injuries to the middle cervical spine segment: an analysis and classification of twenty-five cases. *Am J Sports Med* 1991;19:6–20.

41. White AA, Southwick WO, Panjabi MM. Clinical instability in the lower cervical spine: a review of past and current concepts. *Spine* 1976;1:15–27.

42. Eismont FJ, Arena MJ, Green BA. Extrusion of an intervertebral disc associated with traumatic subluxation or dislocation of cervical facets. *J Bone Joint Surg Am* 1991;73A:1555–1560.

43. Kaye JJ, Nance EP Jr. Cervical spine trauma. *Orthop Clin North Am* 1990;21:449–462.

44. Aebi M, Zuber K, Marchesi D. Treatment of cervical spine injuries with anterior plating: indications, techniques, and results. *Spine* 1991;16:S38–S45.

45. Ripa DR, Kowall MG, Meyer PR, Rusin JJ. Series of ninety-two traumatic cervical spine injuries stabilized with anterior ASIF plate fusion technique. *Spine* 1991;16:S46–S55.

46. Montesano PX, Juach EC, Anderson PA, Benson DR, Hanson PB. Biomechanics of cervical spine internal fixation. *Spine* 1991;16:S10–S15.

47. Gill K, Paschal S, Corin J, Ashman R, Bucholz RW. Posterior plating of the cervical spine: a biomechanical comparison of different posterior fusion techniques. *Spine* 1988;13:813–816.

48. Levine AM. Cervical spine and cord: trauma. In: *Orthopaedic knowledge update 3*. Park Ridge, IL: American Academy of Orthopaedic Surgeons, 1990:395–413.
49. Krag M. Cervical spine: trauma. In: *Orthopaedic knowledge update 4*. Park Ridge, IL: American Academy of Orthopaedic Surgeons, 1993.
50. Herkowitz HN, Rothman RH. Subacute instability of the cervical spine. *Spine* 1984;9:348–357.
51. Stauffer ES. Management of spine fractures C3 to C7. *Orthop Clin North Am* 1986;17:45–53.
52. Schneider RC, Cherry GR, Pantek H. Syndrome of acute central cervical spinal cord injury with special reference to mechanisms involved in hyperextension injuries of the cervical spine. *J Neurosurg* 1954;11:363.
53. Marar BC. Hyperextension injuries of the cervical spine. *J Bone Joint Surg Am* 1974;56A:1655–1662.
54. Goldberg AL, Rothfus WE, Deeb ZL, Frankel DG, Wilberger JE Jr, Daffner RH. Hyperextension injuries of the cervical spine: magnetic resonance findings. *Skeletal Radiol* 1989;18:283–288.
55. Bailes JE, Hadley MN, Quigley MR, Sonntag VKH, Cerullo LJ. Management of athletic injuries of the cervical spine and spinal cord. *Neurosurgery* 1991;29: 491–497.
56. Marks MR, Bell GR, Boumphrey FR. Cervical spine fractures in athletes. *Clin Sports Med* 1990;9:13–29.
57. Micheli LJ. Sports following spinal surgery in the young athlete. *Clin Orthop* 1985;198:152–157.
58. Torg JS. Management guidelines for athletic injuries to the cervical spine. *Clin Sports Med* 1987;6:60.
59. Torg JS, Glasgow SG. Criteria for return to contact activity following cervical spine injury. *Clin J Sport Med* 1991;1:12–26.

Sports Neurology, Second Edition,
edited by Barry D. Jordan.
Lippincott–Raven Publishers, Philadelphia © 1998.

14

Transient Quadriparesis

Robert C. Cantu

Neurological Surgery, Inc.,
John Cuming Building, Suite 820, Concord, Massachusetts 01742

Transient quadriparesis or bilateral neurologic symptoms involving the arms and/or arms and legs after a player is hit in a contact sport raises the specter of spinal cord injury. This condition of spinal cord impairment is to be distinguished from that of a "burner" or "stinger," which is always a unilateral injury that virtually never involves the lower extremities; rather, it involves a single upper extremity and is an injury to either the brachial plexus or the cervical nerve root in the neuroforamen. Thus, if symptoms are bilateral and/or involve the legs, a spinal cord injury must be assumed. Usually, with transient quadriparesis there is not immediate significant neck pain or limitation of neck movement. After minutes or hours, however, neck stiffness is not uncommon and may last for days or weeks. Usually, the motor and sensory symptoms are more profound in the upper extremities than the lower extremities or are confined entirely to the upper extremities and clear within seconds to minutes.

Three such cases of transient quadriparesis seen in consultation by this author are presented later when criteria for return to play after transient quadriparesis are discussed.

EVALUATION AND MANAGEMENT OF TRANSIENT QUADRIPARESIS

All patients who have had an episode of transient quadriparesis should be removed from the athletic playing field on a fracture board with the head and neck immobilized unless the symptoms have been extremely brief and all neurologic symptoms have cleared by the time the attending medical personnel have reached the fallen athlete. Definitive evaluation of an athlete with transient quadriparesis should include not only a detailed neurologic examination, best done initially on the playing field, but also subsequent follow-up at a medical facility with full neuroradiologic diagnostic capabilities. Among the neuroradiologic studies, in addition to cervical spine radiographs with flexion–extension views, should be imaging with magnetic resonance scanning. In some athletes, spinal stenosis may be a contributing factor. Although radiographic bone measurements showing a canal height of 13 mm or less may suggest the presence of spinal stenosis, physicians are cautioned against making the diagnosis of spinal stenosis with radiographs alone. Instead, the diagnostic technologies that image the spinal cord and its surrounding cerebrospinal fluid—magnetic resonance imaging (MRI), contrast positive computed tomography (CT), or myelography when needed—should be employed. Only these imaging modalities can determine whether the spinal cord has a normal functional reserve of cerebrospinal fluid around it to provide a protective cushion between the cord and the spinal canal's interior walls lined by bone, disc, and ligament (Fig. 1). In addition, unlike cervical spine radiography, these techniques can determine whether the nerve tissue is deformed by an abnormality such as a herniated disc, bony osteophyte, or posterior buckling of the ligamentum flavum (Figs. 2 and 3).

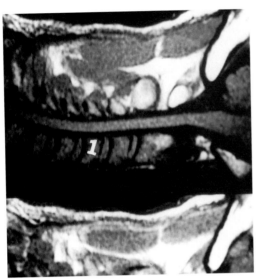

FIG. 1. Normal magnetic resonance image showing wide area of cerebrospinal fluid (functional reserve) around the spinal cord (*dark area above 1*).

PAVLOV–TORG RATIO CONTROVERSY

In the past (1,2), it was proposed that radiographs corrected for magnification error showing sagittal cervical spinal canal heights of 15 mm or more were normal, whereas sagittal canal heights of 12 to 13 mm or less were felt to show spinal stenosis (3,4). To eliminate the need to correct for magnification error, Torg et al. (5) in 1986

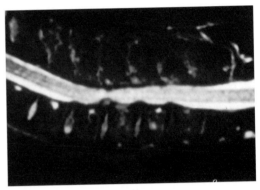

FIG. 3. Spinal cord deformity caused by disc ruptured into an already functionally spinal stenotic (note no cerebrospinal fluid around the cord) canal.

and Pavlov et al. (6) in 1987 proposed a ratio method to assess cervical spinal stenosis radiographically. The ratio method compares the height of the spinal canal from the midpoint of the posterior surface of the vertebral body to the spinolaminar line (numerator) with the height of the corresponding midvertebral body (denominator). The authors concluded that significant spinal stenosis was present when the ratio of canal to vertebral body was 0.8 or less (Fig. 4).

In the past several years, serious doubts have been raised about the accuracy of the ratio method in diagnosing true cervical spinal stenosis. In 1990 Odor et al. (7) reported that 33% of the professional football players they studied had stenosis by the ratio method. In 1991, Herzog

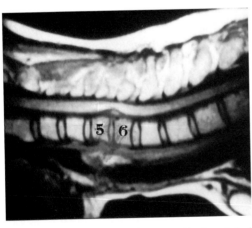

FIG. 2. Functional stenosis caused by herniated disc at C5-6. Note deformity of spinal cord.

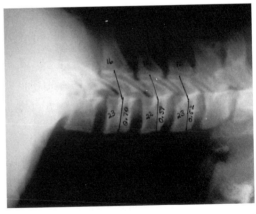

FIG. 4. Lateral cervical spine showing abnormal Torg ratios at C-4, C-5, and C-6.

et al. (8) in a study of 80 asymptomatic professional football players demonstrated that the Torg ratio was less than 0.8 in 49% of the players studied, whereas they found that the true incidence of spinal stenosis was only 12%. Herzog et al. theorized that the Torg ratio therefore had many false positives (88% of the time) and attributed this to the large vertebral bodies of the football players skewing the ratio even though spinal canal heights were of normal or large size. A ratio also raises accuracy concerns because radiographs alone do not assess the size of the spinal cord relative to the size of the spinal canal. The size of the spinal cord has been variably reported to be between 5 and 11.5 mm (9,10). Thus true stenosis may be present with low normal canal measurements and a large spinal canal. Furthermore, the ratio method using radiographs alone does not allow one to appreciate deformity of the spinal cord that may occur as a result of a protruding or herniated disc, significant osteophyte, or marked inward buckling of the ligamentum flavum, all of which may themselves produce spinal stenosis.

Because of these concerns, this author has written several papers advocating the concept of functional spinal stenosis to determine whether true spinal stenosis is present (11,12). "Functional" spinal stenosis is defined as a loss of cerebrospinal fluid around the spinal cord or, in more extreme cases, deformation of the spinal cord documented by MRI, contrast positive CT, or myelography. Functional spinal stenosis may be due exclusively to congenital spinal stenosis or may be contributed to as well by a herniated disc, osteophyte, or buckling of the ligamentum flavum (see Figs. 2 and 3).

DEFINITIVE EVALUATION OF TRANSIENT QUADRIPARESIS

When an athlete has bilateral symptoms suggestive of spinal cord injury, evaluation should include radiographs of the cervical spine looking specifically for subluxation or fracture as well as other possible degenerative changes. For all patients with symptoms suggestive of spinal cord involvement, transient quadriparesis, burning hands syndrome, or other bilateral motor or sensory symptoms, the physician should order MRI after obtaining the initial radiographs.

Contrast positive CT and myelography are useful for defining the degree of spinal stenosis; however, both techniques are invasive and are usually not needed. Contrast positive CT is more sensitive than MRI for fracture and bone abnormalities, and myelography provides a better view of spinal cord compression than MRI.

CRITERIA FOR RETURN TO PLAY

When asked whether I advocate using MRI to screen all athletes who play contact sports for spinal stenosis, my answer is no. This would not be cost effective, and we do not have the data to suggest that it would be appropriate to screen people in this manner.

However, when a player has spinal cord symptoms after an injury, MRI can be very useful in defining who should and should not return to play. I believe strongly that those who have had spinal cord symptoms resulting from sports injuries and are shown to have true spinal stenosis on MRI should not be allowed to return to contact sports. Although it is true that no large, statistically significant, double-blind prospective study substantiates this opinion with unquestioned scientific validity, the reality is that the legal and moral consequences of a controlled trial would be too serious to allow it to be done. A body of literature in the fields of sports medicine, neurology, and radiology indicates that spinal stenosis predisposes a patient to spinal cord injury (2,13–18). Matsuura et al. (15), for example, compared the spinal dimensions of 100 control subjects with those of 42 patients who had spinal cord injuries. They found that the control group had significantly larger sagittal spinal canal diameters than the patients who had spinal cord injuries.

Furthermore, in the National Center for Catastrophic Sports Injury Research in Chapel Hill, North Carolina experience between 1989 and 1994 (R.C. Cantu, unpublished data), no individuals with fracture dislocation of the spinal canal who also had spinal stenosis made a complete neurologic recovery. In contrast, 12 individuals with fracture dislocation of the spinal canal

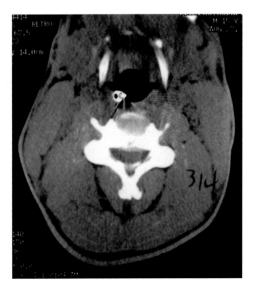

FIG. 5. Computed tomographic scan showing severe spinal stenosis at C3-4 (note flat, narrow height of canal).

and initial quadriplegia who did not have spinal stenosis ultimately made a complete neurologic recovery. In the National Center experience an individual who had an initial episode of transient quadriplegia went on to have a severe permanent spinal cord injury (see case 3). In addition, an individual in the National Center registry had severe spinal stenosis (Fig. 5) and resultant quadriplegia without fracture or dislocation.

CASE STUDIES

Case 1

The first case is that of a National Football League linebacker who incurred an axial load injury during a game while making a tackle that was so forceful that it dented the front of his football helmet. He was quadriplegic for 4 minutes on the football field and over the next half-hour regained full neurologic function.

A neurologic examination performed at the hospital was normal. Radiographic studies including lateral–flexion views documented normal spinal canal heights with all levels being greater than

15 mm. Other than for straightening of his cervical spine, his cervical spine radiographs were normal. Because his vertebral bodies were large, the Torg ratio was abnormal at multiple levels. A cervical magnetic resonance imaging study was normal, as was a cervical CT scan. Both studies documented a normal functional reserve of cerebrospinal fluid at all levels.

Disposition

With no spinal stenosis or other cervical pathology documented, after this individual had complete resolution of his neurologic symptoms and had returned to full range of cervical spine motion and normal neck strength, he was allowed to return to professional football and has since played for several years without further symptoms. This is an individual who would be classified as being at low risk for quadriplegia as his spinal canal anatomy is normal.

Case 2

A National Hockey League center received a blow to the crown of the helmet with the neck flexed that caused several minutes of transient quadriplegia. When he was seen 2 weeks later, his neurologic examination was normal, as were cervical spine radiographs including cervical lordotic curvature and flexion–extension views. MRI and subsequently myelography–contrast positive CT documented a small disc bulge at C3-4 but cerebrospinal fluid still around the cord at this level. Therefore, functional spinal stenosis was not present.

Disposition

This patient, in view of the abnormal disc at C3-4, was counseled that he was at increased, perhaps moderate risk for further spinal cord symptoms. Although discouraged from returning to play, he was told that he did not have true spinal stenosis and therefore absolute return was not contraindicated. The patient has elected to retire from professional hockey and is currently coaching hockey.

Case 3

A high school junior sustained a hyperextension neck injury after making a head-up tackle during a game. He was quadriplegic for 2 minutes and then was able to rise and walk off the field with "spaghetti legs." He did not receive any workup at that time!

Three weeks later he was seen because he had persistent neck pain and rigidity. Cervical spine radiographs at that time showed that his spinal canal height was extremely narrow (12 mm), and he had an extremely abnormal Torg ratio. No further workup was carried out at that time. The patient returned to football 2 weeks later and played the remainder of his junior year and all of his senior season without further neck injury.

During his freshman year in college, a head tackle during a scrimmage rendered him permanently quadriplegic. Magnetic resonance imaging suggested that a disc in his cervical spine had herniated into the narrow stenotic canal, producing not simply radicular nerve root symptoms but also a severe spinal cord injury. Severe cervical spinal cord edema was seen over three levels on his initial MRI. This individual has remained hemiparetic to this date.

PREVENTION

Transient quadriparesis can occur in extremes of flexion and extension, but in most instances, as is true of quadriplegia, transient quadriparesis occurs with the axial load "spearing" type of impact so well described by Torg et al. (5). The incidence of transient quadriparesis increases as the sport becomes increasingly violent and aggressive, as is true of head and neck injury in general. Improperly conditioned neck muscles and lack of knowledge of the proper technique of the sport puts an athlete who sustains a blow to the head at significantly greater risk for spine injury. Although recognition of these features has resulted in a dramatic reduction in catastrophic athletic spine injury, there is no absolute prevention for transient quadriparesis or other serious spine injury. For the reasons discussed earlier, however, if an athlete has had a previous episode of spinal cord symptoms and has been shown to have functional spinal stenosis by MRI, contrast positive CT, or myelography, the athlete should be counseled against returning to contact collision sports (19,20).

At present, there are no good guidelines to help the sports physician manage an athlete with a narrow, asymptomatic cervical spinal canal. When such an abnormality is documented in the process of evaluating an athlete for other than spinal cord injury, management must be individualized according to the patient's symptoms, the degree of canal stenosis, and the perceived risk of permanent neurologic injury.

REFERENCES

1. Boijsen E. The cervical spinal canal in intraspinal expansive processes. *Acta Radiol* 1954;42:101.
2. Wolfe BS, Khilnani M, Malis L. The sagittal diameter of the bony cervical spinal canal and its significance in cervical spondylosis. *J Mt Sinai Hosp* 1956;23:283.
3. Epstein JA, Carras R, Hyman RA, et al. Cervical myelopathy caused by developmental stenosis of the spinal canal. *J Neurosurg* 1979;51:362–367.
4. Ladd AL, Scranton PE. Congenital cervical stenosis presenting as transient quadriplegia in athletes: report of two cases. *J Bone Joint Surg Am* 1986;68:1371–1374.
5. Torg JS, Pavlov H, Genuano SE, et al. Neuropraxia of the cervical spinal cord with transient quadriplegia. *J Bone Joint Surg Am* 1986;68A:1354–1370.
6. Pavlov H, Torg JS, Robie B, et al. Cervical spinal stenosis: determination with vertebral body ratio method. *Radiology* 1987;164:771–775.
7. Odor JM, Watkins RG, Dillin WH, Dennis S, Saberi M. Incidence of cervical spinal stenosis in professional and rookie football players. *Am J Sports Med* 1990;18:507–509.
8. Herzog RJ, Weins JJ, Dillingham MF, Sontag MJ. Normal cervical spine morphometry and cervical spinal stenosis in asymptomatic professional football players: plain film radiography, multi-planar computed tomography, and magnetic resonance imaging. *Spine* 1991;16(6 Suppl):S178–S186.
9. Lamont AC, Zachary J, Sheldon PW. Cervical cord size in metrizamide myelography. *Clin Radiol* 1981;32:409–412.
10. Thijssen HO, Keyser A, Horstink MW, et al. Morphology of the cervical spinal cord on computed myelography. *Neuroradiology* 1979;18(2):57–62.
11. Cantu RC. Functional cervical spinal stenosis: a contraindication to participation in contact sports. *Med Sci Sports Exerc* 1993;25:316–317.
12. Cantu RC. Transient quadriplegia: to play or not to play. *Sports Med Dig* 1994;16:1–3.
13. Alexander MM, Davis CH, Field CH. Hyperextension injuries of the cervical spine. *Arch Neurol Psychiatr* 1958;79:146.

14. Eismont FJ, Clifford S, Goldberg M, et al. Cervical sagittal spinal canal size in spinal injury. *Spine* 1984;9: 663–666.

15. Matsuura P, Waters RL, Adkins RH, Rothman S, Gurbani W, Sie I. Comparison of computerized tomography parameters of the cervical spine in normal control subjects and spinal cord–injured patients. *J Bone Joint Surg Am* 1989;71:183–188.

16. Mayfield FH. Neurosurgical aspects of cervical trauma. In: *Clinical neurosurgery,* vol II. Baltimore: Williams & Wilkins, 1955.

17. Nugent GR. Clinicopathologic correlations in cervical spondylosis. *Neurology* 1959;9:273.

18. Penning L. Some aspects of plain radiography of the cervical spine in chronic myelopathy. *Neurology* 1962; 12:513–519.

19. Cantu RC. Cervical spinal stenosis: challenging an established detection method. *Phys Sports Med* 1993; 21(9):57–63.

20. Cantu RV, Cantu RC. Guidelines for return to contact sports after transient quadriplegia. *J Neurosurg* 1994; 80:592–594.

Sports Neurology, Second Edition,
edited by Barry D. Jordan.
Lippincott–Raven Publishers, Philadelphia © 1998.

15

Injuries to the Thoracic Spine

Robert G. Watkins

University Hospital, 1510 San Pablo South 700, Los Angeles, California 90033

Thoracic spine injuries are more likely to occur in certain sports, particularly those involving torsional throwing, because the thoracolumbar junction is the section of the spine with the greatest involvement in the dynamics of throwing. It is found very infrequently in nonthrowing sports. For example, a study of 93 spinal injuries sustained in rugby football (1), a sport in which there is practically no throwing of the ball for any distance, recorded only one thoracic injury between the years 1956 and 1993 in South Africa, New Zealand, and Australia. The rest were cervical spine injuries, and the one thoracic injury occurred only after a game in which the player fell down a set of stairs.

In North America, thoracic spinal pain can be found most commonly among such ball-throwing athletes as baseball pitchers and football quarterbacks. (Exceptions to this are the thoracic fractures that occur in the sports of football and ice hockey as a result of being slammed or tackled from behind, not of throwing a ball.)

TYPES OF INJURIES

Muscle Fatigue and Strain

Pain in the interscapular area, commonly associated with fatigue problems in an upper extremity and postural abnormalities of the cervical spine and upper thoracic lumbar spine, may be evidenced by tenderness on the spinous process. There is little radiation of the pain, which is paraspinous through the medial scapular border and tips of the spinous processes.

A typical workup includes any test used for mechanical or nonmechanical axial pain. This could include a bone scan and/or magnetic resonance imaging (MRI), although these tests would, in general, be more useful when there is a constant, unrelenting pain rather than clearly fatigue-related, postural pain.

Treatment for muscle strain in this area is typically the same as that used in handling cervical strains: trunk stabilization, joint mobilization, exercises for local modalities, and upper extremity shoulder-strengthening exercises. Posture correction, encouraging a chest-out stance, is central to curing interscapular pain, whether it is referred cervical pain or pain originating in the thoracic muscle insertion.

The costovertebral and costotransverse joints have been successfully resected by certain surgeons in cases not receptive to nonoperative care, but performing such an operation on a high-performance athlete would be most unusual.

T-4 Syndromes

Interscapular pain and high thoracic pain of the T1-7 area is typically associated with upper extremity function, whereas thoracolumbar junction problems are generally associated with lower extremity function and torsional activities. Referred to as the T-4 syndrome, localized tenderness and pain of the T-4 spinous process characterize this common clinical manifestation of chronic postural strain.

The combined muscle function of shoulder elevators and depressors produces a significant tendinous strain and localized inflammation over the proximal T-4 spinous process. Treatment should consist of trunk stabilization (2), strengthening of upper body and local modalities through exercise, and taking appropriate environmental measures to take strain off the shoulders and elbows to relieve chronic pulls and strains on this interscapular area. An example of one such change might be adding arms to the patient's working chair and car seat.

Costicartilage and Rib Injuries

Midthoracic or thoracolumbar junction complaints of the torsional athlete typically occur unilaterally on the side opposite the throwing arm and are definitely related to rotation in the lower thoracic area. Because of the necessary pull of the lateral oblique musculature on the side opposite the throwing arm, costicartilage and rib injuries in this area are common (3). They are the outcome of damage done to the ribs, as well as to the soft tissue and cartilage of the rib cage, produced by the intense pull of the lateral oblique musculature on the side opposite the throwing arm. This is sometimes serious enough to produce a major disability (4).

Selective blocks of these specific structures can be of some benefit, although not until thoracic radicular pain has been eliminated as a potential etiology. Relief of pain through local injection can better demonstrate costicartilage injury, such as that found at the tip of the eleventh and twelfth ribs. Bone scan reveals the rib stress fractures that throwing athletes commonly suffer, typically on the side opposite their throwing arm. Bone scan also shows any costicartilage crepitus.

Spondylitic defects can occur in the thoracic spine, especially in the immature athlete, producing radiating intercostal pain. Bone scanning, which is also instrumental when diagnosing stress fractures in this area, is called for.

Thoracic Spondylosis

In a throwing athlete, a foraminal spur producing radicular symptoms is not an uncommon pathology. (*Non*radicular pain of the thoracic spine, on the other hand, can be produced by the same sources that create similar results in the lumbar spine, intervertebral disc, and facet joints.) Symptoms may indicate a rib stress fracture, a costovertebral articulation problem, torn soft tissues of the muscle or fascia, or injury to the cartilaginous tip of the rib. Because of the tremendous pull produced by the opposite-side abdominal oblique muscles, local modalities, physical therapy, rehabilitation, and antiinflammatory medications seldom, if ever, provide relief.

Bone scan should be performed to rule out possible stress fracture, and MRI should be ordered to eliminate the possibility of thoracic disc herniation or a lumbar spine problem. If thoracic spondylosis is indeed the problem, myelography and contrast computed tomography (CT) may demonstrate calcification.

A nerve root block of the affected area provides pain relief for this problem, but a foraminotomy may be necessary for long-term relief.

Costovertebral Joint Injuries

Additional structures in the thoracic spine include the costotransverse and costovertebral joints. Costovertebral joint pain is an enigma. Certainly, provocative selective blocks of these joints can provide some relief. But, because of cross-innervation of different levels, it would still be difficult to localize the specific level of the problem when the symptoms involve axial pain only.

Thoracic Disc Herniation

Thoracic disc herniations can involve the spinal cord or thoracic nerve. So, even though thoracic disc herniation has an incidence of one in a million (5) and accounts for only 0.15% to 0.80% of all surgery for disc herniations, it is probably the most critical diagnosis to make in thoracic radicular pain.

Up to half of all patients diagnosed with thoracic disc herniation at some centers present with significant spinal cord injury (6,7). If the exiting thoracic nerve is damaged, pressure at that level produces pain in the chest and back and carries the grave risk of permanent cord injury (7,8). A thoracic disc herniation can result in paraplegia with weakness and numbness in the legs and complete loss of bowel, bladder, sexual, and leg function. Because of this risk, a full, complete history should be taken and a thorough physical examination should be performed before a course of treatment is determined.

Accurate gathering of the history and recording of the physical form will usually reveal to the diagnostician whether or not there is radicular pain. Such pain in the thoracic area follows a basic dermatomal pattern extending around laterally and anteriorly on the chest or abdominal wall.

High thoracic disc herniations at T-1 or T-2 may present with one or more symptoms (9):

- Spastic presentation of an upper thoracic disc herniation and/or
- Presentation with symptoms of a cervical spine problem—radiating arm pain, with pain radiating to the medial aspect of the arm, hand and shoulder, with possible intrinsic hand weakness and/or Horner's syndrome (10).

Herniated lower thoracic discs may present with the signs and symptoms of neurogenic claudication or sciatica (11) and show a flaccid neurologic loss mimicking that in lumbar spine disease (6,7).

The nonoperative treatment of radicular pain is similar to the treatment of lumbar pain and starts with a proper trunk stabilization program. Indications for surgery include progressive myelopathy and unrelenting radiculopathy. Relative indications are intermittent thoracic radiculopathy and a large, although asymptomatic, thoracic disc herniation which, if allowed to expand, could produce myelopathy under the kind of heavy loading conditions faced by most athletes.

Compression Fractures

Compression injuries, including fractures, are seen commonly in the seated sports, such as auto racing, horseback riding, motorcycling, bicycling, luge, and bobsled (Fig. 1). The energy of the repeated axial load on the spine is only partially dissipated by the buttocks and pelvis (12). When there is a sudden and severe axial load, is in a sudden stop, compression fracture may result.

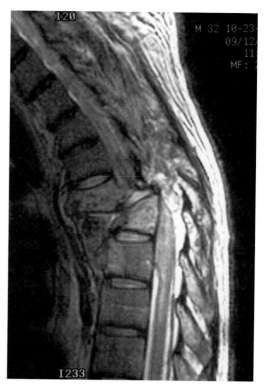

FIG. 1. The thoracolumbar fracture dislocation in this professional motorcycle racer produced bilateral hemopneumothoraces and complete T-6 paraplegia. Open-reduction internal fixation was carried out for spinal alignment, stability, and fusion.

A study of spine and spinal cord injuries in downhill skiers by Prall et al. (13) found that the most common fracture pattern was compression (38%), and the most commonly fractured levels were C-6, T-12, and L-1. Those with thoracolumbar injuries were much more likely to sustain torso and extremity trauma than those with cervical injuries. Compression fractures may also occur among surfers, more commonly body surfers than board surfers, when they go under a wave and are tumbled about violently.

Although the compression fracture most typically occurs in the cervical spine, there are also instances of thoracolumbar compression fractures, which result, for example, when a racing car collides head-on into a barrier at a speed high enough to lift the car's rear wheels off the ground. When the rear wheels slam down, an axial load is produced that is transmitted to the driver's pelvis, buttocks, and thoracolumbar spine.

DIAGNOSIS

For the physician, the thoracic spine can frequently be a most puzzling and difficult area because pain in this area can indicate any of a number of problems. For example, although sometimes seen in other parts of the spine, *flexion–rotation fracture dislocations* may be most commonly found anywhere within the thoracic spine, occurring most typically in the thoracolumbar area. We also see, at times, traumatic back pain resulting from a *compressive load* applied disproportionally upon the thoracolumbar junction. *Disc degeneration* is another possible source of pain; it and other discogenic changes in this area have a higher incidence among elite gymnasts than among the general populace (8). Many of these conditions can be treated nonsurgically, but others require more radical approaches.

The initial workup is much like that used to diagnose cervical spine complaints in that the examiner must determine whether it is a radiculopathy, a myelopathy, a musculoskeletal joint complaint, a referred cervical pain, posterior penetrating duodenal ulcer, renal colic, or other internal medical problem. The key to accurate diagnosis of injury to the thoracic spine is to use a standardized history and physical form that provides sufficient detail to enable a good review of systems, as well as an extensive neurologic examination.

The examiner must be particularly alert to signs and symptoms of neurologic dysfunction, because thoracic disc herniations can cause permanent paraplegia; every effort must be directed toward making this diagnosis when the pathology is present. If there is any suggestion of a neurologic dysfunction, MRI of the thoracic spine can usually provide sufficient detail of a quality necessary to diagnosis a thoracic disc herniation. Thoracic radiculopathy, radiating pain, and intercostal pain, with or without associated sensory loss, can be evaluated by MRI. A thoracic myelogram and contrast CT, which provides the greatest detail of the thoracic intervertebral foramina,

can provide additional information, should MRI leave some questions unresolved.

A number of patterns of neurologic deficit may be seen in patients with spinal cord injuries. Neurogenic shock is seen in the period immediately after complete injury at the T-6 level and above (14). These are areflexia, loss of sensation and flaccid paralysis below the level of the lesion, a flaccid bladder with retention of urine, and a lax anal sphincter (15). In patients with thoracic fractures and dislocations specifically, complete spinal cord injuries are the rule because the spinal canal in that region is small in relation to the size of the spinal cord (16–19). The difference between complete and partial injury is important, as those with partial injury may regain all or part of their neurologic function, no matter how severe the initial neurologic deficit; those with complete injury seldom recover function to any significant degree.

For musculoskeletal joint problems of the thoracic spine, a bone scan can be helpful if the stress fracture, inflamed arthritic joint, or bone tumor of the thoracic spine can be identified and the scan provides sufficient detail.

Radiculopathy

Tingling, numbness, dysesthesias, or weaknesses in various distributions reported by athletes could be manifestations of radiculopathies in the cervical, thoracic, or lumbar spine. However, a number of potential peripheral nerve entrapments can mimic radiculopathy (20). What may appear to be a radiculopathy at the thoracic level, with paresthesias and/or dysesthesias, for example, may actually be herpes zoster. Understanding the anatomy of peripheral nerves and their dermatomal distributions can lead to more effective evaluation of athletes with suspected radiculop-athy (21) (Fig. 2).

Myelopathy

Every patient evaluated for thoracic spine injury must also have an examination to rule out myelopathy, because subtle findings and changes in myelopathy are often not obvious to the patient. If myelopathy is present, a MRI scan or myelogram with contrast CT scan should be

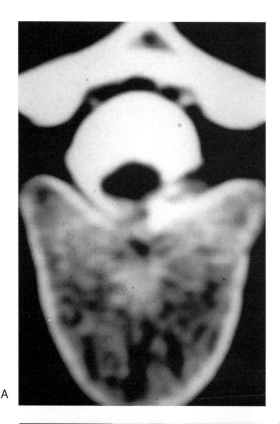

A

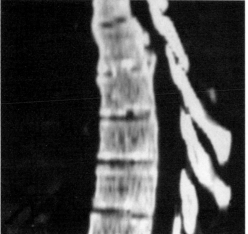

B

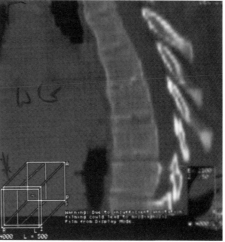

C

FIG. 2. A blow from behind during a game produced intense thoracic radiculopathy but no thoracic myelopathy in this professional athlete. **A:** A calcified extruded fragment of the intervertebral disc can be seen in this contrast computed tomographic (CT) scan. **B:** A parasagittal section of the plain CT scan shows a calcified extruded fragment from the T6-7 disk space extruding upward behind the body of T-6. **C:** With the patient placed on a regimen of aggressive trunk stabilization, chest-out posture correction, and body reconditioning, the intense radiculopathy slowly resolved and he was able to return to his sport 90 days from the onset of conditions. He was able to perform at full function for the rest of the season. This parasagittal section shows the affected area 90 days after the onset of the intense radiculopathy.

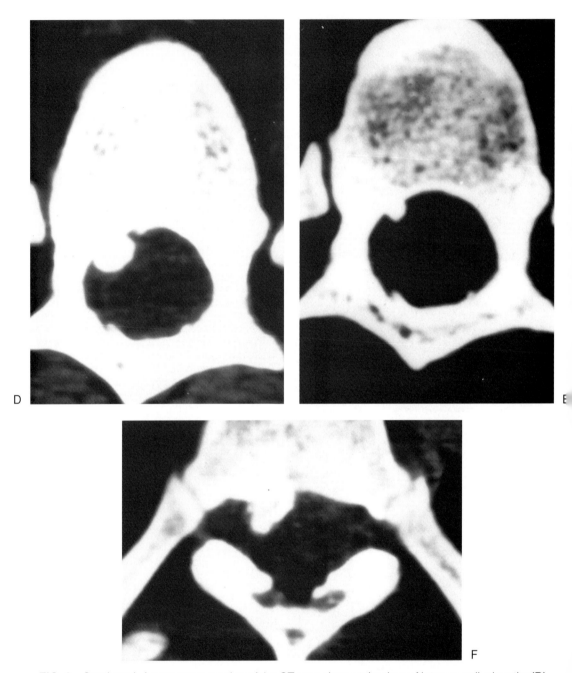

FIG. 2. *Continued*. A transverse section of the CT scan done at the time of intense radiculopathy **(D)** and 90 days later **(E). F:** A large, calcified, extruded fragment.

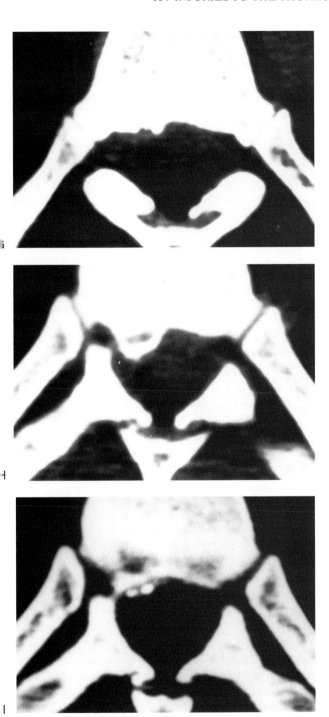

FIG. 2. *Continued.* **G:** Resolution of that fragment. Another section of the extruded fragment **(H)** and its resolution **(I)**. This herniation was an extrusion of an intradiscal calcification that was resorbed by a combination of pulsations of the thoracic cord and healing of the injured area.

obtained. If no myelop-athy is present and the patient has radiating thoracic pain in a dermatomal pattern, an MRI scan or a myelogram and contrast CT scan is still the preferred test. MRI may demonstrate a thoracic disc herniation, but the intervertebral foramen of the thoracic spine is probably best evaluated by a contrast CT scan (22).

TREATMENT

In summary, the key to dealing with thoracic area pain is as follows:

* Identify postural strain syndromes and use posture-correcting techniques.
* Identify radicular syndromes and order the appropriate diagnostic tests.
* Institute a therapeutic technique as aggressive as possible to prevent potential cord or nerve injury to the patient.
* Always check for myelopathy.
* Initiate a prompt diagnostic and therapeutic plan when thoracic myelopathy is suspected or diagnosed.

Nonoperative Care of the Thoracic Disc Herniation

Few studies allow direct comparison of the productiveness of operative versus conservative treatment. Alho (23) noted that no study shows conclusively that operative treatment is preferable to conservative care with regard to neurologic status, because each has its own particular complications. However, it appears that operative treatment is less likely to lead to neurologic deterioration and that the patient's return to mobility, which is faster after operative treatment, leads to improved psychologic and social rehabilitation. Also, according to Alho, patients who have undergone thoracolumbar spinal surgery are less likely to experience postoperative back pain.

There are significant opportunities and indications for proper nonoperative care of thoracic disc herniations when symptoms are minimal and thoracic disc herniations are asymptomatic. It is quite possible that many of the athletic rib injuries and radicular chest pain injuries physicians see intermittently may actually be due to thoracic disc her-

niations that heal quite well nonoperatively. (There may be a much higher incidence of thoracic disc herniation among athletes than we think.)

The mere presence of a herniation does not in itself necessitate surgery (24). When Brown et al. (24) reviewed 55 patients with 72 thoracic disc herniations to determine the natural history of the disease, they found that only 27% of these patients eventually required surgery. The majority did not require surgery and continued to perform activities of everyday life, even participating in such sports as skiing with no paraneurologic deficit. Herniated thoracic discs do not always lead to major neurologic compromise, and appropriate rehabilitation and careful observation are a course of action that can be well within reason. Certainly, any return to function that is brought about nonoperatively should come only after a detailed, comprehensive nonoperative rehabilitation program in a less demanding sport. The rehabilitation used is a modified trunk stabilization program in which all of the usual neural position and ball exercises are done through the five level Watkins-Randle scale (2). The exception is to deemphasize situps, rotations, and crunches that may cause abnormal thoracic motion.

Operative Treatment: Surgical Approaches and Care

Indications for surgery in thoracic disc herniation are (a) significant progressive cervical myelopathy and (b) unrelenting cervical radiculopathy. Intermittent thoracic radiculopathy is a relative indication for surgery, depending on the amount of morbidity of the patient. A large, asymptomatic thoracic disc herniation of already significant size that continues to expand could produce myelopathy under heavy loading situations—and heavy loading situations can certainly be anticipated in an athlete—that can be a relative indication for surgery.

Of the surgical approaches available for excision of a thoracic disc herniation, a standard thoracic laminectomy through a *posterior* approach is felt to be nonacceptable because there is a high incidence of neurologic deficit concomitant with it (25,26). It requires at least some degree of spinal cord manipulation. In one study the posterior approach resulted in some element of neurologic loss in all 23 patients (27) and, reviewing posterior approaches in 1969, Perot and Monroe (28) reported that, of 91 patients, 40 were not improved and 16 were permanently paralyzed by the operation.

Evolution of the *posterolateral* or *lateral rhachiotomy* approach has been popularized in the treatment of tuberculosis (29). Positioning the patient properly on the table to permit a lateral view in a prone oblique position is important in this approach from the intervertebral foramina to the anterior half of the body. The posterolateral approach gives the surgeon access to the thoracic disc prolapse under visual guidance without retraction of the dura, and surgery can be accomplished in any of several manners, such as resecting the last section of the rib and the costovertebral articulation or resecting these structures plus the transverse process and a portion of the pedicle. Introduction of the microscope to better visualize structures has improved the outcomes of this approach.

However, most spinal surgeons now recommend an anterior disc excision, with or without fusion (30). The *antero-lateral transthoracic* approach to intervertebral disc surgery, as described by Ransohoff et al. (29) has proved to be a safe, effective method for resecting thoracic disc herniation. Anterior thorascopic discectomy is quickly becoming the preferred anterior technique.

There is some degree of controversy over an anterior versus posterior approach to fractures of the thoracic spine. Some hold that a posterior approach is safer because (a) the thoracic cage offers additional inherent stability in this approach, (b) the major intrathoracic injury that is frequently associated with patients who have suffered high-energy violence to the thoracic spine further complicates anterior surgery, (c) greater loss of blood is incurred in anterior vertebrectomy, and (d) an anterior approach brings the surgeon into contact with vital structures and often involves invading the chest cavity or crossing the diaphragm, both of which can greatly increase immediate postoperative morbidity (31).

PROGNOSIS AND RETURN TO PLAY

Trunk control, including control of the rectus abdominis, internal and external oblique, and spinal extensor muscles, is affected by the level of thoracic spinal cord injury. The more caudal the injury, the greater the likelihood the patient will readapt to activities requiring controlled and coordinated trunk muscle activity.

As Chapman and Anderson (32) have pointed out, the prognosis of patients with thoracolumbar spine fractures and neurologic deficit has improved in terms of survival and quality of life since the principles of timely fracture reduction, decompression, and stabilization have been implemented.

Postoperative therapy is instrumental in getting the player back into the game in the shortest time possible. The initial phase of therapy consists of motivating the patient to overcome pain mentally and to move despite the pain, followed by increasing the range of motion in muscles and joints and then increasing muscle strength and endurance and the strength and stability of the cardiovascular system. A typical exercise program begins with walking and progresses to gentle stretching and then to strengthening activities, all of which are accompanied by the application of ice and heat to affected joints and muscles (33).

Virtually without exception, full recovery after surgical treatment of the thoracic spine is not complete until a graduated, continuing program of postoperative stabilization training is in place. Stabilization, which in its basic form can be described as using the diaphragm and stomach muscles to maintain the spine in a neutral and balanced position through a broad range of motions, is frequently thought of as a series of exercises. In actuality, trunk stabilization is more than that: it is an athletic endeavor in itself and a way of life (34). As with any other athletic program, it requires that patterns of movement be repeated until they become finely tuned natural motions, basic reflex mechanisms that require no conscious thought to perform. These include patterns of movement that are specific to the sport in which the athlete competes.

Returning the athlete in rehabilitation to his or her sport should be accomplished as soon as it is feasible provided that it is a carefully watched gradual and graduated return to each of the activities that constitute the sport.

REFERENCES

1. Silver JR, Stewart D. The prevention of spinal injuries in rugby football. *Paraplegia* 1994;32:442–453.
2. Watkins RG. Spinal exercise program. In: Watkins RG, ed. *The spine in sports*. St. Louis: Mosby, 1995:283–301.
3. Watkins RG, Dennis S, Schebel B, Schneiderman G. Dynamic EMG evaluation of trunk musculature in professional baseball players. *Spine* 1989;14:404.
4. Watkins R, Dennis S, Schnebel B, Schneiderman G. Dynamic EMG evaluation of trunk musculature in professional baseball players. *Spine* 1989;14(NASS 1988 meeting edition)14:3.
5. Carson J, Gumpert J, Jefferson A. Diagnosis and treatment of thoracic intervertebral disc protrusion. *J Neurol Neurosurg Psychiatry* 1971;34:68–77.
6. Bohlman H, Zdeblick T. Anterior excision of herniated thoracic discs. *J Bone Joint Surg Am* 1988;70A:1038–1047.
7. Dommisse GF. The arteries, arterioles, and capillaries of the spinal cord. Surgical guidelines in the prevention of postoperative paraplegia. *Ann R Coll Surg Engl* 1980; 62:369–376.
8. Sward L, Hellstrom M, Jacobsson B, Nyman R, Peterson L. Disc degeneration and associated abnormalities of the spine in elite gymnasts: a magnetic resonance imaging study. *Spine* 1991;16:437–443.
9. Balague F, Fankhauser H, Rosazza A, Waldburger M. Unusual presentation of thoracic disc herniation. *Clin Rheum* 1989;8:269–273.
10. Alberico A, Sahni KS, Hall JA, Young HF. High thoracic disc herniation. *Neurosurgery* 1986;19:449–451.
11. Morgenlander J, Massey EW. Neurogenic claudication with positionally dependent weakness from a thoracic disc herniation. *Neurology* 1989;39:1133–1134.
12. Farfan HF. Biomechanics of the spine in sports. In: Watkins RG, ed. *The spine in sports*. St. Louis:Mosby, 1995:13–20.
13. Prall JA, Winston KR, Brennan R. Spine and spinal cord injuries in downhill skiers. *J Trauma* 1995;39:1115–1118.
14. Guttman L. *Spinal cord injuries: comprehensive management and research*. Oxford: Blackwell Scientific, 1973.
15. Chiles BW III, Cooper PR. Acute spinal injury. *N Engl J Med* 1996;334:514–520.
16. Bauer RD, Errico TJ. Thoracolumbar spine injuries. In: Errico TJ, Bauer RD, Waugh T, eds. *Spinal trauma*. Philadelphia: JB Lippincott Co, 1991:195–269.
17. Bohlman HH. Treatment of fractures and dislocations of the thoracic and lumbar spine. *J Bone Joint Surg Am* 1985;67:165–169.
18. Bohlman HH, Freehafer A, Dejak J. The results of treatment of acute injuries of the upper thoracic spine with paralysis. *J Bone Joint Surg Am* 1985;67:360–369.
19. Roberts JB, Curtiss PH Jr. Stability of the thoracic and lumbar spine in traumatic paraplegia following fracture or fracture-dislocation. *J Bone Joint Surg Am* 1970;52: 1115–1130.
20. Hirasawa Y, Sakakika K. Sports and peripheral nerve injury. *Am J Sports Med* 1983;11:420.
21. Press JM, Young JL, Herring SA. Electrodiagnostic evaluation of spinal problems. In: Watkins RG, ed. *The spine in sports*. St. Louis: Mosby, 1995:61–70.
22. Hedge S, Staas WE. Thoracic disc herniation and spinal cord injury. *Am J Phys Med Rehabil* 1988; 228–229.
23. Alho A. Operative treatment as a part of the comprehensive care for patients with injuries of the thoracolumbar spine. A review. *Paraplegia* 1994;32:509–516.
24. Brown CW, Deffer PA Jr, Akmakjian J, Donaldson DH, Brugman JL. The natural history of thoracic disc herniation. *Spine* 1992;17:S97–102.
25. Stillerman CB, Weiss MH. Management of thoracic disc disease. *Clin Neurosurg* 1992;38:325–352.
26. Fidler WM, Goedhart ZD. Excision of prolapse of thoracic intervertebral disc: a transthoracic technique. *J Bone Joint Surg Br* 1984;66B:4.
27. Otani K, Yoshida M, Fujii E, Nakai S, Shibasaki K. Thoracic disc herniation: surgical treatment in 23 patients. *Spine* 1988;13:1262–1267.
28. Perot PL Jr, Munro DD. Transthoracic removal of midline thoracic disc protrusions causing spinal cord compression. *J Neurosurg* 1969;31:452–458.
29. Ransohoff J, Spencer F, Siew F, Gage L Jr. Case reports and technical notes: transthoracic removal of thoracic disc—report of three cases. *J Neurosurg* 1969;31:459–461.
30. Hamilton MG, Thomas HG. Intradural herniation of a thoracic disc presenting as flaccid paraplegia: case report. *Neurosurgery* 1990;27:482–484.
31. Hamilton A, Webb JK. The role of anterior surgery for vertebral fractures with and without cord compression. *Clin Orthop Relat Res* 1994;300:79–89.
32. Chapman JR, Anderson PA. Thoracolumbar spine fractures with neurologic deficit. *Orthop Clin North Am* 1994;25:595–612.
33. Steffanus RW. Exercise therapy program after prolonged disability: In: Watkins RG, ed. *The spine in sports*. St. Louis: Mosby, 1995:260–263.
34. White AH. Rehabilitation of athletes with spinal pain. In: Watkins RG, ed. *The spine in sports*. St. Louis: Mosby, 1995:264–265.

Sports Neurology, Second Edition,
edited by Barry D. Jordan.
Lippincott–Raven Publishers, Philadelphia © 1998.

16

Injuries of the Lumbar Spine in the Athlete

Baron S. Lonner, *Frank P. Cammisa, Jr., and *Patrick F. O'Leary

*Spine and Scoliosis Service, Long Island Jewish Medical Center, 270-05 76th Avenue,
New Hyde Park, New York 11040; *The Hospital for Special Surgery,
535 East 70th Street, New York, New York 10021*

The athlete, because of exposure to various repetitive activities and trauma, is subject to injury of the lumbar spine. Repetitive lifting, pulling, twisting, and exposure to vibration have all been shown to increase the risk of low-back pain (1). So-called weekend, recreational athletes who may be poorly conditioned and who often suddenly increase their level of exercise or training are particularly prone to injury. On the other hand, a number of traits attributable to the athlete may have a protective effect, diminishing the incidence of back complaints and injury. The level of fitness of an individual has been associated with the risk of back pain. Individuals with a poor level of conditioning have been found to have a higher risk of chronic low-back pain and disability as well as a longer period of recovery from back pain episodes than an individual who is well conditioned (2–5). In addition to being generally physically fit, athletes are less likely to smoke, another risk factor for back pain and degenerative disc disease (1). The athlete commonly has a heightened sense of well-being and benefits from the stress-reducing effects of exercise and sports activities. Depression and poor state of mind are associated with an increased incidence of low-back pain (1). Furthermore, particularly in the high-level athlete, who has little secondary gain to be derived from a long-term back disability and whose motivation is high, psychosocial forces favor rapid recovery from injury (6).

Also, the athletic individual may be adept at avoiding injury because of heightened agility and skill in performing sports activities. Nevertheless, sports are characterized by repetitive activities that place load on the lumbar spine. When this loading is excessive, breakdown and injury may result.

Back pain is a symptom with a number of associated etiologic and modifying factors. In the clinical setting, the health care professional must find a pathologic basis for an individual's symptoms in order to coordinate treatment on the basis of scientific reasoning rather than trial and error. For this reason, a thorough knowledge of functional anatomy and pain generators in the lumbar spine is essential. At times, the diagnosis is self-evident. At other times the underlying cause of back pain is more elusive.

Personal and physical traits of the athlete as well as the nature of athletic activities make the management of lumbar injuries in this group both challenging and rewarding. In college and professional sports, there are pressures to return the athlete to play quickly. It is important that this is timed appropriately, with the primary concern being the individual's well-being and avoidance of worsening an injury that has not fully healed.

This chapter focuses on the diagnosis and basic management of lumbar spine injuries in the athlete with emphasis on anatomic classification of injury. Appropriate timing of return to play is also addressed.

FUNCTIONAL ANATOMY

The lumbar spine has evolved to its present form to function as a load-bearing structure supporting bipedal locomotion. It also serves to protect vital structures and as a framework from which muscles and tendons have their origins and insertions to permit motion.

There are five lumbar vertebrae articulating with the 12 thoracic vertebrae cranially and the sacrum caudally. The vertebral bodies, pedicles, laminae, and spinous and transverse processes are stout and structurally larger than their more cephalad counterparts. This provides a weight-bearing structure capable of supporting the upper body mass as well as protecting the neural elements that course through the spinal canal. The lumbar facets are oriented in the sagittal plane and are essential in determining normal physiologic motion in the lumbar spine (7). Flexion–extension of 10° to 20° per level is permitted in the lumbar spine. Lateral bending and axial rotation are restricted to below 10° at each level because of the sagittal orientation of the facets. The lumbar spine is aligned with a normal lordosis ranging from 30° to 60° (8).

The basic unit of function, the functional spinal unit (FSU) or motion segment, consists of two adjacent vertebrae, the intervening disc, the facet joints, and the supporting ligaments. The main ligamentous structures are the anterior and posterior longitudinal ligaments, the ligamentum flavum, and the interspinous and supraspinous ligaments. The facet capsules also contribute to the stability of the FSU. The stability of the spinal column as a whole relies on the integrity of each individual FSU and the surrounding muscles and fascial structures. Motions in the spine consist of rotation and translation in three axes, six degrees of freedom of motion, as described by White and Panjabi (90). Spinal motions are coupled so that an intentional motion in one plane is always coupled with a secondary motion in a second plane. From this simplified discussion of the biomechanics of the lumbar spine, it can be appreciated that relatively small alterations in structure may lead to significant functional manifestations.

NEUROANATOMY AND PAIN

Fundamental knowledge of the neuroanatomy and innervation of spinal structures is essential for understanding the clinical expression of spinal injury. The spinal cord, bathed in cerebrospinal fluid and contained by the thecal sac, terminates in the conus medullaris most consistently at the L1-2 level. The cauda equina consists of the collection of nerve roots transmitted caudally in the spinal canal to form the spinal nerves that exit inferior to their respective pedicles (7). Each segmental spinal nerve is composed of ventral (motor) and dorsal (sensory) nerve roots, which merge at the level of the dorsal root ganglion in the intervertebral foramen (IVF). It is also at this level that the meningeal coverings of the nerve roots (root sleeves) give rise to the perineurium and epineurium of the peripheral nerve. Cerebrospinal fluid (CSF) bathes the nerve roots to this junction (10). It is this anatomic relationship that allows visualization of the nerve roots to the level of the lateral extent of the IVF but, normally, not beyond on myelography. The dorsal root ganglion is not completely surrounded by CSF as are the nerve roots (10). The ganglion appears to be sensitive to mechanical stresses and pressure increases caused by edema and compression and is probably at least partially responsible for the onset of radicular pain (11–13).

The spinal nerve divides to form dorsal and ventral primary rami after exiting the IVF. Before this division, the sinuvertebral nerve arises and is joined by a sympathetic branch from the ramus communicans. This nerve then reenters the intervertebral foramen (Fig. 1). The sinuvertebral nerve branches to anastomose with nerves on the contralateral side and cephalad and caudad to form an extensive neural network. This network innervates the posterior longitudinal ligament, the outer third of the annulus fibrosus, the anterior epidural venous plexus (Batson's plexus), the anterior dura mater, the root sleeves, and the posterior vertebral periosteum (10,14–16). The dorsal primary ramus divides into medial and lateral branches. The medial portion supplies the facet capsule, ligamentum flavum, lamina, spinous process, interspinous and supraspinous ligaments, and the medial spinal musculature. The lateral division supplies the intertransverse and iliolumbar ligaments, the lateral spinal musculature, and the skin, posteriorly. The ventral

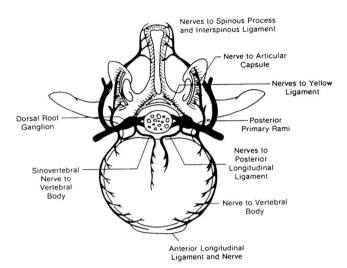

FIG. 1. The three-joint complex receives pleurisegmental innervation by a combination of nerves.

primary ramus provides motor and sensory innervation to the lower extremities in a segmental fashion (17).

The nociceptive response in the patient with nerve root compression is not solely dictated by ongoing mechanical compression of neural structures. This is illustrated in one study in which compression of a nerve root persisted on imaging studies despite resolution of pain (18). Chemical mediators probably play an important role in pain pathways. These include neurotransmitters such as substance P and neurokinin A, with further modulation occurring through inflammatory products of tissue destruction including various prostaglandins, bradykinin, and histamine (19,20).

EPIDEMIOLOGY

Athletes, like all individuals in the general population, are likely to develop low-back pain at some time during their lives. The lifetime cumulative prevalence of low-back pain is between 60% and 80% (21–24). The lumbar spine is subjected to repetitive forces over many years, which eventually leads to degeneration, a normal part of aging (25). The athlete's spine is exposed to many cycles of mechanical load that may lead to acute injury and onset of symptoms. On the other hand, factors associated with low-back pain and degenerative disc disease, (e.g., sedentary lifestyle, poor conditioning, and smoking) are generally absent in the athletic individual, as previously mentioned (26,27). In fact, as a result of aerobic and muscular conditioning, the athlete may have advantages in maintaining the lower back and recovering more quickly from injury (28,29).

A number of sports have a clear association with low-back injuries. These include gymnastics, football, weight lifting, wrestling, dance, and rowing (30–34). No sport is spared of the potential to produce low-back injuries. Sports in which jumping and twisting are common, such as basketball and volleyball, place increased stresses on the lumbar spine (35). Various studies have reported low-back injury in basketball (36), tennis (37), figure skating (38), and golf (39), as well as in other sports. In one study, a 7% incidence of lumbar injuries was noted in intercollegiate athletes involved in football or gymnastics, with low-back strains being the most common diagnosis (40).

There are numerous reports in the literature on the incidence of spondylolysis and spondylolisthesis in the athletic population. The incidence of this entity is increased in sports in which hyperextension of the lumbar spine occurs repetitively, as in gymnastics, football (lineman), weight lifting, and rowing (30,41–43). Jackson (43) found that 40% of athletes with back pain for more than 3 months had abnormalities of the pars interarticularis in the lumbar spine. In another study, 15.2% of college football players had spondylolysis, with only a small percentage being symptomatic (44). This is in comparison with an incidence of 6% in the general population.

An increased incidence of lumbar Scheuermann's disease (45), which may lead to disabling back pain, is seen in weight lifters, swimmers, rowers, gymnasts, and divers.

DIAGNOSTIC EVALUATION

History

Much information is obtained through a complete history. Often, a diagnosis can be made on the basis of thorough questioning and confirmed by physical examination and imaging studies.

The history is tailored according to the nature of the injury. In the event of an acute injury, the chief complaint may be obvious and the diagnosis self-evident from the physical examination and radiographs. In other patients, the onset of symptoms may be more insidious and may require a more extensive history.

A chief complaint should be elicited. Onset, location, intensity, and radiation of pain should be assessed. An acute traumatic event may be associated with low-back strain, contusion, or fracture. The mechanism and energy associated with an injury are also important. For example, a hyperextension injury in a football lineman may be associated with an acute pars interarticularis fracture. A high-energy injury such as a fall of a downhill skier or an accident in automobile racing may result in a burst fracture. Severe pain is associated with acute disc herniation or fracture, whereas milder pain may be associated with chronic degenerative disc disease or low-back strain. Radiation of pain into the foot suggests a herniated disc, and pain that is referred to the buttocks, thigh, and groin may be associated with stenosis or nondiscogenic sources of pain. Factors that exacerbate and relieve symptoms should be sought. Pain that worsens with cough-

ing, sneezing, or bowel movements is commonly related to disc pathology. Symptoms that are brought on by ambulation and relieved by rest or a forward-flexed posture are consistent with spinal stenosis and neurogenic claudication. This is usually seen in the older athlete or the younger individual with a congenitally narrowed canal. Previous back trouble, such as a history of back pain followed by sudden onset of leg pain, is a common presentation for disc herniation. A long history of intermittent low-back complaints in a gymnast may point to an underlying spondylolysis or spondylolisthesis.

In addition, it is important to inquire about previous treatment the patient has undergone as well as response to the treatment rendered. A patient with a previous spinal fusion may be at risk for the development of degeneration and symptoms above or below the arthrodesis (46,47). The patient's past medical history is important. A history of tumor, infection, or scoliosis, for example, may be relevant to the patient's current symptoms. A history of inflammatory bowel disease; joint pain; cardiac, ocular, or pulmonary problems; and urethral discharge may point to one of the seronegative spondyloarthropathies as the underlying diagnosis. Abnormal vaginal bleeding, hematuria, and blood in the stool all suggest the possibility of referred pain from an extraspinal source. Pathology of any of the visceral structures and especially the retroperitoneal organs such as the kidneys, ovaries, and uterus can mimic that of spinal disease. In summary, a plethora of information can be gathered from a comprehensive history.

Physical Examination

A thorough examination is essential for accurate diagnosis of injuries to the lumbar spine. The patient is first asked to stand up and walk if possible. Fluidity of motion and posture are assessed. A patient who leans to one side may have muscle spasm or a sciatic list. The individual who is unable to stand fully erect may have a stenotic spine with symptoms exacerbated by extension due to infolding of hypertrophied ligamentum flavum. Asymmetry, preexisting scoliosis, or sagittal plane abnormalities (e.g., kyphosis, lordosis) should be assessed. Gait is then evaluated. An antalgic (short-strided) gait is likely to be associated with nerve root irritation, marked back pain, and tight hamstrings. A normal gait indicates a lesser degree of dysfunction. The spine is palpated for regions of tenderness. Spinous process tenderness is consistent with fracture or contusion, whereas paraspinal tenderness is secondary to reflex muscle spasm commonly seen in a host of conditions. Spinal mobility is assessed next. Again, the fluidity of motion is observed as the patient is asked to forward flex, extend, lateral bend, and twist to both sides. A hand is placed on the spine to feel for any abnormal motion or crepitus. Pain on forward flexion is consistent with discogenic disease, fractures, or spinal instability. Symptoms on extension indicate pathology in the posterior elements such as spondylolysis or facet-related pain. Pain on lateral bend or rotation is also seen in disc herniation with nerve root involvement or muscle spasm.

Careful neurologic assessment is necessary to localize levels of neurologic deficit. Motor and sensory testing of specific myotomes and dermatomes, respectively, is performed. Motor power must be carefully graded between zero and five. Reflexes, including deep tendon reflexes, plantar responses (Babinski), and ankle clonus, are also assessed. Hyperreflexia and the latter two upper motor neuron signs suggest an injury to the conus medullaris or a more cephalad level of the spinal cord. Tension signs, indicative of nerve root irritation, as caused by disc herniation should be assessed. These include Lasègue sign, straight-leg raising, contralateral straight-leg raising, bowstring signs, and femoral stretch tests (48–50).

Finally, the hips should be assessed as a possible source of pain. Pain in the lower extremities may be due to radiculopathy, direct injury, or osteoarthritis. Leg lengths should also be evaluated. Leg-length inequality can be a source of back pain resulting from the resultant asymmetric load distribution on the lumbar spine.

Radiographic Evaluation

Initial imaging should consist of a standing anteroposterior (AP) and lateral radiograph of the lumbosacral region. Fractures, spondylolisthesis, marked degenerative changes (i.e., disc space narrowing, osteophytes, degenerative scoliosis), deformity, and underlying disease processes such as ankylosing spondylitis are clearly elucidated on these radiographs. On the basis of this initial evaluation, further imaging studies may be warranted. Oblique projections delineate the region of the pars interarticularis and facet joints (Fig. 2). Spondylolysis, facet fractures and arthrosis, and foraminal stenosis may be visualized. In a patient with mechanical back pain and possible segmental instability caused by degenerative disease or trauma, lateral flexion–extension views are helpful in assessing spinal stability (51). Findings that are suggestive of instability include sagittal plane translation, disc space collapse, and facet subluxation. Translation of more than 4.5 mm or 15% of the AP diameter of the vertebral body on flexion–extension views is indicative of instability (52).

Technetium bone scanning is a useful adjunct for detecting occult lesions such as spondylolysis,

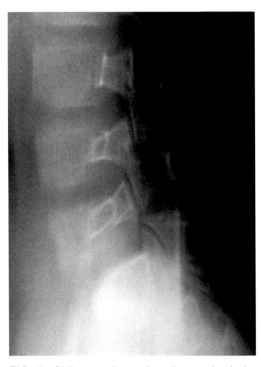

FIG. 2. Oblique radiographs allow optimal visualization of the pars interarticularis. The oblique tomogram illustrates a spondylolytic defect in an 11-year-old boy with back pain.

tumor, or infection that is suspected but not visualized on a plain radiograph. This modality is also valuable for detecting stress fractures of the pars interarticularis region. Single-photon emission computed tomographic (SPECT) scanning has enhanced the physician's ability to localize occult lesions (53). It is also useful in assessing the acuity of a pars interarticularis fracture. Magnetic resonance imaging (MRI) is the ideal noninvasive modality for revealing neural compression and delineating soft tissue structures. It is useful in assessing disc degeneration by showing morphology as well as water content. Infection and subtle bone injuries causing marrow edema as well as ligamentous injuries may be diagnosed with MRI. A high percentage of asymptomatic individuals have been noted to have degenerative findings on MRI, including disc herniation in approximately 20% of individuals under the age of 60 (54). It is for this reason that one must carefully correlate the patient's symptoms with findings on imaging studies before embarking on treatment.

Computed tomography is an excellent modality for assessing bone detail. When combined with myelography, this is highly effective in delineating neural compression. Myelography can be combined with flexion–extension lateral views providing information on the dynamic nature of neural compression. For example, neural element compromise is usually more severe with the spine extended in the individual with spinal stenosis. The disadvantage of myelography is that it is an invasive test that can result in spinal headache, nausea, vomiting, and back pain. This test should be reserved for individuals for whom surgery is planned and MRI is not sufficient.

Discography may be useful in delineating symptomatic levels in patients with low-back pain and more than one degenerative segment. The study is performed by percutaneously injecting radiopaque contrast material into the substance of the intervertebral disc space. A positive test is associated with extravasation of dye from a rent in the annulus fibrosus or filling of a protruding disc accompanied by reproduction of concordant symptoms, that is, the same pain experienced by the patient clinically. This study can also be used to determine levels for fusion in the lumbar spine. If an individual has a clear indication for fusion, based on spinal instability, for example, and there are a number of degenerative segments, discography may define symptomatic levels that should be included in the fusion. The utility of this diagnostic modality remains controversial (55,56).

Electromyography and nerve conduction studies provide further confirmation or clarification of clinically significant neural compression. For example, in a patient with neurogenic claudication related to spinal stenosis without a static neurologic deficit and in whom severe stenosis is clearly seen at one level but moderate stenosis is present at other levels, these studies reveal levels of significant neural compression, guiding the surgeon to the appropriate levels to decompress (57,58). Both somatosensory evoked potentials and dermatosensory evoked potentials have a role in demonstrating preoperative neural compression as well as the adequacy of intraoperative decompression (59,60).

SPECIFIC INJURIES AND DISORDERS

Sprains and Strains

These musculoligamentous injuries are commonly seen in the athletic population. The athlete who has sustained a back injury with local paraspinal tenderness and no neurologic deficit most likely has a sprain or strain. Gradual resolution of symptoms over a 1- to 2-week period can be expected. Local measures, including ice followed by heat, rest, and nonsteroidal anti-inflammatory medications, are the mainstay of treatment. Muscle spasm is often a major component of symptoms. Early treatment with a muscle relaxant such as a benzodiazepine (e.g., Valium) or cyclobenzaprine (Flexeril) helps control symptoms. Contusion resulting from a direct blow to the lower back similarly falls into this category and should respond to the same treatment. The athlete is gradually returned to sports activities as symptoms abate.

Herniated Nucleus Pulposus

Radiculopathy caused by a herniated disc is often preceded by a period in which back pain alone is experienced. This corresponds to a weakening of the annulus fibrosus with bulging of the nucleus pulposus. The onset of leg pain related to frank disc herniation can be insidious or arise suddenly from an event that increases intradiscal pressure such as bending and twisting or lifting (61).

Disc herniation is most common in individuals in the third and fourth decades of life. Herniation is much less common in the adolescent athlete but does occur, frequently in association with avulsion of the posterior ring epiphysis (Fig. 3) (62,91).

Radiculopathy secondary to disc herniation is characterized by pain, paresthesias, or anesthesia along a specific dermatomal distribution with or without weakness of muscles supplied by the affected nerve root. The most commonly involved levels are L4-5 and L5-S1, resulting in L-5 and S-1 radiculopathy, respectively. Disc herniation usually occurs through a weakened portion of the annulus fibrosus just lateral to the centrally located posterior longitudinal ligament. This results in displacement and compression of the nerve root that obliquely traverses the disc space, such as L-5 in L4-5 herniations. A far lateral herniation may occur in the area of the intervertebral foramen or lateral to the foramen. In this instance, compression of the nerve root exiting below the corresponding pedicle is affected (e.g., L-4 in L4-5 herniations). Alternatively, a large central disc herniation may occur, resulting in an acute cauda equina syndrome with loss of bowel and bladder function, saddle anesthesia, and variable neurologic findings in the lower extremities. This constitutes a surgical emergency requiring immediate decompression.

Neurologic findings in individuals with significant nerve root compression are variable. Tension signs are positive in over 95% of patients (63). Lasègue's sign (supine straight-leg raising with the addition of ankle dorsiflexion) and seated straight-leg raising are highly sensitive for disc herniation as indicated earlier. Contralateral straight-leg raising, positive when symptoms are reproduced in the affected limb with elevation of the unaffected extremity, is a highly specific sign for disc herniation but is present in only 20% of patients with the pathology (63). The femoral nerve stretch test, flexion of the knee performed with the patient in the prone position, is positive with disc herniations

cephalad to the L4-5 level. MRI is the imaging modality of choice for confirming suspected disc herniation (Fig. 4).

Nonoperative management of symptomatic disc herniation is successful in more than 90% of patients. No more than 2 to 3 days of bed rest is recommended. Prolonged bed rest is associated with a greater loss of workdays without additional therapeutic benefit over a brief period of bed rest (64). Analgesia with a nonsteroidal antiinflammatory medication is provided. Narcotics are added as necessary. In selected situations, a tapering regimen of an oral corticosteroid preparation may be administered in an attempt to control symptoms caused by an inflammatory process. Muscle relaxants are helpful in reducing pain due to muscle spasm.

If symptoms in the acute period do not respond to the preceding regimen of medication and rest, epidural steroid injections or selective nerve root injection may be considered. The antiinflammatory effects of a locally injected steroid preparation such as methylprednisolone results in improvement in 25% to 75% of patients (65,66). Complications of epidural steroid injections are not common but include meningitis, epidural abscess, dural cutaneous fistula, and development of Cushing's syndrome secondary to excessive glucocorticoid administration, a rare complication (67). Spinal headache can result from intrathecal needle placement.

Other modalities such as physical therapy, spinal manipulation, ultrasonography, transcutaneous electrical nerve stimulation, corsets, and traction do not have proven benefit, although temporary relief may be experienced with these methods, allowing improved mobilization (68).

For the athlete who has failed a conservative regimen and has continued difficulty with activities of daily living and/or inability to engage in sports activities, surgery is indicated. In addition, for the individual presenting with a profound neurologic deficit, such as a footdrop, a progressive deficit, or cauda equina syndrome, surgery must be performed urgently. A surgical success rate of 90% or more can be expected with current microsurgical techniques in which spinal stability is preserved (69). In patients who did not have an absolute indication for surgery, a comparison

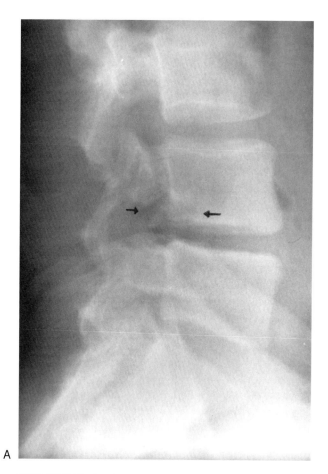

A

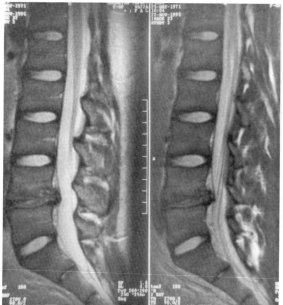

B

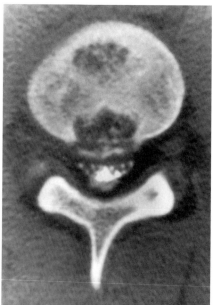

C

FIG. 3. Avulsion of posterior ring apophysis. **A:** Lateral radiograph demonstrating avulsion of posterior ring apophysis (*arrows*). Note defect in posterior inferior corner of vertebral body and bone avulsion within canal. **B:** Magnetic resonance image demonstrates lesion of bone with associated disc material. **C:** Axial computed tomographic image obtained after myelography demonstrating defect in vertebral body with retropulsion into canal, with resultant stenosis.

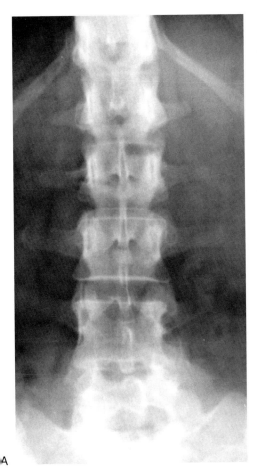

A

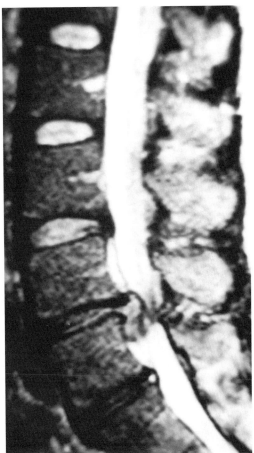

B

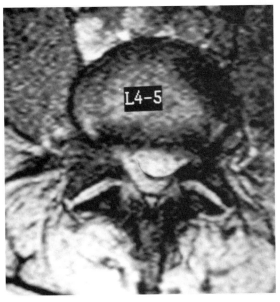

C

FIG. 4. Magnetic resonance imaging is the ideal modality for diagnosing disc herniation. **A:** The plain antero-posterior radiography of this 38-year-old male with acute onset of leg pain reveals no abnormalities. **B:** The sagittal magnetic resonance image reveals a large disc herniation at L4-5 that protrudes to the left side, compressing the fifth lumbar nerve root as seen on the axial image (**C**).

of results obtained with nonoperative and operative treatment showed improved results in the operative group at 1 year with no difference in outcome between the two groups at 4 and 10 years (70). Thus, for the patient to whom early return to athletics and work is important, more rapid results can be expected with surgery.

Spinal Stenosis

Lumbar spinal stenosis represents the end stage of a continuum of degenerative pathology. Kirkaldy-Willis (71) elucidated the concept of progressive degeneration of the three-joint complex—the intervertebral disc and the two facet joints—through the phases of spinal dysfunction, instability, and finally stabilization. The last phase is characterized by disc space narrowing, facet subluxation, often low-grade spondylolisthesis, and facet hypertrophy and osteophyte formation. Bone pathology, hypertrophy and infolding of the ligamentum flavum, and bulging or herniation of the intervertebral disc all contribute to stenosis. Stenosis occurs centrally in the spinal canal, in the lateral recesses, or commonly in combination. Symptoms depend on the locale of neural compression. The clinical expression of this problem is a result of vascular congestion and local inflammatory responses in addition to pure mechanical compression leading to chronic neural changes (72).

Spinal stenosis is more common in the older athlete but is also seen in younger individuals with congenitally narrowed spinal canals. Neurogenic claudication is the clinical expression of this pathology. Symptoms of pain or paresthesias in the buttocks, thigh, and groin and occasionally below the knee occur with walking and upright posture. Relief of symptoms occurs with leaning forward (shopping cart sign), sitting, or lying down. There is often a paucity of physical findings with no neurologic deficits present with the patient at rest. Tension signs are usually negative. Spinal flexion is usually excellent, although extension is often limited by pain and facet joint arthrosis.

Plain radiographs should be obtained to assess for degenerative scoliosis, spondylolisthesis, and lateral listhesis as well as overall spinal alignment. Spondylosis may be advanced or seemingly minor on radiographs. MRI serves as a good screening

study for visualizing neural compression (Fig. 5). For patients in whom surgery is contemplated, computed tomography (CT)–myelography provides the added benefit of good visualization of bone anatomy. Electromyographic and nerve conduction velocity studies or dermato-sensory evoked potential may assist in surgical decision making as well.

The initial management of the athlete with spinal stenosis is similar to that of the patient with an acute disc herniation. An oral steroid taper has been found to be helpful in some of our patients with acute, severe symptoms. Epidural steroid injections or selective nerve root blocks are often employed; however, success rates may be as low as 20% to 30% (73,74).

For patients who fail to respond to nonoperative management, including a course of as many as three injections, surgery is recommended. Surgery is directed at the specific pathology. In an individual with unilateral lateral recess and foraminal stenosis, laminotomy and foraminotomy with or without disc excision are all that is required. In a patient with central stenosis, complete laminectomy is necessary. Care must be taken to preserve the facet articulations to maintain spinal stability. Concomitant arthrodesis has been found to improve the success rate in patients with associated spondylolisthesis (75). Fusion is also performed for patients with degenerative scoliosis and/or lateral listhesis in whom laminectomy is required or patients in whom adequate decompression destabilizes the spine.

Spondylolysis and Spondylolisthesis

Wiltse et al. (76) have classified the causes of spondylolisthesis into five types. Two types are traumatic in origin and are relevant to this chapter. An acute trauma or repetitive stress over time may lead to overt fracture or microfractures in the pars interarticularis. Spondylolysis when associated with displacement may lead to spondylolisthesis. So-called isthmic spondylolisthesis, then, is divided into three subtypes: acute fracture, lytic, and elongated types (Fig. 6). Fracture of other portions of the vertebrae such as the facet may also lead to vertebral translation (traumatic spondylolisthesis).

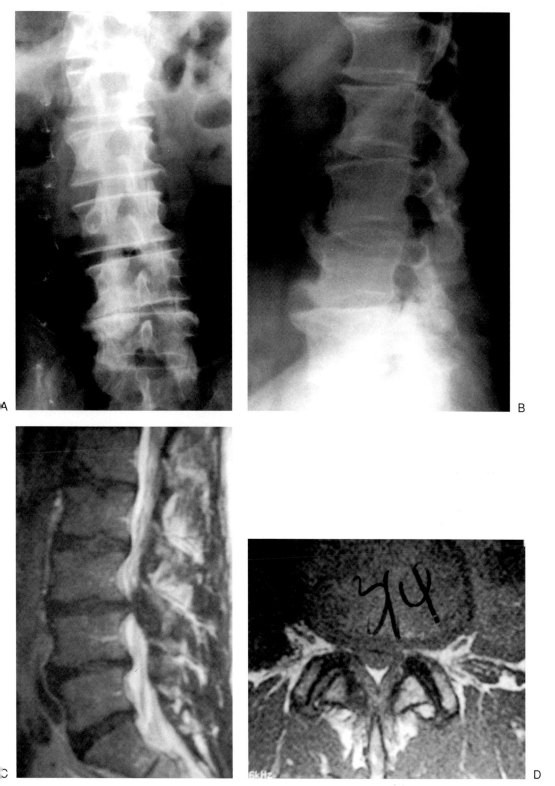

FIG. 5. A 58-year-old avid downhill skier presented with symptoms of neurogenic claudication. Skiing is well tolerated by the patient due to the forward-flexed posture characteristic of this sport. **A:** The anteroposterior radiograph reveals degenerative scoliosis. **B:** A lateral radiograph depicts disc space collapse, retrolisthesis, and osteophyte formation. **C:** Sagittal magnetic resonance image shows multilevel stenosis most marked at the L3-4 level as illustrated in the axial image **(D)**.

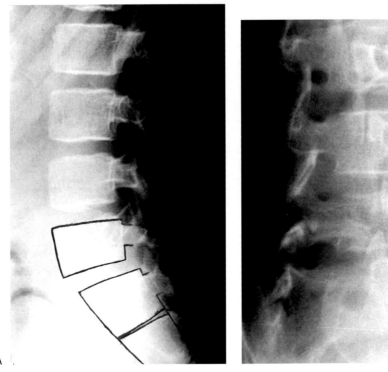

A   B

FIG. 6. An 11-year-old boy presented with back pain after an injury sustained during a hockey game. **A:** The lateral standing radiograph reveals a grade I spondylolisthesis of L-5 on S-1. **B:** The oblique view points to the etiology of the slip, a spondylolytic defect of the pars interarticularis of the fifth lumbar vertebra.

Spondylolytic defects occur most commonly in individuals engaged in repetitive hyperextension activities, as mentioned previously. In the adult athlete, spondylolysis or spondylolisthesis may be found incidentally on radiographs and is often an asymptomatic lesion. In these individuals, back pain caused by a muscle strain resolves with a brief period of rest. On the other hand, acute fractures and high-grade slips may be symptomatic and require more aggressive treatment.

Spondylolisthesis is graded by the percentage of slip of the vertebra on the one below. Grade I, II, III, and IV lesions denote 0% to 25%, 25% to 50%, 50% to 75%, and 75% to 100% slippage, respectively (92). Spondyloptosis refers to a vertebra that is completely displaced and migrated caudal to the superior end plate of the vertebra below. The slip angle, the angulation of the cephalad vertebra on the caudad one, most commonly L-5 on S-1, is also measured.

Spondylolysis is the most common bone injury in the young athlete's spine. Physical findings include localized midline bone tenderness and pain with extension of the spine that loads the posterior elements. Spondylolisthesis is often associated with hamstring tightness accompanied by a characteristic short-strided gait. The Phalen-Dickson sign denotes the typical gait of the patient with tight hamstrings who walks with the knees and hips slightly flexed (77). In patients with advanced slips, obvious sagittal deformity may be observed. Pain may be referred to the buttocks, thigh, and groin. In some individuals, radicular symptoms occur. This is commonly caused by impingement on the exiting nerve root by fibrocartilaginous tissue that forms in an attempt to heal the defect.

In a patient with a nondisplaced lesion or early stress reaction, radiographic visualization may be difficult. Oblique views allow direct evaluation of the pars interarticularis region. A bone scan is helpful in localizing an early injury. Single-photon emission computed tomography gives greater detail (78). Tomograms provide excellent visualization of bone detail and may be performed in oblique projections. Computed tomography is also helpful and results in less radiation exposure than with tomography.

The treatment of the athlete with an acute spondylolytic defect consists of casting or bracing of the lumbar spine in a hypolordotic or straightened position to decrease the stresses on the pars interarticularis caused by a pincer mechanism from the inferior facet of the vertebra above and the superior facet of the vertebra below the lesion. Assessment of acuity of the fracture is assisted by imaging modalities. Radiographs revealing a fracture with jagged edges and no reactive sclerosis combined with a positive bone scan point to an acute fracture. A chronic defect is characterized by bone resorption or sclerosis with rounded edges and a negative bone scan. In a patient with an acute fracture without displacement, healing of the fracture may occur with immobilization for 3 to 6 months (79,80). A unilateral fracture is more likely to heal. In the patient with a chronic injury with acute pain, a brief period of rest with modification of offending activities usually results in resolution of symptoms. Physical therapy consists predominantly of a flexion program and stretching of the lumbodorsal fascia and hamstrings to make them more supple, minimizing forces in the lumbar spine that occur with forward flexion. Antilordotic bracing may be instituted for patients who are refractory to this management (79). If this fails to alleviate symptoms, a spinal fusion may be indicated. In patients with neurologic deficits related to nerve root impingement, fusion should be combined with the appropriate decompression. Direct repair of minimally displaced spondylolytic defects cephalad to L-5 may be attempted in some patients (81).

In the skeletally immature athlete with a grade I or II spondylolisthesis, the foregoing approach is followed. Activity modification is indicated for individuals with symptomatic grade I or II involvement. For the child who demonstrates progression of slip, with or without onset of neurologic findings or back pain, or for the skeletally immature patient with a grade III or IV slip, fusion is indicated. For the asymptomatic adult, observation alone is all that is required. Progression is unlikely. The adolescent female patient during the growth spurt is most likely to exhibit progression (82,83). Patients must be observed with serial standing lateral radiographs of the lumbar spine. The issue of reduction of high-grade slips when performing an arthrodesis is controversial. It is generally accepted that in patients with sagittal plane decompensation and imbalance, slip angle greater than 30°, or severe cosmetic deformity, reduction is warranted. More important than anatomic reduction is the correction of the slip angle to approach 0° (84). Reduction is associated with a significant rate of neurologic complications including cauda equina syndrome.

Fractures

Fractures of the lumbar spine are often associated with high-energy injuries. Various fractures or fracture-dislocations may occur in sports such as skiing or automobile racing. A widely used classification scheme has been introduced by Denis (85). This classification is based on a three-column model of the spine. The anterior column is composed of the anterior longitudinal ligament and the anterior half of the vertebral body. The middle column consists of the posterior portion of the vertebral body and the posterior longitudinal ligament. The posterior column is composed of the posterior elements including the pedicles, laminae, facets, and spinous and transverse processes.

Damage to one column results in a stable injury, whereas involvement of two or more columns results in a potentially unstable injury. In general, stable fractures may be managed nonoperatively and unstable injuries require arthrodesis with or without decompression. Neurologic "stability" must also be factored into the decision on whether or not to perform surgery. For example, burst fractures occurring at the thoracolumbar junction involving only the anterior and middle columns in a neurologically stable patient can be effectively managed with a total contact orthosis or cast. Such treatment of this injury has been found to result in healing with maintenance of alignment and no neurologic deterioration (86). In patients with progressive neurologic deficits or incomplete neurologic injuries, arthrodesis with decompression is indicated.

The following specific injuries have been defined by Denis (85) and are discussed briefly. Management of these individual fracture types is outlined in the accompanying table (Table 1).

Compression fractures are caused by a flexion mechanism resulting in decreased height in the anterior column. This is a common fracture in the elderly and in others with osteoporosis. In the young patient with normal bone mineral density, a higher magnitude of trauma is necessary to cause this type of injury. In these patients, the middle column may act as a fulcrum about which the vertebra rotates, resulting in posterior column ligamentous disruption and a potentially unstable injury.

Burst fractures are caused by axial compression. By definition, the anterior and middle columns are involved. There is often significant retropulsion of bone fragments into the spinal canal. This injury is often associated with neurologic deficits. The posterior column may also be involved with fractures of the laminae and/or facets. This may lead to dural laceration and nerve root entrapment (87).

A flexion–distraction mechanism causes the so-called Chance fracture. In the past, this was caused by a sudden deceleration in an automobile in which the injured patient was restrained by the now-outlawed lap-type seat belt. The injury is caused by flexion around an axis just anterior to the vertebral body with a distraction moment arising in the posterior column and proceeding anteriorly. This may be a pure bone injury, ligamentous injury, or mixed bone and ligamentous injury. The nature of the injury determines the mode of treatment (88).

Finally, a fracture-dislocation results from shear and torsional forces causing dislocation of a motion segment. This is a highly unstable injury that must be treated with operative stabilization.

RETURN TO PLAY

For the majority of athletes afflicted with a lumbar injury, return to the previous activity level is possible. The timing of the return to play is governed by the nature of the injury and treatment required.

In patients with contusions and strains, gradual return to full activity is allowed as symptoms abate. It is helpful to enroll patients in a physical therapy program emphasizing abdominal and postural muscle strengthening, flexibility and stretching exercises, as well as aerobic conditioning (89). Appropriate protective padding and instruction on prevention of injury in specific sports are important to minimize future injuries.

Return to the preinjury level of sports participation is variable in athletes who have undergone spinal surgery. Timing of rehabilitation must be

TABLE 1. *Management of specific fracture types*

Injury	Nonoperative	Operative
Compression fracture	Rigid orthosis	Posterior instrumentation and fusion for two-column injury with posterior ligamentous failure
Burst fracture	Rigid orthosis for patients without neurologic deficits or complete deficits and minimal deformity	Posterior instrumentation with indirect decompression, anterior decompression and fusion with instrumentation, or combined anterior and posterior approach for progressive or incomplete neurologic deficits, significant deformity, and/or three-column injuries
Chance fracture	Rigid orthosis or cast for bone injury	Posterior instrumentation and fusion for predominantly ligamentous injury
Fracture-dislocation		Posterior instrumentation and fusion

tailored to the individual. Patients who have had discectomy may begin a graduated physical therapy program at 4 to 6 weeks, whereas those who have undergone arthrodesis should not begin rehabilitation until fusion is complete. A single-level arthrodesis in the lumbar spine carries a better prognosis for return to sports than a multi-level fusion in which nonfused adjacent motion segments are placed under significantly increased loads. Furthermore, although it is possible, return to full contact sports after spinal fusion is generally not advisable.

For most individuals, some degree of sports participation is possible following lumbar spine injuries. Modification of previous levels of activity may be necessary to minimize chronic symptoms and prevent further injury. Unfortunately, for the professional athlete, this may signify the end of a career.

SUMMARY

The successful diagnosis and long-term management of injuries to the lumbar spine in the athlete rely on a pathoanatomic approach to these conditions. This approach allows matching of appropriate treatment modalities with specific diagnostic entities. Treating spinal disorders in the athlete who is uniquely exposed to repetitive injuries is often rewarding because of the athlete's psychosocioeconomic predisposition to obtaining maximal improvement. The individual's preinjury level of conditioning and general health as well as motivation promote optimal functional recovery.

REFERENCES

1. Frymoyer JW, Pope MH, Clements JH, et al. Risk factors in low back pain. *J Bone Joint Surg Am* 1983;65A:213.
2. Cady LD, Bischoff DP, O'Connell ER, et al. Strength and fitness and subsequent back injuries in fire fighters. *J Occup Med* 1979;21:269–272.
3. Nachemson A, Eck C, Lindstrom IL, et al. Chronic low back disability can largely be prevented: a prospective randomized trial in industry. AAOS 56th Annual Meeting, Feb 1989, Las Vegas.
4. Kelsey JL. An epidemiological study of acute herniated lumbar intervertebral discs. *Rheumatol Rehabil* 1975;14:144–159.
5. Svensson, HO, Andersson GBJ, Johansson S, Wilhelmsson C, Vedin A. A retrospective study of low back pain in 38- to 64-year-old women. Frequency of occurrence and impact on medical services. *Spine* 1988;13:548–552.
6. Fordyce WE. Behavioral factors in pain. *Neurosurg Clin North Am* 1991;2:749–759.
7. Bullough PG, Boachie-Adjei O. Descriptive anatomy: gross and microscopic. In: *Atlas of spinal diseases.* Philadelphia: JB Lippincott Co, 1988:10–33.
8. Bernhardt M, Bridwell KH. Segmental analysis of the sagittal plane alignment of the normal thoracic and lumbar spines and thoracolumbar junction. *Spine* 1989;14:717–721.
9. White AA, Panjabi MM. *Clinical biomechanics of the spine.* Philadelphia: JB Lippincott Co, 1978.
10. Hollingshead WH. Anatomy for surgeons, vol 3. *The back and limbs,* 3rd ed. Philadelphia: Harper & Row, 1982:167–193.
11. Howe JF, Loeser JD, Calvin, WH. Mechanosensitivity of dorsal root ganglia and chronically injured axons: a physiologic basis for the radicular pain of nerve root compression. *Pain* 1977;3:25–41.
12. Rydevik B, Myers RR, Powell HC. Pressure increase in the dorsal root ganglion following mechanical compression. Closed compartment syndrome in nerve roots. *Spine* 1989;14:574.
13. Vanderlinden RG. Subarticular entrapment of the dorsal root ganglion as a cause of sciatic pain. *Spine* 1984;9:19–22.
14. Edgar MA, Ghadially JA. Innervation of the lumbar spine. *Clin Orthop* 1976;115:35.
15. Hirsch C, Ingelmark B, Miller M. The anatomical basis for low back pain. *Acta Orthop Scand* 1963;1:33.
16. Bogduk N. The innervation of the lumbar spine. *Spine* 1983;8:286–293.
17. Hoppenfeld S. Nerve root lesions by neurologic level. In: *Orthopaedic neurology.* Philadelphia: JB Lippincott Co, 1977:45–72.
18. Garfin SR, Rydevik BL, Brown RA. Compressive neuropathy of spinal nerve roots: a mechanical or biological problem? *Spine* 1991;16:162–166.
19. Aimone LD. Neurochemistry and modulation of pain. In: Sinatra RS, Hord AH, Ginsberg B, Preble LM, eds. *Acute pain: mechanisms and management.* St. Louis: Mosby–Year Book, 1992:29–43.
20. Marx JL. Brain peptides: is substance P a transmitter of pain signals? *J Sci* 1979;205:886–889.
21. Hult L. Cervical, dorsal, and lumbar spinal syndromes. *Acta Orthop Scand* 1954;24:174–175.
22. Horal J. The clinical appearance of low back disorders in the city of Gothenburg, Sweden. *Acta Orthop Scand Suppl* 1969;118:1–109.
23. Lawrence JS. Disc degeneration. Its frequency and relationship to symptoms. *Ann Rheum Dis* 1969;28:121–138.
24. Kelsey JL, White AA. Epidemiology and impact of low back pain. *Spine* 1980;5:133.
25. Frymoyer JW. Epidemiological studies of low back pain. *Spine* 1980;5:419.
26. Brigham CD, Schafer MF. Low back pain in athletes. *Adv Sports Med Fitness* 1988;1:145.
27. Frymoyer JW. Spine radiographs in patients with low back pain: an epidemiological study in men. *J Bone Joint Surg Am* 1984;66A:1048.
28. Cady LD, Thomas PC, Karwasky RJ. Program for increasing health and fitness of firefighters. *J Occup Med* 1985;27:110.

29. Plowman SA. Physical activity, physical fitness, and low back pain. In: Holloszy JO, ed. *Exercise and sports sciences review,* vol 20. Philadelphia: Williams & Wilkins, 1992.

30. Hoshina H. Spondylolysis in athletes. *Phys Sports Med* 1980;8:75.

31. Jackson DW. Low back pain in young athletes: evaluation of stress reactions and discogenic problems. *Am J Sports Med* 1979;7:364.

32. Micheli LJ. Back injuries in gymnastics. *Clin Sports Med* 1985;4:85.

33. Micheli LJ. Back injuries in dancers. *Clin Sports Med* 1983;2:473.

34. Stanitski CL. Low back pain in young athletes. *Phys Sports Med* 1982;10:77.

35. Schultz A. Loads on the lumbar spine. *J Bone Joint Surg Am* 1982;64A:713.

36. Henry JH, Lareau B, Neigut D. The injury rate in professional basketball. *Am J Sports Med* 1982;10:16.

37. Feeler LC. Racquet sports. *Spine* 1990;4:337.

38. Fortin JP, Roberts D. Competitive figure skating injuries. *Arch Phys Med Rehabil* 1987;68:642.

39. Duda M. Golf injuries: they really do happen. *Phys Sports Med* 1987;15:191.

40. Keene JS, Albert MJ, Springer SL, Drummond DS, Clancy WG Jr. Back injuries in college athletes. *J Spinal Disord* 1989;2:190–195.

41. Ferguson PJ, McMaster MC, Stanitski CL. Low back pain in college football linemen. *J Bone Joint Surg Am* 1979;56A:1300.

42. Jackson DW, Wiltse LL, Cirincione RJ. Spondylolysis in the female gymnast. *Clin Orthop* 1981;117:68.

43. Jackson DW. Low back pain in young athletes: evaluation of stress reactions and discogenic problems. *Am J Sports Med* 1979;7:364.

44. McCarroll JR, Miller, JM, Ritter MA. Lumbar spondylolysis and spondylolisthesis in college football players: a prospective study. *Am J Sports Med* 1986;14:404.

45. Wilcox PG, Spencer CW. Dorsolumbar kyphosis in Scheuermann's disease. *Clin Sports Med* 1986;5:343.

46. Dekutoski MB, Schendel MJ, Ogilvie JW, et al. Comparison of in-vivo and in-vitro adjacent segment motion after lumbar fusion. *Spine* 1994;19:1745–1750.

47. Lee CK, Langrana NA. Lumbosacral spinal fusion. *Spine* 1984;9:574.

48. Troup JDG. Straight leg raising and the qualifying tests for increased root tension. Their predictive value after back and sciatic pain. *Spine* 1981;6:526–527.

49. Kosteljanetz M, Bang F, Schmidt-Olsen F. The clinical significance of straight leg raising (Lasègue's sign) in the diagnosis of prolapsed lumbar disc. *Spine* 1988;13:393–395.

50. Estridge MN, Rouhe SA, Johnson NG. The femoral stretch test: a valuable sign in diagnosing upper lumbar disc herniations. *J Neurosurg* 1982;57:813–815.

51. Kirkaldy-Willis WH, Hill RJ. A more precise diagnosis for low back pain. *Spine* 1979;4:102–107.

52. Posner I, White AA, Edwards WT, et al. A biomechanical analysis of the clinical stability of the lumbar and lumbosacral spine. *Spine* 1982;7:374–389.

53. Collier BD, Johnson RP, Carrera GF, et al. Painful spondylolysis or spondylolisthesis studied by radiography and single-photon emission computed tomography. *Radiology* 1985;154:207–211.

54. Boden SD, Davis DO, Dina TS, et al. Abnormal magnetic resonance scans of the lumbar spine in asymptomatic patients: a prospective investigation. *J Bone Joint Surg Am* 1990;72A:403–408.

55. Nachemson A. Lumbar discography—where are we today? *Spine* 1989;14:555–557.

56. Walsh TR, Weinstein JN, Spratt KF, et al. Lumbar discography in normal subjects: a controlled prospective study. *J Bone Joint Surg Am* 1990;72A:1081–1088.

57. Eisen A, Hoirch M. The electrodiagnostic evaluation of spinal root lesions. *Spine* 1983;8:98–106.

58. Johnsson KE, Rosen I, Uden A. Neurophysiologic investigation of patients with spinal stenosis. *Spine* 1987;12:483–487.

59. Gepstein R, Brown MD. Somatosensory-evoked potentials in lumbar nerve root decompression. *Clin Orthop* 1989;245:69–71.

60. Heron LD, Trippi AC, Gonyeau M. Intraoperative use of dermatomal somatosensory-evoked potentials in lumbar stenosis surgery. *Spine* 1987;12:379–383.

61. Nachemson A, Morris JM. In vivo measurements of intradiscal pressure. *J Bone Joint Surg Am* 1964;46A:1077.

62. Takata K, Inoue S, Takahashi K, et al. Fracture of the posterior margin of a lumbar vertebral body. *J Bone Joint Surg Am* 1988;70A:589–594.

63. Spangfort EV. The lumbar disc herniation: a computer-aided analysis of 2,504 operations. *Acta Orthop Scand* 1972;142(Suppl):1–95.

64. Deyo RA, Diehl AK, Rosenthal M. How many days of bedrest for acute low back pain? A randomized clinical trial. *N Engl J Med* 1986;315:1064–1070.

65. Benzon H. Epidural steroid injections for low back pain and lumbosacral radiculopathy. *Pain* 1986;24:277–295.

66. Berman AT, Garbarino JL, Fisher SM, et al. The effects of epidural injection of local anesthetics and corticosteroids on patients with lumbosciatic pain. *Clin Orthop* 1984;188:144.

67. Tuel SM, Meythaler JM, Cross LL. Cushing's syndrome from epidural methylprednisolone. *Pain* 1990;40:81–84.

68. Deyo RA. Fads in the treatment of low back pain. *N Engl J Med* 1991;325:1939–1940.

69. Wiskneski RJ, Rothman RH. Microdiscectomy techniques. *Semin Spine Surg* 1989;1:54–59.

70. Weber H. Lumbar disc herniation: a controlled prospective study with ten years of observation. *Spine* 1983;8:131–140.

71. Kirkaldy-Willis WH. Pathology and pathogenesis of lumbar spondylosis and stenosis. *Spine* 1979;3:319.

72. Jayson MIV. The role of vascular damage and fibrosis in the pathogenesis of nerve root damage. *Clin Orthop* 1992;279:40.

73. Cuckler JM, Bernini P, Wiesel S, et al. The use of lumbar epidural steroids in the treatment of lumbar radicular pain—a prospective, randomized, double-blind study. *J Bone Joint Surg Am* 1985;67A:63–66.

74. Rosen C. A retrospective analysis of the efficacy of epidural steroid injections. *Clin Orthop* 1988;288:270–272.

75. Herkowitz HN, Kurz LT. Degenerative lumbar spondylolisthesis with spinal stenosis: a prospective study comparing decompression with decompression and intertransverse process arthrodesis. *J Bone Joint Surg Am* 1991;73A:802–808.

76. Wiltse LL, Newman PH, MacNab I. Classification of spondylolysis and spondylolisthesis. *Clin Orthop* 1976;117:23.

77. Phalen GS, Dickson JA. Spondylolisthesis and tight hamstrings. *J Bone Joint Surg Am* 1961;43A: 505–512.

78. Bellah RD, Summerville DA, Treves ST, Micheli LJ. Low back pain in adolescent athletes: detection of stress injury to the pars interarticularis with SPECT. *Radiology* 1991;180:509–512.

79. Micheli LJ, Hall J, Miller E. Use of modified Boston brace for back injuries in athletes. *Am J Sports Med* 1980;8:351–356.

80. Steiner ME, Micheli LJ. Treatment of symptomatic spondylolysis and spondylolisthesis with the modified Boston brace. *Spine* 1985;10:937–943.

81. Bradford DS, Iza J. Repair of the defect in spondylolysis or minimal degrees of spondylolisthesis by segmental wire fixation and bone grafting. *Spine* 1985;10: 673–679.

82. Seitsalo S, Osterman K, Hyvarinen H, et al. Severe spondylolisthesis in children and adolescents. *J Bone Joint Surg Br* 1990;72B:259–265.

83. Seitsalo S, Osterman K, Hyvarinen H, et al. Progression of spondylolisthesis in children and adolescents: a longterm follow-up of 272 patients. *Spine* 1991;16:417–421.

84. Boxall D, Bradford DS, Winter RB, Moe JH. Management of severe spondylolisthesis in children and adolescents. *J Bone Joint Surg Am* 1979;61A:479–495.

85. Denis F. Spinal instability so defined by the three-column concept in acute spinal trauma. *Clin Orthop* 1984;189:65.

86. Cantor JB, Lebwohl NH, Garvey T, Eismont FJ. Nonoperative management of stable thoracolumbar burst fractures with early ambulation and bracing. *Spine* 1993;18:971–976.

87. Cammisa FP Jr, Eismont FJ, Green BA. Dural laceration occurring with burst fractures and associated laminar fractures. *J Bone Joint Surg Am* 1989;71A:1044–1052.

88. Gertzbein SD, Courtney-Brown CM. Flexion–distraction injuries of the lumbar spine: mechanisms of injury and classification. *Clin Orthop* 1988;27:52–60.

89. Jackson CD, Brown MD. Analysis of current approaches and a practical guide to prescription of exercise. *Clin Orthop* 1983;179:46.

90. White AA, Panjabi MM. The basic kinematics of the human spine—a review of past and current knowledge. *Spine* 1978;3:12–20.

91. Hashimoto K, Fugita K, Kojimoto H, et al. Lumbar disc herniation in children. *J Pediatr Orthop* 1990;10:394–396.

92. Meyerding HW. Spondylolisthesis. *Surg Gynecol Obstet* 1932;54:371.

Sports Neurology, Second Edition,
edited by Barry D. Jordan.
Lippincott–Raven Publishers, Philadelphia © 1998.

17

Head Injuries in Sports

Julian E. Bailes

Division of Neurosurgery, Osceola Regional Medical Center,
Orlando, Florida 32801

Of all sports injuries, trauma to the brain is fortunately not common, although in every sport, head impact resulting in scalp and facial lacerations, minor ocular injuries, mandibular and dental trauma, and other cranial injuries occur. Severe brain injury is fortunately relatively rare. Despite its rarity, the possibility of major brain injuries and even death remains a constant concern in nearly every sport.

Certain sports, by their design, are more likely to result in the occurrence of severe head injuries. These include the contact sports such as football, boxing, ice hockey, rugby, soccer, and the martial arts. Head injuries in sports may be considered in two broad categories. The first is severe head injuries that result in major skull fracture, intracranial bleeding, and diffuse axonal injuries. Along with the development of posttraumatic hydrocephalus or posttraumatic epilepsy, these are the major entities seen in this group. Although rare, they constitute a reproducible number of cases of severe neurologic impairment and death on an annual basis in the United States. Minor head injuries, exemplified by cerebral concussion, do not appear on first consideration to be of such importance. However, we are now appreciating that they may have an even more profound impact in sports medicine. This is due to the absolute number of players, particularly in football, who sustain cerebral concussions, which makes this a large public health issue. In addition, we are now realizing that the cumulative effects of repeated minor head blows and concussions may have long-term sequelae and vast ultimate importance in chronic injury.

The return of the athlete to contact sport participation following minor head injury has been the source of considerable debate. We are currently still evolving in our knowledge of minor head injuries in sports, in particular the effects of cumulative injury. The recommendations for resuming contact sport participation are based on a gradation of the severity and number of concussions.

HEAD INJURY

The incidence and severity of head injury and its impact on the player's role in the contest vary greatly with the sport involved. Considering the classification of recreational, nonorganized versus organized, sanctioned sports helps us to analyze the frequency and degree of involvement of head injury. In recreational athletic activities, head injuries occur at one of the highest rates in downhill skiing. Many of these are serious injuries, occurring as a result of collision, often at high speed, with trees, boulders, other skiers, and so forth. Head injury is the leading cause of fatality at most large Alpine skiing resorts (1). Most of these traumatic lesions are extraaxial hematomas, often with associated parenchymal damage, cerebral edema, skull fractures, and resultant brain herniation syndromes. Most other sports involve only sporadic head injuries, cycling, equestrian sports, and race car driving being important exceptions. In diving mishaps, intracranial injury is very unusual (2).

Football ranks first in frequency and incidence of head injuries in organized athletics. Of the nearly 1.5 million annual participants in contact football, it has been estimated that approximately 15% sustain a minor head injury each season. A small number suffer either cumulative minor head injuries or serious head injuries annually. Currently, there are approximately ten deaths annually in the United States from head injuries in football (3). The frequency of football head injuries is undoubtedly related to the nature of the game, in which collisions with opponents are intentional and occur with every play. Often the head initiates the impact, and the involved activities are usually blocking or tackling.

Schneider pioneered great advances in the reduction of head injuries in football in the 1960s. These improvements were made primarily through alterations in helmet design and associated rule changes. Schneider observed that vertex impact could transmit energy through the neural axis in a rostral–caudal direction, resulting in foramen magnum herniation or obliteration of the subarachnoid space, lateral sinuses, and bridging veins. He noted that the upper cervical spinal cord is relatively fixed by the dentate ligaments and that the brain is freely movable when pathologically displaced caudally by high-velocity forces. This movement can result in distortion of the upper cervical cord and lead to hemorrhage within it. This mechanism was believed to be the cause of death in several of his reported cases of football players. He labeled "spearing" or "stick-blocking," the direct use of the cranium to tackle or block an opponent, as a main cause of these injuries. He also suggested that helmets may actually have caused some cervical hyperextension injuries as the rear of the helmet struck the cervical spine, which he referred to as the guillotine effect. This latter mechanism has subsequently been refuted as it has not been borne out in experience. With severe central nervous system football injuries, most have been shown to have an axial compression mechanism. Schneider frequently commented that the football field was where one could watch, record, and thus study neurologic trauma and represented a clinical trauma laboratory (4).

Schneider's work contributed to replacing the old leather football helmets with synthetic covering and inner suspension headgear (Fig. 1). In the 1960s and 1970s, several manufacturers made further improvements with the development of thick foam padding suspended inside the helmets. Helmets came to be made of a hard polycarbonate shell with a "birdcage" face mask (iron bars covered with rubber) and suspension systems made of pneumatic, web, and hydraulic features. This was soon followed by the four-point attachment chin strap, which further improved stability and safety. Suggestions that football adopt helmets made of a highly absorptive material similar to rubber have been rejected because it would not be consistent with the desired collisions or "hits" of the sport. More important, the biomechanics involved in redesigning helmet shape and material are complex (Fig. 2). Helmet use in ice hockey has been unequivocally shown to have reduced the incidence of severe brain injury.

The incidence of serious head injuries declined in football with the improvement in helmet design and the addition of the face mask. However, there was a simultaneous increase in serious cervical spine fractures and spinal cord injury. This was due to the instinct of the players to use their protective helmet as a battering ram. Collisions occurred in which the player would strike a charging opponent with the crown of his protected head, placing his straightened cervical spine at risk for fracture or dislocation. This mechanism has been demonstrated with studies of impact on the helmeted heads of cadavers. The studies showed that much greater strain was produced in the cervical spine when the neck was flexed and received a vertex impact. Forces directed to the top of the head transferred more traumatic energy to the cervical vertebrae than did impact to the areas of the head located farther forward (6). Between 1971 and 1975, 54% of the quadriplegic injuries in football were caused by spearing techniques or making contact with the vertex of the helmet. In high school and college players, 72% and 78%, respectively, sustained quadriplegia while making a tackle (7). In 1976, the National Federation of State High School Association (NFSHSA) and the National Collegiate Athletic Association (NCAA) made rule changes prohibiting making initial contact with an opponent with the top of the head, the so-called

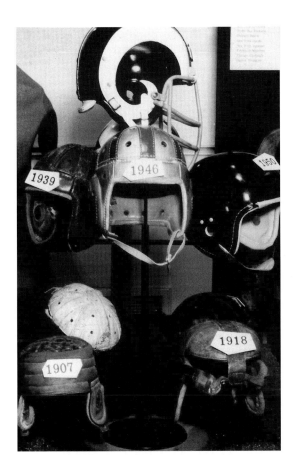

FIG. 1. The evolution of the football helmet is shown here with the original leather cap type being replaced with more rigid and protective helmets. (Courtesy of the Professional Football Hall of Fame, Canton, OH.)

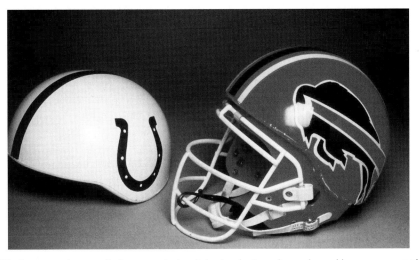

FIG. 2. Efforts are under way to improve helmet design but are incumbered by many complexities of the game and by the biomechanics involved. The Procap utilizes a polyurethane cover placed over the football helmet in an effort to mitigate the effects of a head impact. Its effectiveness is under study.

spearing technique. Although this was not always enforced, it is believed that it had a positive impact on reducing the previous upward trend of catastrophic cervical spine injuries in football.

Owing to the violent nature of the game and the constant head impacts that occur, there is still a risk of serious head injury in football participation. In the ten-year reporting period 1975 through 1984, there were 132 football players with intracranial hemorrhages. The apparent increase is somewhat related to improved detection of clots with the advent and widespread use of computed tomographic (CT) scanning during that period. During this period the fatality rate from intracranial injuries in U.S. football averaged eight per year, which on an exposure basis is small but nonetheless significant (8). All medical attendants at football contests, especially at the high school and college level, where significant high-velocity impacts occur, should be cognizant that severe head injury may still occur. Despite improvements in equipment and rule changes, every unconscious player must be considered a candidate for serious head injury, similar to the consideration of possible cervical fracture.

BIOMECHANICS

The pathophysiology of brain injury has been divided into focal and generalized brain trauma. A focal brain injury is one that often results from a direct blow or penetration of the brain and tearing of cerebral substance or vessels. This results in a localized area of bleeding (hematoma) or impact of the brain against bony irregularities of the inner surface of the skull. These result in macroscopic lesions that are hemorrhagic in nature. These injuries include cortical or subcortical brain contusions, hematomas in an extraaxial location, and intracerebral hematomas. These focal brain lesions result in the most serious form of neurologic dysfunction. Patients may present with a wide spectrum of neurologic deficits ranging from mild focal neurologic deficits to severe brain injury, which results in many cases of death and neurologic disability annually.

Diffuse brain injuries occur as a consequence of widespread or global interruption of neurologic function. These injuries exist along a spectrum from physiologic dysfunction only, known as cerebral concussion, to severe, white matter shearing injuries. These injuries are generally considered to be microscopic or physiologic and do not represent a major anatomic disruption or hemorrhage. Each of these types of brain trauma is considered in greater detail in the following discussion.

Diffuse brain injury is in contrast to focal brain injury and indicates that there has been a global insult to cerebral function and/or structure usually resulting in widespread dysfunction. Diffuse brain injury exists along a continuum from mild concussion to more severe forms of concussion with alteration of consciousness. Diffuse brain injury also occurs with diffuse axonal injury, a clinical entity characterized by shearing of white matter fiber tracts as they course through the cerebral tissue from the cortex to the midbrain and brainstem to enter the spinal cord. Often at sites of relative tethering such as the corpus callosum and brainstem, shearing of white matter tracts occurs, especially with rotational energy forces. This leads to disruption of axons at these levels, sometimes marked by small areas of hemorrhage visualized on CT scanning. In its most severe form, diffuse brain injury consists of so-called shear injuries, in which the patient is rendered deeply and often permanently comatose. There are associated severe cognitive memory and motor deficits as well as greater than 50% mortality with severe shearing injury.

Forces imparted to the cranium are generally considered to be of two types: acceleration–deceleration and rotational. The first is acceleration–deceleration injury, also considered as translational (linear) impact. This mechanism most commonly occurs when the subject's body and head are traveling at a particular speed and strike a solid object. Likewise, a stationary cranium may be struck by a moving object. The resultant injury causes linear, tensile, and compressive strains that disrupt the cerebral cytoarchitecture. The brain, housed in a protective bony skull and bathed by a layer of cerebrospinal fluid (CSF), has freedom of movement before it abuts against the skull. Particularly in the anterior and middle cranial fossae, bone irregularities project at the undersurface of the frontal and temporal lobes and lead to the development of focal injuries. In addition, as the cerebral tissue shifts within the cranium, a vacuum phenomenon may occur, particularly in polar regions, leading to microscopic tearing of small vessels and capillaries that may result in formulation of localized bleeding and hematoma.

Rotational (angular) movements are also a frequent etiology of cerebral injury. This occurs because of the fixation of the brain at the foramen magnum and craniospinal junction and the relative tethering of the midbrain and brainstem as they pass through the tentorial hiatus. Energy directed to the cranium may cause transmission of force in a rotatory direction. This often leads to diffuse brain injuries in which shearing of the white matter fiber tracts can occur. Rotational energy input is associated with diffuse white matter brain injuries, including those along the entire spectrum from concussion to the severe form of shearing injury.

Head injuries in sports thus occur as a result of both acceleration–deceleration (translational, linear) and rotational (angular) factors. It is also possible for both of these pathogenetic mechanisms to coexist in a single patient's injury. However, usually one mechanism dominates. Contact sports, especially football, ice hockey, and boxing, have a high degree of acceleration–deceleration energy input. These occur within the framework of the rules and often within a single contest. The same individual may be subjected to numerous insults during the course of one contest. Activities such as blocking and tackling, checking, jabs, cross-punches, and many others predominantly deliver acceleration–deceleration or linear energy vectors to the contestant. On the other hand, mechanisms exemplified by the boxing hook punch impart rotatory forces to the mandible and cranium. It is believed that the rotary component of cranial impacts contributes most directly to injuries that include loss of consciousness, including the etiology of many football cerebral concussions.

The maintenance of the conscious state implies that the person is awake and alert with the ability to interact with the environment. A normal level of consciousness is dependent on a complex interaction of cortical, subcortical, and brainstem nuclei. Alteration of the state of con-

sciousness occurs when the integrity of this neurophysiologic functional unit has been interrupted. The reticular activating system extending throughout the brainstem must interact with the hypothalamus and cerebral hemispheres in a normal feedback loop mechanism for consciousness to be maintained. Any alteration of this circuitry and feedback produces an alteration of the state of consciousness. This may be secondary to an anatomic disruption such as hematoma, contusion, swelling, or other focal injury. Diffuse brain injuries are believed to interrupt neurophysiologic function on a more widespread or global basis involving mild, moderate, or severe cerebral dysfunction and injury.

SEVERE HEAD INJURY

Epidural Hematoma

Epidural hematoma is a collection of blood localized between the dura and skull. The dura becomes detached and blood accumulates beneath the skull and outside the dura. It dissects until the point of dural attachment to the overlying cranium. This results in the classic CT appearance of a biconvex or lenticular shape of the hematoma (Fig. 3). Epidural hematoma is caused by head impact, usually of the acceleration–deceleration type, and may result in inward deformity of the cranium leading to dural detachment from the inner table of the skull. Epidural hematomas are often associated with skull fractures that lead to laceration of the middle meningeal artery or vein. In addition, bleeding may occur from the actual bone fragments or diploic space, leading to collection of blood in the epidural location. A skull fracture is present in approximately 75% of patients who sustain an epidural hematoma (9,10).

An important factor in epidural hematoma is that this is usually an isolated injury to the skull, dura, and dural vessels that leads to the collection of blood and hematoma formation. In most of these acceleration–deceleration injuries, the skull has taken the brunt of the forces and absorbed the energy of the impact. There is often an associated loss of consciousness because the heavy force delivered to the cranium has disrupted the physiologic substrate of conscious-

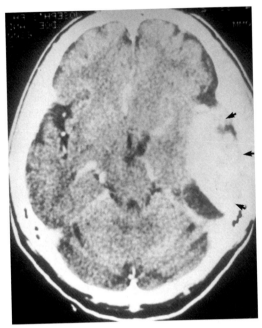

FIG. 3. Computed tomographic scan showing the typical appearance of an epidural hematoma (*arrows*). The blood, located between the skull and dura, is limited by dural attachments in its ability to spread, resulting in the typical bioconvex or lenticular appearance.

ness. In contrast to other injuries such as subdural hematoma, in which the brain often sustains primary and massive injury, epidural hematoma is often not associated with substantial primary brain injury.

Another important distinguishing feature of this clinical entity is the concept of a lucid interval. The lucid interval occurs when a substantial blow has been transmitted to the cranium and causes loss of consciousness. After awakening, the patient may appear asymptomatic and have a normal neurologic examination. The problem arises when an injury to the skull and/or dural vessels leads to a slow accumulation of blood in the epidural space. This hematoma outside the brain may remain relatively asymptomatic until it reaches a critically large size and can cause compression of the underlying brain. The compression may be transmitted to the brainstem and rapidly progress to neurologic dysfunction, brain herniation, and possibly death. Any patient or athlete who has sustained a significant head impact

should be observed in the awakened state and not allowed to retire for sleep until the longer lasting effects of the head impact are known. Any patient with a significant loss of consciousness (minutes) or neurologic abnormality should have a more thorough medical evaluation including CT scanning. The clinical manifestations of epidural hematoma depend on the type and amount of energy transferred, the time course of the hematoma formation, and the presence of simultaneous brain injuries. In addition to a lucid interval, patients with an epidural hematoma may present with no loss of consciousness, persistent unconsciousness, or any variation of these.

Subdural Hematoma

This lesion has been divided into acute subdural hematoma, which presents within 48 to 72 hours after injury, and chronic subdural hematoma, which occurs in a later time frame with more variable clinical manifestations. Acute subdural hematoma is perhaps the most common major head injury seen and leads to severe neurologic disability and death in many cases. Acute subdural hematoma results from bleeding within the subdural space as a result of stretching and tearing of the veins located in the subdural space. These veins drain from the cerebral surface and connect to the dura or dural sinuses. In many people, especially older patients with brain atrophy, these veins are stretched and more easily subjected to a traumatic tear. Rupture of these venous channels results in blood escaping into the subdural space. With no subdural structure to apply tamponade to this flow of blood, this area accommodates formation of a subdural hematoma. In addition, the bone irregularities of the middle cranial fossa, sphenoid bone, and frontal fossa form a rough surface over which inferior cortical surface contusions may form, resulting in hemorrhage to the subdural space.

A subdural hematoma may occur as an isolated collection of blood within the subdural space or as a more complicated hematoma associated with brain parenchymal injury (11). Many patients with complicated acute subdural hematomas sustain diffuse irreversible brain damage and do not improve after evacuation of the hematoma, the latter being something of an epiphenomenon in the injury process. Therefore, the outcome of subdural hematoma is influenced by the extent of parenchymal brain injury more than the subdural hematoma collection per se.

The clinical presentation of a patient with acute subdural hematoma may vary and include those awake and alert with no focal neurologic deficits, but, typically, patients with any sizable acute subdural hematoma have a significant neurologic deficit. This may consist of alteration of consciousness, often to a state producing coma or focal neurologic deficit. Skull fracture is much less commonly associated with subdural hematoma than epidural hematoma (11,12). One case has been reported and the author knows of another in which a football player with two mild concussions without loss of consciousness, separated by 7 and 10 days, resulted in acute subdural hematomas (13). Emergent CT scan diagnosis is mandatory for expeditious and successful treatment of patients with acute subdural hematoma (Fig. 4).

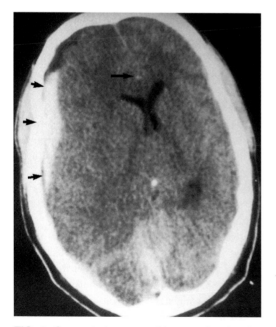

FIG. 4. Computed tomographic scan showing the typical appearance of a left subdural hematoma, with the blood spreading around the convexity giving a crescentic shape to the clot (*arrows*). A considerable mass effect and brain shift due to concomitant left hemispheric injury (*large arrow*) are also seen.

Chronic subdural hematoma is defined as a hematoma present 3 weeks or more after a traumatic injury. The pathogenesis of chronic subdural hematoma involves an injury that results in bleeding into the subdural space. Initial hemorrhage may be a small amount that fails to generate significant brain compression. However, bleeding or oozing of blood into the subdural space may continue. After 1 week a chronic subdural hematoma involves infiltration of fibroblasts to organize into an outer membrane. Subsequently, an inner membrane may form, and this capsulated hematoma may become a dynamic osmotic membrane that interacts with the production and absorption of cerebrospinal fluid. Effusion of protein may occur, setting up an active process within the membrane.

The diagnosis of chronic subdural hematoma is often difficult because of the protean clinical manifestations. Patients may have clinical symptoms suggestive of increased intracranial pressure, mental disturbance such as personality change or even dementia, symptoms with focal transient neurologic deficits similar to transient ischemic attacks, a meningeal syndrome with nuchal rigidity and photophobia, a clinical course with a slow progression of neurologic signs reminiscent of cerebral neoplasm, or a progressive and severe headache syndrome only. Although not common in athletes, a chronic subdural hematoma must always be the differential diagnosis, especially in those presenting with a remote history of head impact. The diagnosis is confirmed by CT scanning demonstrating the extraaxial low-density fluid collection in the subdural space.

Cerebral Contusion

This represents a heterogeneous area of brain injury that consists of hemorrhage, cerebral infarction, necrosis, and edema. Cerebral contusion is a frequent sequela of head injury and in some studies represents the most common traumatic lesion of the brain visualized on radiographic evaluation (14). Contusions occur most often as a result of acceleration–deceleration mechanisms as a result of the inward deformation of the skull at the impact site. This results in transient compression of the brain against the skull and the focal area of parenchymal injury. This energy is conducted to the underlying brain, resulting in cerebral contusion, the degree of which depends on the energy transmitted, the area of contact, the involved area of the cranium, and other factors.

Contusions may vary from small localized areas of injury to large extensive areas of involvement. There may also be evolution of a cerebral contusion injury of which the size and hemorrhagic nature evolve over the hours and days after the injury. Multiple small areas of contusions may coalesce into a large area resembling a lesion more accurately classified as intraparenchymal hemorrhage (Fig. 5). In addition, injuries remote from the site of impact may occur. The direct or coup lesion results from injury at the impact site and the remote or contrecoup lesion occurs as the opposite pole of the brain rebounds against the skull or because of vacuum phenomena being set up within the parenchyma at that location. This leads to a hemorrhagic lesion in the area diametrically opposed to the impact site (Fig. 6). The inferior surfaces of the frontal and temporal lobes are the areas most commonly seen with this type of injury.

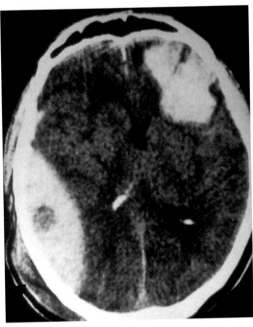

FIG. 6. Computed tomographic scan showing a coup–contrecoup injury. The point of direct injury (impact) is inferred from the scalp swelling (*arrow*).

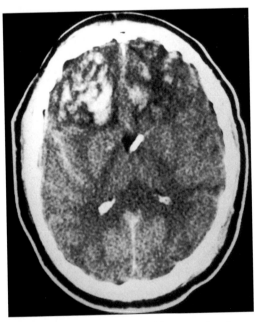

FIG. 5. Computed tomographic scan showing a large, hemorrhagic, coalesced cerebral contusion in both frontal lobes.

Contusions are often multiple and frequently associated with other extraaxial and intraaxial hemorrhagic lesions. Skull fracture is present in approximately 70% of patients with cerebral contusion.

The clinical course of patients with cerebral contusion is greatly variable, depending on the location, number, and extent of the hemorrhagic contusion lesions. The patient may present with essentially normal function or may experience any type of neurologic deterioration, including coma. Frequently, behavioral or mental status changes are apparent because of the common involvement of the frontal or temporal lobes. The diagnosis of cerebral contusion is firmly established by CT scanning, which is also useful for following patients as the lesions evolve throughout their clinical course.

An intracerebral hematoma is parenchymatous and is often similar in pathophysiology and radiographic appearance to a cerebral contusion. An intracerebral hematoma represents a localized collection of blood within the brain. In this context, as a result of cranial trauma, the distinction between a hemorrhagic contusion and intra-parenchymal hematoma depends on the latter being recognized as a confluent area of homogeneous bleeding within the brain. Intracerebral hematomas usually present with a focal neurologic deficit but may progress to further neurologic deterioration including coma and death resulting from brain herniation syndromes. Diagnosis is readily achieved by CT scanning, which shows a hyperdense localized collection of blood. Intracerebral hematomas have been, along with subdural hematomas, the most common cause of sports-related lethal brain injuries.

Another entity, delayed traumatic intracerebral hematoma, is a clot that forms hours to days after the initial trauma. Although most frequently seen in the older population, it must always be borne in mind when evaluating and attending to any patient who has sustained a significant head impact. The athlete is also at risk because these hematomas are seen more commonly when there has been rotational head trauma. Delayed traumatic hematomas are believed to be due to later bleeding into an already contused region of the brain, vascular injury, or the development of a coagulopathy (15–17).

Skull Fracture

Cranial injury resulting in fracture of the skull is a common occurrence in sports, especially sports in which helmets are not regularly employed. Any recreational or sporting activity in which planned or inadvertent head impact occurs may result in skull fracture. Skull fractures are considered in two categories, linear and depressed. Linear skull fractures are common entities involving the frontal, parietal, temporal, or occipital bones. They may occur in conjunction with an overlying scalp laceration, in which case they are considered to be compound fractures. Linear skull fractures occur as a result of a direct blow to the skull and a fracture without malalignment of the bone edges. Most linear fractures are uncomplicated and, per se, not serious. They are more important as a harbinger of the patient sustaining an underlying cerebral injury and thus serve as a marker for potentially serious neurologic damage. When they occur over the major

venous sinuses or particularly in the temporal fossa overlying the groove for the middle meningeal artery and vein, they may indicate that an underlying bleeding source exists. Most linear skull fractures do not require specific treatment other than the necessary observation for neurologic dysfunction. They usually heal within several months to a year and often do not prevent the athlete from resuming participation, even in contact sports.

Depressed skull fractures ordinarily require a relatively small object or contact point that results in depression of the underlying bone. The bone fragments separate and are driven into the dura or penetrate the dura to touch or invade the brain surface. Many patients with depressed skull fractures do not have significant brain injury, although underlying hematoma, cerebrospinal fluid leakage, or infection may occur. In addition, laceration leading to hemorrhage or thrombosis of a major dural venous sinus may be a concomitant injury. In contrast to linear skull fractures, depressed fractures often require treatment based on the location, degree of depression, contamination, cosmetic appearance, and other features. The diagnosis is made with skull radiographs and confirmed with CT scanning. The latter is necessary to ascertain the degree of cerebral abnormality.

Epilepsy

Posttraumatic seizures have been thought to be present in approximately 5% of all patients with cranial cerebral trauma and are increased in those with severe head injuries, occurring in approximately 15%. Patients with an intracerebral lesion such as a contusion or hematoma, those with a depressed skull fracture impinging on the dural or cortical surface, and those experiencing seizures later than the first week post trauma are felt to have a higher incidence of posttraumatic epilepsy.

Posttraumatic epilepsy is generally considered in several forms. Impact seizures occur immediately at the time of the trauma and are believed to result from the direct impact producing deranged electrochemical conductance. Immediate seizures occur within the first 24 hours after trauma. Early seizures occur within the first week after trauma and are believed to be acute reactions to trauma and not prognostic of the future development of epilepsy. Late seizures occur at a time remote from the initial injury and can be more accurately considered as posttraumatic epilepsy. Prophylactic anticonvulsants have been administered to patients who are believed to be at high risk for posttraumatic epilepsy or to those who experience convulsions. Research has found that phenytoin reduced the incidence of seizures in the first week post trauma but not subsequently. This suggests that prophylactic anticonvulsants are not helpful after the first week after trauma.

The management of late posttraumatic seizures follows the guidelines for treatment of patients with epilepsy. Phenytoin has been the antiepileptic most commonly employed for treatment of posttraumatic epilepsy but at times is not as effective for late-onset seizures. Phenobarbital has been commonly employed as a second agent; however, its sedative side effect is often a liability in recovering head-injured patients. When seizures have occurred, anticonvulsants are continued for a minimum of 1 year in most cases. The subsequent discontinuance of anticonvulsants would be done on an individualized basis (see Chapter 22).

Posttraumatic Hydrocephalus

After the occurrence of head trauma, enlargement of the cerebral ventricular system can occur. This usually requires that a significant head injury has occurred. This instance of posttraumatic ventriculomegaly has been reported to range from 30% to 86% (18). It is always necessary to attempt to discern whether this anatomic ventricular enlargement represents ventriculomegaly alone or symptomatic hydrocephalus.

After head trauma, especially in patients with severe head injury, it is not uncommon to have permanent cerebral injury. This results in loss of cerebral tissue, which can be visualized on CT or magnetic resonance imaging (MRI) scanning in the posttraumatic period as areas of porencephaly, areas of arterial or venous infarction, or atrophy. As this loss of cerebral tissue ensues, there can be a passive dilatation of the ventricular system, in part to occupy the area of brain loss. As the ventri-

cles expand to fill a void, this condition has been termed hydrocephalus ex vacuo. In patients with significant head injuries, injuries such as subarachnoid hemorrhage, posterior fossa hematomas, supratentorial hematomas, and meningitis may all cause disturbance in the normal CSF obstructive pathways. As the inexorable production of CSF continues at approximately 450 mL daily, the fluid accumulates and can result in ventricular dilatation. This active ventricular enlargement would be considered symptomatic and has been estimated to occur in approximately 18% of those with posttraumatic ventricular enlargement (19).

In a comatose patient, the diagnosis of hydrocephalus is usually difficult to make on a clinical basis. At times, although unusual enough to be an isolated phenomenon in the posttraumatic period, hydrocephalus may produce an altered level of consciousness, even coma. Funduscopic examination may reveal blurring of the disc margins or papilledema in these patients. In these cases, the diagnosis is made most readily with radiologic imaging. Enlargement of the lateral ventricles and frontal and temporal horns, periventricular edema, and effacement of the cerebral sulci are all seen with CT scanning or MRI. The diagnosis of hydrocephalus in an awake patient is characteristically made with symptoms of aggressive mental status changes and dementia, sphincteric incontinence, and gait apraxia. It is also not uncommon to see posttraumatic hydrocephalus present as a leveling off of neurologic improvement in the rehabilitation phase of head injury. The majority of patients with posttraumatic hydrocephalus improve after the placement of a CSF diversion device, most commonly a ventriculoperitoneal shunt (20). Because of the delicate and intricate function of a ventricular shunt, the active, constant production of CSF within the brain, and the shunt dependence and potential for rapid neurologic demise in those who suffer an acute shunt malfunction, this author believes that the participation of athletes with an indwelling ventricular shunt in contact sports should generally be prohibited.

Intracranial Hypertension

Elevated intracranial pressure is a common sequela in the pathophysiology of severe head injury. Because the brain is housed in the cranium, which acts as a closed, rigid box, processes that lead to cerebral swelling can come to be associated with high intracranial pressure. The unyielding skull causes pressure to be turned within and directs displacement of CSF and blood as compensatory mechanisms. When this compensation is exhausted, brain tissue begins to shift, resulting in brain herniation syndromes as the brain is expelled through the tentorial hiatus and/or foramen magnum. This leads to severe brainstem dysfunction and/or death. The pressure of the CSF that surrounds and nourishes the brain is normally below 10 mm Hg. In certain disease states including traumatic injury, the normal homeostatic mechanism is deranged, which can often lead to increases in intracranial pressure, referred to as intracranial hypertension. The Monroe-Kellie hypothesis helps explain the pathophysiologic state that occurs in intracranial hypotension. When the compensatory mechanism of intracranial volume displacement has been exhausted, a linear and rapid increase in intracranial pressure occurs (Fig. 7). Dramatic increases in pressure result in brain tissue displacement (herniation) and insufficient cerebral blood flow leading to ischemia.

Intracranial hypertension may exist in patients who have intracranial mass lesions. These become space-occupying masses that, together with a surrounding edematous brain reaction, lead to increases in intracranial pressure. It is also possible to have severe generalized cerebral edema without intracranial mass lesions, and this also results in intracranial hypertension. The management of patients with intracranial hypertension involves strict adherence to set guidelines for minimizing the systemic insults (hypoxia, hypotension) and optimizing cerebral perfusion. This constant management is facilitated by monitoring of intracranial pressure through one of various modalities such as ventricular catheters or subdural and epidural monitoring devices. Careful surveillance of intracranial pressure levels is necessary so that treatment may be instituted to reduce intracranial pressure and optimize the cerebral perfusion pressure. The cerebral perfusion pressure equals the mean systemic arterial blood pressure minus the jugu-

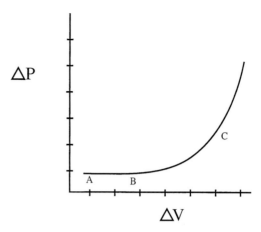

FIG. 7. An intracranial dynamic volume–pressure curve illustrates three phases. "A" shows the normal, equilibration state of intracranial pressure (ICP) for a normal volume of intracranial contents. In "B" the volume has risen (e.g., a small intracranial hemorrhage or edema) but compensation has occurred, allowing the ICP to be controlled. In "C" the increase in intracranial content volume has exceeded the brain's compensatory capacity, resulting in a state of dysequilibrium and rising ICP. If it is allowed to continue to rise, compensatory failure and brain herniation syndrome occur.

lar venous pressure, and the latter parameter is replaced by intracranial pressure whenever there is intracranial hypertension. Efforts are always made to maintain the cerebral perfusion pressure at a level greater than 50 mm Hg. Numerous medical modalities, such as osmotic diuretics and hyperventilation, are employed to optimize the cerebral perfusion pressure by minimizing and controlling intracranial pressure.

The pathophysiologic processes that occur with cerebral injury may be termed primary and secondary injuries. The primary injury is that which occurs at the moment of impact, leading to physical, anatomic injury and structural damage to the brain. This results in formation of hematomas, such as parenchymal hematomas and contusions, or to diffuse trauma resulting in diffuse axonal injury or shear injury. Surgical treatment is often necessary to improve the patient's condition and subsequent clinical course by removing the primary injury if it is hematoma compression, depressed skull fragments, or foreign body.

Secondary cerebral injury begins momentarily after the primary injury and consists of a series of biochemical steps that are set in motion by the primary injury. Secondary neurologic injury involves a cascade of hypoxic and ischemic cellular events beginning with loss of membrane integrity by the Na^+,K^+- ATPase-driven ionic pump. This subsequently leads to passive movement of ions following concentration gradients, generation of electrical potential and activation of the voltage-dependent calcium channels, influx of calcium, breakdown of the cellular membrane, cellular swelling, and death. As clinicians, we can only intervene and minimize the degree of secondary brain injury. This involves treatments aimed at controlling hypoxia, hypotension, temperature, and other features of the patient's initial response to the injury. Pharmacologic intervention may play a greater role in the future in minimizing the degree of secondary injury.

MINOR HEAD INJURY

(CONCUSSION)

In athletic injuries, concussion is the most common form of head injury. The classical cerebral concussion is defined as a posttraumatic state that results in loss of consciousness. This state is associated with retrograde and posttraumatic amnesia. The patient regains full consciousness within 24 hours, and this condition may be accompanied by microscopic neuronal abnormalities. However, in clinical terms, cerebral concussion has been defined as physiologic without anatomic disruption of cerebral function. The concept of minor head injury is usually synonymous with concussion.

Confusion has been considered to be the hallmark of concussion. Although consciousness is preserved, there is dysfunction of cerebral processes whereby orientation, higher thought processes, and memory are affected. This syndrome is completely reversible and, unless repetitive, is believed not to be associated with neurologic sequelae. Various classification schemes have been devised to categorize and help understand and treat concussion. The gradation of severity of concussion has been especially pertinent for treating the athletic injury and for prognostication regarding return to play (Table 1). Cerebral concussion has been defined in various ways but generally means an alteration of cerebral function without associated pathologic changes in brain structure. Experimental evidence has suggested, however, that reactive axonal swelling is seen on electron microscopy after even mild head injury. Concussion has also been defined as an "immediate and transient impairment of neural function such as alteration of consciousness, disturbance of vision, equilibrium and other similar symptoms" (21). Concussion has been defined, especially for athletic purposes, as "a traumatically induced alteration of mental status." In the United States, it is estimated that there are approximately 250,000 concussions yearly in football alone (22).

Concussion has been categorized into three types or grades for clinical purposes. Other classification schemes have also been proposed (Tables 2 and 3). A mild concussion (grade 1) is most common; it involves no loss of consciousness, and confusion is the hallmark sign. This type of concussion is often seen in football games

TABLE 1. *Colorado Medical Society guidelines for management of concussion in sports*

Grade	Action	Return
1 (mild)	Remove from contest, examine immediately and every 5 minutes.	Return to contest if no symptoms for 20 minutes.
2 (moderate)	Remove from contest, examine immediately and every 5 minutes.	Return to practice after one full week without symptoms.
3 (severe)	Transport from field to nearest appropriate hospital, complete neurologic examination, CT scan, overnight admission and observation.	Return to practice after 2 weeks without symptoms.

From ref. 24, with permission.

TABLE 2. *Cantu grading scale for concussion*

Grade	Symptoms
1 (mild)	No loss of consciousness, posttraumatic amnesia less than 30 minutes in duration
2 (moderate)	Loss of consciousness less than 5 minutes in duration or posttraumatic amnesia longer than 30 minutes but less than 24 hours in duration
3 (severe)	Loss of consciousness for more than 5 minutes or posttraumatic amnesia for more than 24 hours

From ref. 22, with permission.

and occurs to at least one player in nearly every game, if thoroughly searched for. It may be stated that the player was "dinged." The athlete, who is awake and alert, may be able to function unnoticed during the course of the athletic contest. Management entails removing the player, who is sometimes identified by teammates because of his confusion or difficulty remembering plays, from the field of competition for 20 to 30 minutes. If significant disorientation, confusion, memory disturbance, dizziness, headache, or any neurologic abnormality persists after this observation period, the athlete should not be allowed to return. Otherwise, he may be considered for return to play following a mild concussion if these features are absent. One should keep in mind that concussion may be present and significant even without loss of consciousness. Ommaya and Gennarelli (23) showed in their animal model that three of six grades of concussion do not involve loss of consciousness. They postulated that, unless shearing forces reached the reticular activating system, cortical and subcortical structures could be affected to produce amnesia and confusion but not loss of consciousness.

TABLE 3. *Colorado concussion classification*

Severity of concussion	Symptoms
Grade 1	Confusion without amesia No loss of consciousness
Grade 2	Confusion with amnesia No loss of consciousness
Grade 3	Loss of consciousness

From ref. 24, with permission.

The athlete who has been withheld from play because of a mild concussion should be examined as soon as possible by the team physician. With a single mild concussion, the athlete may return to competition within 1 week if none of the foregoing symptoms are present. The athlete who is still symptomatic should be withheld further until the symptoms abate and a head CT scan is obtained. With a second mild concussion in the same season, the athlete should be withheld from contact sports for 2 weeks and consideration given to CT scanning, especially if the concussions come in short succession. A normal neurologic and CT scan examination must be obtained and the athlete must be asymptomatic before being allowed to return. Most experts recommend terminating the athlete's season if a third concussion occurs in a single season. Appropriate neurodiagnostic tests are then indicated.

A moderate or grade 2 concussion is associated with the development of amnesia either initially or during the period of observation. There is no loss of consciousness. The athlete is removed from competition and not to be allowed to return. The athlete should be examined as soon as possible by the team physician and consideration given to consultation with a neurologic or neurosurgical specialist, especially if disturbances in level of consciousness or other neurologic signs develop. Brain radiologic imaging studies (e.g., CT or MRI) are performed in all athletes who have neurologic abnormalities, headaches, or other associated symptoms that either worsen or persist for more than 1 week. We recommend allowing return only after one full week without symptoms. We have found a "provocative exertional" practice session, in which the athlete participates fully in sports with the exception of avoiding head impacts, to be helpful in deciding whether the athlete is ready for competition. An athlete with a second moderate concussion in one season should be withheld for 1 month and have a normal CT scan prior to returning. A third moderate concussion would be grounds for terminating the season. Some suggest that at this point consideration should be given to not allowing return to contact sports.

A severe or grade 3 concussion is associated with loss of consciousness. It requires emergent transport to the nearest facility with CT scanning, and consideration should be given for neurosurgical consultation. The possibility of concomitant cervical spine injury must always be considered in an unconscious patient and transport performed with cervical immobilization and maintenance of an adequate airway (Fig. 8). Often, unless the loss of consciousness has been very brief (i.e., less than 30 seconds), the athlete is admitted to the hospital overnight for observation and treated according to standard accepted procedure for closed-head injury. Caretakers should be aware of the phenomenon of the "lucid interval" (serious, sometimes fatal brain hematomas are preceded by hours of an apparently clear mental state as described earlier). This phenomenon has also been described in baseball players and golfers struck on the head by a high-velocity ball.

With loss of consciousness, neurologic and CT examination is required. If both are normal and there are no symptoms, it is felt that the athlete may return to competition within 2 weeks of being asymptomatic if the length of unconsciousness was less than 1 minute. With loss of consciousness for more than 1 minute, implying significant interruption of cerebral function, it is recommended that return be withheld for 1 month. A second severe concussion will terminate the athlete's season and consideration should be given to ending participation in any contact sport. These recommendations are based on our experience and that of others and are reinforced by neuropsychologic testing. With a single incident of minor athletic head injury, abnormalities on neuropsychologic testing usually resolve by 1 month; however, with a second concussion, they may be present for up to 6 months.

The problem is not only concussion per se but the cumulative effects of multiple cerebral impacts. Repeated concussions, especially within a short time span, may lead to headaches, visual disturbances, vertigo, and other symptoms typical of postconcussive syndrome. However, permanent injuries are also possible, such as neuropsychologic abnormalities, cerebral atrophy, and even fatalities. Cumulative effects of concussion may lead to cerebral edema and death, similar to the reactive hyperemia resulting from autoregulatory dysfunction seen in some pediatric head trauma cases. Children, adolescents, and young adults appear to be susceptible to this phenomenon of pathologic vascular congestion. Kelly et al. (24) described a 17-year-old high school football player who sustained a loss of consciousness a week before being struck again on the left side of his helmet during a game. He subsequently collapsed on the field, never regained consciousness, and expired 15 hours later. Detailed investigation showed cerebral

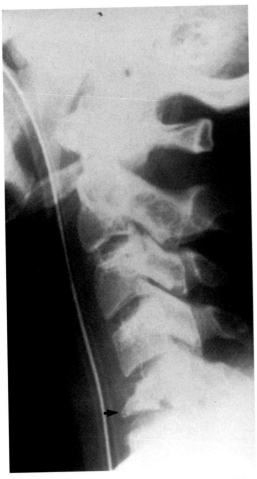

FIG. 8. Cognizance must always be taken of the possibility of a coexistent cervical spine and head injury. Every downed or unconscious athlete must have proper spinal immobilization to prevent further injury and in case cervical fracture exists as illustrated here (*arrow*).

edema on a CT scan and uncontrolled intracranial hypertension. Necropsy findings were of cerebral edema. This patient demonstrated that serious, fatal injury can result from repeated concussions without loss of consciousness or any obvious preceding abnormality of the athlete (24). The previously concussed athlete is at perhaps a fourfold greater risk of sustaining another minor head injury. Gronwall and Wrightson (25) studied 20 young adults and found that information processing capacity is reduced to a greater degree and for a longer time after a second concussion. Multiple concussions caused an increased interval before normal cerebral function returned. They concluded that the mechanism of concussion of all grades of severity involves neuronal damage.

SECOND IMPACT SYNDROME

The occurrence of a catastrophic and fatal brain injury after a relatively minor injury has been documented in contact sports. Originally believed to be recognized in football players and reported by Schneider, the second impact syndrome continues to occur and has been reported in boxers and ice hockey players. Ordinarily, a football player has received a relatively minor blow to the head and suffered a mild concussion. In a short time frame, usually within 1 week after the initial impact, the player sustains a second cranial energy input that results in rapid neurologic demise and death usually within several hours. Autopsy studies have demonstrated cerebral contusion and/or parenchymal hematomas. However, the overwhelming pathophysiologic abnormality is diffuse cerebral edema with brain herniation. Saunders and Harbaugh (26) reported the case of a 19-year-old college football player who was involved in a fistfight and received a blow to the head resulting in a brief loss of consciousness. Four days later he was involved in a football game and, despite receiving no unusual head impact, collapsed on the field. He died 4 days later with diffuse and uncontrollable cerebral edema. They postulated that loss of vasomotor tone allows increased intracranial vascular volume, provoking large increases in intracranial pressure and failure of intracranial compliance with a sec-

ond, minor head impact during the susceptible time.

POSTCONCUSSION SYNDROME

A postconcussion syndrome is not an uncommon problem after closed-head injury. It is most commonly seen in patients after motor vehicle accidents. It may also be seen in athletes, especially those with repeated or successive concussions during the course of one season. A multitude of common complaints occur with postconcussion syndrome, including persistent headache, irritability, inability to concentrate, dizziness, vertigo, memory impairment, and generalized fatigue. Many factors, including motivation, psychological factors, pending litigation, educational level, and degree of injury, influence the duration, extent, and number of postconcussion syndrome complaints (Table 4).

Postconcussion syndrome consists predominantly of deficits in cognition, the sense of physical well-being, and mood. This results in diminished memory and concentration, fatigue, dizziness, depression, anxiety, and irritability. Headaches are also a common symptom in these patients. It appears that the incidence of postconcussion syndrome is highest for patients who have suffered mild head injuries. Mild head injury has been defined quantitatively by a Glasgow Coma Scale score of 13 to 15. However, the

TABLE 4. *Postconcussion syndrome*

Cognitive
  Memory
  Attention
  Problem solving
Language
  Receptive
  Expressive
  Word finding
  Fluency
Personality
  Sleep disturbance
  Depression
  Lassitude
  Mood changes
  Motivation
Somatic
  Headaches
  Dizziness
  Photophobia

use of such a scale alone may be misleading in that it does not consider factors related to prior cortical function such as orientation and memory. It is suggested that certain athletes involved in contact sports who have received repeated cerebral concussions may be at risk for developing a prolonged postconcussion syndrome. Most studies of postconcussion syndrome patients have involved a single episode of minor or at times severe head injury. The potential for repeated cerebral concussion and minor head injury is almost unique to athletes who participate in contact sports. Whether they can develop a prolonged postconcussion syndrome or suffer cumulative effects is at present incompletely defined and under study.

It is believed that most of these symptoms run a self-limited and benign course, usually resolving by 6 to 8 weeks after the accident. Neuropsychologic testing documents recovery in 1 to 6 months post injury in most patients (who are nonathletes). Neurologic examination as well as radiographic workup is usually normal. Neuropsychologic evaluation with a formal testing battery may be the best objective measure for documentation and serial follow-up in these patients and is invaluable for athletes who must, in addition, perform at maximal physical levels.

NEUROPSYCHOLOGIC TESTING

In most instances, radiographic tests (CT, MRI) of athletes with concussion do not show evidence of intracranial hemorrhage, contusion, or other anatomic abnormalities. In addition, the neurologic examination is often within normal limits. In the days and weeks following a cerebral concussion in the athlete, it has traditionally been difficult to obtain a measure of the degree of persistent cognitive and mental status dysfunction. However, with the implementation of a neuropsychologic test battery, we have the ability to measure, quantify, and follow persistent and evolving cognitive and higher cortical function modalities in these patients. Even mild abnormalities on a formal neuropsychologic evaluation indicate that there are persistent and ongoing brain effects of the prior concussion. The work of Lovell et al. (27) at the NFL level has demonstrated the ability of neuro-

TABLE 5. *Neuropsychologic testing: areas to evaluate*

Orientation (person, place, date, time)
Attention and concentration
Information processing
Memory (particularly short term)
Speech fluency
Visual scanning
Hand speed

psychologic testing to quantitate the extent of abnormalities following concussion.

Effective neuropsychologic testing must be brief to administer, be reproducible, and be somewhat tailored for the examination. The importance of a baseline examination done in the preseason cannot be overemphasized. Orientation, attention, memory, information processing, and other modalities are the basis for neuropsychologic testing of the athlete (Table 5). Since 1990, we have employed a neuropsychologic test battery with the Pittsburgh Steelers football team members (Table 6). This assessment has proved to be reliable, reproducible, and efficient. It has been helpful in many cases involving following athletes with postconcussion symptoms and deciding when it would be safe to return to play. It has also been utilized successfully at the collegiate and high school football level (Fig. 9).

Neuropsychologic examination provides an objective measuring stick to use for documenta-

TABLE 6. *Pittsburgh Steelers project: neuropsychological test battery*

Test	Ability assessed
Orientation Questionnaire	Orientation, posttraumatic amnesia
Digit Span Test	Attention span
Stroop Test	Mental flexibility, complex attention
Trail Making Test	Visual scanning, mental flexibility
Symbol Digit Modalities	Visual scanning, visual motor coordination
Controlled Oral Word Association Test	Word fluency
Hopkins Verbal Learning Test	Verbal memory (word list)
Grooved Pegboard Test	Motor speed and coordination

From ref. 27, with permission.

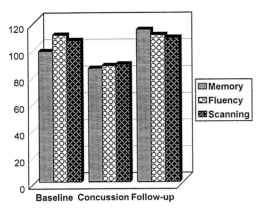

FIG. 9. A composite graph illustrates the baseline, time of concussion, and 2-week follow-up neuropsychologic testing results of three professional football players following cerebral concussions. An approximately 20% reduction in memory, word fluency, and visual scanning is characteristic of even mild to moderate cerebral concussion effects in the presence of an otherwise normal neurologic examination.

tion of true brain dysfunction when all other tests, including physical and neurologic examinations, are normal. As the effects of the concussion resolve, reliable improvement in the neuropsychologic battery occurs. This objective demonstration of cognitive and mental status abnormality is valuable for the athletes, team physicians, trainers, coaches, officials, and parents in understanding and following the extent of the injury.

NEUROLOGIC EXAMINATION

When evaluating the athlete for possible head injury, the neurologic assessment follows an abbreviated but definite examination. Any player who is downed or unconscious must be addressed with the basic principles of cardiopulmonary resuscitation in mind. As always, any unconscious player, who is thus unable to manifest signs or verbally report symptoms of spinal cord or spinal column injury, must be treated as having a possible cervical spine fracture or dislocation. Therefore, there is meticulous attention to spinal alignment during the on-field evaluation and in moving or transporting the athlete. Maintenance of the airway and ensuring adequate ventilation for air movement are of paramount im-

portance. When a player is unconscious, there is no immediate treatment more important than maintaining good spinal alignment and guaranteeing adequate ventilation. In most athletes, the period of unconsciousness is very short, lasting from seconds to only a few minutes. It is therefore unusual for a prolonged loss of consciousness to occur. If there is a prolonged period of unconsciousness, arrangements should be made for rapid evacuation to a center that has appropriate trauma services and resources to deal with acute neurosurgical emergencies.

Even with an unconscious or semiconscious athlete, important information may be gleaned from the neurologic examination that will subsequently assist in determining the degree of injury and formulating an appropriate treatment plan. The neurologic examination for suspected head injury in the athlete should begin with an assessment of the level of consciousness. For any patient who has an altered level of consciousness, a determination should be made of the degree of response to verbal, tactile, and painful stimulation. The Glasgow Coma Scale has improved our ability to quantitate the response of a patient who is comatose or has an altered level of consciousness and in addition ultimately allows prognostication (Table 7). When the level of consciousness and degree of interaction of the patient with the environment have been determined, an examination of cranial nerve function should be carried out.

TABLE 7. *Glasgow Coma Scale*

Response	Score
Verbal	
None	1
Incomprehensible sounds	2
Inappropriate words	3
Confused	4
Oriented	5
Eye opening	
None	1
To pain	2
To speech	3
Spontaneously	4
Motor	
None	1
Abnormal extension	2
Abnormal flexion	3
Withdraws	4
Localizes	5
Obeys	6

The movement and conjugate deviation of the eyes should be assessed. The pupillary position and reaction to light and accommodation are very important signs in patients with head injury. The pupillary assessment can be carried out quickly and reproducibly. In conscious patients, the reported visual acuity, facial movement and sensation, degree of hearing, and tongue movement complete the cranial nerve examination. The patient's motor function in all limbs is assessed, with voluntary function noted in conscious patients and involuntary and reflex activity noted in unconscious patients. A brief sensory examination and reflex assessment complete the cursory neurologic assessment of the athlete on the field. A more detailed and formal neurologic examination is carried out when the patient has been transported to a definitive care facility.

With patients who are being considered for cerebral concussion, the examination centers around mental status changes. The patient's orientation to person, place, and time is first acknowledged. Next, a measure of memory for immediate, recent, and remote facts is obtained. The ability to perform simple calculations and abstract reasoning and to solve simple practical problems can be assessed within 2 minutes. We have found it particularly useful to quiz the player on particular game day assignments, as these have been added to recent memory and serve as a good benchmark for cerebral concussion. In addition, players have been found to be unable to remember key components of assignments and therefore would be unable to contribute adequately to the team effort. In a matter of minutes, such a brief mental status and neurologic examination provides a reproducible and accurate assessment of the athlete's cerebral function, assists in appropriate triage for further medical diagnosis and care, and assists in making decisions regarding future return to competitive participation (Table 8).

Any patient with serious head injury, including those with grade 3 concussion, requires hospitalization and appropriate diagnostic evaluation. The ultimate treatment plan is dictated by the pathophysiologic processes that are discovered. Mass lesions of significant size, such as epidural or subdural hematomas, usually require emergent evacuation. In patients with elevated intracranial pressure, monitoring is used to help guide in selecting and administering therapy.

TABLE 8. *Sideline assessment of concussion: general guidelines*

Area	What to do
Orientation	Check for orientation to person, time, place
Attention	Repetition of digits in backward order or months of year backward
Retrograde amnesia	Memory for previous plays, what player was doing at time of injury and just before
Anterograde amnesia	Memory for three objects, immediately and after 5 minutes
General appearance	Dazed or blank expression, mumbling or incoherent speech, change in emotional status (e.g., inappropriate laughter)

From ref. 24, with permission.

REFERENCES

1. Harris JB. Neurological injuries in winter sports. *Phys Sports Med* 1983;11:110–122.
2. Bailes JE, Herman JM, Quigley MR, Cerullo LJ, Meyer PR Jr. Diving injuries of the cervical spine. *Surg Neurol* 1990;34:155–158.
3. Wilberger JE, Maroon JC. Head injuries in athletes. *Clin Sports Med* 1989;8:1–9.
4. Schneider RC. Serious and fatal neurosurgical football injuries. *Clin Neurosurg* 1966;12:226–236.
5. Roberts AH. *Brain damage in boxers.* London: Pittman, 1969.
6. Hodgson VR, Thomas LM. Mechanisms of cervical spine injury during impact to the protected head. In: *24th Stapp Car Crash Conference.* Detroit: Society of Automotive Engineers, 1980:15–42.
7. Torg JS, Quedenfeld TC, Burstein A, et al. National Football Head and Neck Injury Registry report on cervical quadriplegia 1971–1975. *Am J Sports Med* 1977; 7:127–132.
8. Torg JS, Vegso JJ, Sennett B, Das M. The National Football Head and Neck Registry: 14 year report on cervical quadriplegia, 1971 through 1984. *JAMA* 1985; 254:3439–3443.
9. Kvarnes TL, Trumpy JH. Extradural hematomas. Report of 132 cases. *Acta Neurochir* 1978;41:223–231.
10. Phonprasert C, Suwanwela C, Hongsaprabhas C, et al. Extradural hematoma: analysis of 138 cases. *J Trauma* 1980;20:679–683.
11. Jamieson KG, Yelland JDN. Surgically treated traumatic subdural hematomas. *J Neurosurg* 1972;37:137–149.
12. Richards T, Hoff J. Factors affecting survival from acute subdural hematoma. *Surgery* 1974;75:253–258.
13. Shell D, Carico GA, Patton RM. Can subdural hematoma result from repeated minor head injury? *Phys Sports Med* 1993;21:74–84.

14. Sweet RC, Miller JD, Lipper M, et al. Significance of bilateral abnormalities on the CT scan in patients with severe head injury. *Neurosurgery* 1978;3:16–20.

15. Fukamachi A, Kohno K, Nageseki Y, et al. The incidence of delayed traumatic intracerebral hematoma with extradural hemorrhages. *J Trauma* 1985;25: 145–149.

16. Gudeman SK, Kishare P, Miller J, et al. The genesis and significance of delayed traumatic intracerebral hematoma. *Neurosurgery* 1979;5:309–313.

17. Kaufman HH, Moake JL, Olson JD, et al. Delayed and recurrent intracranial hematomas related to disseminated intravascular clotting and fibrinolysis in head injury. *Neurosurgery* 1980;7:445–449.

18. Katz RT, Brander V, Sahgal V. Updates on the diagnosis and management of posttraumatic hydrocephalus. *Am J Phys Med Rehabil* 1989;68:91.

19. Gudeman SK, Kishare PRS, Becker DP. Computed tomography in the evaluation of incidence and significance of post-traumatic hydrocephalus. *Neuroradiology* 1981; 141:397.

20. Cardoso, ER, Galbraith S. Posttraumatic hydrocephalus: a retrospective review. *Surg Neurol* 1985;23:261.

21. Committee on Head Injury Nomenclature of the Congress of Neurological Surgeons. *Clin Neurosurg* 1966; 12:386–394.

22. Cantu RC. Guidelines for return to contact sports after a cerebral concussion. *Phys Sports Med* 1986;14: 75–83.

23. Ommaya AK, Gennarelli TA. Cerebral concussion and traumatic unconsciousness: correlation of experimental and clinical observations on blunt head injuries. *Brain* 1974;97:633–654.

24. Kelly JP, Nichols JS, Filley CM, Lillenhei KO, Rubinstein D, Kleinschmidt-DeMasters BK. Concussion in sports. Guidelines for the prevention of catastrophic outcome. *JAMA* 1991;266:2867–2869.

25. Gronwall D, Wrightson P. Cumulative effect of concussion. *Lancet* 1975;2:995–997.

26. Saunders RL, Harbaugh RE. The second impact in catastrophic contact sports head trauma. *JAMA* 1984; 252:538–539.

27. Lovell MR, Maroon JC, Bailes JE, Norwig J. Neuropsychological assessment following minor head injury in professional athletes. In: Bailes JE, Lovell MR, Maroon JC, eds. *Sports-Related Concussion.* St. Louis, MO: Quality Media Publishing, 1998 (*in press*).

Sports Neurology, Second Edition,
edited by Barry D. Jordan.
Lippincott–Raven Publishers, Philadelphia © 1998.

18

Headache in Sports

Alexander Mauskop and Boris Leybel

New York Headache Center, 30 East 76th Street, New York, New York 10021

Chronic headaches afflict over 40 million Americans. In addition to headaches observed in the general population, athletes can experience headaches that are specific to their sports. A survey of 178 medical students and 190 physical education students (1) showed that 35% of both groups suffered from sport- and exercise-related headaches. Among men, more physical education students suffered from headaches, probably because of the high frequency of trauma-related headaches in contact sports. The widely accepted International Headache Society (IHS) classification (2) often does not distinguish between various subtypes of sports-related headaches. This usually indicates lack of sufficient data about a particular headache type that prevents proper classification. Because IHS diagnostic categories are widely used, we will use both the commonly used term as well as the IHS classification (Table 1).

Clues to the correct diagnosis and effective treatment of an athlete with headaches lie in the detailed history. It is necessary to establish circumstances surrounding the onset of pain; possible precipitating factors; character of the pain (e.g., throbbing, pressure-like, sharp, stabbing, exploding); location of the pain; and preceding and accompanying symptoms, such as nausea, vomiting, diarrhea, vertigo, nasal congestion, lacrimation, weakness, sensory symptoms, dysarthria, confusion, scintillating scotomas, and other visual disturbances. Other factors that must be considered include history of non–sports-related headaches, family history of headaches, prior and current illnesses, excessive caffeine intake, psy-chosocial factors, and substance abuse. In addition to a thorough neurologic evaluation, a majority of athletes with headaches need to have a magnetic resonance imaging (MRI) scan of the brain. Rooke (3) reported that of 103 patients with exertional headaches, 10 had an organic lesion that was responsible for the headaches (Table 2). Assessment of possible traumatic brain injury in a patient with posttraumatic headache is also best done with an MRI scan.

HEADACHE SYNDROMES

Benign Exertional Headache

Exertional and effort-induced headaches are grouped together in the IHS classification and they do have many features in common; however, there are some clear differences. Exertional headache appears to be a response to lifting, pushing, pulling, or a similar activity as well as sexual activity, coughing, sneezing, or straining at stool. The Valsalva maneuver is one common denominator among all of these activities.

Paulson (4) reported five cases of weight lifter's headache in which the headache was mostly occipital with neck and back pain. We also find that in a large number of our patients a strain of neck muscles and spasm is responsible for this type of headache. This putative etiology is supported by findings of muscle spasm and tenderness in the occipital and paraspinal cervical regions. These patients do well with trigger point injections or occipital nerve blocks when pain is prolonged. They can often return to the headache-

TABLE 1. *International Headache Society Classification*

1. Benign exertional headache (4.5)[a]
   Weight lifter's headache (4.5)
   Effort-induced (4.5)
   Walker's, runner's, swimmer's headache (4.5)
2. Trauma related
   Head
     A. Acute posttraumatic headache (5.1)
       a. With significant head trauma and/or confirmatory signs (5.1.1)
       b. With minor head trauma and no confirmatory signs (5.1.2)
       Footballer's migraine (5.1.2.1)
       Tension-type headache (5.1.2.2)
       Cluster headache (5.1.2.3)
     B. Chronic posttraumatic headache (5.2)
       a. With significant head trauma and/or confirmatory signs (5.2.1)
       b. With minor head trauma and no confirmatory signs (5.2.2)
   Neck (11.2)
     A. Cervical spine (11.2.1)
3. Headache associated with vascular disorders
   Acute ischemic cerebrovascular disease (6.1)
   Intracranial hematoma (6.2)
     Intracerebral hematoma (6.2.1)
     Subdural hematoma (6.2.2)
     Epidural hematoma (6.2.3)
   Subarachnoid hemorrhage (6.3)
   Unruptured vascular malformation (6.4)
   Carotid or vertebral artery pain (6.6)
     Carotid or vertebral dissection (6.6.1)
   High cerebrospinal fluid pressure (7.1)
     Posttraumatic high-pressure hydrocephalus (7.1.2)
   Low cerebrospinal fluid pressure (7.2)
     Cerebrospinal fluid fistula headache (7.2.2)
4. External compression headache (4.2)
     A. Swim-goggle, helmet, headband headache (4.2)
5. Environmental
   Hypoxia (10.1)
   High-altitude headache (10.1.1)
   External application of cold stimulus headache (4.3.1)
   Divers' headache
   High humidity, heat
   Scuba divers' headache

[a] The numbers in parentheses indicate the code from the "Classification and diagnostic criteria for headache disorders, cranial neuralgias, and facial pain" published by the IHS (2).

TABLE 2. *Organic lesions in 103 patients with exertional headache originally diagnosed as "benign"*

Type	Cases
Arnold-Chiari deformity	3
Platybasia	2
Basilar impression	1
Subdural hematoma	
Chronic (duration, 20 years)	1
Subacute (duration, 1 month)	1
Brain tumor	
Parietal glioma	1
Cerebellar hemangioendothelioma	1
Total	10

inducing activity after a period of isometric neck-strengthening exercises. A typical occipital neuralgia in a football player that was relieved by a nerve block has been reported (5). Absence of a typical neuralgia does not preclude the use of occipital nerve blocks in patients with a headache and occipital tenderness. A positive clinical response to such block does not necessarily establish the etiology of the headache as being an occipital nerve compression.

Exertional headaches are seen in a variety of sports. They are not necessarily in response to maximal physical effort; very often a headache occurs at submaximal activity and even at the beginning of exercise. In such cases it is important to pay attention to predisposing metabolic factors.

Exertional headache can often be prevented by taking aspirin or another nonsteroidal antiinflammatory drug (NSAID) an hour prior to the activity. Prolonged exertional headache was reported to respond to indomethacin in 13 of 15 patients (6).

Effort-Induced Headache

This type of headache is described by several authors as a response to aerobic activities such as running or swimming (7). The majority of these patients have a headache of migraine type (three or more of the following features: throbbing, unilateral, moderate, or severe pain that is worsened by physical activity, accompanied by nausea, photophobia, and phonophobia). A possible mechanism of effort-induced headaches is hyperventilation leading to vasoconstriction that triggers a reactive vasodilatation with a resultant migraine headache. In addition to the classical contributing factors such as tyramine-rich foods, red wine, chocolate, and others, athletes may have predisposing circumstances such as dehydration, hypoglycemia, and overheating. We have found that low serum ionized magnesium levels may be a contributing factor in some patients with migraines (8).

North and Davies (9) described a postmenopausal woman with postexercise headache who had a headache only when she had a transdermal estrogen patch and never when taking an oral estrogen. The authors explained this by increased absorption of estrogen from the skin during exercise and a vascular headache precipitated by estrogen "bolus."

A warm-up regimen may also prevent an effort-induced migraine (10). Because the headache usually begins after the exercise, a prolonged cool-down period may also help.

Posttraumatic Headaches

Collision and contact sports inherently can cause a head injury and posttraumatic headaches. Frequently it is a mild trauma that produces long-lasting headaches. It seems that there is an inverse correlation between the severity of the head trauma and the likelihood of a posttraumatic headache (11). In cases of subdural, epidural, intraventricular, subarachnoid, or parenchymal hemorrhages, severe headaches occur along with other neurologic symptoms such as changes of mental status, neck stiffness, nausea, vomiting, and focal neurologic findings. Such cases usually do not present diagnostic difficulties. The incidence of headaches after a concussion in football players in one study was found to be as high as 96% (12). However, prolonged postconcussion headaches appear to be less common in athletes than in the general population. In nonathletes, the unexpected nature of the head injury, emotional stress surrounding the injury, and to a lesser extent litigation may all predispose to prolonged posttraumatic headaches.

Another type of trauma-related headache is an acute migraine induced by a head injury (13–17). In some patients a single trauma causes recurrent migraines (17,18). It appears that migraines without aura induced by an initial trauma are different from nontraumatic migraines because of a different risk for migraines among first-degree relatives (18). Cluster-like headaches have been reported to occur after a head injury (19,20).

Beta-blockers are effective for migraine and cluster headaches; however, they may impair athletes' performances by limiting the heart rate increase necessary for strenuous activities. Calcium channel blockers such as verapamil are preferred for migraine and cluster headache prophylaxis. Abortive treatment of a migraine or cluster attack begins with NSAIDs. NSAIDs are often ineffective, and combination drugs that contain butalbital and caffeine (Fiorinal, Fioricet, Esgic) or ergotamine and caffeine (Wigraine tablets, Cafergot suppositories) can be used. The amount of these drugs should be limited to no more than 15 to 20 tablets a month. Excessive caffeine intake, including dietary caffeine and caffeine in over-the-counter drugs (Anacin, Excedrin) can cause refractory rebound headaches.

In some athletes, posttraumatic headache fits the criteria for a tension-type headache (nonpulsatile; not severe; bilateral and not associated with nausea, photophobia, or phonophobia).

Management of prolonged headaches of this type is similar to that in nontraumatic cases. Tricyclic antidepressants are effective, although they can produce somnolence and dry mouth, which can interfere with athletic performance. Newer antidepressants of selective serotonin reuptake inhibitor (SSRI) type can be effective with fewer side effects, although controlled studies in headache patients have not been done.

Neck injury frequently accompanies head trauma and the neck itself can be a source of severe headaches. Cervical roots C-2 and C-3 can produce a shooting, neuralgic-type headache in the occipital area similar to a headache produced by greater occipital nerve entrapment.

Headache due to traumatic carotid artery dissection is described mostly in contact sports (21), but one case in a scuba diver has been reported (22). This is an uncommon condition that can easily go undiagnosed and therefore constant awareness of this possibility is necessary for early detection. By the time neurologic signs appear, an infarction may have occurred. Doppler ultrasound studies, magnetic resonance angiography, or conventional angiography can establish the diagnosis. Prompt treatment with anticoagulation and sometimes surgery can prevent infarction and permanent neurologic damage.

In the evaluation of an athlete with a posttraumatic headache it is critical not to miss any underlying organic pathology. Neurologic examination should include a mental status examination, appropriate neuropsychologic tests, and an MRI scan of the head and, if indicated, the neck area. An athlete should be allowed to return to competitive sports not earlier than 1 week after the resolution of headache and neurologic abnormalities. The 1-week period is intended to avoid the most catastrophic and often unpredictable second impact syndrome (23–25). This syndrome occurs when an additional blow to already existing minor trauma may precipitate brain swelling and a catastrophic increase in intracranial pressure with brainstem herniation and death within minutes.

Sport Device–Triggered Headache

Headache triggered by constricting equipment was described in swimmers experiencing pressure from their goggles (26) and in hockey players with pressure from their helmets. This type of headache is usually dull and located in temporal and occipital areas, but sometimes it can have features of a migraine headache with all typical manifestations including an aura. Loosening goggles can also stop a headache. A muscle contraction headache was ascribed to the gripping of a mouthpiece, which could be due to strain of facial and cervical muscles. A case of supraorbital neuralgia caused by goggles has been described (27).

Environmentally Triggered Headache

Jokl (28) described a migraine-like headache in runners at the 1968 Olympics in Mexico City (7000 feet above sea level), in spite of absence of headache in these well-trained athletes at sea level. Usually, headache begins from 3000 m above sea level. The mildest mountain sickness syndrome also includes nausea, vomiting, and fatigue. The headache is throbbing in character, increases with any physical activity, occurs after 6 to 96 hours of exposure, and can resolve with acclimatization or may require treatment. Above 5000 m, patients can develop acute cerebral edema and may need prompt medical intervention with immediate, rapid descent, oxygen, and steroids. A single report suggested the efficacy of sumatriptan (29), and a randomized, double-blind trial showed that ibuprofen but not sumatriptan was effective for high-altitude headache (30). Acetazolamide can be used prophylactically 3 days prior to ascent, and at least 1 week of acclimatization at 3000 to 5000 m is needed to prevent serious complications. Low oxygen tension usually triggers migraines in these athletes. High-altitude headache is seen in mountain climbers and skiers. Dysbaric air embolism and decompression sickness in scuba divers can also present with a headache. Dysbaric air embolism usually occurs within minutes, not only with a headache but with focal neurologic signs as well. Neurologic injury resulting from decompression often involves the spinal cord. Early diagnosis is crucial because of different treatment of dysbaric air embolism and decompression sickness. Divers can also develop a vascular headache due to accumulation of CO_2 and headache induced by a cold stimulus.

REFERENCES

1. Williams SJ, Nukada H. Sport and exercise headache: Part 1. Prevalence among university students. *Br J Sport Med* 1994;28(2):90–95.
2. Headache Classification Committee of the International Headache Society. Classification and diagnostic criteria for headache disorders, cranial neuralgia, and facial pain. *Cephalalgia* 1988;8(Suppl 7):1–96.
3. Rooke ED. Benign exertional headache. *Med Clin North Am* 1968;52:801–809.
4. Paulson GW. Weightlifters headache. *Headache* 1983; 23:193–194.
5. Rifat SF, Lombardo JA. Occipital neuralgia in a football player: a case report. *Clin J Sport Med* 1995;5(4):251–253.
6. Diamond S. Prolonged benign exertional headache: its clinical characteristics and response to indomethacin. *Headache* 1982;22:96–98.
7. Massey EW. Effort headache in runners. *Headache* 1982;22:99–100.
8. Mauskop A, Altura BT, Cracco RQ, Altura BM. Intravenous magnesium sulfate relieves migraine attacks in patients with low serum ionized magnesium levels: a pilot study. *Clin Sci* 1995;89:633–636.
9. North K, Davies L. Postexercise headache in menopausal women. *Lancet* 1993;341:972.
10. Lambert RW Jr, Burnet DL. Prevention of exercise induced migraine by quantitative warm-up. *Headache* 1985;25:317–319.
11. Kelly RE. Post-traumatic headache. In: Vinken PJ, Bruyn GW, eds. *Handbook of clinical neurology*, vol 48. Amsterdam; Elsevier, 1986:383–390.
12. Maddocks DL, Dicker GD, Saling MM. The assessment of orientation following concussion in athletes. *Clin J Sport Med* 1995;5(1):32–35.
13. Matthews WB. Footballers' migraine. *Br Med J* 1972; 2:326–327.
14. Bennett DR, Ruenning SI, Sullivan G, et al. Migraine precipitated by head trauma in athletes. *Am J Sports Med* 1980;8:202–205.
15. Kalanak A, Petro DJ, Brennan W. Migraine secondary to head trauma in wrestling. *Am J Sports Med* 1978;6: 112–113.
16. Morris AM. Footballer's migraine. *Br Med J* 1972;2: 769–770.
17. Ashworth B. Migraine, head trauma, and sport. *Scott Med J* 1985;30(4):240–242.
18. Russell MB, Olesen J. Migraine associated with head trauma. *Eur J Neurol* 1996;3:424–428.
19. Bracker MD, Rothrock JF. Cluster headache among athletes. *Physician Sports Med* 1989;17(2):147–158.
20. Reik L Jr. Cluster headache after head injury. *Headache* 1987;27:509–510.
21. Li MS, Smith BM, Espinosa J, Brown RA, Richardson P, Ford R. Nonpenetrating trauma to the carotid artery: seven cases and a literature review. *J Trauma* 1994; 36(2):265–272.
22. Nelson EE. Internal carotid artery dissection associated with scuba diving. *Ann Emerg Med* 1995;25(1): 103–106.
23. Saunders RL, Hahaugh RE. The second impact in catastrophic contact sports head trauma. *JAMA* 1984;252: 538–539.
24. McQuillen JB, McQuillen EN, Morrow P. Trauma, sport, and malignant cerebral edema. *Am J Forensic Med Pathol* 1988;9(1):12–15.
25. Cantu RC. Second impact syndrome: immediate management. *Physician Sports Med* 1992;20(9):55–66.
26. Pestronk A, Pestronk S: Goggle migraine. *N Engl J Med* 1983;308:1363.
27. Jacobson RI: More "goggle headache": supraorbital neuralgia. *N Engl J Med* 1983;308:1363.
28. Jokl E. Olympic medicine and sport cardiology. *Ann Sports Med* 1984;1:149.
29. Bartsch P, Maggi S, Kleger G, Ballmer PE, Baumgartner RW. Sumatriptan for high-altitude headache. *Lancet* 1994;344:1445.
30. Burtscher M, Likar R, Nachbaner W, Schaffert W, Philadelphy M. Ibuprofen versus sumatriptan for high-altitude headache [Letter]. *Lancet* 1994;344:1445.

Sports Neurology, Second Edition,
edited by Barry D. Jordan.
Lippincott–Raven Publishers, Philadelphia © 1998.

19

Peripheral Nerve Injury

Mark Hallett

National Institute of Neurological Disorders and Stroke, National Institutes of Health, Building 10,
Room 5N226, 10 Center Drive, MSC 1428, Bethesda, Maryland 20892-1428

Although much of sports injury involves bone or soft tissue injury, radiculopathy, and spinal cord or brain injury, the peripheral nerves can also be affected. There is no good epidemiologic information concerning the incidence or prevalence of the different conditions. In one survey from an orthopedic clinic in Japan, 66 of 1167 cases (5.7%) of peripheral nerve injuries were due to sports (1). The nerves most commonly involved in order of frequency were the brachial plexus, radial, ulnar, peroneal, and axillary nerves. The most common sports causes of injury were mountain climbing, gymnastics, and baseball, which is undoubtedly related to the popularity of different sports in Japan.

There are several ways in which a nerve might be injured. One is direct, acute trauma. This might be due to a blow to a nerve or to concomitant injury together with a fracture. A second way is "microtrauma" resulting from repetitive stress of the soft tissues leading to "overuse" with either direct nerve involvement or indirect involvement related to remodeling of collagenous tissues and nerve entrapment (2).

This chapter is modified and updated from Chapter 16 of *Entrapment Neuropathies,* 2nd edition, by D. M. Dawson, M. Hallett, and L. H. Millender, Little Brown, Boston, 1990 (2), and large portions are repeated unchanged with permission of the publisher. It was originally written by Dr. Hallett as a syllabus for a course at the American Association of Electrodiagnostic Medicine and revised for many course syllabuses subsequently.

NERVE INJURIES

There are three main classes of nerve injury (2).

Neurapraxia is segmental block of axonal conduction. In this situation, the axon is intact and a nerve can conduct actions potentials above and below the involved region but not across the region. The phenomenon is due to a focal region of demyelination of the nerve.

Axonotmesis refers to loss of continuity of nerve axons with continuity of the connective tissue sheath. Such injury leads to wallerian degeneration of the distal part of the nerve, but regeneration is possible because the connective tissue sheath serves as a road map for the regrowth of the axon.

Neurotmesis refers to damage of nerve with loss of continuity of the axons and the nerve sheath. Regrowth is much less likely in this circumstance. The nerve attempting to grow may form a neuroma.

Acute trauma may cause any of these three types of nerve injuries; microtrauma is likely to cause only the first two types. How nerve entrapment damages a nerve is only partly understood, and there are likely to be a number of mechanisms. Pressure, stretch, angulation, and friction are physical injuries that entrapment might cause. An early entrapment might cause only neurapraxia but then progress to axonotmesis over time.

Symptoms of nerve injury include those related to loss of function, sensory loss, and weakness. Ectopic generation of impulses in damaged sensory fibers might give rise to paresthesias such as a pins-and-needles sensation. Pain can also be present either at the site of the nerve injury or in the distribution of the nerve. Clearly, these symptoms can be very detrimental to the athlete trying for an optimal performance.

EVALUATION OF THE PATIENT AND ELECTRODIAGNOSIS

Clinical evaluation should include careful analysis of motor and sensory function. Sites of possible entrapment and all sites of local pain should be examined. Often it is useful to evaluate movements performed by patients in their sports. A good example is in the tennis player with elbow pain. The technique of the patient's backhand should be observed. A tennis lesson might well accompany medical advice!

To confirm clinical suspicion of nerve involvement, electrodiagnosis is often useful. Electrodiagnosis includes a number of tests; the most commonly used are nerve conduction studies and electromyography (EMG).

Nerve conduction studies give information about the number of nerve fibers in a nerve and the condition of the myelin. Nerve injuries, including entrapments, might damage only the myelin in the region of the injury, giving rise to an area of neurapraxia with focal conduction block or slowing of conduction. If there is axonotmesis or neurotmesis, there will be loss of fibers.

Focal slowing of nerve conduction can be detected with studies of segmental conduction velocity. This observation can be made with either sensory or motor nerve conduction. With motor conduction, conduction velocity cannot be measured in the most distal segment, and the distal latency is measured instead. The classic example of focal motor slowing is focal compression of the median nerve at the wrist in the carpal tunnel syndrome. Sensory conduction across the wrist is slowed and the distal latency of motor conduction is prolonged, while there is normal sensory and motor conduction in other segments.

Loss of nerve fibers is identified by loss of amplitude of the sensory nerve action potential (SNAP) or the compound muscle action potential (CMAP). Such observations are much more reliable with sensory nerve conduction studies than with motor nerve conduction studies. The reason for this is that the SNAP is a direct measure of the sensory axons whereas the CMAP is a measure of the muscle response. Thus, the CMAP is indirect. If motor axons are lost but there is complete reinnervation of the muscle by collateral sprouting, the CMAP could still be normal. Hence, the CMAP may give a false-negative result.

EMG studies are most useful in looking for denervation in the territory of the nerve suspected of being injured. Studies of this sort should also explore other territories to confirm that muscles innervated by other nerves are normal. EMG findings of fibrillation and positive sharp waves indicate acute denervation, and large-amplitude and long-duration motor units indicate reinnervation and chronic denervation. Decreased recruitment of numbers of motor units (spatial recruitment) is also indicative of a nerve injury.

In some circumstances, nerves cannot be examined by electrodiagnosis. In some pain syndromes in which a nerve entrapment is suspected, block of the nerve with local anesthetic might help confirm the diagnosis. This is useful, for example, in the analysis of heel pain, as discussed later.

THE THROWING MOTION AND ITS INJURIES

The throwing motion is common to many sports. The best studied is the pitch in baseball, but the same basic motion is seen with the tennis serve, throwing a football or a javelin, and serving overhand in volleyball. Pain at the medial side of the elbow and damage to the ulnar nerve at the elbow are a common problem. The biomechanics of the throwing motion have been studied in detail and can explain the disorder. More recently described is an injury to the infraspinatus branch of the suprascapular nerve. This is somewhat more controversial in origin. Lastly, the pronator syndrome has been described in pitchers, but this appears to be rare.

There are three phases of the throwing motion (Fig. 1) (3–5).

1. Cocking phase: The shoulder is abducted to 90° and the humerus is brought into hyper-

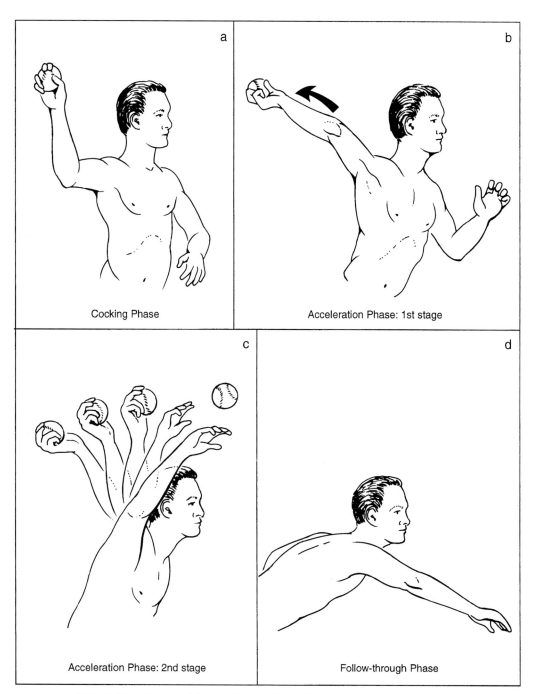

FIG. 1. The phases of the pitching motion. (From ref. 5, with permission.)

extension and extreme external rotation. The elbow is flexed approximately 45° and the wrist is fully extended. In this phase the deltoid, supraspinatus, and infraspinatus are active. This phase is slow and great forces are not necessary.

2. Acceleration phase, first stage: The body and shoulder are brought forward, leaving the forearm and hand behind. If the body gets too far ahead of the arm, this "opening up" too soon is called rushing.

   Acceleration phase, second stage: This phase lasts only about 50 msec and is the time of maximal forces and stress. The humerus is whipped into maximal internal rotation with a torque estimated to be about 14,000 inch-pound. This is accomplished by the internal rotators including the latissimus dorsi, pectoralis major, and teres major. The serratus anterior becomes active to pull the scapula forward. This motion has about four times the kinetic energy of the kicking foot. In addition, the wrist is rapidly flexed to add speed to the ball. In this phase, the shoulder rotates with peak velocities averaging 6180 deg/sec and the elbow extends with peak velocities averaging 4595 deg/sec (6).

3. Follow-through phase: Begins with release of the ball and is characterized by completion of extension of the elbow and full horizontal flexion and internal rotation of the shoulder. This phase requires deceleration of both the internal rotation and elbow extension. Muscle activity is seen in the biceps, deltoid, supraspinatus, and infraspinatus. Activity in the serratus anterior continues.

Medial Elbow Stress Syndrome and Injury to the Ulnar Nerve at the Elbow

It is in the acceleration phase that there is maximal stress on the medial side of the elbow (5,7). In the first stage the elbow is forced into extreme valgus, and in the second stage contracting wrist flexors in the forearm pull on the medial epicondyle on the humerus where they insert. It is more efficient and less stressful for the hand to be close to the vertical plane during acceleration; sidearm delivery and "snaps" add to the stress.

Such forces stress the medial collateral ligament of the elbow, which can be sprained or ruptured. In addition, the medial epicondyle of the humerus can be avulsed. The forearm flexors can be strained or ruptured. Chronically, the medial collateral ligament becomes stretched and scarred, leading to medial joint laxity. Professional pitchers show hypertrophy of the forearm flexor muscles and have a flexion contracture of the elbow and an increased valgus angle.

Ulnar nerve lesions are the most common nerve injuries in pitching. The ulnar nerve passes the medial side of the elbow and is subject to injury there (8,9). The ligaments holding the nerve may become lax or rupture, leading to subluxation or dislocation. The collateral ligament may become inflamed or calcified, leading to entrapment of the nerve. There can be traction on the nerve because of irregularity of the ulnar groove resulting from osteoarthritis or loose bodies or because of a severe valgus deformity. At the entrance to the cubital tunnel, the origin of the flexor carpi ulnaris, there can be inflammation or a contricting band.

Of course, ulnar nerve lesions at the elbow are common even without the severe medial elbow stress syndrome. There may be other causes of ulnar nerve damage. One case of ulnar entrapment in a pitcher was due to an anomalous muscle, the epitrochleoanconeus, which runs from the medial epicondyle to the medial olecranon (10). In two published cases of entrapment by this muscle, the symptoms seemed related to exercise (11), so it might be that even in this circumstance the act of pitching played an etiologic role.

Symptoms of an ulnar nerve lesion at the elbow include numbness and tingling on the medial side of the hand and in the fifth finger and the medial side of the fourth finger. There is weakness of intrinsic muscles of the hand sparing only the thenar muscles, which are largely supplied by the median nerve. Local pain may be present at the elbow. Pressure on the elbow may lead to increased paresthesias.

Various surgical options are available for ulnar nerve lesions at the elbow. In the professional athlete, this is a delicate situation, because the surgery must not only correct the problem but also not cause any new problems. Surgery with anterior transfer of the nerve and placement of the nerve deep to the flexor muscles can be successful treatment and may be the best option (12). The verification that such an operation can be successful is that postoperatively professional pitchers have won games in World Series competition.

Infraspinatus Branch
of the Suprascapular Nerve

Suprascapular neuropathy is a classic entrapment neuropathy. Typically, entrapment is at the suprascapular notch by the suprascapular ligament and there is weakness of both the supraspinatus and infraspinatus muscles. A number of cases have been reported in which there appeared to be isolated involvement of just the infraspinatus muscle. A well-studied case of isolated infraspinatus weakness in a fencer was reported by Aiello et al. (13). In this circumstance, the nerve was entrapped by hypertrophy of the inferior transverse scapular ligament. This ligament, also called the spinoglenoid ligament, is present in 50% of persons and runs from the lateral border of the spine to the scapular neck or scapulohumeral joint capsule. It covers the spinoglenoid notch at the lateral border of the spine of the scapula through which the nerve branch to the infraspinatus travels. The ligament is present in only 50% of women but in 87% of men (14). The variation of the distance between the ligament and the bone is greater in men than in women. These two facts should make this disorder more likely in men than women. The patient reported by Aiello et al. improved after operation. A similar case has been reported by Jerosch et al. (15). Bryan and Wild (16) have described the sudden onset of posterior shoulder pain and isolated infraspinatus weakness after a hard throw.

Ringel et al. (17) have described two cases of pitchers with shoulder pain and involvement of the suprascapular nerve. One had atrophy of the infraspinatus and weakness of abduction and external rotation of the shoulder. Electrodiagnostic evaluation revealed abnormalities in the supraspinatus and infraspinatus. Operation on this case did not reveal obvious entrapment at the suprascapular notch, but the superior transverse scapular ligament was resected and the patient gradually improved. The other case had isolated involvement only of the infraspinatus on clinical and electrodiagnostic grounds. In this case there was entrapment at the suprascapular notch, but only the branch to the infraspinatus went through the notch; innervation of the supraspinatus came from a branch before the notch. These authors also examined six pitchers with nerve conduction studies before and after a baseball season. All were asymptomatic, but one showed an increase of the distal latency to infraspinatus from Erb's point of 3.2 to 4.7 msec. In a detailed study of a cadaver with the shoulder in horizontal abduction and external rotation, these authors identified three sites of possible trauma in addition to the suprascapular notch and the spinoglenoid notch: in the fascia of the scalene muscles, in the fascia of the subclavius and omohyoid muscles, and within the supraspinous fossa between the base of the coracoid process and the supraspinatus muscle. They raised the possibility that damage to the nerve could result from intimal damage to the axillary or suprascapular artery and subsequent production of microemboli that become trapped in the vasa nervorum of the suprascapular nerve.

A study of volleyball players is relevant to this issue. Ferretti et al. (18) had noted isolated weakness of the infraspinatus in several volleyball players and conducted a survey. Of 96 players, 12 had asymptomatic weakness of the infraspinatus only on the dominant side. Three of three had denervation on EMG. The authors blamed the serve for this disorder, and, as noted earlier, the volleyball serve is a similar motion to throwing. (Spiking may also be important because it is a similar motion and possibly more abrupt and powerful.) They pointed out that the nerve branch to the infraspinatus makes an acute angle as it goes around the lateral edge of the spine in 30% of persons. During external rotation of the shoulder (the cocking phase), the terminal branches of the nerve are shifted medially, which tenses the nerve against the spine. A similar event occurs at the end of the serve (the follow-through phase) when the infraspinatus fires eccentrically to brake the arm. Confirming the importance of this nerve injury, in a more recent survey of 66 high-performance volleyball players, 22 had either clinical or electrophysiologic evidence of suprascapular neuropathy (19). The authors of this study thought the most common site of injury was the suprascapular notch.

The pathophysiology of this disorder has not been settled. A mechanical analysis of the nerve at the suprascapular notch during the throwing motion has not been reported. Some of these patients have posterior shoulder pain and others have no pain. Ferretti et al. (18) suggested that isolated involvement of the nerve to the infraspinatus might well be painless because there are no sensory branches.

Pronator Syndrome

The pronator syndrome involves entrapment of the median nerve as it passes between the superficial and deep head of the pronator teres in the upper forearm. Throwing the fastball involves vigorous contraction of the pronator teres and the median nerve can be entrapped by hypertrophy of this muscle. Additional mechanisms of entrapment in the same region include thickened lacertus fibrosus, a fibrous band within the pronator teres, and a tight fibrous arch of the flexor digitorum superficialis. All of these events are uncommon. A case treated successfully by fascial release was described by Barnes and Tullos (7). Another case was treated with steroid injection (20).

Radial Nerve Injury

Radial nerve injury may also be a result of the throwing motion, although the biomechanical stresses on this nerve have not been worked out in detail. This may have been reported first by Gowers (21), who saw such a case after throwing a stone with energy. Cases have been described after throwing a discus (22) and serving in tennis (23).

Two cases of radial nerve injury in different sites have been described in competitive softball pitchers who throw with a "windmill" pitching motion (24). One site was in the brachial plexus and the other was at the spiral groove. Both patients had surgery where severe injury was found, and the patients experienced only limited improvement. In both cases, the authors suggested that trauma to the radial nerve was the re-

sult of the rapid acceleration phase of the pitch, in which the arm is brought downward and forward from behind, which is associated with elbow extension, forearm supination, and shoulder rotation.

A number of cases of radial nerve injury have occurred with just strong muscular effort and not with rapid motion (25–27). Thus, the mechanism of radial nerve injury might be the contraction of the muscles themselves. Injury to the musculocutaneous nerve has been reported after vigorous upper extremity resistive exercise, and the mechanism has also been thought to be entrapment by muscular contraction, in this case by the coracobrachialis (28).

INJURIES WITH RUNNING

Running is common to many sports and is the central activity in jogging, which is becoming increasingly popular. Foot pain is a common complaint, and although the cause is often orthopedic, a number of nerve syndromes should be recognized.

A detailed study was done of 25 runners to see if frequent running damaged the nerves in the feet (29). None of these subjects had symptoms or routine clinical signs of neuropathy. Minimal changes in quantitative sensory thresholds and nerve conduction velocities, however, were found. The investigators concluded that minor nerve damage in the feet does occur, but it does not appear to be of significance. On the other hand, many individual nerve entrapments may occur.

Heel Pain

Probably the most important clinical syndrome to understand is that of heel pain, because it is so common. In one series, 19% of runners' complaints concerning the feet related to heel pain (30). Orthopedic conditions are common and include plantar fasciitis and tuber calcanei pain. There are three neurologic considerations (Fig. 2).

Tarsal tunnel syndrome. This well-described syndrome is entrapment of the tibial nerve at the ankle. It is not particularly common. In athletes it may be present after ankle injury.

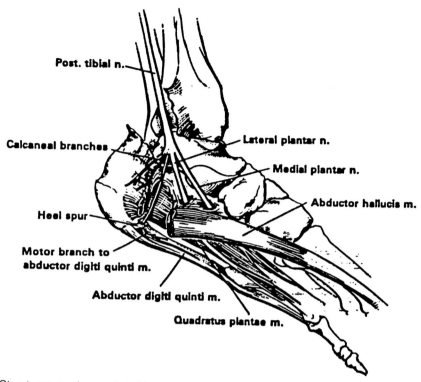

Post. tibial n.

Calcaneal branches

Lateral plantar n.

Medial plantar n.

Abductor hallucis m.

Heel spur

Motor branch to
abductor digiti quinti m.

Abductor digiti quinti m.

Quadratus plantae m.

FIG. 2. Structures on the medial side of the ankle. Potential causes of heel pain are entrapment of the (posterior) tibial nerve, the (medial) calcaneal branches, and the first branch of the lateral plantar nerve. The deep fascia of the abductor hallucis muscle has been incised, exposing more of the course of the lateral plantar nerve. (From ref. 34, with permission.)

Plantar surface paresthesias or a burning pain may occur. A Tinel sign behind the medial malleolus may be present.

Medial calcaneal neuritis. A branch of the tibial nerve at the ankle is the medial calcaneal branch, which supplies sensation to the medial side of the heel. Pain with entrapment is localized to the medial heel area (30). There may be numbness or paresthesias over the medial heel.

Entrapment of the first branch of the lateral plantar nerve. The lateral plantar nerve is one of the terminal branches of the tibial nerve. This nerve itself has three branches, the first to the medial process of the calcaneal tuberosity, the second to the flexor digitorum brevis, and the third to the abductor digiti minimi. Schon and Baxter (31) claimed that entrapment of this nerve is re-sponsible for chronic unresolving heel pain in 10% to 15% of athletes. The entrapment occurs between the deep fascia of the abductor hallucis muscle and the medial caudal margin of the quadratus plantae muscle. The syndrome is of pain, either dull or sharp, that is aggravated by running. There is no numbness of the heel or foot. There may be tenderness over the nerve deep to the abductor hallucis muscle. In Baxter and Pfeffer's (32) series of 69 operations, 89% had good or excellent results and 83% had complete resolution of pain.

In separating these neurologic conditions, nerve conduction studies may be useful, but a selected abnormality of the first branch of the lateral plantar nerve will not be identified in this way. Selective nerve blocks may be useful (30).

Morton's Toe

Entrapment of the interdigital nerves of the toes is called Morton's toe (31). This is due to trauma of the nerves at the intermetatarsal ligament. Symptoms include plantar or forefoot pain and numbness or tingling of the affected toes.

Peroneal Nerve

Seven runners and one soccer player were reported with peroneal compression neuropathy (33). Running produced pain, numbness, and tingling on the lateral side of the leg. Examination after running revealed muscle weakness and a Tinel sign. Nerve conduction were abnormal in five cases in which it was studied. Seven of eight had marked improvement after surgery. Specific entrapment of the superficial peroneal branch or the deep peroneal branch at the level of the ankle has also been described (31). These conditions are often posttraumatic. Tight-fitting shoes may also be responsible.

Medial Plantar Nerve (Jogger's Foot)

Entrapment of the medial plantar nerve has been designated jogger's foot (31,34,35). Patients complain of aching or shooting pain in the medial aspect of the arch. Deep to the abductor hallucis muscle, the medial plantar nerve runs along the plantar surface of the flexor digitorum longus tendon and passes through the master knot of Henry, where the entrapment occurs. The master knot of Henry is the medial investing fascia of the flexor hallucis longus and the calcaneonavicular ligament (Fig. 3).

Miscellaneous Nerves

Cases of involvement of the lateral femoral cutaneous nerve (producing meralgia paresthetica) (36) and sural nerve have been described (31).

BACKPACKING

The fact that mountain climbing is the most common cause of sport nerve injury in Japan is suggestive that it is more popular in Japan than in the United States (1). "Backpack paralysis" was the most common such injury. Either the brachial plexus, the axillary nerve, the suprascapular nerve, the accessory nerve, the long thoracic nerve, or the radial nerve can be damaged by a heavy pack and its straps and pads.

Two cases of tarsal tunnel syndrome were seen and ascribed to repeated dorsal and plantar flexion of the ankle joint (1).

BASEBALL

The most common nerve syndromes seen in baseball players have already been described in relation to throwing and running, but there are a few more that have been described.

The axillary nerve (or the posterior humeral circumflex artery) is subject to compression in the quadrilateral space (quadrangular space) (37). This space is bounded by the teres minor superiorly, the capsule of the glenohumeral joint and humerus laterally, the long head of the triceps medially, and fascia and adipose inferiorly. Two cases of the quadrilateral space syndrome have been described in baseball pitchers (38,39). The symptoms are pain in the anterior aspect of the shoulder exacerbated by abduction and external rotation of the humerus. Paresthesias can be present on the shoulder and in the upper arm. Diagnosis can be made with subclavian arteriography performed with the arm in abduction and external rotation (38). The etiology is generally thought to be abnormal fibrous strands in the quadrilateral space, although excessive muscle hypertrophy might lead to nerve entrapment. Surgery with lysis of the abnormal strands can be helpful (37,38).

In addition, the axillary nerve might be damaged by an osteophyte on the posterior aspect of the glenoid fossa as suggested by Bennett (40). Analysis by Barnes and Tullos (7) has cast doubt on that mechanism.

A traumatic neuroma of the ulnar digital nerve to the thumb was described in a batter (41). This is a common problem in bowling and is called bowler's thumb (see below). Trauma to the digital nerves of the index finger can occur with catching (H. S. Tullos, personal communication, 1988).

Carpal tunnel syndrome and thoracic outlet syndrome may well occur in baseball players, but it is not clear that these problems are due to the

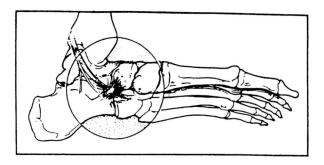

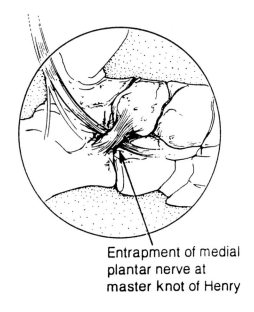

Entrapment of medial
plantar nerve at
master knot of Henry

FIG. 3. The medial plantar nerve is shown compressed at the master knot of Henry. (From ref. 34, with permission.)

baseball. For example, a reported thoracic outlet syndrome in two athletes was due in both cases to a cervical rib. Similarly, isolated cases of a musculocutaneous nerve lesion (A. Pappas, personal communication) and a long thoracic nerve lesion (H. S. Tullos, personal communication, 1988) are not clearly due to the baseball.

BICYCLING

One of the classic sports neuropathies is compression of the ulnar nerve at the wrist, in the canal of Guyon, associated with pressure of the hands on the handlebars of a bicycle (42). Compression of the ulnar nerve at this site due to occupational trauma is sometimes called the Ramsay Hunt syndrome. A callus over the base of the palm may be a clue to this disorder.

Etiologic factors include the use of worn-out gloves, unpadded handlebars, riding a poorly fitted bicycle, receiving vibration from rough roads, and prolonged grasping of the dropped handlebars (43,44). Less well known is the fact that the median nerve might also be affected by a similar injury (43).

There has been a case report of bilateral "sciatica" (associated with traumatic urethritis) following prolonged use of a unicycle (45). The presumed mechanism was pressure from the unicycle seat in the perineal area. A case of sciatic nerve damage with low back pain with radiation into the hip and leg, proved electrodiagnostically, was dubbed "pedal pusher's palsy" (46). This was associated with use of an exercise bicycle with pressure from the seat in the region of the sciatic notch. We have seen a patient with perineal numbness including penile numbness that lasted for several days after a long bicycle trip, again presumably caused by pressure from the seat on the pudendal nerve. Solomon and Cappa (47) have reported a case with a tight sensation of the head of the penis and impotence with the same presumptive mechanism.

BOWLING

A neuroma of the digital nerve to the thumb is referred to as bowler's thumb (48). Clinically, skin atrophy or callus can be seen over the neuroma, and Tinel's sign is typically positive. Pathologically, there is not true neuroma formation but a proliferation of fibrous tissue and nerve atrophy.

FOOTBALL

One of the most controversial neurologic syndromes is the "burner" or "stinger" of the football player. It is a common disorder and may affect as many as half of the members of a football squad (49–51). On the other hand, only about 30% of incidents are reported (52), probably because the players are concerned that if they report the symptom, they might not be allowed to play. The symptom is that of a sudden sensation of burning or stinging in the arm after a tackle or other jolt to the head. The pain extends from the shoulder to the hand. Typically, the burning lasts about 3 to 10 seconds (51). Weakness in the arm lasts 1 to 2 minutes but may be more persistent, particularly with repeated episodes. Weakness may be seen in shoulder abductors, shoulder external rotators, and forearm flexors. The trauma may include depression of the ipsilateral shoulder and/or deviation of the head back or toward the opposite shoulder. The controversy is whether the lesion is in the plexus, nerve root, or even spinal cord.

Advocates of a brachial plexus origin point out that the provocative movement should stretch the upper trunk of the plexus. With EMG studies of 10 patients, Robertson et al. (51) have found that arm muscles including supraspinatus, infraspinatus, biceps, and deltoid showed denervation, but paraspinal muscles were normal.

DiBenedetto and Markey (53) found proximal conduction slowing in 16 of 18 patients; they emphasized that conduction studies with nerve root stimulation were helpful as well as studies with stimulation at Erb's point to find these abnormalities. Slowing was seen in the musculocutaneous nerve in 62%, suprascapular nerve in 53%, axillary nerve in 43%, and accessory nerve in 47%. Fibrillation was also seen in some limb muscles (most commonly the deltoid), but paraspinal muscle fibrillation was seen in only one patient, who had a clinical radiculopathy. In Wilbourn's experience (54) also, fibrillations are uncommon.

Some of the EMG findings have suggested nerve root involvement. Poindexter and Johnson (55) found fibrillation in cervical paraspinal muscles in 6 of 12 football players without denervation in the arm. Rockett (56) reported improvement of burner symptoms in a patient who underwent cervical laminectomy and noted scarring of C-5 and C-6 roots at surgery. Some players certainly may have a ruptured cervical disc. The physical examination of a patient should take this into account. A positive Sperling test, increased pain with neck extension, and tilt toward the painful side would favor an abnormal cervical disc.

Some patients may have transient spinal cord symptoms and signs including transient quadriparesis (57). Such patients should not be allowed to return to play while still symptomatic and should not continue the sport if their cervical spine is abnormal on magnetic resonance imaging (57). Maroon (58) has reported two cases of patients with "burning hands," both of whom had fracture and dislocation of the cervical spine and central cord injury. Clearly, patients with this condition need to be examined carefully.

A narrow spinal canal might predispose to burners and certainly to spinal cord injury. A Torg ratio, the AP canal to the AP vertebral body, of less than 0.8 may be somewhat predictive (59).

The proper medical advice to patients with burners is not settled. Some would advocate not returning to play with persistent symptoms, and others would advocate caution if stingers are frequent. Both views seem reasonable, but it is not always possible to get the players to agree. Certainly, an abnormal cervical spine would be a clear contraindication to return to play. Some investigators have promoted orthoses, which limit neck motion, to prevent stingers, and these have had some success (52,60).

As an additional syndrome in football players, trauma to the axillary nerve in the quadrilateral space can occur (49).

TENNIS

Tennis elbow is a classic sports medicine syndrome, but there is some confusion about it. The "classic" symptom is pain in the region of the lateral epicondyle of the elbow. In one survey of complaints of tennis players, however, pain was more common on the medial side of the elbow than on the lateral side (61). The medial pain was associated most commonly with serving and the mechanism would seem to be similar to that of the medial elbow problems of baseball pitchers. A special syndrome of pain in the region of the cubital tunnel appears to be due to the spin serve. In this situation the spin is partly conveyed to the ball by flexion and ulnar deviation of the wrist, both movements being functions of the flexor carpi ulnaris (61).

The lateral elbow pain was associated most commonly with ground strokes, especially the backhand. Strong contraction of the wrist extensors is clearly needed in this circumstance. The incidence of symptoms has been correlated with technique in detailed biomechanical investigations (62). In good backhand technique the elbow is in extension and the movement is mainly that of external rotation of the shoulder. In poor technique, labeled the "leading elbow," the elbow is partly flexed with the olecranon pointed to the net and the power is generated by abduction at the shoulder and extension at the elbow.

In one view, the pain of tennis elbow is due to damage to the muscles or tendons that insert on the lateral (or medial) epicondyle. Coonrad and Hooper (63) found macroscopic tears of the tendon of origin during operation in 28 of 39 patients and scar tissue in another 9 of the patients. In some patients calcification can be seen with radiographs in the extensor aponeurosis (64). In the series of operations of Nirschl (64), scarring

was also commonly seen, but some cases were apparently normal. This trauma might lead to inflammation, and the term lateral epicondylitis has been applied.

In a second view, another possible source of lateral elbow pain is entrapment of the posterior interosseus nerve. Possible entrapment sites include the extensor carpi radialis brevis, the arcade of Frohse at the entrance to the supinator, and the supinator itself. The region from the arcade of Frohse through the supinator is called the radial tunnel. This syndrome is called the resistant tennis elbow syndrome. Clinically, the entrapment should be recognized by pain when patients forcefully supinate the forearm to resist passive pronation or forcefully extend the wrist or middle finger to resist passive flexion. There should be tenderness over the radial nerve and not over the lateral epicondyle itself. Electrodiagnostic studies in the resistant tennis elbow syndrome have been controversial, with some authors finding abnormalities and others not. A comprehensive study by Rosen and Werner (65) showed that motor conduction in the posterior interosseous nerve might be abnormal if studied during forceful supination. In addition, they found denervation in the extensor digitorum communis.

In a number of series, surgical release of the posterior interosseous nerve has provided good relief of symptoms (66,67). Capener (68) operated on six cases of "tennis elbow" with release of the posterior interosseous nerve and obtained relief in all. Jalovaara and Lindholm (69) decompressed the posterior interosseous nerve in 111 cases and reported results after a median follow-up of 5 years; 85% showed improvement, and 30% were almost completely relieved of symptoms. The authors concluded that only the 30% who had the best improvement really had nerve compression. They cautioned that there is no good technique for being certain of nerve compression preoperatively and that some improvement after operation does not prove that nerve compression was responsible for the symptoms.

Another syndrome seen uncommonly in many different athletes, but most commonly in tennis players, is a long thoracic neuropathy (70). The onset is often insidious, but it can develop acutely together with shoulder pain after vigorous activity. The etiology may be stretch. Conservative treatment typically leads to significant improvement.

OTHER SPORTS

Occasional entrapments of nerves occur in other sports, but these are not very common and typically described only in single case reports. A relatively complete list has been published (2).

REFERENCES

1. Hirasawa Y, Sakakida K. Sports and peripheral nerve injury. *Am J Sports Med* 1983;11:420–426.
2. Dawson DM, Hallett M, Millender LH. *Entrapment neuropathies,* 2nd ed. Boston: Little, Brown and Company, 1990:434.
3. Jobe FW, Moynes DR, Tibone JE, Perry J. An EMG analysis of the shoulder in pitching. A second report. *Am J Sports Med* 1984;12:218–220.
4. Jobe FW, Tibone JE, Perry J, Moynes D. An EMG analysis of the shoulder in throwing and pitching. A preliminary report. *Am J Sports Med* 1983;11:3–5.
5. Woods GW, Tullos HS, King JW. The throwing arm: elbow joint injuries. *J Sports Med* 1973;1:43–47.
6. Pappas AM, Zawacki RM, Sullivan TJ. Biomechanics of baseball pitching. A preliminary report. *Am J Sports Med* 1985;13:216–222.
7. Barnes DA, Tullos HS. An analysis of 100 symptomatic baseball players. *Am J Sports Med* 1987;6:62–67.
8. Del Pizzo W, Jobe FW, Norwood L. Ulnar nerve entrapment syndrome in baseball players. *Am J Sports Med* 1977;5:182–185.
9. Indelicato PA, Jobe FW, Kerlan RK, Carter VS, Shields CL, Lombardo SJ. Correctable elbow lesions in professional baseball players: a review of 25 cases. *Am J Sports Med* 1979;7:72–75.
10. Hirasawa Y, Sawamura H, Sakakida K. Entrapment neuropathy due to bilateral epitrochleoanconeus muscles: a case report. *J Hand Surg* 1979;4:181–184.
11. Hodgkinson PD, McLean NR. Ulnar nerve entrapment due to epitrochleo-anconeus muscle. *J Hand Surg Br* 1994;19:706–708.
12. Glousman RE. Ulnar nerve problems in the athlete's elbow. *Clin Sports Med* 1990;9:365–377.
13. Aiello I, Serra G, Traina C, Tugnoli V. Entrapment of the suprascapular nerve at the spinoglenoid notch. *Ann Neurol* 1982;12:314–316.
14. Kaspi A, Yanai J, Pick CG, Mann G. Entrapment of the distal suprascapular nerve. An anatomical study. *Int Orthop* 1988;12:273–275.
15. Jerosch J, Hille E, Schulitz KP. Selective paralysis of the infraspinatus muscle, caused by compression of the infraspinatus branch of the suprascapular nerve. *Sportverletz Sportschaden* 1987;1:231–233.
16. Bryan WJ, Wild JJ Jr. Isolated infraspinatus atrophy. A common cause of posterior shoulder pain and weakness in throwing athletes? *Am J Sports Med* 1989;17:130–131.
17. Ringel SP, Treihaft M, Carry M, Fisher R, Jacobs P. Suprascapular neuropathy in pitchers. *Am J Sports Med* 1990;18:80–86.
18. Ferretti A, Cerullo G, Russo G. Suprascapular neuropathy in volleyball players. *J Bone Joint Surg Am* 1987; 69A:260–263.
19. Holzgraefe M, Kukowski B, Eggert S. Prevalence of latent and manifest suprascapular neuropathy in high-performance volleyball players. *Br J Sports Med* 1994; 28:177–179.
20. Khurana RK, Schlagenhauff RE, Zwirecki RJ. The pronator syndrome (a case report and reappraisal). *Neurology (Bombay)* 1975;23:46–48.
21. Gowers WR. *A manual of diseases of the nervous system.* London: Churchill, 1892.
22. Woltman HW, Kernohan JW, Goldstein NP. Diseases of peripheral nerves. In: Baker AB, ed. *Clinical neurology.* London: Hoeber-Harper, 1965:1816–1848.
23. Prochaska V, Crosby LA, Murphy RP. High radial nerve palsy in a tennis player. *Orthop Rev* 1993;22:90–92.
24. Sinson G, Zager EL, Kline DG. Windmill pitcher's radial neuropathy. *Neurosurgery* 1994;34:1087–1089.
25. Lotem M, Fried A, Levy M, Solzi P, Najenson T, Nathan H. Radial nerve palsy following muscular effort. *J Bone Joint Surg Br* 1971;53B:500–506.
26. Mitsunaga MM, Nakano K. High radial nerve palsy following strenuous muscular activity. A case report. *Clin Orthop* 1988;234:39–42.
27. Streib E. Upper arm radial nerve palsy after muscular effort: report of three cases. *Neurology* 1992;42:1632–1634.
28. Braddom RL, Wolfe C. Musculocutaneous nerve injury after heavy exercise. *Arch Phys Med Rehabil* 1978; 59:290–293.
29. Dyck PJ, Classen SM, Stevens JC, O'Brien PC. Assessment of nerve damage in the feet of long-distance runners. *Mayo Clin Proc* 1987;62:568–572.
30. Ludder LD. Surgical decisions in athletes' subcalcaneal pain. *Am J Sports Med* 1986;14:481–485.
31. Schon LC, Baxter DE. Neuropathies of the foot and ankle in athletes. *Clin Sports Med* 1990;9:489–509.
32. Baxter DE, Pfeffer GB. Treatment of chronic heel pain by surgical release of the first branch of the lateral plantar nerve. *Clin Orthop* 1992;279:229–236.
33. Leach RE, Purnell MB, Saito A. Peroneal nerve entrapment in runners. *Am J Sports Med* 1989;17:287–291.
34. Murphy PC, Baxter DE. Nerve entrapment in the foot and ankle in runners. *Clin Sports Med* 1985;4:753–763.
35. Rask MR. Medial plantar neurapraxia (jogger's foot): report of three cases. *Clin Orthop* 1978;134:193–195.
36. Massey EW, Pleet AB. Neuropathy in joggers. *Am J Sports Med* 1978;6:209–211.
37. Cahill BR, Palmer RE. Quadrilateral space syndrome. *J Hand Surg* 1983;8:65–69.
38. Cormier PJ, Matalon TAS, Wolin PM. Quadrilateral space syndrome: a rare cause of shoulder pain. *Radiology* 1988;167:797–798.
39. Redler MR, Ruland LJI, McCue FCI. Quadrilateral space syndrome in a throwing athlete. *Am J Sports Med* 1986;14:511–513.
40. Bennett GE. Shoulder and elbow lesions distinctive of baseball players. *Ann Surg* 1947;126:107–110.
41. Belsky M, Millender LH. Bowler's thumb in a baseball player. *Orthopedics* 1980;3:122–123.
42. Noth J, Dietz V, Mauritz KH. Cyclists's palsy. *J Neurol Sci* 1980;46:111–116.

43. Rettig AC. Neurovascular injuries in the wrist and hands of athletes. *Clin Sports Med* 1990;9:389–417.

44. Richmond DR. Handlebar problems in bicycling. *Clin Sports Med* 1994;13:165–173.

45. Gold S. Unicyclist's sciatica—a case report. *N Engl J Med* 1981;305:231–232.

46. Haig AJ. Pedal pusher's palsy. *N Engl J Med* 1989;320:63.

47. Solomon S, Cappa KG. Impotence and bicycling. A seldom-reported connection. *Postgrad Med* 1987;81:99–102.

48. Dobyns JH, O'Brien ET, Linschied RL, Farrow GM. Bowler's thumb—diagnosis and treatment: a review of seventeen cases. *J Bone Joint Surg Am* 1972;54A:751–755.

49. Cofield RH, Simonet WT. The shoulder in sports. *Mayo Clin Proc* 1984;59:157–164.

50. Meyer SA, Schulte KR, Callaghan JJ, et al. Cervical spinal stenosis and stingers in collegiate football players. *Am J Sports Med* 1994;22:158–166.

51. Robertson WC, Eichman PL, Clancy WG. Upper trunk brachial plexopathy in football players. *JAMA* 1979; 241:1480–1482.

52. Sallis RE, Jones K, Knopp W. Burners: offensive strategy for an underreported injury. *Physician Sports Med* 1992;20:47–55.

53. DiBenedetto M, Markey K. Electrodiagnostic localization of traumatic upper trunk brachial plexopathy. *Arch Phys Med Rehabil* 1984;65:15–17.

54. Wilbourn AJ. Electrodiagnostic testing of neurologic injuries in athletes. *Clin Sports Med* 1990;9:229–245.

55. Poindexter DP, Johnson EW. Football shoulder and neck injury: a study of the "stinger." *Arch Phys Med Rehabil* 1984;65:601–602.

56. Rockett FX. Observations on the "burner": traumatic cervical radiculopathy. *Clin Orthop* 1982;164:18–19.

57. Jordan BD, Warren RF, Tsairis P, Ghelman B. How to evaluate transient quadriparesis. *Physician Sports Med* 1992;20.

58. Maroon JC. "Burning hands" in football spinal cord injuries. *JAMA* 1977;238:2049–2051.

59. Torg JS, Sennett B, Pavlov H, Leventhal MR, Glasgow SG. Spear tackler's spine. An entity precluding participation in tackle football and collision activities that expose the cervical spine to axial energy inputs. *Am J Sports Med* 1993;21:640–649.

60. Markey KL, DiBenedetto M, Curl WW. Upper trunk brachial plexopathy. The stinger syndrome. *Am J Sports Med* 1993;21:650–655.

61. Preist JD, Jones HH, Nagel DA. Elbow injuries in highly skilled tennis players. *J Sports Med* 1974;2: 137–149.

62. Bernhang AM, Dehner W, Fogarty C. Tennis elbow: a biomechanical approach. *J Sports Med* 1974;2:235–260.

63. Coonrad RW, Hooper R. Tennis elbow. Its course, natural history, conservative and surgical management. *J Bone Joint Surg Am* 1973;55A:1177–1185.

64. Nirschl RP. The etiology and treatment of tennis elbow. *J Sports Med* 1975;3:308–323.

65. Rosen I, Werner CO. Neurophysiological investigation of posterior interosseous nerve entrapment causing lateral elbow pain. *Electroencephalogr Clin Neurophysiol* 1980;50:125–133.

66. Lister GD, Belsole RB, Kleinert HE. The radial tunnel syndrome. *J Hand Surg* 1979;4:52–59.

67. Roles NC, Maudsley RH. Radial tunnel syndrome: resistent tennis elbow as a nerve entrapment. *J Bone Joint Surg Br* 1972;54B:499–508.

68. Capener N. Biomechanical studies. *Br Med J* 1960;2:130.

69. Jalovaara P, Lindholm RV. Decompression of the posterior interosseous nerve for tennis elbow. *Arch Orthop Trauma Surg* 1989;108:243–245.

70. Schultz JS, Leonard JAJ. Long thoracic neuropathy from athletic activity. *Arch Phys Med Rehabil* 1992; 73:87–90.

Sports Neurology, Second Edition,
edited by Barry D. Jordan.
Lippincott–Raven Publishers, Philadelphia © 1998.

20

Skeletal Muscle Injuries and Disorders

Peter Tsairis

Hospital for Special Surgery, 535 East 70th Street, New York, New York 10021

Injury to skeletal muscle can be the result of a direct or indirect insult. Direct injuries may cause muscular strains, contusions, hematomas, and lacerations and may evolve into myositis ossificans or rhabdomyolysis. All of these injuries result in destruction of all or part of an individual muscle, the degree of loss being directly proportional to the severity of the insult. Diagnosis and treatment of these injuries are based on a solid understanding of anatomy, physiology, and healing of skeletal muscle.

Following trauma, skeletal muscle has been shown to have a limited capacity for regeneration and repair in response to a direct insult (1,2). Injured muscle fibers degenerate back from the injured area for a short distance. After injury, muscle fibers release proteolytic enzymes, which in turn initiate degradation of lipid and protein structures in the injured muscle cell (3). The breakdown of damaged muscle fibers in connective tissue is accompanied by diffusion of intracellular components into the interstitial space and plasma. Many of these substances, including prostaglandins, attract neutrophils, macrophages, and monocytes (3). Necrotic muscle tissue is then removed by the macrophages and other phagocytic cells. During the injury phase and depending on the severity of injury, there is an influx of fluid into the muscle resulting in an elevation of intramuscular pressure (4). In addition, Friden et al. (5) have demonstrated individual muscle fiber swelling and an inflammatory response following excentric exercise. They believe that fiber swelling may be one of the factors associated

with the development of delayed-onset muscle soreness in a structured compartment. Armstrong (6) suggested that group IV sensory neurons that terminate in the endomysium between myofibers are sensitive to increased osmotic pressure and may carry the sensation of dull diffuse pain associated with delayed-onset muscle pain after injury (7).

Activation of reserve myoblasts then provides a period of rapid self-proliferation in the injured muscle. In most injuries, regeneration of muscle fibers follows a process that parallels embryotic development of muscle. For example, muscle forms by condensation of the mesenchyma to form myoblasts. The synthesis of contractile proteins leads to fusion of these individual myoblasts into elongated multinucleated myotubes that ultimately fuse to reform the muscle. These myotubes then produce more contractile proteins, which aggregate into myofilaments. The individual cell nuclei are then squeezed peripherally, leading to mature muscle cells. Small mononucleated satellite cells develop and lie between the sarcolemma around the myofibrils and the basilaminae of the muscle cell. These satellite cells are felt to be precursors for the reparative process. Although the repair process is a complicated one, it is capable of bridging only small local injuries. The repair process in larger insults of muscle is primarily by the formation of scar tissue (1).

Therefore, in the healing process of skeletal muscle injury there are two competing events occurring simultaneously: regeneration of disrupted muscle fibers and production of connective tissue that leads to scar formation. Excessive scar formation is capable of inhibiting complete regeneration of the muscle because it acts as a mechanical barrier. During the formation of granulation tissue, the reactive collagen is gradually reabsorbed, but if inflammation persists, the amount of collagen remains high, which in time leads to fibrosis (1).

Indirect muscle injuries occur as a result of either neurologic or vascular insults. Neurologic compromise is secondary to either an upper or lower motor neuron lesion causing muscle weakness or paralysis and eventually muscle disuse. Vascular occlusion or insufficiency of an extremity may result in diffuse ischemia of the skeletal muscle leading to muscle death and necrosis. Both of these types of indirect injury, depending on the severity, reduce the capacity for skeletal muscle to regenerate and repair itself (2).

Warming up before muscular exercise increases flexibility and thus decreases the potential for muscular injury.

Magnetic resonance (MR) imaging is now considered the primary imaging modality for detecting muscle injury and for determining the type of injury and the degree of muscle involvement (8). This technique has been found to be highly sensitive in detecting muscle edema, hemorrhage, denervation, and ossification (9) and therefore can be an invaluable tool in the evaluation of muscle injury of any cause.

MUSCULAR CONTUSIONS

Usually, contusions result from a blunt injury to soft tissues or muscle and, depending on the severity of the external force, damage and partial disruption of muscle fibers can occur (10). Frequently, capillary rupture and an infiltrative type of bleeding with intramuscular hematoma formation are observed (11). The visible ecchymosis is usually followed internally by edema and an intense inflammatory reaction resulting in local superficial and deep swelling. Local prostaglandin production stimulates the phagocytic process to remove necrotic tissue. During this process there is connective tissue proliferation with a variable amount of scar formation. The speed of tissue repair is directly related to vascular ingrowth during the repair process.

Contusions can be classified as mild, moderate, and severe. A mild contusion usually results in near-normal joint range of motion or no alteration of gait and minimal tenderness. Moderate contusions are characterized by swollen tender muscles and usually affect joint range of motion to some degree and produce an antalgic gait. A severe contusion presents with a marked swelling and tenderness with less than 50% joint range of motion and a severe limp (10).

Treatment of these injuries consists of limiting the range of motion of the affected extremity to minimize further hemorrhage. This is accomplished through rest, elevation of the limb, ice, and compression (12). This treatment is followed by restoration of active assisted range-of-motion exercises and may be augmented with heat, ultrasound, and whirlpool therapy. Reinjury during rehabilitation is a significant factor in prolonging disability and increasing the severity of the contusion. However, prolonged immobilization may lead to longer periods of disability, so a common ground has to be found in treating these injuries.

MUSCULAR HEMATOMAS

Intramuscular hemorrhage can result not only from direct blunt trauma but also from penetrating wounds, rupture of blood vessels, or coagulation defects. Muscle fibers are damaged by pressure from the hematoma and from the accompanying inflammatory reaction (11). The collection of blood within a relatively close space is usually painful, leading to reduced muscle strength as a result of pain. The presence of fluctuance is pathognomonic but may be difficult to detect deep in a large muscle mass.

Treatment consists of evacuation of the hematoma and protection of the muscle mass while healing takes place. Prevention of further bleeding is also important if this occurs as a result of coagulation defect.

MYOSITIS OSSIFICANS

Severe traumatic injury to muscle in association with considerable hemorrhage may result in deposition of fibrous tissue and ectopic bone formation within the muscular origin on the bone. In some, the development of myositis ossificans can occur after a muscle strain or tear or a mild contusion (10,11). The etiology of this condition is unknown, but it is theorized that ectopic muscular calcification or actual ossification is secondary to ossification of a muscular hematoma (13). A calcified lesion of myositis ossificans can be associated with significant pain and restricted motion that may preclude continued athletic activity. Although this condition can occur in any muscle, it is seen most commonly in the quadriceps and brachialis (14).

MR or computed tomographic (CT) imaging may be useful in the early detection and management of this condition. Ossification or calcification may not become apparent until 3 to 5 weeks after the muscle injury. Radiographic differential diagnosis of an expanding heterotopic bone mass includes osteogenic sarcoma.

Myositis ossificans can be prevented if the muscle injuries are managed properly. Once a muscle injury is diagnosed, the sporting activity should be discontinued and the injured muscle should not be stretched. Cryotherapy should be applied to the muscle area to reduce local swelling and hemorrhaging. Local whirlpool therapy may be initiated after the pain and swelling have abated, and care should be taken to avoid exercise drills until there is painless full range of motion (15,16). There is no place for operative treatment in the early stages of myositis ossificans. Surgical excision in the early phases of ossification is contraindicated, as increased morbidity and increased reossification are likely. Although heterotopic bone formation may result completely in time, it will usually shrink in size and form an exostosis on the normal bone. Surgical excision of mature symptomatic heterotopic bone is indicated after decreased activity is seen on MR scanning (17). In general, if an athlete who suffers from muscle contusion or strain does not regain significant passive motion of the joint associated with the injured muscle within 3 weeks, MR or CT imaging should be obtained to rule out myositis ossificans.

EXERTIONAL RHABDOMYOLYSIS AND MYOGLOBINURIA

Any disease or trauma that results in rapid destruction of a large mass of skeletal muscle can precipitate rhabdomyolysis (18). In exertional rhabdomyolysis, the injury or insult to the skeletal muscle is secondary to excessive muscular contractions. The severe trauma or excessive exercise results in rapid alterations of the integrity of the cell membrane, which allows the escape of cellular contents including enzymes and myoglobin into the extracellular fluid, resulting in myoglobinuria (19). This condition may be quite severe and lead to renal failure and death in some individuals.

Other causes of rhabdomyolysis include severe ischemia and necrosis of muscle, toxins, drugs, metabolic abnormalities, primary muscle diseases, hereditary or familial muscle diseases, and polymyositis (Table 1).

The usual clinical presentation in athletes with exertional rhabdomyolysis includes exertional effort followed by diffuse myalgias, decreased range of motion, a profound weakness, and the passage of dark, reddish urine (20). In some cases there may be elevated compartment pressures. Laboratory abnormalities include increased levels of creatine phosphokinase, lactate dehydrogenase, blood urea nitrogen, creatinine, and myoglobin.

Complications of rhabdomyolysis include anuric acute renal failure, which is secondary to mechanical obstruction of precipitated myoglobin, and compartment syndromes. In those with acute renal failure, hemodialysis may be necessary in conjunction with alkalinization of the urine to prevent deposition of the myoglobin casts in the kidney (21). Patients with com-

TABLE 1. *Causes of myoglobinuria*

Trauma or ischemic muscle injuries
Muscle overactivity or overtraining (i.e., in marathon runners, heat exhaustion syndrome with cramps)
Water and electrolyte depletion or imbalance
Infections (viral or bacterial with or without fever)
Drugs (clofibrate, barbiturates)
Toxins (snake venom, alcohol)
Disorders of muscle energy metabolism
Glycogen/glucose: myophosphorylase deficiency (McArdle's disease), phosphoglycerate kinase deficiency, phosphoglycerate mutase deficiency
Lipids: carnitine palmityltransferase deficiency, carnitine deficiency
Idiopathic rhabdomyolysis

partment syndromes are treated with appropriate fasciotomies.

METABOLIC MYOPATHIES

These myopathies are disorders of muscle energy production that result in skeletal muscle dysfunction, pain, weakness, cramping, and myoglobinuria. Cardiac and systemic metabolic dysfunction may coexist. The symptoms are often intermittent and provoked by exertion or changes in supply of lipid and carbohydrate fuels.

Type II carnitine palmitoyltransferase deficiency is the most common cause of exercise-induced rhabdomyolysis, myoglobinuria, and proximal muscle weakness and pain in young adults or athletes (22). Carnitine palmitoyltransferase deficiency is unusual but not rare and is often detected by finding elevated creatine phosphokinase (CPK) levels in a routine blood chemistry profile. A lack of this enzyme impairs mitochondrial oxidation of long-chain fatty acids, leading to myoglobinuria and possible renal failure.

Myophosphorylase deficiency (McArdle's disease) is the next most frequent cause of similar symptoms. The patient who has a defect of this enzyme is unable to utilize glycogen as a source of energy, resulting in predictable difficulties during heavy or intensive short-term exercise (23,24). This illness is inherited as an autosomal recessive or rarely as an autosomal dominant, is more common in males than females, and usually begins before the age of 10. Children with the illness complain of fatigue and inability to keep up with their peers. As children progress into adolescence and become more active physically, they develop aching or cramping in their legs, which may be provoked by nothing more than the mildest of exertion. Every bout of exercise is accompanied by painful muscle cramps, which may last for several hours, even overnight. In some cases the patient may pass dark brown urine because of the attendant myoglobinuria. As the years progress with repeated bouts of muscle pain and cramping, a permanent weakness in the proximal distribution may develop.

The ischemic forearm exercise test was one of the first tests to be designed with the specific aim of testing for myophosphorylase deficiency. The absence of this enzyme leads to a predictable absence of lactate in the venous circulation from exercising muscle. The forearm is used because it is convenient to obtain blood from the antecubital vein and the exercise of repetitive gripping utilizes all the muscles in the forearm (25).

MUSCLE WEAKNESS

It is important to assess muscle weakness from several angles. Is it organic or functional? Often the physician finds it difficult to determine a cause of a patient's weakness on the basis of the history alone. A vague description of generalized weakness should raise suspicion about its authenticity. These patients may have "neurasthenia" related to psychological or neurotic conditions. On the other hand, difficulty in climbing stairs, squatting, or unscrewing bottle tops is usually indicative of a genuine muscle disorder. In examining patients with muscle weakness it is important to determine the anatomic distribution of the weakness, for example, whether it is proximal or distal and also whether there is associated cranial nerve involvement.

Selective proximal weakness is usually characteristic of neuromuscular disease. Neurogenic disorders (anterior horn cell disease or peripheral neuropathies) should be suspected if there is a history or finding on examination of distal focal muscle atrophy, fasciculations, dysautonomia, or concomitant sensory dysfunction (Table 2).

Selective distal muscle weakness is manifested by difficulty in buttoning shirts or turning door knobs or keys, stumbling over small objects, or twisting an ankle. In most instances this pattern of weakness indicates a neurogenic disease. Several primary muscle disorders, for example, myotonic dystrophy or atrophy, distal myopathies of the dystrophic type, congenital hypotonias, adult-onset (rod body) nemaline myopathy, inclusion body myositis, and the scapuloperoneal type of fascioscapulohumeral dystrophy, present with or characteristically show predominant distal weakness.

The time course of development of muscle weakness is also important. Weakness evolving over a short period of time may be the presentation

TABLE 2. *Causes of muscle weakness*

Anterior horn cell disease
  Spinal muscle atrophy
  Polio
Neuropathies
  Landry-Guillain-Barré syndrome
  Diabetic amyotrophy
  Lumbosacral or brachial plexopathies
  Paraneoplastic neuropathies
  Porphyria
  Drugs and toxins[a]
Junctional disorders
  Myasthenia gravis[a]
  Eaton-Lambert syndrome
Myopathic diseases
  Polymyositis
  Limb-girdle dystrophy
  Endocrine myopathy
  Disorders of lipid metabolism
  Ethanol abuse
  Steroid toxicity
  Sarcoid disease[a]
  Acid maltase deficiency

[a] Cranial nerve involvement may be present.

of a number of neuromuscular disorders, for example, myasthenia gravis, botulism, tick paralysis, Guillain-Barré syndrome, periodic paralysis, carnitine deficiency, and alcoholic myopathy. Most of these disorders begin with symmetrical proximal weakness and can usually be distinguished and differentiated on the basis of associated clinical manifestations and laboratory abnormalities. Diseases of the spinal cord, particularly in the cervical or thoracic region as a result of compression or intrinsic disease, may also present acutely with painless symmetrical weakness. This type of weakness in conjunction with sphincter incontinence, increased tendon reflexes, clonus, or Babinski signs with or without sensory dysfunction should alert you to a spinal cord lesion.

Athletes who experience exercise-induced muscle weakness and/or fatigue may have a neuromuscular junction disorder. Those who complain of muscle weakness that comes on later in the day or after exercise with or without extraocular muscle dysfunction are most likely to have myasthenia gravis. Weakness that is greatest on arising in the morning and improves with minimal exercise is usually a manifestation of a neuromuscular junction disorder called the Lambert-Eaton syndrome (myasthenic syndrome sometimes associated with bronchogenic carcinoma).

MUSCLE CRAMPS

Muscle cramps are not uncommon in normal people and perhaps are the most common of the neuromuscular complaints of an athlete. Nearly every athlete has them at one time or another. For the most part they are of a benign nature. Muscle cramping represents a sudden powerful involuntary contraction of muscle associated with painful shortening of the muscle and attended by visible knotting of the affected muscle. Sometimes this leads to abnormal posturing of an affected joint. Other common causes of muscle cramps are vascular changes related to tight shoes or stockings and unaccustomed muscle strain. Temperature changes may also play a part. Cramps commonly occur during the night when the feet are cold. A thorough warm-up and stretching exercises before competition are effective preventive measures. In fact, warming up before muscular exercise has been shown to increase flexibility and decrease muscular injury and cramping. Relief of tight clothing, massage and stretching, or even rest of the muscle may help during the cramped phase. Other causes of muscle cramps are covered below.

HEAT ILLNESS

Heat illness occurs in three stages: heat cramps, heat exhaustion, and heatstroke (26). Most muscle cramps in athletes follow dehydration in very hot, humid weather. Electrolyte depletion may be an associated factor. Athletes who exercise and sweat on a regular basis can sweat up to 2 liters per hour and the sweat has a very low electrolyte content. In contrast, the unacclimated athlete can sweat up to 0.8 liter per hour and the sweat is very high in sodium chloride. Athletes are more likely to have muscle cramps during the first 2 weeks of athletic activity or competition. As they become more acclimated, the cramping occurs less frequently.

Most muscle cramps occur in the calf and hamstring groups of muscles. Usually the first step is to stretch or rub the affected muscle until the cramp resolves. Rehydration is the next step; water is usually the best replacement fluid during athletic competition. Sports drinks, such as Gatorade, may be helpful early in the training period when electrolyte losses are greater. In addition, these drinks are beneficial in long endurance events, especially when they are held in hot, humid weather. Most athletes, especially long-distance runners, dilute these drinks to improve gastric emptying and absorption.

If heat cramps progress to heat exhaustion, the athlete will experience flulike symptoms and fatigue. The body core temperature may rise to 39.5°C, and the skin becomes moist in this phase because the sweat mechanism is still functional. Treatment in this case should include cooling with compresses, moving the athlete into a shaded area, and rehydrating him or her with oral fluids. Intervenous fluid and salt supplementation may be considered if appropriate facilities are available. Sometimes symptomatic relief of a cramp is accomplished only with medication, for example, intravenous or oral diazepam or quinine sulfate.

Heatstroke is dangerous and usually occurs when the body core temperature exceeds 40°C. In this state the athlete becomes confused and agitated and the skin becomes dry as the sweat mechanism ceases to function. Patients with heatstroke should be hospitalized for observation and intravenous fluid therapy.

In the pathologic sense, spontaneous or exercise-induced cramps may be symptoms of motor neuron disorders (spinal muscular atrophy, amyotrophic lateral sclerosis, and familial peripheral neuropathies) and may also occur in hypothyroidism or disorders of muscle energy metabolism such as glycogen and lipid disorders of muscle as described before. Cramps may also be a manifestation of malignant hyperthermia during the acute phase of this disorder. Clinical examination and on occasion electromyography are important in differentiating pathologic from benign muscle cramps.

MYALGIAS AND SORENESS

In most cases these are nonspecific symptoms of muscle strain or overuse. However, these symptoms even without associated muscle weakness may indicate some pathologic disorder. Myalgias in conjunction with soreness and tender muscles may represent a form of inflammatory or toxic-

induced myopathy, for example, polymyositis or alcohol-induced myopathy, respectively. These symptoms may also be indicative of electrolyte disorder, for example, potassium deficiency secondary to drug use or intestinal disease with diarrhea. Several acute neuropathies or denervating disorders may present with significant myalgias and soreness. For example, painful or sore muscles, particularly in the shoulder girdle or arms, followed after short intervals by proximal or diffuse weakness should alert you to the condition of acute brachial plexopathy.

Diabetic amyotrophy may produce a similar painful syndrome, but this disorder usually affects one or both proximal lower extremities, particularly the quadriceps group. Electromyographic studies are extremely useful for differentiating all of these conditions.

EOSINOPHILIC FASCITIS AND MYOSITIS

This condition was described in the mid-1970s (27) and since then there have been reports of over 100 patients with this entity (28,29). In most of these cases the onset of the disease follows unaccustomed physical exertion. It is considered a disease of adults, although it has also been reported in children. The upper extremities are the commonest site of affliction but the thighs and legs may also be involved, and the condition is usually symmetrical. On examination the skin may be dimpled and taut and appear to be bound down to underlying muscle, giving the appearance of an orange peel.

An elevated sedimentation rate and hypergammaglobulinemia have been reported in a high proportion of patients. A skin and muscle biopsy may show eosinophilic infiltrates. On some occasions eosinophils may be missing from the inflammatory response in the fascia. They are, however, noted in over 90% of patients when the peripheral blood smear is evaluated.

In 1977 Layser et al. (30) reviewed the problem of eosinophilic polymyositis. Each case is presented with an inflammatory myopathy as part of a systemic hypereosinophilic syndrome which had associated cardiac and pulmonary involvement, skin changes (fasciitis), peripheral neuropathy, and encephalopathy. The myositis component was manifested by a localized tender swelling in either calf or thigh muscle. This condition needs to be distinguished from trichinosis and from other parasitic infections of skeletal muscle. Its relationship to eosinophilic fasciitis is uncertain, although the two conditions are probably closely related. Most of these cases respond to treatment with steroids.

MUSCLE STIFFNESS AND/OR RIGIDITY

Muscle stiffness and/or rigidity in association with decreased limb mobility is usually indicative of a central nervous system disorder, for example, pyramidal or extraparamidal neuronal dysfunction or frontal lobe apraxia. These individuals should be examined for signs of spasticity and/or muscular rigidity resulting from basal ganglia disease. Muscle stiffness may also be a manifestation of myotonic muscle disorders or hypothyroid myopathy. Muscle stiffness in association with boardlike muscles, particularly the axial muscles, should lead one to suspect the diagnosis of stiff-man syndrome, an illness first described by Moersch and Woltman (31).

Muscle stiffness in association with muscle cramps and contractures may be seen in a rare disorder called the syndrome of continuous muscle fiber activity (neuromyotonia or Isaacs syndrome) (32). This condition is characterized by limb stiffness, muscle twitching (myokymia), hyperhidrosis, focal muscular hypertrophy, and distal muscle contractures. Myokymia reflects the constant rippling activity seen in the skin overlying affected muscles. These movements may be disturbing because the patient is always aware of them and may be kept awake at night. There may be difficulty in relaxing the muscle after a voluntary contraction. Stiffness is severe and may impede movement. The disease occurs sporadically and at any age. The abnormal tone in myokymia does not disappear during sleep. The movements are not altered during spinal block, during pentothal anesthesia, or by proximal nerve blocks, indicating that the defect is in the distal part of the motor unit. A motor point infiltration of muscle with xylocaine reduces the activity although it does not abolish it completely. Curarization abolishes the spontaneous activity (33).

Treatment of this disorder is with diphenyl-hydantoin (Dilantin), which has been successful in abolishing most of the symptoms. Carbamazepine (Tegretol) and dantrolene sodium (Dantrium) have been reported to be of some benefit.

Lastly, there is a congenital disorder in which chondrodystrophy and epiphyseal dysplasia are superposed on an abnormality of continuous muscle fiber activity that resembles myotonia. This condition is called the Schwartz-Jampel syndrome (chondrodystrophic myotonia) (34). Children with this disorder are short statured and have short necks, facial dysmorphism with micrognathia, narrowed palpebral fissures, low-set ears, dental abnormalities, and intellectual impairment. Their muscles are often enlarged and firm and have myotonia-like contractions causing dimpling of the chin and blepharospasm. Contractures of joints may be present. Careful electromyography usually differentiates the spontaneous activity from true myotonia (35). No specific treatment has proved useful.

REFERENCES

1. Lahto M, Jarvinen M, Nelimarkka O. Scar formation after skeletal muscle injury. *Arch Orthop Trauma Surg* 1986;104:366–370.
2. Garrett WE, Best TM. Anatomy, physiology and mechanics of skeletal muscle. In: Simon SR, ed. *AAOS orthopaedic basic science.* Chicago: AAOS Press, 1994: 89–125.
3. Armstrong RB. Initial events in exercise-induced muscular injury. *Med Sci Sports Exerc* 1990;22:429–434.
4. Friden JP, Sfakianos PN, Hargens AR. Muscle soreness and intramuscular fluid pressure: comparison between excetric and concentric loads. *J Appl Physiol* 1986; 61:2175–2179.
5. Friden JP, Sfakianos PN, Hargens AR, Akeson WH. Residual muscular swelling after repetive excentric contractions. *J Orthop Res* 1988;6:493–498.
6. Armstrong RB. Mechanisms of exercise-induced delayed onset muscle soreness: a brief review. *Med Sci Sport Exerc* 1984;16:529–538.
7. Mense S, Schmidt RF. Activation of group IV afferent units from muscle by algesic agents. *Brain Res* 1974; 72:305–310.
8. Steinbach LS, Fleckenstein JL, Mink JH. Magnetic resonance imaging of muscle injuries. *Orthopaedics* 1994; 17:1991–1999.
9. Kransdorf MJ, Meis JM, Jelinek JS. Myositis ossificans: MR appearance with radiographic–pathologic correlation. *Am J Radiol* 1991;157:1243–1248.

10. Jackson DW, Feagin JA. Quadripceps contusions in young athletes. *J Bone Joint Surg Am* 1973;55-A:95–105.

11. Rothwell AG. Quadriceps hematoma: a prospective clinical study. *Clin Orthop* 1982;171:97–103.

12. McMaster WC. A literary review of ice therapy in injuries. *Am J Sports Med* 1977;5:124–126.

13. Hait G, Boswick JA, Stone JJ. Heterotopic bone formation secondary to trauma (myositis ossificans traumatica). *J Trauma* 1970;10:405–411.

14. Huss CD, Puehl JJ. Myositis ossificans of the upper arm. *Am J Sports Med* 1980;8:419–424.

15. Moxley RT. Muscle and muscle-like complaints associated with sports: potential outpatient problems for the neurologist. *Semin Neurol* 1981;1:324–333.

16. Danchik JJ, Yochum TR, Aspegren DD. Myositis ossificans traumatica. *J Manip Physiol Ther* 1993;9:605–614.

17. Lipscomb AB, Thomas ED, Johnston RK. Treatment of myositis ossificans traumatica in athletes. *Am J Sports Med* 1976;4:111–120.

18. Gabow P, Keaney W, Kelleager S. The spectrum of rhabdomyolisis. *Medicine (Baltimore)* 1982;61:142–152.

19. Rowland LP, Penn AS. Myoglobinuria. *Med Clin North Am* 1972;56:1233–1261.

20. Ritter WS, Stone MJ, Willerson JT. Reduction in exertional myoglobinuria after physical conditioning. *Arch Intern Med* 1979;139:644–647.

21. Ralph D. Rhabdomyolisis and acute renal failure. *J Am Coll Emerg Phys* 1978;7:103–106.

22. Faigel HC. Carnitine palmityl transferase deficiency in the college athlete: a case report and literature review. *J Am Coll Health* 1995;44(2):51–54.

23. McArdle B. Myopathy due to a defect in muscle glycogen breakdown. *Clin Sci* 1951;10:13–33.

24. Engel WK, Eyerman EL, Williams HE. Late onset type of skeletal muscle phosphorylase deficiency. *N Engl J Med* 1963;268:135–141.

25. Munsat TL. A standardized forearm eschemic exercise test. *Neurology* 1970;20:1171–1178.

26. Murphy RJ. Heat illness in the athlete. *Am J Sports Med* 1984;12(4):258–261.

27. Shulman LE. Diffuse fascitis eosinophilia: a new syndrome. *Arthritis Rheum Suppl* 1976;19:205–217.

28. Moore TL, Zucker J. Eosinophilic fascitis. *Semin Arthritis Rheum* 1980;9:228–235.

29. Michet CJ, Doyle JA, Ginsburg WW. Eosinophilic fascitis. *Mayo Clin Proc* 1981;56:27–34.

30. Layser RB, Shearn MA, Satya-Murti S. Eosinophilic polymyositis. *Ann Neurol* 1977;1:65–70.

31. Moersch FP, Woltman HW. Progessive fluctuating muscular rigidity and spasm (stiff man syndrome). *Proc Staff Meet Mayo Clin* 1956;31:421–427.

32. Issacs H. A syndrome of continuous muscle fiber activity. *J Neurol Neurosurg Psychiatry* 1961;24:319–325.

33. Wallis WE, Van Poznak A, Plum F. Generalized muscular stiffness: fasciculations in myokymia of peripheral nerve origin. *Ach Neurol* 1970;22:430–439.

34. Edwards WC, Root AW. Chondrodystrophic myotonia (Schwartz-Jampel syndrome): report of a new case and follow-up with patients initially reported in 1969. *Am J Med Genet* 1982;13:51–56.

35. Jableki C, Schult P. Single muscle fiber recordings in Schwartz-Jampel syndrome. *Muscle Nerve* 1982;5:S64–69.

Sports Neurology, Second Edition,
edited by Barry D. Jordan.
Lippincott–Raven Publishers, Philadelphia © 1998.

21

Thermal Injuries in Sports: Neurologic Aspects

Ludwig Gutmann

*Department of Neurology, Robert C. Byrd Health Sciences Center, West Virginia University,
Morgantown, West Virginia 26505-9180*

The human body requires that its temperature be maintained within a fairly narrow range. Both hyperthermia and hypothermia lead to serious dysfunction of various human bodily functions and, if untreated, ultimately lead to death.

Despite the rather narrow window of acceptable physiologic core (rectal) temperatures, it is not unusual for athletic and recreational endeavors to be carried out in temperatures between 0° and 100°F (−17.8° and 37.8°C). The effect of the ambient temperature is further influenced by rain, wind, and sunshine; whether these have a moderating or exacerbating effect depends on the temperature at that moment. For example, bright sunshine exacerbates the effect of heat, and cloud cover and rain have a moderating effect. As the environment deviates from relatively ideal ambient temperatures, it becomes increasingly difficult for the body to maintain an acceptable core temperature. Physiologic mechanisms involved in temperature maintenance include heat production, acquisition, conservation, and dissipation.

TEMPERATURE REGULATION AND EXERCISE

Physical activity requires the increased utilization of energy-producing substances. The amount required is dependent on the level of exertion. This can be illustrated by the example of a 70-kg person jogging a distance of 1 mile, which requires approximately 100 cal irrespective of the speed (1). The faster one runs the mile, however, the more quickly the 100 cal are utilized. This translates into the expenditure of 400 cal/h for a slow jogger and 1200 cal/h for a well-trained runner during a marathon. A heavier individual utilizes more calories for each mile, and a lighter individual utilizes fewer.

The heat generated during the utilization of calories increases core temperature. The rostral hypothalamus is exposed to heated blood and initiates heat dissipation by dilation of skin blood vessels and sweating. Mean core temperature in the normal steady state is 37°C (98.6°F), and skin temperature is approximately 33°C (91.4°F). The closer the ambient temperature of the outside environment is to the skin temperature, the less effective are the heat loss mechanisms of radiation, convection, and conduction and the more the body relies on sweating for heat dissipation (2).

During physical exertion the body establishes a new temperature steady state, usually in the range of 39° to 41°C (102.2° to 105.8°F) (3). An exception is when a sports event is carried out in a sufficiently cold environment and when the athlete is wearing light clothing, allowing a fall in core temperature. The actual new steady state during the sports event depends on the ambient temperature, the body's ability to dissipate or conserve generated heat, the degree of physical exertion, and the acclimatization of the athlete. The process is illustrated in Fig. 1. In this case, an athlete ran 8 miles in a comfortable fashion during a 65-minute period on a warm midsummer day.

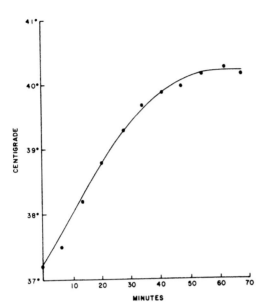

FIG. 1. Core temperature changes during an uneventful 8-mile run.

Both training and heat acclimatization of the individual exercising in a hot environment improve cardiovascular function and the efficient dissipation of heat. Training results in an increased maximal cardiac output, a decrease in resting and peak heart rates, and an increase in stroke volume. This facilitates the delivery of heated blood to the body surface, where heat can be dissipated. The enhanced utilization of carbohydrates and oxygen occurs in response to training, and there is an associated increase in skeletal muscle vascular supply. The increased oxidative capacity of human muscle with training is manifested by an increase in the activity of oxidative enzymes associated with an increase in the protein content of the mitochondrial fraction as well

There was no fluid intake, and no adverse symptoms were experienced. The new steady state of 40.2°C (104.4°F) was reached in approximately 45 minutes. The core temperatures at the completion of several additional training runs of 65 minutes on subsequent similar afternoons (Fig. 2) reached a range of 39.4° to 40.2°C (103° to 104.4°F). A weight loss of 2.5 to 5.0 pounds (mean, 3.2 pounds) occurred during these 65-minute periods and therefore involved a loss of 1.25 to 2.5 quarts of fluid as a result of sweating to maintain the new steady state and to prevent further temperature increases that might have serious sequelae.

A number of physiologic events occur during physical exertion in a warm environment that result in a decreased plasma volume. These include sweating, intracellular movement of water, and shunting of blood flow into exercising muscles and dilated skin vessels. The concomitant decrease in splanchnic blood flow is insufficient to compensate for these losses (4). The net result is a decrease of venous return to the heart, an increased heart rate, a decreased stroke volume, and ultimately a decrease in cardiac output (5).

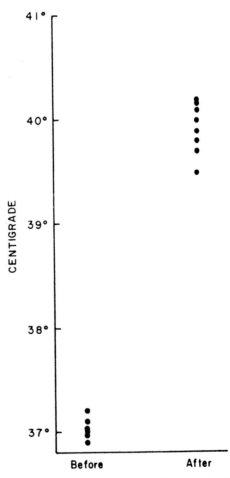

FIG. 2. Core temperatures before and after several 8-mile training runs.

as morphologic evidence of increased mitochondrial volume (6).

Endurance exercise is a powerful stimulus for capillary proliferation in human skeletal muscle. Various studies have revealed higher capillary densities in the skeletal muscles of trained individuals compared with untrained individuals. The study by Andersen and Henriksson (7) revealed a 50% increase in the number of capillaries per fiber in the vastus lateralis muscle after 2 months of training. This proliferation of the skeletal muscle vascular supply further facilitates the delivery of nutrients and oxygen to muscle as well as the removal of the generated heat.

Heat acclimatization produces a significant change in the amount and quality of sweat, resulting in a smaller increase in core temperature with a given quantity of physical exertion. In the heat-acclimatized individual, sweating and vasodilation begin at a lower body temperature, sweating is increased in amount, and the sodium concentration of sweat is diminished (3,8,9).

Certain medications and illnesses may have an adverse effect on temperature regulation. Drugs with a cholinergic effect (e.g., trihexyphenidyl hydrochloride, atropine, and amitriptyline) impair sweat production. Amphetamine usage by athletes may result in physical overactivity resulting from an exaggerated sense of well-being. In a hot environment this may lead to hyperthermia (4,10). Antihistamines and phenothiazines alter body temperature control by impairing sweating mechanisms and may also lead to hyperthermia (11). Parkinson's disease is an example of a chronic illness that places the patient at risk for heat exhaustion and heat stroke when he or she is exposed to a hot environment. This is related to the increased motor activity, altered autonomic nervous system function, and impaired sweat production that are due in part to the use of anticholinergic drugs in the treatment of Parkinson's disease (12).

HYPERTHERMIA

Hyperthermia may result in heat exhaustion and heat stroke.

Heat Exhaustion

Heat exhaustion is the most common clinical syndrome complicating physical exertion in warm or hot weather. Both the degree of environmental heat and the intensity of the physical activity play an important role. Intense physical exertion in moderately warm weather may be as dangerous in this regard as moderate exertion in hot weather. Heavy sweating resulting in dehydration, excessive hyperthermia, and failing cardiovascular functions causes the clinical symptoms of heat exhaustion. Rapid recognition and treatment of heat exhaustion are necessary to avoid progression to the much more serious and devastating entity of heatstroke.

Two forms of heat exhaustion have been described (4). One is related primarily to water depletion and the other to salt depletion. Although both phenomena may be expected to play some role in most patients, water depletion plays the most important role in athletes. Here heat exhaustion usually arises after a relatively short period of intense physical exertion. Examples include several hours of football practice, cycling, or even shorter periods of running.

Heat exhaustion may be expected to occur when the core temperature approaches or exceeds 41°C (105.8°F). Factors such as inadequate fluid intake and subsequent dehydration and lack of training and heat acclimatization increase the likelihood of heat exhaustion (4,13). Serum electrolyte levels during marathons and other long runs show a rise, rather than a fall, in serum potassium of 6% to 15% in most individuals. This probably reflects an efflux of potassium ion from intracellular stores and the lower ion concentration of sweat compared with that of serum. A mild increase in serum sodium usually also occurs, partly for the same reason (14). Prolonged physical exertion in a hot environment may ultimately result in hyponatremia, however, especially if liberal amounts of free water are being consumed. This was well illustrated by the occurrence of a hyponatremic encephalopathy in ultramarathon runners after completing 80 and 100 km in the 1983 American Medical Joggers Association Ultra-Marathon Race in Chicago. The hyponatremia in these cases was caused primarily by increased intake and retention of dilute fluids in conjunction with excessive sodium loss through sweat (15). This syndrome of heat exhaustion produced primarily by water depletion may occur in well-trained and acclimatized athletes performing at maximal intensity, often under intense competition.

Signs and symptoms of heat exhaustion from water depletion include hypotension, nausea, tachycardia (often 180 beats/min or greater), irritability, disorientation, anxiety, and confusion. Hyperventilation syndrome, hysteria, and psychotic behavior may occur. Anhidrosis is often present, but sweating may still occur with heat exhaustion, especially in the well-trained acclimatized athlete. Despite the occurrence of mild mental symptoms in heat exhaustion the patient remains conscious, which distinguishes this syndrome from the more serious heatstroke (16).

The heat exhaustion that is due predominantly to salt depletion usually occurs in periods of prolonged heat exposure during which large volumes of sweat are replaced with adequate amounts of water but inadequate electrolytes. Intracellular water is usually increased, whereas interstitial fluid is decreased. Symptoms consist of weakness, fatigue, lightheadedness, anorexia, nausea, vomiting, diarrhea, and muscle cramps; the last of these is similar to the syndrome of muscle cramps (discussed later). Hypotension and tachycardia often occur, and body temperature may not be elevated.

Heatstroke

Heatstroke is a catastrophic event with a mortality rate that may exceed 50% (17). It is the outcome of uncontrolled hyperthermia, decreased plasma volume, electrolyte abnormalities, and cardiac decompensation. High temperatures in the presence of failing metabolic machinery result in damage to a number of organs. It is characterized by hyperpyrexia with rectal temperatures higher than 41°C (105.8°F) and sometimes as high as 45°C (113°F). This is combined with delirium, coma, and often anhidrosis.

Heatstroke is a much less common event than heat exhaustion. A number of factors increase the likelihood of heatstroke. These include cardiovascular disease and such chronic illnesses as diabetes mellitus, malnutrition, alcoholism, and cystic fibrosis (4,13). These conditions are usually not present in young athletes but may be present in older sports participants.

Heatstroke in the athlete may occur after a few hours of intense activity in a hot environment. It may occur in healthy, highly acclimatized, trained athletes when they become unable to dissipate endogenously produced heat effectively. In the past, heatstroke in athletes occurred primarily in unacclimatized football players and military recruits. In recent years, however, it has increasingly occurred among runners (especially novice runners) and cyclists during hot-weather races (18). Heatstroke is nevertheless uncommon among athletes. This is related, in part, to the appropriate physiologic adaptations in trained and heat-acclimatized athletes, the scant clothing worn especially by runners, protective measures encouraged by coaches and race directors (e.g., fluid replacement), and the steady pace of the runner, which allows efficient aerobic metabolism. In contrast, Hanson and Zimmerman (18) described four runners who collapsed with hyperthermia after increasing their pace at the conclusion of a race. Symptoms of their heat illness occurred within 5 to 10 minutes of the onset of increased effort. The additional energy demand may have required anaerobic metabolism. It is probable that the homeostatic mechanisms of these four runners were overwhelmed by the additional heat production coinciding with inevitable dehydration.

Pathologically, heatstroke is associated with widespread hemorrhagic necrosis involving the muscles, myocardium, liver, kidneys, and brain (4,19). Thrombocytopenia, endothelial damage, and disseminated intravascular coagulation play important roles in the development of hemorrhages. Myocardial damage occurs commonly with subendocardial hemorrhages, scattered myocardial necrosis, and frank myocardial infarction (often in the absence of coronary artery occlusion). These contribute to the signs of cardiac failure and hypotension that are so commonly seen. Kidney damage is common, and clinical manifestation ranges from mild proteinuria to acute renal failure, the latter occurring in 25% of cases of heatstroke among athletes. In most patients who survive, the renal abnormalities are reversible (4).

Damage to the central nervous system occurs in all fatal cases. The expected changes in the brain are edema, diffuse petechial hemorrhages, pyknotic nuclei, chromatolytic changes, and swollen dendrites (19). The most striking changes are in the cerebellum, but changes may occur in the cerebral cortex, striatum, thalamus, and sometimes the hypothalamus. In the cerebellum there is marked loss of Purkinje cells, and damage to skeletal muscle and liver is a frequent concomitant. Liver damage is reflected by myoglobinuria and significant elevation of prothrombin time and liver and muscle enzymes (4,13).

The most important neurologic manifestations include delirium and coma, which occur in virtually all cases. Focal or generalized seizures occur in 60% of patients. Cerebellar symptoms may occur and include limb ataxia and dysarthria. Decorticate posturing, hemiparesis, diminished stretch reflexes, and fecal incontinence are expected findings. Extensor plantar signs are present in most patients (20).

After aggressive therapy the patient may recover from heatstroke uneventfully, but sequelae are frequent (2). There may be intolerance to heat reflecting some permanent damage to heat-dissipating hypothalamic mechanisms, but permanent anhidrosis is unusual. Personality changes with emotional lability and irritability have been described. Permanent cerebellar symptoms occur and include incoordination, ataxia, dysmetria, and dysarthric speech. A residual motor neuron syndrome has been described (16,21).

The various changes in serum potassium levels that may occur in heatstroke and the implications of these changes deserve special attention (4,22). As noted earlier, mild hyperkalemia is often present immediately after strenuous exercise. Hypokalemia is at times the case early in acute heatstroke during hot-weather athletic endeavors, however. This is due to the intracellular movement of potassium associated with hyperventilation-induced respiratory alkalosis, which is a frequent accompaniment of acute heatstroke. Although there has been loss of potassium in urine and sweat, the hypokalemia in this circumstance does not have a serious prognosis. On the other hand, hypokalemia associated with a metabolic acidosis does reflect a significant deficiency of potassium. This is because the metabolic acidosis is expected to cause a mild hyperkalemia through a shift of potassium from intracellular to extracellular areas. In this case, the hypokalemia occurs after many days of training in hot weather and inadequate replacement of potassium. The hypokalemia associated with metabolic acidosis early in acute heatstroke increases the patient's susceptibility to rhabdomyolysis. Once cellular destruction has supervened, hyperkalemia occurs and may be of such severity as to result in fulminating potassium intoxication and death.

Treatment of Heat Exhaustion and Heatstroke

Prompt recognition and treatment of heat exhaustion is essential to avoid its evolution to heatstroke. The patient should be immediately moved to an air-conditioned or shaded environment. Removal of clothes allows optimal heat dissipation. Cooling the patient with cold water, fans, and ice massages and packs is useful. Rehydration with water in association with commercially available electrolyte solutions given orally is usually sufficient. Intravenous electrolyte solutions are at times needed. Treatment should always begin at the site of the athletic endeavor; if treatment is sufficiently prompt, the patient may not require transportation to a medical facility.

Prompt cooling and rehydration are even more crucial once heatstroke has occurred. The body temperature should be rapidly lowered with cooling blankets, ice packs, and cold water in an air-conditioned environment. Immersion of the patient in a tub of cold water is also effective, although this method is less comfortable and creates potential problems should the patient have a tonic-clonic seizure. The hypotension that occurs with heatstroke may respond to cooling alone once peripheral vasodilation subsides. The use of large quantities of saline or plasma expanders to treat the hypotension while the patient is still hyperthermic may result in acute pulmonary edema because of an overload of the circulation once cooling occurs. If hypotension persists after cooling, volume expansion with saline may be necessary. Vasopressive drugs must be used with great caution because intense peripheral vasoconstriction may reestablish hyperthermia. Should shivering occur before the patient reaches the desired physiologic temperature, small doses of chlorpromazine and diazepam may be given. Seizures may be controlled with intravenous diazepam. Lactic acidosis is treated with sodium bicarbonate. Potassium levels must be monitored carefully. As already noted, hypokalemia occurs early in acute heatstroke as a result of the intracellular movement of potassium associated with hyperventilation-induced respiratory alkalosis. If hypokalemia is present in association with a metabolic acidosis, however, potassium should be judiciously administered because this circumstance increases the patient's susceptibility to rhabdomyolysis. Hyperkalemia may result from rhabdomyolysis and renal failure. Serum creatine kinase; lactate dehydrogenase, and glutamic-oxaloacetic transaminase levels should be monitored because they are sensitive indicators of cellular damage. Disseminated intravascular coagulation and thrombocytopenia are treated with heparin anticoagulation. Acute renal failure must be treated appropriately and may require dialysis (2,4,13,17).

Heat-Related Syndromes

Heat cramps are brief, intermittent, painful cramps in skeletal muscle that has undergone sustained intense activity during hot weather (4). They are especially common in athletes whose physical condition and heat acclimatization are excellent. Heat cramps result from an acute deficiency of sodium incurred by sweating. Typically, they occur toward or at the end of physical activity. A number of factors predispose to heat cramps. The acclimatized individual produces large amounts of

sweat and, during intense physical activity, usually consumes adequate amounts of water to replace fluid loss. It is after the completion of the athletic event, when the plasma volume again expands, that the decreased total body sodium level develops into evident hyponatremia and the resulting heat cramps develop. A less dramatic form of the same syndrome is the fasciculations that may occur in the exercised muscles after exertion. Treatment involves the use of oral (and only rarely intravenous) saline solutions.

Myoglobinuria after excessive physical activity occurs most commonly in association with hyperthermia (4,10). It occurs in otherwise normal individuals without any underlying disorder of carbohydrate or lipid metabolism. The untrained individual is especially at risk. The condition has been reported in long-distance runners, military recruits, ice skaters, and skiers.

Rhabdomyolysis, resulting in myoglobinuria, may occur independent of heat stroke. The duration and intensity of exercise and the associated degree of ischemia are important determinants of the development of rhabdomyolysis. Rhabdomyolysis results in hyperkalemia, hyperphosphatemia, and hypocalemia. The hyperkalemia may be sufficiently severe to provoke serious cardiac dysrhythmias. Hypocalcemic tetany has also been reported.

As noted earlier, increased core temperatures further increase the risk of myoglobinuria, as does potassium depletion. Carbohydrate loading, a fashionable premarathon technique thought to improve performance, has been suggested as a further predisposing factor for myoglobinuria (23). Acute renal failure is a serious complication. High elevations of serum creatine kinase are expected with myoglobinuria (4,10).

Hyperthermia and Other Neurologic Disorders

Hyperthermia, whether the result of exogenous environmental heat or such heat combined with physical activity, may have a deleterious effect in the presence of other neurologic disorders. It is well recognized that neurologic symptoms of multiple sclerosis may worsen with even mild degrees of hyperthermia. Patients develop varying degrees of muscle weakness when pyramidal tract involvement is present. Other neurologic symptoms, including defects of visual acuity and visual scotoma, may become more prominent with hyperthermia; this is referred to as Uhthoff's sign. This is thought to be due to a decreased safety factor for nerve conduction in demyelinated nerves when their temperature is increased, which results in a conduction block in the demyelinated axons (24). Symptoms worsen when this condition occurs in a significant number of axons.

The following case report illustrates Uhthoff's sign in dramatic fashion. The patient, a 30-year-old engineer, was a dedicated athlete, having been involved in swimming, biking, and running for many years. He was captain of his college swim team, and his race times for 10 km were excellent (as fast as 34 minutes). In the spring of 1985 he noticed the development of a left foot drop about 6 miles into a training run. This prevented him from planting his left foot properly, causing him to trip. If he walked for 50 yards this symptom would improve, and he would be able to run for a short period of time before it occurred again. It was at this time that he also noted mild weakness in the left leg when spending any significant time in a jacuzzi. During the summer of 1986 he noted that much of the left leg would be weak once he had run 1.5 miles. This prompted him to give up running, and he concentrated on swimming and biking. Swimming was not a problem, and he could swim strenuously for as long as 3 hours without any neurologic symptoms. When biking 20 to 30 miles, however, he noted symptoms when dismounting, when he had mild difficulty with balance and left ankle clonus for a short period of time. All his neurologic symptoms were associated with profuse sweating. He experienced no neurologic symptoms at any other time.

Neurologic examination showed that the cranial nerves, gait, coordination, strength, and sensory examination were all normal. Deep tendon reflexes were slightly brisker in the left arm than in the right, and knee jerks were mildly hyperactive bilaterally. Unsustained clonus was present bilaterally in the ankles, and an extensor toe sign was present on the right.

Brainstem auditory evoked potential studies showed an absent wave 3 and an increase in the I-V interval on the left side. Visual evoked potentials were normal. A magnetic resonance scan showed multiple areas of increased signal intensity involving the white matter and basal ganglia of the brain bilaterally. A cerebrospinal fluid study showed an immunoglobulin G content of 21.5% and 10 oligoclonal bands.

The patient was presumed to have multiple sclerosis on the basis of all the clinical and laboratory data available. The most extraordinary feature of the case was that he was entirely asymptomatic except at times when he had a significant increase in his core temperature, which gave rise to Uhthoff's sign.

Increased weakness has also been documented in patients with myasthenia gravis in the presence of hyperthermia. Hyperthermia lowers the safety factor of neuromuscular transmission in patients with myasthenia gravis and results in increased extremity and bulbar weakness. This mechanism may be one of the factors producing myasthenic crisis in the presence of a febrile illness (25).

HYPOTHERMIA AND COLD-RELATED SYNDROMES

Hypothermia

Although many athletic endeavors are carried out in cold environments, hypothermia is a less common problem than hyperthermia. Nonetheless, it represents a serious potential risk in a number of athletic and recreational activities including hiking, camping, mountain climbing, ice fishing, skiing, long-distance swimming in cold water, and long runs in cool or cold weather. Old age and number of medical problems (including alcohol abuse, myxedema, hypoglycemia, sedative overdose, Addison's disease, head trauma, and pituitary insufficiency) may predispose an individual to hypothermia.

Hypothermia in otherwise healthy individuals develops when heat loss in a cool or cold environment exceeds the body's rate of heat production. This can be a particular problem among runners during marathons. A fall in ambient temperature or clothes wet from sweat or rain facilitate rapid heat loss. Hypothermia is more likely to occur in inexperienced marathon runners who frequently run the second half of the race much more slowly than the first half. These runners are able to maintain their core temperature initially, but with the slower pace on a cool, wet, or windy day they are at risk for hypothermia (16).

Early signs and symptoms of hypothermia include shivering, euphoria, mild disorientation, and slurred speech. Shivering ceases at body temperatures less than 29.4° to 32°C (85° to 90°F), and muscle stiffness supervenes. Varying degrees of lethargy are followed by unconsciousness when core temperature falls to less than 26.7°C (80°F). Pupils often respond sluggishly but may become fixed. The patient is usually cold and pale with slow, shallow respiration, bradycardia, and hypotension. Hemoconcentration, uremia, and metabolic acidosis may occur; the last is due in part to hypoxic peripheral tissues. Hypoglycemia or hyperglycemia may also occur. Various cardiac dysrhythmias may occur, including atrial or ventricular fibrillation. Eye movement abnormalities and extensor plantar responses do not occur with increasing frequency with progressively decreasing temperatures. Severe hypothermia is associated with marked depression in cerebral blood flow and oxygen requirement, reduced cardiac output, and decreased arterial pressure. Patients may appear to be clinically dead as a result of the marked depression of brain function. Peripheral pulses may be difficult to detect because of bradycardia and vasoconstriction (26–29).

The diagnosis of hypothermia can be missed. Its signs and symptoms may be misleading. Standard thermometers read only as low as 34.4°C (94°F); glass thermometers that read as low as 23.8°C (75°F) must be used in this circumstance (28). Knowing that the patient has been using drugs or detecting the smell of alcohol may further mislead the physician into not considering hypothermia.

Excessive amounts of alcohol may play a major contributing role in the development of hypothermia. Its peripheral vasodilating effect produces a feeling of warmth but leads to further heat loss. Despite conventional folk wisdom, alcohol is not useful in the treatment of hypothermia and should be avoided.

Mild hypothermia can easily be treated by placing the patient in a warm environment, removing wet clothes and replacing them with warm dry ones, and administering warm liquids. In young healthy individuals, dramatic recoveries may occur. Even patients appearing dead after prolonged exposure to cold temperatures should not be considered dead until they are near-normal core temperature and are still unresponsive to cardiopulmonary resuscitation. It may be difficult to detect the presence of vital signs in severely hypothermic patients, and a full minute or more may be required to find them. Severe hypothermia requires vigorous treatment, but patients whose hearts are still beating and who have respirations, however slow, should not be subjected to unnecessary resuscitative procedures. If the patient has not gone into cardiac arrest, various physical manipulations (e.g., endotracheal and nasogastric intubation or temporary pacemaker or pulmonary artery flow-directed catheter insertion) may precipitate ventricular fibrillation. Such procedures should not be witheld if urgently needed, however. Endotracheal intubation may be necessary in the unconscious hypothermic patient with inadequate ventilation. This allows effective ventilation with warmed humidified oxygen and may help in preventing aspiration. Prior ventilation with 100% oxygen may lessen the likelihood of precipitating ventricular fibrillation during the procedure. Once an airway has been established, monitoring of blood gases and treatment of hypoglycemia and metabolic acidosis with glucose and sodium bicarbonate, respectively, are in order. Blood volume may require expansion.

External warming is appropriate primarily in mild hypothermia. Patients with rectal temperatures of 29.5° to 32.5°C (85° to 90.5°F) and a stable cardiac status should be warmed slowly but actively with heated blankets, warm intravenous fluids, and heated humidified oxygen. When the core temperature is less than 29.5°C (85°F), the patient is at high risk for cardiac dysrhythmias. The patient should be warmed with warm enemas, warm intravenous solutions, hemodialysis with warm blood, and peritoneal dialysis with warm dialysate. The use of external warming in the severely hypothermic patient may divert blood from the body's core as a result of dilation of peripheral blood vessels (23,24,28,30).

Hypothermia and frostbite are associated with an increased incidence of rhabdomyolysis and myoglobinuria. This is largely related to ischemia and crush injury and not just to cooling (10,31). Typically, myoglobinuria occurs when an individual has been lying immobile for prolonged periods in snow, an ideal circumstance to crush and damage muscle (muscle crush syndrome). In addition, ischemia to muscle (and other tissues) may occur with frostbite. Circulation of blood ceases as vessels become necrotic and occluded by thrombi (32). Infarction of muscles as a cause of myoglobinuria has also been documented in other entities (e.g., thrombotic or embolic arterial occlusion).

Cold-Related Syndromes

Frostbite

Frostbite occurs when tissue freezing produces major tissue damage. The combination of cold and high winds is especially dangerous and increases the risk of frostbite. The parts of the body most likely to suffer frostbite are those farthest from the trunk and large muscles (e.g., nose, earlobes, cheeks, fingers, and toes). The exposure of bare hands to cold metal or gasoline (e.g., skiers placing skis on ski racks or skimobile drivers spilling gasoline) may precipitate frostbite.

Prompt warming of the frostbitten area may prevent serious tissue injury. When frostbite is especially early and mild, no residual damage may occur. Mild residual numbness of the tips of the digits may occur and probably reflects damage to nerve endings or terminal digital nerves. Warming of severely frostbitten areas should be carried out as promptly as possible but should be witheld if there is a risk of refreezing. The frostbitten extremity should be warmed in a water bath at 40° to 42°C (104° to 108°F). The subsequently thawed extremity is quite susceptible to trauma and infection, requiring a number of medical and surgical therapies (33). Residual Raynaud's phenomenon may occur after either mild or serious frostbite (32).

Cold Muscle Syndrome

The cold muscle syndrome, which occurs whenever muscle is cooled, is characterized by weakness, stiffness, and clumsiness of the involved muscles (26,27). This is due to alterations in excitation–contraction coupling in muscle. At muscle temperatures of 25° to 28°C (77° to 82°F), there is a prominent prolongation of both the action potential and the contraction time of muscle. Clinically, the duration of deep tendon reflexes in cold extremities is prolonged, as is the case in myxedema (34). The slurred dysarthric speech that occurs in hypothermic patients may, in part, be a result of this.

Hypothermia or just cold muscles may have an adverse effect on muscle function in several neuromuscular disorders. These include hypokalemic and hyperkalemic periodic paralysis, myotonic dystrophy, and paramyotonia congenita. People with these disorders quickly learn to avoid cold-weather recreational activities.

PREVENTION OF THERMAL INJURIES IN SPORTS

Hyperthermia

The trained and heat-acclimatized athlete is in a much better position to deal with the stresses of a warm environment than an untrained individual. Serious sequelae arising from hyperthermia can be prevented by maintaining plasma volume as close to its normal level as possible during athletic endeavors in the heat. Carrying out athletic endeavors during relatively cooler periods of the day (usually morning and evening) decreases the amount of sweating required to maintain body temperature at the new steady state. Wearing light clothing facilitates heat dissipation and minimizes sweating. This obvious precaution is, surprisingly, overlooked by novice athletes and poorly informed coaches. The use of various types of suits to facilitate sweating is thought to promote weight loss. This may have disastrous results, however.

The amount of fluid lost can be minimized in several ways. Much has been written about the types of replacement fluids that are most effective. Currently, a number of commercially prepared drinks containing various electrolyte mixtures are available. As mentioned earlier, studies of serum electrolyte levels during marathons show an increase in serum sodium and potassium reflecting the efflux of potassium ions from intracellular stores and the lower ion concentration of sweat compared with that of serum. In view of this, consumption of water alone is recommended during marathons; electrolytes need to be replaced after the completion of the activity, when rehydration occurs (14). An exception is the prolonged physical exertion in the ultramarathon in a hot environment that may ultimately result in hyponatremia, especially if liberal amounts of water are being consumed (15). In this special circumstance, the use of a commercially prepared electrolyte mixture late in the activity helps prevent hyponatremia.

Although normal glucose levels should be maintained during physical activity, glucose content of replacement fluids should be low because sugar acts as an osmotic gradient to slow gastric absorption of liquids, a process already compromised by the decrease in splanchnic blood flow (35). The use of salt tablets is deleterious because it results in a high concentration of sodium chloride in the gastrointestinal tract, producing an osmotic gradient and causing further dehydration.

It is important to monitor athletes carefully during strenuous athletic activities in a hot environment. Especially during the summer months, race directors need to schedule events early in the day or in the late afternoon. Participants need to moderate their physical exertion during hot periods. Racing or maximal physical effort in hot weather is especially dangerous. Facilities need to be available at the athletic event to deal promptly and effectively with the heat-exhausted athlete to avoid the more devastating problem of heatstroke (26).

Hypothermia

Some sort of warming facility is usually available for many winter athletic and recreational activities, including downhill skiing and winter road racing. Athletes not near such facilities or who expect to be outdoors for long periods must take great care to have sufficient warm and dry clothes to prevent heat loss. Wet clothes, whether from rain, snow, or sweat, lose much of their in-

sulating quality; this is especially true of down. Adequate clothing involves multiple layers that trap air. Particular care must be taken to protect susceptible areas from cold or frostbite. The amount of susceptibility depends on the athletic endeavor. For example, the cold-weather runner does not develop cold feet because large amounts of warm blood circulate through the distal portion of the legs. Cold feet are an important problem for downhill skiers, however, because their feet are constricted by ski boots. Cold hands and earlobes are a common problem and require the proper use of gloves or mittens and head coverings. A common problem among cold-weather male runners is cold urethritis, which can be avoided by utilizing appropriate extra insulation (such as a folded washcloth).

Sweating may be minimized by regulating the insulating quality of clothing. Being able to zip or unzip jackets and to remove or add extra sweaters can be especially helpful.

Finally, it is important to recall the chilling effect of wind. For example, at temperatures of −6°C (21°F), a wind of 45 miles/hour results in a wind chill temperature of −40°C (−40°F). For the runner and skier, this may result in wide fluctuations in effective temperature, depending on whether he or she is moving into the wind or with the wind. In this circumstance, the availability of zippered jackets is of particular importance to minimize sweating (16).

REFERENCES

1. Sander N. Light at the end of the run. *Runner's World* 1979;14:96–103.
2. Haymaker W, Anderson E. Disorders of hypothalamus and pituitary gland. In: Baker AB, Baker LH, eds. *Clinical neurology.* Hagerstown, MD: Harper & Row, 1980:1–78.
3. Nadel ER, Wenger CB, Roberts MF, et al. Physiological defenses against hyperthermia of exercise. *Ann N Y Acad Sci* 1977;301:98–109.
4. Knochel JP. Environmental heat illness. *Arch Intern Med* 1974;133:841–864.
5. Gold J. Development of heat pyrexia. *JAMA* 1960; 173:1175–1182.
6. Salmons S, Henriksson J. The adaptive response of skeletal muscle to increased use. *Muscle Nerve* 1981; 4:94–105.
7. Andersen P, Henriksson J. Capillary supply of the quadriceps femoris muscle of man: adaptive response to exercise. *J Physiol (Lond)* 1977;270:677–690.

8. Dill DB, Hall FG, Edwards HT. Changes in composition of sweat during acclimatization to heat. *Am J Physiol* 1938;123:412–419.

9. Costill DL. Sweating: its composition and effects on body fluids. *Ann N Y Acad Sci* 1977;301:160–175.

10. Penn AS. Myoglobin and myoglobinuria. In: Vinken PJ, Bruyn GW, eds. *Handbook of clinical neurology.* Amsterdam: Elsevier–North Holland,1979;41:259–285.

11. Zelman S, Quillan R. Heat stroke in phenothiazine-treated patients: a report of three fatalities. *Am J Psychol* 1970;126:1787–1790.

12. Litman RE. Heat stroke in parkinsonism. *Arch Intern Med* 1952;89:562–567.

13. Wyndham CH. Heat stroke and hyperthermia in marathon runners. *Ann N Y Acad Sci* 1977;301:128–138.

14. Cohen I, Zimmerman AL. Changes in serum electrolyte levels during marathon running. *S Afr Med J* 1978; 49:449–453.

15. Frizzell RT, Lang GH, Lowance DC, et al. Hyponatremia and ultramarathon running. *JAMA* 1986;255:772–774.

16. Gutmann L. Temperature-related problems in athletic and recreational activities. *Semin Neurol* 1981; 1:242–252.

17. Clowes GHA, O'Donnell TF. Heat stroke. *N Engl J Med* 1974;291:564–567.

18. Hanson PG, Zimmerman SW. Exertional heat stroke in novice runners. *JAMA* 1979;242:154–157.

19. Malamud N, Haymaker W, Custer RP. Heat stroke: a clinicopathologic study of 125 fatal cases. *Mil Surg* 1946;99:397–449.

20. Gottschalk PG, Thomas JE. Heat stroke. *Mayo Clin Prac* 1966;41:470–482.

21. Mehta AC, Baker RN. Persistent neurological deficits in heat stroke. *Neurology* 1970;20:336–340.

22. Knochel JP. Potassium deficiency during training in the heat. *Ann N Y Acad Sci* 1977;301:175–182.

23. Bank WJ. Myoglobinuria in marathon runners: possible relationship to carbohydrate and lipid metabolism. *Ann N Y Acad Sci* 1977;301:942–948.

24. Rasminsky M. The effects of temperature on conduction in demyelinated single nerve fibers. *Arch Neurol* 1973; 28:287–292.

25. Gutmann L. Heat-induced myasthenic crisis. *Arch Neurol* 1980;37:671–672.

26. Duquid H, Simpson RG, Stowers JM. Accidental hypothermia. *Lancet* 1970;2:1213–1219.

27. Tolman KG, Cohen A. Accidental hypothermia. *Can Med Assoc J* 1970;103:1357–1361.

28. Treatment of hypothermia. *Med Lett* 1983;25:9–11.

29. Fishbeck KH, Simon RP. Neurologic manifestations of hypothermia. *Neurology* 1981;31(Suppl):46.

30. Zell SC, Kurtz KJ. Severe exposure hypothermia: a resuscitation protocol. *Ann Emerg Med* 1985;14: 339–345.

31. Kulka JP. Histopathologic studies in frostbitten rabbits. In: Ferrer MI, ed. *Cold injury.* New York: Josiah Macy Jr Foundation, 1956:97–151.

32. Blair JR. Follow-up study of cold injury cases from the Korean war. In: Ferrer MI, ed. *Cold injury.* New York: Josiah Macy Jr Foundation, 1956:9–35.

33. Treatment of frostbite. *Med Lett* 1980;22:112–114.

34. Lambert EH, Underdahl LO, Beckett S, et al. A study of the ankle jerk in myxedema. *J Clin Endocrinol* 1951; 11:1186–1205.

35. Costill DL, Saltin B. Factors limiting gastric emptying during rest and exercise. *J Appl Physiol* 1974;37: 679–683.

Sports Neurology, Second Edition,
edited by Barry D. Jordan.
Lippincott–Raven Publishers, Philadelphia © 1998.

22

Epilepsy and the Athlete

Salah M. Mesad and Orrin Devinsky

Department of Neurology,
New York University-Hospital for Joint Diseases,
301 East 17th Street, New York, New York 10003

Epileptic seizures are the clinical manifestations of excessive and hypersynchronous, usually self-limited, abnormal cortical activity. The behavioral features of an epileptic seizure reflect the cerebral cortical areas where the abnormal neuronal activity originates and spreads (1). Epilepsy is a condition characterized by two or more unprovoked recurrent seizures. Epilepsy and seizures are among the most common neurologic problems. By age 20, about 1% of the population of the United States have epilepsy, and this cumulative incidence increases to 3% to 4% at age 80 years (2,3). The annual incidence of epilepsy is about 50 per 100,000 population (2–4). This increases to 65 per 100,000 if single unprovoked seizures are included and up to 85 per 100,000 if afebrile reactive seizures are added (2,3). The prevalence of epilepsy ranges from 4 to 8 per 1000. Of those afflicted, 75% experience their first seizure before the third decade of life (5), the crucial time period for teaching and enjoying the benefits of physical exercise, developing one's athletic abilities, and experiencing the challenge and excitement of team sports. In 1981, the number of patients with epilepsy in the United States in the age group 5 to 24 years was estimated to be approximately 375,000 (6).

People with epilepsy often have limited involvement in exercise and sports programs (6). The lack of participation, particularly during high school, is largely based on unfounded fears and misconception by parents, school athletic policies, and physicians. These critical developmental years witness a peak in peer pressure. For students with epilepsy, restrictions of sports activity can contribute to isolation and stigma and can worsen psychologic problems. The medical and lay communities need to address this problem. Sports activities should be pursued to the degree that safety permits. Most queries to the family physician address whether a patient with epilepsy can participate in a physical conditioning program or recreational sport rather than team activities. Team sports in which collision (e.g., football, rugby, hockey, lacrosse) or contact (e.g., baseball, soccer, basketball, wrestling) is likely must be pursued more cautiously by patients with epilepsy. However, many of these patients can compete successfully in collision or contact sports. Because epilepsy affects each person differently, the approach to sports and epilepsy must be considered on a patient-by-patient basis. The seizure type, frequency, loss of consciousness or motor control, warning and its duration, postictal symptoms, and type of medication and its side effects as well as the nature of safety precautions and supervision must all be considered (7). A number of important questions should be addressed in considering the appropriateness of sports activity for the person with epilepsy:

1. Will exercise adversely affect seizure control?
2. What is the risk of a seizure during an athletic activity?
3. Will antiepileptic medications increase the risk for injury?

The medical debate on whether patients with epilepsy can engage in physical fitness programs and recreational or competitive sports, particularly those involving collision or contact, has existed for many years. The major reasons against participation are that physical exercise may precipitate a seizure and adversely affect seizure control through head trauma and that if a seizure occurred during a sporting activity, physical injury would occur. These sports activities may increase the risk of serious injury (6). The major reason for participation is inclusion and allowing children and adults with epilepsy to pursue a fuller and more active life. Restriction and isolation foster low self-esteem, dependence, and helplessness. This chapter reviews the issue of seizures and physical exercise and tries to answer the preceding three questions.

CLASSIFICATION OF SEIZURES

A seizure is not a diagnosis; it is a symptom. Phenotypically, seizures can result from different underlying cerebral processes. In some cases, seizures are the sole manifestation of the disorder; in others, they represent only a minor component. Certain seizures affect patients in a restricted age group and produce a characteristic clinical and electroencephalographic (EEG) profile but have no

known cause. The International League Against Epilepsy classifies epileptic seizures on the basis of clinical symptoms and EEG features (see Tables 1 and 2) (8,9). Definition of the seizure type and the epilepsy syndrome is extremely important, taking into the account the individual seizure type(s) as well as the natural history, clinical and neurologic findings, family history, and EEG and neuroimaging studies. Defining the syndrome helps determine whether medication is necessary, the likelihood of complete response to antiepileptic drug treatment, and the duration of treatment. This classification subdivides epileptic seizures into two major categories: partial and generalized. Partial seizures have clinical or electroencephalographic evidence of a focal onset from one or more cortical areas. Generalized seizures begin in both sides of the brain simultaneously and may arise in subcortical pacemaker regions (e.g., thalamus). Partial seizures are subdivided into simple partial seizures (i.e., without impairment of consciousness) and complex partial seizures (i.e., with impairment of consciousness). Simple partial seizures may evolve to complex partial seizures, and both types may evolve into generalized tonic–clonic (grand mal) seizures. Auras are simple partial seizures.

Generalized seizures can be further categorized as convulsive or nonconvulsive. The typical convulsive generalized seizure is the tonic–clonic

---

TABLE 1. *Outline of the International Classification of Epileptic Seizures (8)*

I. Partial (focal, local) seizures
  A. Simple partial seizures
  • With motor signs
  • With special sensory or somatosensory symptoms
  • With autonomic symptoms or signs
  • With psychic symptoms
  B. Complex partial seizures
  • Simple partial onset followed by impairment of consciousness
  • With impairment of consciousness at onset
  C. Partial seizures evolving to secondarily generalized seizures
  • Simple partial seizures evolving to generalized seizures
  • Complex partial seizures evolving to generalized seizures
  • Simple partial seizures evolving to complex partial seizures evolving to generalized seizures
II. Generalized seizures (convulsive or nonconvulsive)
  A. Absences seizures
  • Typical absences
  • Atypical absences
  • Myoclonic seizures
  B. Clonic seizures
  C. Tonic seizures
  D. Tonic–clonic seizures
  E. Atonic seizures astatic seizures
III. Unclassified epileptic seizures

TABLE 2. *Outline of the International Classification of Epilepsies and Epileptic Syndromes (9)*

1. **Localization-related (focal, local, partial)**
   - **1.1 Idiopathic (primary)**
     - Benign childhood epilepsy with centrotemporal spikes
     - Childhood epilepsy with occipital spikes
     - Primary reading epilepsy
   - **1.2 Symptomatic (secondary)**
     - Temporal lobe epilepsies
     - Frontal lobe epilepsies
     - Parietal lobe epilepsies
     - Occipital lobe epilepsies
     - Chronic progressive epilepsia partialis continua of childhood
       - Syndromes characterized by seizures with specific modes of precipitation
   - **1.3 Cryptogenic,** defined by:
     - Seizure type
     - Clinical features
     - Etiology
     - Anatomic localization
2. **Generalized**
   - **2.1 Idiopathic (primary)**
     - Benign neonatal familial convulsions
     - Benign neonatal convulsions
     - Benign myoclonic epilepsy in infancy
     - Childhood absence epilepsy (pyknolepsy)
     - Juvenile absence epilepsy
     - Juvenile myoclonic epilepsy (impulsive petit mal)
     - Epilepsies with grand mal seizures (GTCS) on awakening
     - Other generalized idiopathic epilepsies
       - Epilepsies with seizures precipitated by specific modes of activation
   - **2.2 Cryptogenic or symptomatic**
     - West syndrome (infantile spasms, Blitz-Nick-Salaam Kraempfe)
     - Lennox-Gastaut syndrome
     - Epilepsy with myoclonic astatic seizures
     - Epilepsy with myoclonic absences
   - **2.3 Symptomatic (secondary)**
     - Nonspecific etiology
       - Early myoclonic encephalopathy
       - Early infantile epileptic encephalopathy with suppression bursts
       - Other symptomatic generalized epilepsies
     - Specific syndromes
       - Epileptic seizures may complicate many disease states
3. **Undetermined epilepsies**
   - **3.1 With both generalized and focal seizures**
     - Neonatal seizures
     - Severe myoclonic epilepsy in infancy
     - Epilepsy with continuous spike-waves during slow-wave sleep
     - Acquired epileptic aphasia (Landau-Kleffner syndrome)
     - Other undetermined epilepsies
   - **3.2 Without unequivocal generalized or focal features**
4. **Special syndromes**
   - **4.1 Situation-related seizures (Gelegenheitsanfälle)**
     - Febrile convulsions
     - Isolated seizures or isolated status epilepticus
     - Seizures occurring only when there is an acute or toxic event due to factors such as alcohol, drugs, eclampsia, nonketotic hyperglycemia

seizure. Some convulsive seizures may be characterized by only clonic or only tonic or myoclonic (i.e., single or series of jerks) manifestations. The major group of generalized nonconvulsive seizures is absence epilepsy characterized by brief lapses of consciousness. Absences that last less than 10 seconds, are associated with bilaterally synchronous 3-Hz spike-and-wave complexes on EEG, and have no postictal EEG or behavioral disturbances are referred to as typical. Those that last longer, have slower or more irregular EEG correlates, or are followed by varying periods of postictal dysfunction are referred to as atypical. Absence seizures may be accompanied by minor motor activity, such as eye blinking or lip movements.

CAUSES OF EPILEPSY

Epileptic seizures have many causes. In approximately 50% of cases, no specific cause is identified. Most others have a single cause such as genetic or environmental (e.g., head trauma) factors. Some patients have more than one underlying disturbance, that is, a multifactorial etiology. Any injury to the brain can cause epilepsy, including infections, head trauma, stroke, and tumors. These can occur at any age but have age-related predilections (e.g., infections, highest in children; trauma, in young adults; stroke and degenerative disorders, in the elderly). Many patients with epilepsy secondary to structural causes, particularly if the damage is extensive, have other mental or neurologic handicaps that limit their participation in active sports programs. Seizures in the patient with extensive brain damage may be multiple in type and are often difficult to control with medications. Nonspecific predisposing factors (e.g., missed medications, sleep deprivation, intercurrent illnesses, especially with fever, stress, alcohol or illicit drugs, hormonal changes) determine differences in individual susceptibility to generating epileptic seizures, whereas specific (e.g., flashing light, reading) predisposing factors can provoke reflex epileptic seizures in susceptible individuals. Precipitating factors are endogenous or exogenous perturbations capable of acutely evoking epileptic seizures in persons with chronic epilepsy and, in some cases, reactive seizures in nonepileptic individuals.

Head trauma increases the risk for seizures and epilepsy in proportion to the severity of the injury. The occurrence of seizures is highest in the first few years after injury. In patients with penetrating head injuries or loss of consciousness for more than 24 hours, the risk of seizures remains 5 to 15 times above the population rate for 15 years or more following the injury (10). Early seizures, those occurring within the first week following injury, occur in approximately 5% of individuals with brain trauma. Early seizures are associated with an increased risk of later epilepsy in adults but not children.

Seizures occur in 10% to 15% of patients with acute stroke, especially in patients with cortical infarcts. Epilepsy develops in 15% to 20% of stroke survivors. Seizures in the week following stroke are associated with an increased risk for epilepsy when compared with stroke patients without early seizures (10).

Individuals with encephalitis or bacterial meningitis have a four- to sixfold risk for epilepsy compared with the general population (3,11). The risk for meningitis patients is increased only in the presence of persistent neurologic deficits suggesting structural brain damage. About 5% of patients have seizures at the time of infection. Patients with aseptic meningitis have no subsequent discernible increase in risk for epilepsy.

Intracranial tumors can cause epilepsy, particularly among adult patients. Seizures are frequently the presenting manifestation of a tumor. Although seizures occur in approximately 30% of individuals with brain tumors, they account for less than 5% of new cases of adult-onset epilepsy. Epilepsy related to brain tumors occurs at all ages but has its greatest proportionate impact in the age group 25 to 64 (12).

Ten percent to 15% of patients with Alzheimer's disease experience unprovoked seizures in the course of their illness, a rate 10 times or more than expected in the general population older than 60 years (13). Multiple sclerosis increases the risk of epilepsy threefold. Approximately 5% of patients with multiple sclerosis have seizures or epilepsy (14).

Seizures that occur during abstinence or reduced alcohol intake are well recognized as alcohol withdrawal seizures. Risk increases with increasing consumption: persons who drink less than 50 g of alcohol daily are not at increased risk, but the risk of epilepsy is 20 times greater than expected in individuals who drink more than 300 g of alcohol daily. Chronic alcoholism was the only factor identified in 20% of adults with newly diagnosed epilepsy (10).

Epilepsy occurs in approximately 10% of children with mental retardation (MR) or with cerebral palsy (CP). For those with either MR or CP alone, the risk for epilepsy is increased in proportion to the severity of mental retardation or physical handicap. When the two conditions coexist, seizures occur in 50% or more of patients (15,16).

Children with febrile convulsions have an increased risk of developing epilepsy. This averages sixfold but strongly depends on the characteristics of the initial seizure (17). There is controversy about whether prolonged febrile convulsions are a marker for or contribute to the development of mesial temporal sclerosis and chronic temporal lobe epilepsy.

DIAGNOSTIC APPROACH TO THE PATIENT WITH SUSPECTED EPILEPTIC SEIZURES

The diagnosis of epilepsy is clinical and is based on a detailed description of events experienced by the patient before, during, and after a seizure and, more important, on an eyewitness account. EEG is a single valuable tool in evaluating patients with suspected seizures. Three questions need to be answered when a clinician is evaluating a patient with possible epileptic seizures: Is it epilepsy? What kind of epilepsy? and What is the etiology of the patient's epilepsy?

The EEG can provide supportive evidence for the clinical diagnosis of epilepsy by demonstrating epileptiform discharges, although normal studies do not exclude the occurrence of seizures. EEG aids in the classification of seizures, in the selection of appropriate antiepileptic agents (AEDs), and in following the response of the disorder to therapy. Magnetic resonance imaging (MRI) and computed tomography (CT) of the brain complement electrophysiologic studies by identifying structural brain lesions that may be causally related to epilepsy. MRI is more sensitive than CT in detecting cerebral lesions related to epilepsy, such as cortical heterotopias or mesial temporal sclerosis, hamartomas, and low-grade gliomas. Some abnormalities, such as calcified or bone abnormalities, may be easier to interpret on CT than MRI. Positron emission tomography (PET) and single-photon emission computed tomography (SPECT) are less readily obtainable but can identify areas of cerebral hypometabolism or hypoperfusion interictally (PET, SPECT) or ictally (SPECT) in patients with partial epilepsy, even when MRI and CT results are normal.

Differential diagnosis of epileptic seizures from other paroxysmal nonepileptic events is a common problem. Reviewing all conditions that resemble epileptic seizures is beyond the scope of this chapter. Instead we will review syncope, as it can occur at any age, it may be induced by physical exercise, and it usually requires prompt recognition and treatment.

Syncope is a sudden transient loss of consciousness resulting from a reduction of cerebral blood flow and is associated with a loss of postural tone with spontaneous recovery. The diagnosis of syncope is supported if episodes (a) are precipitated by anxiety or pain (e.g., venipuncture) or assumption of the upright position; (b) exclusively occur while standing or sitting; (c) are associated with pallor and diaphoresis; (d) are not associated with sustained tonic or clonic movements, bladder incontinence, or tongue or cheek bites; and (e) are not followed by postepisode confusion, lethargy, muscle soreness, and headache. Although incontinence strongly suggests an epileptic seizure, if the bladder is unusually full when syncope occurs, there may be incontinence. Although seizures often cause tachycardia and rarely cause tachy- or bradyarrhythmias, loss of consciousness with documented bradycardia or tachyarrhythmias should be considered a primary cardiac disorder until proved otherwise. Prodromal symptoms such as abdominal sensations (e.g., "butterflies" or nausea), flushing and warmth, dizziness and lightheadedness, bilateral paresthesia, and feeling of fear and unreality occur with both syncope and epileptic seizures. Symptoms such as formed visual or auditory hallucinations, olfactory hallucinations, déjà vu, or focal sensory or motor phenomena strongly suggest partial seizures. A prodrome lasting several seconds followed by loss of consciousness for 15 to 60 seconds followed by a rapid return to a normal level of attentiveness is typical of syncope. The greatest source of error in distinguishing seizures and syncope is failure to recognize that brief tonic or clonic movements often occur in syncope (18). Witnesses often observe these movements and their duration and intensity may be exaggerated.

Convulsive syncope refers to an episode in which the diminution of blood flow to the brain is more severe or prolonged (19). In such cases, the person, most often a child, has a tonic–clonic seizure due to cerebral hypoxia (20). Convulsive syncope often occurs when a person is maintained in the upright or sitting position. The physical examination of patients with possible syncope includes a brief survey of general medical and neurologic systems and, specifically, palpation of the pulse and thyroid, measurement of orthostatic heart rate, and examination of lungs and neck. Electrocardiography may help detect abnormalities such as arrhythmias and conduction blocks. The QT interval must be measured. Patients with prolonged QT syndrome often present with syncope and later die during a subsequent attack (21).

DRUG TREATMENT OF EPILEPSY

Once the diagnosis of epilepsy has been confirmed, long-term treatment with an AED is usually recommended, with the goal of complete seizure control with a minimal or no adverse drug effects. In approximately one-third of patients, any single drug or combinations of drugs cannot adequately control seizures (22). Until recently, the major AEDs were barbiturates, carbamazepine, ethosuximide, phenytoin and valproate (Table 3). Most of the established AEDs were developed before 1980 and generally act on sodium or calcium channels or γ-aminobutyric acid type A (GABA-A) receptors. Although their mechanisms of action have not been fully established, all appear to decrease membrane excitability. With decreased membrane excitability, the tendency of neurons to produce abnormal, high-frequency, repetitive action potentials is reduced: Such patterns of firing are associated with epilepsy and may serve as a trigger or a source of entrainment for further abnormal electrical activity in the nervous system.

Benzodiazepines and barbiturates act at the GABA-A receptor, enhancing the inhibitory action of GABA. Valproate may also have GABAergic activity. Phenytoin, carbamazepine, and possibly valproate enhance the inactivation of sodium channels, thereby decreasing the high-frequency, repetitive firing of action potentials. Ethosuximide and possibly sodium valproate act by reducing the low-threshold (T-type) calcium channel current, thereby affecting the neuron's excitability.

There are newer AEDs approved by the Food and Drug Administration or in late stages of clinical development. Many are approved only for adults or as add-on therapy but are currently used for children, and their use as monotherapy is gradually expanding. Gabapentin is an effective add-on drug for patients with partial epilepsy with or without secondary generalization (23). Although it is structurally similar to GABA, gabapentin does not act directly on the GABA system but may do so indirectly. Gabapentin is usually well tolerated, has no significant hepatic metabolism, lacks protein binding, and has minimal interactions with other drugs. Lamotrigine is approved for adults with partial epilepsy with or without secondary generalization (24) but is also used for primary generalized epilepsy. Lamotrigine decreases the sustained high-frequency, repetitive firing of voltage-dependent sodium action potentials, an action that may preferentially decreased release of presynaptic glutamate. Lamotrigine is well tolerated, although headache, nausea and vomiting, dizziness, and ataxia are common side effects. Approximately 5% of patients develop a rash when treated with lamotrigine, but in many cases the rash disappears during continued therapy. However, in 1% to 2% of patients, the rash represents a more serious allergic reaction and occasionally patients develop the Stevens-Johnson syndrome. Concomitant use of lamotrigine with valproate can increase the likelihood of a serious rash, especially if lamotrigine is added to valproate therapy and the dose is increased rapidly. The plasma half-life of lamotrigine when administered alone is approximately 25 hours. However, drugs such as carbamazepine, phenytoin, and phenobarbital, which induce liver enzymes, can decrease the half-life of lamotrigine by 50%, necessitating a higher dose of lamotrigine. In contrast, valproic acid slows the metabolism of lamotrigine and prolongs it half-life (70 hours), necessitating a lower dose. Felbamate was introduced in the United States in August 1993, and within 1 year approximately 100,000 people had taken it. It is effective for partial seizures with or without secondary generalization

TABLE 3. *List of antiepileptic agents*

AED	Seizure type[a]	Half-life (h)	Dose (mg/kg/d)	Common adverse reactions	Idiosyncratic reactions[b]
Carbamazepine Tegretol	P, SGTC, PGTC	12	10–25	Dizziness, nystagmus, diplopia, drowsiness, hyponatremia, headache, skin rash	Granulocytopenia, aplastic anemia, hepatotoxicity, SJS
Clonazepam Klonopin	Myoclonic, absence	30	0.1–2.5	Fatigue, drowsiness, dizziness, ataxia, agitation, tolerance	
Divalproex sodium Depakote	PGE, GTC, P	10	10–60	Nausea, vomiting, hair loss, weight loss, weight gain, tremor, drowsiness	Acute pancreatitis, hepatotoxicity, thrombocytopenia, SJS
Ethosuximide Zarontin	Absence, myoclonic	48	15–60	Nausea, vomiting, anorexia, lethargy, headache	Agranulocytosis, SJS, dermatitis, SLE
Felbamate Felbatol	LGS, P, SGTC, myoclonic	20	15–60	Nausea, vomiting, headache, insomnia, weight loss	Aplastic anemia, fulminant hepatotoxicity
Gabapentin Neurontin	P, SGTC	6	10–30	Drowsiness, fatigue, nausea, vomiting	Rash
Lamotrigine Lamictal	P, SGTC, PGE	25	5–10	Skin rash, nausea, vomiting, insomnia, drowsiness	Stevens–Johnson syndrome
Phenobarbiturates Phenobarbital	P, PGTC, SGTC	96	1.5–5	Sedation, hyperactivity (in children), depression, impotence	Hepatotoxicity, frozen shoulder, rash
Phenytoin Dilantin	P, PGTC, SGTC	24	5–10	Nausea, vomiting, ataxia, gum hyperplasia, hirsutism, facial coarsening	Hepatotoxicity, bone marrow suppression, megaloplastic anemia
Primidone Mysoline	P, PGTC, SGTC	12	10–18	Nausea, vomiting, sedation, hyperactivity (in children), impotence	Agranulocytosis, thrombocytopenia, rash
Valproate Depakene	Absence, myoclonic, PGTC, SGTC, P	10	10–60	Nausea, vomiting, drowsiness, weight gain, tremor, peripheral edema	Acute pancreatitis, hepatotoxicity, thrombocytopenia

[a] P, partial seizures; GTC, generalized tonic–clonic; PGE, primary generalized epilepsy; SGTC, secondary generalized tonic–clonic; PGTC, primary generalized tonic–clonic; LGS, Lennox-Gastaut syndrome.
[b] SJS, Stevens-Johnson syndrome; SLE, systemic lupus erythematosus.

and for patients with Lennox-Gastaut syndrome (25). Felbamate often caused nausea, decreased appetite, insomnia, agitation, and headache but was well tolerated by many patients. After felbamate was marketed, aplastic anemia and fulminant hepatic failure were recognized, leading to severe restriction of its use.

Clinician should clearly understand the most common and serious adverse effects of each AED and how best to manage them (Table 3). They should be aware of variation in response in individual patients as well as interactions among all medications (26).

In Table 3 the drugs most commonly used for the treatment of epilepsy are listed. With proper drug selection, dose, and timing of intake, optimal seizure control can be achieved in roughly 75% of patients. As newer AEDs have become available, others, such as phenobarbital, have declined in popularity because of sedative and behavioral side effects. Felbamate, a newer AED, is now seldom prescribed because of its association with bone marrow suppression and hepatic failure.

Several general conclusions can be drawn from studies of other drugs (27–29). Physical exercise inhibits gastric emptying and can delay absorption. Therefore, epilepsy patients should take their medications at least 1 hour before physical activity. Aerobic exercise can accelerate drug metabolism. Therefore, in patients who significantly change the level of physical activity or exercise, AED levels should be checked and interpreted in light of their clinical status (i.e., seizure control, adverse effects).

Maintaining optimal seizure control in the athlete with epilepsy requires close rapport between physician and patient. Noncompliance is a major cause of breakthrough seizures and should be avoided. Patients, coaches, and trainers should be educated about seizures and antiepileptic drugs and their side effects.

For athletes, drug selection should be determined not only by seizure type but also by potential side effects, which might interfere with performance. For example, primidone or phenobarbital should probably not be prescribed because of their sedative effects; high levels of phenytoin, carbamazepine, and lamotrigine (as well as other AEDs) can impair coordination.

Blood levels should be monitored periodically, especially if new complaints are reported.

Patients with epilepsy who are most likely to request clearance to participate in competitive sports are those who are otherwise neurologically and mentally normal or with neurologic or cognitive impairment but do have progressive disorders. In most cases, they can actively participate in exercise and sports programs.

Patients with epilepsy who have breakthrough seizures after a long interval of excellent control or who have an unexplained increase in a previously established seizure frequency should be reevaluated. The following are possible explanations:

1. Poor compliance with medication regimen. This is a common problem with teenagers and can be dealt with by explaining how blood levels are used. Poor compliance is especially common when routines are disturbed, such as at holiday time or on trips. Linking medication to other routines such as tooth brushing is very helpful. Alarm pillboxes are also helpful.
2. Sleep deprivation and fatigue (can occur with team sports and travel).
3. Alcohol and drug abuse, such as cocaine and amphetamines.
4. Intercurrent illnesses, especially with fever.
5. Emotional, mental, or physical stress.
6. Menstrual cycle in certain female patients.
7. Unrecognized intracranial structural problems such as brain tumor or arteriovenous malformation.

SEIZURES AND PHYSICAL EXERCISE

The relationship between seizures and physical exercise is incompletely defined and underinvestigated. Seizures have been reported to occur only rarely during exercise (30). Korczyn (31) reported that only 5 of 250 epilepsy patients aged 10 years and older had seizures while participating in athletic events. Ninety epilepsy patients denied ever having a seizure during physical exertion. Götze et al. (32) reported that seizures were never observed in epilepsy patients during intense physical exertion, particularly swimming, at a German Air Force rehabilitation center during World War II.

These authors (32) also found fewer seizure discharges in the electroencephalograms of 30 epileptics during exercise (deep knee bends) than during hyperventilation or rest. The reasons for this are unclear; however, it may be related to inhibition of the epileptic process by psychic stimuli such as arousal, alertness, concentration, proprioceptive impulses, or biochemical changes, such as metabolic acidosis. Seizures during exercise or in the immediate postexertion period have been infrequently reported. Bennett (6) speculated that the temporal lobe is more sensitive to exercise-induced epileptiform discharges than other cortical areas. He mentioned that if a patient's first seizure occurs during physical exertion, particularly a simple or complex type, a symptomatic cause such as a brain tumor or arteriovenous malformation should be suspected. Ogunyemi et al. (33) reported three patients with exercise-induced seizures (two with tonic–clonic seizures and one with a probable absence seizure) who had generalized epileptiform EEG abnormalities that were activated by exercise. The baseline EEGs of these patients showed no paroxysmal discharges during resting, wakefulness, or hyperventilation. Only one patient showed epileptiform activity during sleep. Kuijer (34) reported increased epileptiform EEG abnormalities during the recovery phase after exercise, particularly after continuous exertion. This correlated with low blood pH values. In an investigation of 43 epilepsy patients, Horyd et al. (35) reported a decrease in EEG discharges during exercise but an increase in 10 of 43 patients during the postexercise period. Bemey et al. (36) reported an increase in EEG epileptiform activity in the immediate postexercise rest period in some patients after strenuous dancing. The subjects who showed this increase were also susceptible to EEG activation by eye opening, hyperventilation, and photic stimulation and were not fully controlled with AEDs. In most studies, clinical seizures are not mentioned. The mechanism underlying the activation or suppression of clinical seizures or EEG epileptiform discharges during exercise or in the immediate postexertion period remains unknown.

Hyperventilation activates absence seizures and less commonly partial seizures. The degree of EEG activation is dependent on the type of exercise (i.e., short- versus long-distance racing) as well as the age, physical condition, and experience of the participitant. Children are more susceptible than adults, particularly in the earlier stages of training when they find it difficult master proper breathing techniques. With exposure to high altitude, increased ventilation occurs because decreased oxygen tension stimulates the peripheral chemoreceptors. This produces respiratory alkalosis, which can lead to seizures. Therefore, epilepsy patients should not be exposed to rapid decreases in barometric pressure. Metabolic changes with physical exercise can inhibit seizures, possibly secondary to lactic acidosis (37). EEG changes were evaluated in 30 adolescents with epilepsy and abnormal EEGs before and after exercise. A significant decrease in slow waves and spike waves was observed.

Many seizures are preceded by an aura, giving patients a brief period to protect themselves from injury. Nevertheless, a brief loss of awareness or concentration, arrest of movement, or loss of tone and reflexes associated with minor attacks could be disastrous during downhill skiing or mountain climbing. In contact or collision sports the athlete with absence or complex partial seizures may be susceptible to injuries because an opponent may not recognize that the person is incapacitated and may level a crushing block or tackle a defenseless player (38).

Whether a regular exercise program can improve seizure control by reducing seizure frequency during inactive times is not known. The U.S. Department of Health, Education and Welfare's Commission for the Control of Epilepsy and Its Consequences stated in its final summary report that "Physical activity also appears to play a role in seizure prevention." The need for activity and physical fitness was documented by data collected by the commission and testimony at the regional hearings. Such activity is important for those with epilepsy because some evidence suggests that activity may, in fact, reduce the likelihood of seizure (39). Clinical data suggest that the incidence of seizures during sports and exercise is reduced. In the cool-down period, however, seizures tend to occur more frequently (40). Before giving advice about the most suitable type of sport, the physician should know the patient's medical history, have good insight into the different types of sports, and be able to judge the role and function of sport for the particular patient. With certain precautions virtually all sports are suitable for most epilepsy patients and therefore are encouraged. However, a small minority of patients with severe epilepsy need the supervision of qualified trainers, coaches, and volunteers (40) and can participate to a limited degree.

MORBIDITY AND MORTALITY

Approximately 7% of epileptic patients die as a result of accidents (41). Only 5% of these deaths, however, can be directly attributed to injuries sustained during a seizure (42). Bathtub drownings account for many of these deaths. Ryan and Dowling (41) retrospectively studied the demographic characteristics and risk factors associated with death from drowning among people with epilepsy. Of 482 deaths from drowning in Alberta during a 10-year period, 25 (5%) were considered by the medical examiner's office to be directly related to seizures. Fifteen (60%) of the 25 deaths occurred while the person was taking an unsupervised bath. Only one patient (4%) died while taking a shower; the remaining deaths occurred on a river lake (16%), in a private pool (8%), in a public pool (8%), and in a jacuzzi (4%). Two people fell out of moving boats while having a seizure; neither was wearing a personal flotation device. Nineteen (83%) of 23 people who had been receiving AED therapy had undetectable or subtherapeutic levels of one or more of the drugs at autopsy. Enhanced seizure control and compliance with AED therapy may have prevented some of these deaths. People with persistent seizures that impair consciousness or motor control should be encouraged to take showers while sitting in the bath instead. The presence of people in the same house who are not directly supervising the person in the bathroom does not protect against drowning. Personal flotation devices should be worn at all times during boating activities.

With the exception of swimming, morbidity and mortality data on sports are lacking. Pearn et al. (43) estimated that the risk of drowning for children with epilepsy while swimming is four times greater than for nonepileptic peers. Proper training and supervision can substantially reduce the risk. However, only 9 of 274 consecutive immersion accidents (3.3%) were caused by seizures, and these patients survived without neurologic deficits (44). With regard to sports-related injuries, patients with epilepsy have injury rates similar to those of their nonepileptic peers (45,46). Most injuries are extremity fractures.

A blow to the head precipitating a seizure or adversely affecting seizure control is a special concern, particularly in patients involved in collision or contact sports. Livingston and Berman (45) had never observed a case of recurrence of seizures related to a head injury in any of their athletes with epilepsy over a 34-year period of experience. Berman, on the basis of an unpublished study, concluded "a history of epilepsy does not indicate a predisposition to a seizure after a blunt head injury" (47). There were nine epilepsy patients and 292 control children with blunt head injuries in the studies. One child with epilepsy had a seizure 1 week after injury. In Jennett's (46) study of early posttraumatic epilepsy (within 7 days of injury), there were nine cases with preexisting epilepsy. Of these, four had been seizure free for prolonged periods. One of these patients experienced a series of generalized seizures immediately after injury. However, this patient had no further seizures over the next 10 years. Of the remaining three patients, two experienced seizures 6 months and 2 years, respectively, after the accident, and the attacks continued. These seizures may have resulted from a new cortical injury. Four of the remaining five patients with early epilepsy had been seizure free for 1 year before the injury. Only one was seen in follow-up. This patient's seizure frequency at that time was unchanged from the pattern before injury. Although incomplete, the data do not suggest that epilepsy patients are more predisposed to immediate or early seizures after head injury than other patients.

There is no evidence that traumatic injuries sustained by epilepsy patients have different sequelae when they occur during physical activity and at other times. The most frequent injuries during generalized tonic–clonic seizures are fractures of the humeral neck, femoral trochanter, clavicle, and ankle (48). The incidence of vertebral fractures in epileptic patients is approximately 15% (49). Shoulder and hip dislocations also result from tonic–clonic seizures, and, less often, cervical spine and serious head injuries may result from falls.

There is no evidence that the sudden death syndrome in epilepsy patients is related to exercise. Most patients with this disorder were found dead in bed (50).

The available data do not suggest an increased risk for injury or death in epilepsy patients participating in supervised recreational and team sports (with the possible exception of swimming).

The natural history of epilepsy and single seizures varies tremendously among patients, so no universal rules or dictums can be applied to all patients who wish to participate in recreational or competitive athletic events. Each case presents different problems. Recommendations must be tailored to meet individual needs, keeping in mind the risk–benefit ratio. Evidence suggests that seizures during exercise are rare and regular exercise may improve seizure control. Exercise does not appear to affect control adversely, except in unusual cases. Morbidity and mortality related to sports are not increased in epilepsy patients (with the possible exception of swimming and other aquatic sports). It is not the seizure type or the sport that determines participation but the seizure frequency. The principal risk of seizures during sports participation is loss of consciousness or confusion. Table 4 shows sports activities ranked according to the risk to the participant. For some activities, such as climbing with multiple individuals connected by a cord, there can be risks to other participants. Table 4 depicts most of the sports activities ranked according to their relative risks for patients with epilepsy.

People with epilepsy should not be prohibited from participating in any recreational or competitive sport, including collision and contact sports (boxing excluded), provided that their seizures are well controlled and there are no toxic effects from the medication. If a seizure was experienced during the sport, it would not endanger the lives of others (automobile racing and mountaineering are exceptions). Patients with epilepsy should not pursue boxing because a seizure in the ring could leave them defenseless and at risk for a serious brain injury. Also, single severe or repeated minor blows to the head, particularly those causing a concussion, could cause cortical injury and increase seizure frequency. Patients with frequent seizures that impair consciousness or motor control should pursue contact or collision sports only after careful consideration of the risks and accommodations to minimize the chance of injury. In many cases, they are wise to pursue less injury-prone sports, such as golf, tennis, or bowling. Paramount in the decision is that the patient and his or her parents, legal guardian, spouse, school officials, and coaches fully support the decision.

In summary, sport and epilepsy are not mutually exclusive, provided the disorder is correctly diagnosed and managed and adequate safeguards are used. Compliance and minimizing lifestyle factors that can provoke seizures should be encouraged.

TABLE 4. *List of sports activities and their relative risks for patients with epilepsy*

High risk	Moderately high risk	Moderately low risk	Low risk
Scuba diving	Football	Baseball	Track and field
Long-distance swimming	Lacrosse	Basketball	Hiking
Hang gliding	Rugby	Gymnastics	Cross-country skiing
Auto racing	Wrestling	Sailing	Crew, rowing
	Boxing	Wind surfing	Golf
	Soccer	Martial arts	Tennis
	Ski racing	Horseback riding	Table tennis
	Hockey		Badminton
			Archery
			Bowling
			Canoeing
			Riflery

REFERENCES

1. Engel J Jr. *Seizures and epilepsy.* Philadelphia: FA Davis Co, 1989.
2. Hauser WA, Annegers JF. Epidemiology of epilepsy. In: Laidaw JP, Reichens A, Chadwick D, eds. *Textbook of epilepsy,* 4th ed. New York: Churchill Livingstone, 1992.
3. Hauser WA, Annegers JF, Kurland LT. Prevalence of epilepsy in Rochester, Minnesota: 1940–1980. *Epilepsia* 1991;32:429–445.
4. Kurtzke JF. Neuroepidemiology. *Ann Neurol* 1984; 16:265–277.
5. Department of Health, Education and Welfare. Plan for nationwide action on epilepsy. DHEW Publication NIH 78-726, 1978:17–26.
6. Bennett DR. Sports and epilepsy: to play or not to play. *Semin Neurol* 1981;1:345–357.
7. Devinsky O. A guide to understanding and living with epilepsy. Philadelphia: FA Davis Co, 1994.
8. Commission on Classification and Terminology of the International League Against Epilepsy. Proposal for revised classification of epilepsies and epileptic syndromes. *Epilepsia* 1989;30:389–399.
9. Commission on Classification and Terminology of the International League Against Epilepsy. Proposal for revised clinical and electroencephalographic classification of epileptic syndromes. *Epilepsia* 1981;22:489–501.
10. Hauser WA, Annegers J. Risk factors for epilepsy. *Epilepsy Res.* 1991 (Suppl 4):45–52.
11. Annegers JF, Hauser WA, Beghi E, Nicolosi A, Kurland LT. The risk of unprovoked seizures after encephalitis and meningitis. *Neurology* 1988;38:1407–1410.
12. Franceschetti S, Battagha G, Lodrini S, et al. Relationship between tumors and epilepsy. In: Groggi G, ed. *The rational basis of surgical treatment of epilepsies.* London: John Libbey and Co, 1988.
13. Hauser WA, Morris ML, Heston LL, et al. Seizures and myoclonus in patients with Alzheimer's disease. *Neurology* 1986;36:1226.
14. Kinnunen E, Wikstrom J. Prevalence and prognosis of epilepsy in patients with multiple sclerosis. *Epilepsia* 1986;27:729.
15. Hauser WA, Nelson KB. Epidemiology of epilepsy in children. *Cleve Clin J Med* 1989; 56 (Suppl pt 2): S185–S194.
16. Goulden KJ, Shinnar S, Koller H, et al. Epilepsy in children with mental retardation: a cohort study. *Epilepsia* 1991;32:690–697.
17. Rocca WA, Sharbrough FW, Hauser WA, Annegers JF, Schoenberg BS. Risk factors for complex partial seizures: a population-based case-control study. *Ann Neurol* 1987;21:22–31.
18. Devinsky O. The differential diagnosis of epilepsy. *Semin Neurol* 1990;10:321–327.
19. Kempster PA, Balla JL. A clinical study of convulsive syncope. *Clin Exp Neurol* 1986;22:53–55.
20. Ziegler DK, Lin J, Bayer WL. Convulsive syncope: relationship to cerebral ischemia. *Trans Am Neurol Assoc* 1978;103:150–154.
21. Pacia SV, Devinsky O, Luciano DJ, Vazquez B. The prolonged QT syndrome presenting as epilepsy: a report of two cases and literature review. *Neurology* 1994;44: 1408–1410.
22. Mattson RH, Cramer JA, Collins JF, Department of Veterans Affairs Epilepsy Cooperative Study No. 264

Group. A comparison of valproate with carbamazepine for the treatment of complex partial seizures and secondarily generalized tonic–clonic seizures in adults. *N Engl J Med* 1992;327:765–771.
23. US Gabapentin Study Group No. 5. Gabapentin as add-on therapy in refractory partial epilepsy: a double-blind, placebo-controlled, parallel-group study. *Neurology* 1993;43:2292–2298.
24. Risner M, the Lamictal Study Group. Multicenter, double-blind, placebo-controlled, add-on, crossover study of lamotrigine (Lamictal) in epileptic outpatients with partial seizures. *Epilepsia* 1994;31:619–620.
25. Faught E, Sachdeo RC, Remler MP, et al. Felbamate monotherapy for partial-onset seizures: an active-control trial. *Neurology* 1993;43:688–692.
26. Pellock JM. Efficacy and adverse effects of antiepileptic drugs. *Pediatr Clin North Am* 1989;36:453–448.
27. Rosenbloom D, Sutton JR. Drugs and exercise. *Med Clin North Am* 1985;69:177–187.
28. Aslaksen A, Aanderudl L. Drug absorption during physical activity. *Br J Clin Pharmacol* 1980;10:383–385.
29. Boel J, Andersen LB, Rasmussen B, et al. Hepatic drug metabolism and physical fitness. *Clin Pharmacol Ther* 1984;36:121–126.
30. Lennox WG, Lennox MA. *Epilepsy and related disorders.* Boston: Little, Brown and Company, 1960;2:823–824.
31. Korczyn AD. Participation of epileptic patients in sports. *J Sports Med* 1979;19:195–198.
32. Götze W, Kubicki ST, Munter M, et al. Effect of physical exercise on seizure threshold (investigated by electroencephalographic telemetry). *Dis Nerv Syst* 1967; 28:664–667.
33. Ogunyemi A, Gomez MR, Klass DW. Seizures induced by exercise. *Neurology* 1988;38:633–634.
34. Kuijer A. Epilepsy and exercise, electroencephalographical and biochemical studies. In: Wada JA, Penry JK, eds. *Advances in epileptology: The Tenth Epilepsy International Symposium.* New York: Raven, 1980: 545.
35. Horyd W, Gryziak J, Niedzielska K, et al. Wplyw wysilku fizyczhego Na wyladowania Napadowe w EEG v chorych Na padaczke. *Neurol Neurochir Pol* 1981; 15:545–552.
36. Bemey TP, Osselton JW, Kolvin I, et al. Effect of discotheque environment on epileptic children. *Br Med J* 1981;282:180–182.
37. Department of Health, Education and Welfare. Plan for nationwide action on epilepsy. DHEW Publication NIH 78–276. Washington: USGPO, 1978: 29–43.
38. Van Linschoten R, Backx FJ, Meinardi H. Epilepsy and sports. *Sports Med* 1990;10(1):9–19.
39. Hauser WA, Annegers JF, Elveback LR. Mortality in patients with epilepsy. *Epilepsia* 1980;21:399–412.
40. Zielinski JJ. Epilepsy and mortality rate and cause of death. *Epilepsia* 1974;15:191–201.
41. Ryan CA, Dowling G. Drowning deaths with epilepsy. *Can Med Assoc J* 1993;148:781–784.
42. Peam J, Nixon J, Wilkey I. Freshwater drowning and near drowning accidents involving children. *Med J Aust* 1976;2:942–946.
43. Peam J, Bart R, Yamaoka R. Drowning risks to the epileptic: a study from Hawaii. *Br Med J* 1978;2: 1284–1285.
44. Aisenson MR. Accidental injuries in epileptic children. *Pediatrics* 1948;2:85–88.

45. Livingston S, Berman W. Participation of epileptic patients in sports. *JAMA* 1973;224:236–238.
46. Jennett BW. Early traumatic epilepsy: incidence and significance after non-missile injuries. *Arch Neurol* 1974;30:394–398.
47. Berman W. Sports and the child with epilepsy [Letter]. *Pediatrics* 1984;74:320–321.
48. Lidgren L, Walloe A. Incidence of fracture in epileptics. *Acta Orthop Scand* 1977;48:356–361.
49. Pedersen KK, Christiansen C, Ahlgren P, Lund M. Incidence of fracture of the vertebral spine in epileptic patients. *Acta Neurol Scand* 1976;54:200–203.
50. Jay GW, Leestma JE. Sudden death in epilepsy. *Acta Neurol Scand* 1981;82(Suppl):1–66.

Sports Neurology, Second Edition,
edited by Barry D. Jordan.
Lippincott–Raven Publishers, Philadelphia © 1998.

23

Stroke in Sports

Daniel MacGowan and *John J. Caronna

253 West 73rd Street, New York, New York 10023;
*Department of Neurology and Neuroscience, Cornell University
Medical College, 520 East 70th Street, New York, New York, 10021

In the United States, about 500,000 individuals have a stroke and 150,000 die from stroke each year, and about 2 million stroke survivors are living in the United States at any one time (1). Despite this, the association between stroke and sporting activity is reportedly rare and restricted to 44 case reports which are listed in Table 1. Nearly all of these are restricted to the population under the age of 45. Hence, this reflects a subsection of causes of stroke in the young. In the Western world, the annual incidence of stroke in those under the age of 45 is estimated as between 2 and 11 per 100,000, which means that 3% to 4% of all ischemic infarctions occur in this group (2,3). There are two interacting factors in the etiology of stroke occurring in sport. First, the sporting activity itself may in some way predispose to stroke through a number of different mechanisms that will be discussed. Second, the sportsperson may have medical risk factors for stroke (usually without his or her knowledge) that increase the stroke risk during exercise when blood pressure and cardiac index both rise. Thus, this chapter will initially discuss the etiology of stroke in the young and then discuss stroke specifically with reference to sport.

STROKE IN THE YOUNG

The incidence of stroke in the young (younger than age 45) is 6 per 100,000 per year in whites but is 2.5 times higher in blacks. In addition, this incidence markedly increases in those older than 40 years to 38 per 100,000 and nearly three times

this in African-American males (4). The largest cohort of young stroke patients has been published (5). It is a group of 329 patients admitted with an arterial ischemic stroke with a mean age of 35 accumulated over 15.5 years. The etiology of stroke differed markedly from that in older populations in that there was less primary atherosclerosis (9.7%) and much more hematologic and cardiac abnormalities (48%). Small vessel occlusion, primarily vasculitic, accounted for 7.9% of causes, and the etiology in the remaining 34.3% was undetermined. This more complex etiologic profile reflects both increased use of new technology [Transesophageal echo-cardiography (TEE), MRI, anticardiolipin antibody, protein C and S, and anti–thrombin III testing] and the wide range of diagnostic possibilities for stroke in the young (Table 2). Stroke secondary to venous sinus occlusion, which was not included in the preceding survey, may be due to blockage resulting from a mass such as a meningioma or a hypercoagulable state, be it congenital or acquired. As listed in Table 2, there are three broad diagnostic categories, cardiac, vascular, and hematologic abnormalities, along with two types of stroke, arterial and venous.

Arterial dissections accounted for 6% of cases. These are often spontaneous but may be related to a history of trauma to the neck as in many of the reported cases of stroke in sports. Some of the causes of stroke in the young remain controversial. Anticardiolipin antibodies are often an epiphenomenon after endothelial injury, particularly the immunoglobulin M (IgM) variant, but

TABLE 1. *Case reports of stroke directly related to sporting activity*

Scenario	Central nervous system findings	Documentation
Baseball pitching (33)	Subclavian artery injury	
	Right hemisphere infarct	Arteriography
Basketball (44)	Internal carotid artery dissection	
	Right hemisphere infarct	Arteriography
Bowling (44)	Right retinal and brain TIAs	Arteriography
Football (58)	Hemisphere infarct	Arteriography
Swimming (44)	Left hemisphere infarct	Arteriography
Water-skiing (46)	Right hemisphere infarct	Arteriography
Skiing (10 cases) (42)	Hemisphere infarcts	MRI, angiography
Scuba diving (45)	Left hemisphere stroke	MRI, angiography
Raquetball (61)	Vertebral artery dissection	
	Left medullary infarct	Arteriography
Skiing (two cases) (42)	Brainstem infarcts	CT, MRI, angiography
Volleyball (62)	Brainstem TIAs	History, MRI
Judo (63)	Left thalamic stroke	CT, MRI
Aerobics/calisthenics (64)	Cervicomedullary infarct	CT, MRI, angiography
Skating	Cerebellar infarct	CT, MRI
Golf (65)	Lateral medullary infarct	MRI
Archery (66)	Right medullary infarct	Arteriography
Calisthenics (67)	Cervical cord infarct	Arteriography
Diving (68)	Right medullary TIAs	Neurologic examination
Football (tackling) (58)	Cervical cord infarct	Neurologic examination
Football (blocking) (69)	Cervical cord infarct	Autopsy
Football (catching) (69)	Brainstem TIAs	Neurologic history
Football (44)	Brainstem infarct	Arteriography
Football (tackling) (70)	Brainstem infarct	Arteriography
Gymnastics (parallel bar) (71)	Cervical cord infarct	Arteriography
Swimming (crawl) (72)	Right cerebellar infarct	CT, MRI, angiography
Wrestling (73)	Brainstem TIAs	Neurologic history
Wrestling (half-Nelson) (74)	Right brainstem infarct	Arteriography
Yoga (71)	Left cerebellar infarct	Arteriography
Yoga (41)	Left brainstem infarct	Arteriography
Yoga (75)	Medulla and cerebellar infarct	Autopsy
Body building with androgen abuse (76)	Basal ganglia infarct	MRI, angiography
Body building with androgen abuse (57)	Hemispheric infarct	CT, angiography
Body building with androgen abuse (77)	Hemispheric infarct	CT, angiography
Body building with androgen abuse (78)	Sagittal sinus thrombosis	MRI, angiography

there seems little doubt that repeated IgG positivity in the clinical setting of stroke or transient ischemic attack (TIA) represents a high vascular risk and these patients should be treated with anticoagulation to an international normalized ratio (INR) value greater than 3 (6). Similarly, free protein S (functional activity) deficiency in the presence of normal total (or antigen) levels reflects increased uptake by complement C4bBP, an acute-phase reactant increased in acutely ill patients (7). However, reduced total levels of protein C and/or S are always significant. The finding of a patent foramen ovale (PFO) with a right-to-left shunt on TEE is difficult to assess, as it is found in up to 30% of autopsies and is associated with a low stroke recurrence risk. Parameters used to assess its significance include its size, the extent of the shunt, and the presence of deep venous thrombosis (8). Despite this, there is little evidence to justify management with anything other than aspirin or low-dose warfarin. Surgical closure does not appear justified. Few patients demonstrate any evidence of deep venous thrombosis. An attractive concept linking this entity with stroke in sports would be the increased likelihood of right-to-left shunt with the Valsalva and increased intrathoracic pressure that occur during physical exercise. However, there are no reported cases of this association.

The relationship between drug use and stroke in the young is relatively firm and established. Thirty of 329 patients in the study mentioned ear-

TABLE 2. *Conditions predisposing to early stroke*

Arterial stroke

Cardiac
  Atrial fibrillation
  Valvular disease (congenital, rheumatic, prosthetic, infectious, or merantic)
  Cardiomyopathy
  Patent foramen ovale (paradoxical embolus)
Vascular disease
  Congenital—Moyamoya, hereditary elastic tissue disorders, (Marfan's, Ehler-Danhos, pseudoxanthoma elas-
    ticum), coarctation of the aorta, and mitochondrial disorders (MELAS)[a]
  Atherosclerotic—hypertension, diabetes, hyperlipidemia, hypertriglyceridemia, homocystinuria, and Fabry's
    disease
  Arteritis—collagen vascular disease, Behçet's. Takayasu's, Wegener's, and cocaine
  Vasospasm—post subarachnoid hemorrhage, migraine, cocaine, amphetamine, phenylpropranolamine
  Dissection—trauma, spontaneous, fibromuscular dysplasia and elastin disorders
  Infectious or parainfectious—syphilitic or tuberculous arteritis, post zoster angiitis, mycotic aneurysm, and
    cerebral malaria
Hypercoagulable states
  Oral contraception, androgens, pregnancy, puerperium, hemoglobinopathies, polycythemia, thrombocytosis,
    DIC, TTP, HUS,[b] antiphospholipid antibodies, deficiencies of proteins C and S and antithrombin III

Venous stroke

Structural
  Occlusion of sinuses by a mass (e.g., meningioma) or thrombosis by a fistula)
Functional
  Hypercoagulable states, as listed above

[a] MELAS, myoclonic epilepsy, lactic acidosis, and strokelike episodes.
[b] DIC, disseminated intravascular coagulation; TTP, thrombotic thrombocytopenic purpura; HUS, hemolytic ure-
mic syndrome.

lier (5) had a history of recent use of drugs most commonly alcohol (9), cocaine and amphetamine (10), phenylpropanolamine (11), and heroin (11). The amphetamines, cocaine, and sympathomimetic alpha-agonists are all occasionally used before sporting activity and all predispose to cerebral infarction resulting from acute hypertension and cerebral vasospasm. Both amphetamine and cocaine can rarely cause an inflammatory cerebral vasculitis that leads to ischemic stroke and/or subarachnoid hemorrhage. The more traditional cocaine hydrochloride causes intracerebral or subarachnoid hemorrhage much more often than infarction, whereas alkaloidal cocaine ("crack") causes hemorrhage and infarction with equal frequency (12). More than 50% of cocaine-induced cerebral or subarachnoid hemorrhages demonstrate an aneurysm or arteriovenous malformation on arteriography (12). Unlike the situation in the middle-aged and elderly (13), heavy acute alcohol consumption (> 40 g within the past 24 hours) appears to be a significant independent risk factor for ischemic stroke in the young (14).

Cigarette consumption, however, was not found to be a siginificant risk factor. In the elderly and middle-aged, moderate alcohol intake protects against ischemic stroke, and heavy alcohol intake is a major risk factor for intracerebral hemorrhage. Arterial hypertension and cigarette consumption are the major risk factors for ischemic stroke in this population.

The oral contraceptive pill appears to double the risk of all stroke in current users, an effect independent of smoking status (15). This risk falls to nonsignificant levels in former users. Finally, there are now four reported cases of stroke associated with anabolic steroid use in bodybuilders, as listed in Table 1. Three are ischemic strokes in the internal or middle cerebral artery distribution and the fourth is a case of extensive superior sagittal, straight, and transverse sinus thrombosis without a complete infarction. The agents used were intramuscular testosterone, metolonone, trembolone, and oral ethylestrenol. The use was prolonged in three cases for 4 to 5 years but in one patient was limited to a 6-week period of 6 to 8 mg of ethylestrenol daily followed by a complete internal carotid artery stroke. Results of detailed laboratory and hematologic testing were all normal, but it is well established that exogenous androgens are thrombogenic by potentiating platelet aggregation in vivo and disturbing the prostacyclin–thromboxane A_2 ratio in favor of the latter (16,17). Arterial and venous stroke complicating androgen therapy for aplastic anemia and hypogonadism is also well described (16). Thus, athletes would be well advised of the risks of thrombotic events before taking performance-enhancing androgens. In addition, a careful inquiry may be necessary to elicit a history of androgen use in young patients with acute vascular events.

Lastly, the prognosis for stroke in the young is clearly better than in the elderly, but there are significant mortality and morbidity. Prospective follow-up over a mean period of 6 years for 296 patients aged 15 to 45 with acute stroke revealed a mortality of 4% and stroke recurrence risk of 9% (3). Overall mortality rose to 18% over the 6 years as a result of recurrent stroke or another vascular event. Outcome was worse in those with a large-vessel stroke and those who had a determined cause of their stroke. Only 49% of patients were still alive, without a recurrent event and not disabled or requiring major vascular surgery, after the 6 years.

Table 3 shows the important historical features, symptoms, and signs in the athlete with an acute stroke. It is important to note that a history of exertional syncope, presyncope, or palpitations is an important predictor of exercise-related deaths and vascular events, as 15% of sports-related sudden deaths have been heralded by these symptoms (18). Careful cardiac and electrocardiographic examination is invaluable in detecting cardiac lesions and conduction abnormalities. Traditionally, it has been felt that as many as 50% of subarachnoid hemorrhages have a preceding history of a sudden warning occipital "sentinel" headache (19). Evidence suggests that this concept may be overestimated (20). A prospective study of 148 patients with acute, severe, "thunderclap" occipital headache showed that 25% were caused by subarachnoid hemorrhage. An additional 12% had another serious

TABLE 3. *Physical signs in the evaluation of the athlete with stroke*

History
Neck pain, neck trauma, drug use, oral contraception, recent purulent infection or dental work, family history, cigarette or alcohol use

Physical signs
Appearance, habitus: obesity, marfanism, joint hypermobility, "chicken pock skin" in axillae (pseudoxanthoma elasticum), cutaneous xanthomata (hyperlipidemia), butterfly malar rash (systemic lupus erythematosus), livedo reticularis (antiphospholipid antibody syndrome), cutaneous angiokeratomata on abdomen (Fabry's disease), Horner's syndrome (carotid dissection)
Pulse, blood pressure: atrial fibrillation, pulsus bisferiens (hypertrophic obstructive cardiomyopathy), inter-limb discrepancy (subclavian stenosis, aortic coarctation), secondary hypertension.
Cardiac examination: thrills or heaves, cyanosis, murmurs or clicks, rubs and "plops"
Neck: bruits, arterial tenderness
Urine: hematuria (subacute bacterial endocarditis), glycosuria (diabetes mellitus), proteinuria (renal disease)

neurologic disorder, and the remaining 63% had migraine and other benign diagnoses. None of these patients developed a subarachnoid hemorrhage or other serious neurologic disorder over the following year. This seemed to downplay the concept of a sentinel headache. The best approach is CT scanning of all patients with acute severe occipital headache and performing a lumbar puncture if the scan is negative and clinical suspicion is still high. There is much retrospective evidence showing that acute, severe exertional headache is a presenting feature of a third of ruptured aneurysms and a quarter of bleeding arteriovenous aneurysms (21). This reflects the increase in systolic, diastolic, and pulse pressures that occurs during exercise (9).

The management and treatment of stroke in the young are more elaborate than in the elderly. A careful cardiac, hematologic, and rheumatologic workup is required, in addition to MRI and magnetic resonance angiography (MRA) of the brain. A cerebral arteriogram is usually performed if vasculitis is suspected, and if it is negative, a biopsy of meninges may be necessary. Serial blood cultures should be obtained if endocarditis is suspected. Traditionally, cardioembolic stroke has been managed with acute heparinization [maintaining partial thromboplastin time (PTT) at 1.5 to 2 times the control value), provided the infarct is not large with a mass effect (22). However, one report contradicts infarct size and clinical severity as risk factors for clinically relevant hemorrhagic conversion (23), finding a PTT greater than twice the control value to be the only significant predictor. Hemorrhagic change occurred at a frequency of 24% but was clinically relevant in only 8% of patients heparinized for cardioembolic stroke. Long-term warfarinization is usually necessary for chronic stroke prophylaxis. Warfarinization to an INR value above 3 is recommended to treat stroke due to anticardiolipin antibody syndrome or protein C, protein S, or antithrombin III deficiency. Cerebral vasculitis with or without a primary connective tissue disorder is best treated with pulse steroids and/or cycophosphamide (24). Plasmapheresis may be useful in the acute setting (24). The management of arterial dissection is discussed later. Stroke related to venous sinus thrombosis presents more insidiously, complicated by encephalopathy, focal signs, seizures, and ultimately herniation caused by massive cerebral edema. It is crucial to commence therapy with heparin before stupor and herniation begin. Prompt heparinization dramatically improves outcome even if the venous infarct is hemorrhagic, as it often is (16). The outcome is usually fatal by the time the patient is stuporous and herniating.

Finally, the advent of multiple experimental trials using thrombolytic, cytoprotective, and other therapies underlines the importance of rapid acute transfer and management of the patient with acute stroke, as the therapeutic window is about 4 to 6 hours (25). The American Heart Association has issued guidelines for the management of acute ischemic stroke and transient ischemic attacks (11).

THE MECHANISMS OF STROKE IN SPORTS

Stroke associated with physical activity may be caused by (a) trauma to the extracranial arteries feeding the brain or (b) the physiologic effects of exercise on patients with any of the underlying

cardiac, vascular, toxic, hematologic, or rheumatologic risk factors already discussed. The risk of intracranial and subarachnoid hemorrhage with physical exertion has also been discussed. There remains a need to discuss the effect of trauma on the neck and intracranial vessels. Arterial trauma of the neck may be external or caused by excessive head turning, flexion, or extension. Strokes have been ascribed to both mechanisms. Both lead initially to hemodynamic effects of occluded flow but may also cause acute arterial dissection. Stroke is a consequence of the latter (26) as it has long been recognised that neck movement leads to significant angiographic reduction of flow without symptoms (27). This is a consequence of the rich primary collateral sources of flow in all directions around the circle of Willis. The reported cases of "sporting stroke" have been listed in Table 1.

Carotid Artery Dissection

The incidence is reportedly 2.6 per 100,000 (28), but with the advent of MRI, this entity is being increasingly recognized. There is usually a history of mild or moderate neck trauma and localized pain just beneath the angle of the jaw (29,30). An ipsilateral Horner syndrome and pulsatile tinnitus are both useful signs. Lower cranial nerve signs and dysgeusia may also occur (31). Oculomotor palsies have been reported as a presenting sign (32). Subsequent transient ischemic attacks are common and may involve both the ipsilateral eye and brain. Visual scintillations and bright sparkles reminiscent of migraine are also common. These TIA's herald acute infarction, which is invariably in the territory of the middle cerebral artery and is either arterioembolic or due to distal propagation of the thrombus. Evidence suggests that only a half of dissections lead to a stroke and the outcome of these strokes is invariably good, as most of these patients are young and have an intact collateral system (28,33–35). Recurrence is unusual, with an annual rate of approximately 1%, and, interestingly, never affects the same artery as before (35). The trauma, usually blunt, leads to an intimal tear and intramural bleeding into the media. This intramural clot expands longitudinally and ultimately compresses the lumen. A pseudoaneurysm may form and may rupture back into the lumen, leading to intraluminal thrombus formation. The thrombus propagates distally and embolizes, leading to cerebral ischemia. The dissection always occurs distal to the carotid bulb at the pharyngeal section and the arteriogram shows a long tapering "string" sign with expansion again intracranially. MRI and MRA are at least as good as arteriography (36) for diagnosis and Doppler ultrasonography is also useful, particularly in prospective monitoring of the dissection (37). Many dissections are spontaneous with no apparent cause apart from mild trauma, but it is important to rule out many predisposing entities: hereditary elastic tissue disorders (38), fibromuscular dysplasia (39), cystic medial necrosis, and carotid arterial loop redundancy (40). There are no prospective trials of anticoagulation, but there is ample retrospective and anecdotal evidence for its efficacy (28,33,34,41). Most authors recommend warfarin until recanalization is complete, which traditionally required repeated arteriography but can now be done using Doppler or MRA (37). Surgical endarterectomy and removal of the clot are rarely required and reserved for patients who have ongoing ischemic events despite heparinization.

The largest report of sporting carotid dissection with stroke was of 10 cases that occurred while skiing (42). The patients had a mean age of 47.1 years with no one under the age of 25, suggesting a predisposing age-related weakness of the arterial wall. All but one of the patients had a fall, with severe trauma in six and moderate to minor trauma in five. An additional two patients had vertebral artery dissections and posterior circulation strokes. The effect of high-altitude hypoxia may increase the likelihood of stroke after dissection. Carotid dissections resulting from sudden or repeated neck movements have been reported during many sporting activities, including football (43), swimming (44), scuba diving (45), bowling (44), and water-skiing (46). Extreme head rotation results in compression of the contralateral internal carotid artery by the transverse process of C-1, and this is the the proposed mechanism for these dissections (Fig. 1). Intracranial dissections of the carotid artery are very rare and may occur in the intrapetrous section of the artery as a complication of head trauma with (47) and without (48) basal skull fractures. Dissections of the supraclinoid internal carotid artery and middle cerebral artery are also very rare but more serious and invariably associated with severe infarction, pseudoaneurysm, and subarachnoid hemorrhage. These patients usually have elastic tissue disorders and the dis-

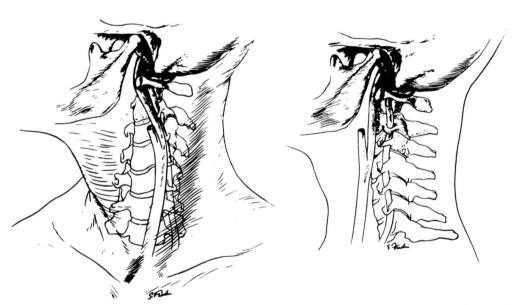

FIG. 1. Extreme head rotation resulting in compression of the contralateral internal carotid artery by the transverse process of C-1.

sections occur spontaneously, affecting both anterior and posterior circulations.

Figure 2 shows an internal carotid artery dissection demonstrated by MRI with an associated stroke.

Vertebral Artery Dissection

Fifty percent of head rotation occurs at the atlantooccipital joint before any at the lower cervical spine (10), and this is the site at which nearly 90% of vertebral artery dissections occur (49). Indeed, rotation of the head is often followed by asymptomatic arteriographic interruption of flow at the level of the atlantooccipital junction (27). At this site the vessels emerge from the transverse process of C-1 and kink backward before entering the suboccipital triangle. They then pierce the atlantooccipital membrane and dura to run up the lateral cervicomedullary spine and join to form the basilar artery at the lower pons. Figure 3 shows the mechanical compression of the contralateral vertebral artery on turning the head. Sometimes head turning leads to brief direction-specific symptoms of vertebrobasilar ischemia (VBI) that are relieved by moving the head out of the incriminating position. It has long been suspected from multiple case reports and anecdote that cervical zygoapophyseal osteophytes (50), anomalous muscle insertions (51), posterolateral disc rupture (52), dysplastic occipital condyles (53), fractures, dislocations, and rheumatoid arthritis (54) may all cause extrinsic vertebral artery compression that leads to symptoms of VBI on head turning. However, these pathologic entities are all common and only rarely associated with these symptoms. Transcranial Doppler (TCD) assessment has managed to elucidate this syndrome and its causes more clearly (55). The P-1 segments of both posterior cerebral arteries (PCAs) were insonated continuously while observing changes in flow on head rotation and flexion. Four patients with severe degenerative cervical spine disease and a clear history of brief direction-specific hemodynamic VBI were compared width 10 patients with more vague, prolonged symptoms without a clear relationship to a specific head motion. Ten normal control subjects showed physiologic reductions in PCA flow by an average of 15% without any symptoms developing. Extension reduced flow the most (24%). All 10 patients with vague symtoms of dizziness and blurred vision showed

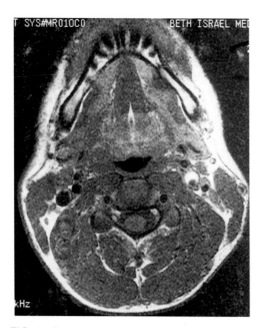 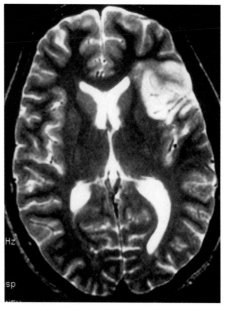

FIG. 2. An internal carotid artery dissection demonstrated by magnetic resonance imaging with an associated stroke.

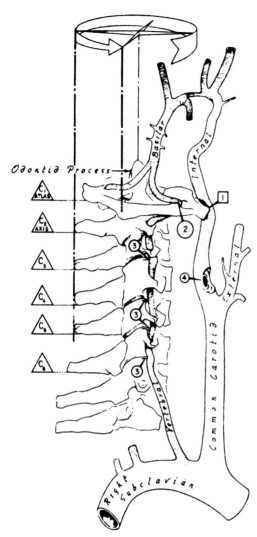

FIG. 3. Mechanical compression of the contralateral vertebral artery on turning the head.

phytes. However, this is a common asymptomatic arteriographic finding, suggesting that for symptoms to occur, contralateral vertebral artery anomalies or disease must occur. Interestingly, all four patients failed to fill the posterior communicating arteries on carotid injection, resulting in a failed anteroposterior compensatory shunt. Thus, it would appear that anomalies or occlusion of the circle of Willis precipitate hemodynamic VBI in these patients. These are all common, in up to 50% of autopsy series (56): vertebral artery hypoplasia, termination of the vertebral artery at the posterior inferior cerebellar branch, posterior communicating artery hypoplasia, and fetal origin of the posterior cerebral artery. Vertebral arteries may also be commonly occluded by atheroma. The transcranial Doppler method is now useful for assessing the significance of these symptoms that are commonly seen in practice and that may occur during sporting activities with excessive neck motion.

However, posterior fossa stroke occurs rarely because the patients move their heads out of the incriminating position. Stroke occurs as a consequence of dissection and thrombus formation at the atlantooccipital level. By far the most common reported cause of this syndrome is chiropractic manipulation (57,58). A review of 39 cases with arteriography showed that 89% had dissection at the atlantooccipital level (57). Infarction is most common in the brainstem and often of the lateral medullary variant. Mortality and severe morbidity (locked-in syndrome) were high at nearly 30%. A remarkable finding is the lack of any of the predisposing comorbid features of hemodynamic VBI discussed earlier. Sometimes there may be an anomaly of the contralateral vertebral artery, but significant cervical spine abnormalities were not present. Neither were there significant vascular risk factors. This correlates with the reported cases of sporting vertebral dissection stroke listed in Table 1, which had no particular risk factors apart from the activity itself. Nearly all were reportedly healthy young adults under the age of 45. Therefore, stroke related to vertebral artery dissection seems to be a difficult entity to predict and prevent. Treatment is invariably medical with anticoagulation as in carotid dissection. Patients refractory to medical therapy may be considered for a by-

no significant difference from controls, whereas the remaining 4 patients with specific VBI symptoms (vertigo, diplopia) showed significant, greater than 50% drops in PCA flow on turning the head to the incriminating side. All these drops in flow were followed by a reactive hyperemic mean increase in flow of 149%, suggesting hemodynamically significant compression and restoration of flow. All four patients showed arteriographic features of rotation-induced vertebral artery occlusion at the level of the transverse foramina by osteo-

pass procedure connecting the occipital and the posterior inferior cerebellar arteries (59). Another option may be to bypass the superficial temporal artery to the posterior cerebral artery.

Subclavian Stenosis and Sports

This has been reported in a baseball pitcher and presumably resulted from recurrent traumatic compression by the first rib (33). The pitcher developed an acute stroke as a consequence of thrombus formation and proximal propagation into the innominate artery with embolization up the internal carotid artery. The subclavian steal syndrome results from a vertebral shunt downward to the subclavian artery with resulting ipsilateral symptoms of VBI on exercise and elevation of the arm. Like all purely hemodynamic VBI, stroke occurs rarely. The subclavian steal syndrome is far more commonly seen as an asymptomatic arteriographic entity (60).

SUMMARY

Stroke complicating sporting activity is a rarely reported event, and most cases involve external trauma or sustained head rotation with resulting dissection of a major extracranial vessel. Ischemic symptoms usually occur within the next few days or hours but have been reported to be delayed by up to a month. Anticoagulation is necessary to prevent further thrombosis and ischemia. Stroke without any history of trauma or precipitation by head motion suggests either a major risk factor for stroke in the young or the use of stimulants or anabolic steroids. The advent of many new experimental therapies for acute stroke requires that these patients be rapidly transferred and assessed within 6 hours.

REFERENCES

1. American Heart Association. The National Health and Nutrition examination survey II, 1976–1980. 1992 Heart and Stroke facts. Dallas 1991.
2. Nencini P, Inzitari D, et al. Incidence of stroke in young adults in Florence, Italy. *Stroke* 1988;19:977–981.
3. Jaap Kappelle L, Adams HP. Prognosis of young adults with ischemic stroke. A long term follow up study assessing recurrent vascular events and functional outcome in the Iowa Registry of stroke in young adults. *Stroke* 1994;25:1360–1365.
4. Kittner SJ, McCarter RJ, et al. Black–white differences in stroke risk among young adults. *Stroke* 1993; (Suppl): 13–15.
5. Adams HP, Jaap Kappelle L, et al. Ischemic stroke in young adults. Experience in 329 patients enrolled in the Iowa Registry of Stroke in Young Adults. *Arch Neurol* 1995;52:491–495.
6. Khamashta MA, Cuadrado MJ, et al. The management of thrombosis in the antiphospholipid-antibody syndrome. *N Engl J Med* 1995;332:993–997.
7. Barinagarrementeria F, Cantu-Brito C, et al. Prothrombotic states in young people with idiopathic stroke. A prospective study. *Stroke* 1994;287–290.
8. Hanna JP, Sun JP, et al. Patent foramen ovale and brain infarct. Echocardiographic predictors, recurrence and prevention. *Stroke* 1994;25:782–786.
9. Carlstein A, Grimby G. The circulatory response to muscular exercise in man. Springfield, IL: Charles C Thomas, 1966.
10. Cailliet R. *Neck and arm pain.* Philadelphia: FA Davis Co, 1964.
11. Adams HP, Brott TG, et al. Guidelines for the management of patients with acute ischemic stroke. A statement for healthcare professionals from a special writing group of the Stroke Council, American Heart Association. *Stroke* 1994;25:1901–1914.
12. Brust JC. Clinical, radiological and pathological aspects of cerebrovascular disease associated with drug abuse. *Stroke* 1993; (Suppl 1):129–133.
13. Gorelick PB, Rodin MB, et al. Is acute alcohol ingestion a risk factor for ischemic stroke? Results of a controlled study in middle aged and elderly stroke patients at three urban medical centers. *Stroke* 1987;18:359–364.
14. Hillbom M, Haapaniemi H, et al. Recent alcohol consumption, cigarette smoking and cerebral infarction in young adults. *Stroke* 1995;26:40–45.
15. Hannaford PC, Croft PR, et al. Oral contraception and stroke. Evidence from the Royal College of General Practitioners' oral contraception study. *Stroke* 1994;25: 935–942.
16. Einhaupl KM, Villringer A, et al. Heparin treatment in sinus venous thrombosis. *Lancet* 1991;338:597–600.
17. Ferenchick GS. Are androgenic steroids thrombogenic? *N Engl J Med* 1990;322:476.
18. Maron BJ, Roberts WC, et al. Sudden death in young adults. *Circulation* 1980;62:218–229.
19. Gillingham FJ. The management of ruptured intracranial aneurysms. *Scott Med J* 1967;12:377–383.
20. Linn FH, Wijdicks EF. A prospective study of sentinel headache in aneurysmal subarachnoid hemorrhage 1994; 344:590–593.
21. Locksley HB. Report on cooperative study of intracranial aneurysms and subarachnoid hemorrhage. Section V, Part I: Natural history of subarachnoid hemorrhage, intracranial aneurysms and arteriovenous malformations. *J Neurosurg* 1966;25:219–239.
22. Hornig CR, Bauer T, et al. Hemorrhagic transformation in cardioembolic cerebral infarction. *Stroke* 1993;24: 465–468.

23. Chamorro A, Vila N, et al. Early anticoagulation after large cerebral embolic infarction. A safety study. *Neurology* 1995;45:861–865.

24. Cohen Tervaert JW, Kallenberg C. Neurological manifestations of systemic vasculitides. *Rheum Dis Clin North Am* 1993;19:913–940.

25. Siesjo BK. Pathophysiology and treatment of focal cerebral ischemia. Part II: Mechanisms of damage and treatment. *J Neurosurg* 1992;77:337–354.

26. Sherman DG, Hart RG. Abrupt change in head position and cerebral infarction. *Stroke* 1981;12:2–6.

27. Bauer R, Sheehan S, et al. Arteriographic study of cerebrovascular disease. II. Cerebral symptoms due to kinking, tortuosity and compression of carotid and vertebral arteries in the neck. *Arch Neurol* 1961;4:119–131.

28. Schievink WI, Mokri B, et al. Internal carotid artery dissection in a community: Rochester, Minnesota, 1987–1992. *Stroke* 1993;24:1678–1680.

29. Fisher CM, Ojemann RJ, et al. Spontaneous dissection of cervicocerebral arteries. *Can J Neurol Sci* 1978;5:9–19.

30. Hart RD, Easton JD. Dissections and trauma of cerebral arteries. *Neurol Clin* 1983;1:155–182.

31. Sturzenneger M, Huber P. Cranial nerve palsies in spontaneous carotid artery dissection. *J Neurol Neurosurg Psychiatry* 1993;56:1191–1199.

32. Schievink WI, Mokri B, et al. Oculomotor nerve palsies in spontaneous disorders of cervical internal carotid artery. *Neurology* 1993;43:1938–1941.

33. Fields WS. Neurovascular syndromes of the neck and shoulders. *Semin Neurol* 1981;1:301–309.

34. Schievink WI, Mokri B, et al. Spontaneous dissections of cervicocephalic arteries in childhood and adolescence. *Neurology* 1994;44:1607–1612.

35. Schievink WI, Mokri B. Recurrent spontaneous cervical-artery dissection. *N Engl J Med* 1994;330:393–397.

36. Klufas RA, Hsu L, et al. Dissection of carotid and vertebral arteries: imaging with magnetic resonance angiography. *AJR* 1995;164:673–677.

37. Steinke W, Rautenberg W, et al. Non-invasive monitoring of internal carotid artery dissection. *Stroke* 1994; 25:998–1005.

38. Schievink WI, Michels VV. Neurovascular manifestations of heritable connective tissue disorders. A review. *Stroke* 1994;25:889–903.

39. Luscher TF, Lie JT, et al. Arterial fibromuscular dysplasia. *Mayo Clin Proc* 1987;62:931–952.

40. Barbour PJ, Castaldo JE, et al. Internal carotid artery redundancy is significantly associated with dissection. *Stroke* 1994;25:1201–1206.

41. Hanus S, Homer T, et al. Vertebral artery occlusion complicating yoga exercises. *Arch Neurol* 1977;34:574–575.

42. Noelle B, Clavier I, et al. Cervicocephalic arterial dissections related to skiing. *Stroke* 1994;24:526–527.

43. Schneider RC. Serious and fatal neurosurgical football injuries. *Clin Neurosurg* 1966;12:226–236.

44. Luken MG, Ascher GF, et al. Spontaneous dissecting aneurysms of the extracranial internal carotid artery. *Clin Neurosurg* 1979;26:353–375.

45. Nelson EE. Internal carotid artery dissection associated with scuba diving. *Ann Emerg Med* 1995;25:103–106.

46. Fields WS. Non-penetrating trauma of the cervical arteries. *Semin Neurol* 1981;1:284–290.

47. Thompson JLG. Traumatic thrombosis of the internal carotid artery in the carotid canal. *Br J Radiol* 1963; 36:840–842.

48. Mastaglia FL, Savas S, et al. Intracranial thrombosis of the internal carotid artery after closed head injury. *J Neurol Neurosurg Psychiatry* 1969;32:383–388.

49. Frisoni GB, Anzola PA. Vertebrobasilar ischemia after neck motion. *Stroke* 1991;22:1452–1460.

50. Nagashima C. Vertebral artery insufficiency and cervical spondylosis. In: Fein JM, Flam ES, eds. *Cerebrovascular surgery.* New York: Springer-Verlag, 1985:529–555.

51. Dadsetan MR, Skerhut H. Rotational vertebrobasilar insufficiency secondary to vertebral artery occlusion from fibrous band of the longus colli muscle. *Neuroradiology* 1990;32:514–515.

52. Budway RJ, Senter HJ. Cervical disc rupture causing vertebrobasilar insufficiency. *Neurosurgery* 1993;33: 745–747.

53. Berciano J, Coria F. Occipitoatlantal instability: a hemodynamic cause of vertebrobasilar ischemia after neck motion. *Stroke* 1992;23:921.

54. Jones MW, Kaufmann JC. Vertebrobasilar insufficiency in rheumatoid atalantoaxial subluxation. *J Neurol Neurosurg Psychiatry* 1976;39:122–128.

55. Sturzenneger M, Newell DW, et al. Dynamic transcranial Doppler assessment of positional vertebrobasilar ischemia. *Stroke* 1994;25:1776–1783.

56. Riggs HE, Rupp CH. Variation in form of the circle of Willis. *Arch Neurol* 1963;8:24–30.

57. Frankle MA, Eichberg R, et al. Anabolic androgenic steroids and a stroke in an athlete: case report. *Arch Phys Med Rehabil* 1988;69:632–633.

58. Schneider RC, Reifel E, et al. Serious and fatal football injuries involving the head and spinal cord. *JAMA* 1961;177:362–367.

59. Sundt TM Jr. *Occlusive cerebrovascular disease: diagnosis and surgical management.* Philadelphia:WB Saunders, 1987.

60. Hennerici M, et al. The subclavian steal phenomenon: a common vascular disorder with rare neurological deficits. *Neurology* 1988;38:669.

61. Tramo MJ, Hainline B. Stroke in sports, In: Jordan B, Tsairis P, Warren R, eds. *Sports neurology.* Rockville, MD: Aspen Publishers, 1989.

62. Behnke DJ, Brady W. Vertebral artery dissection due to minor neck trauma (while playing volleyball). *J Emerg Med* 1994;12:27–31.

63. Lannuzel A, Moulin T, et al. Vertebral artery dissection following a judo session, a case report. *Neuropediatrics* 1994;25:106–108.

64. Pryse-Phillips W. Infarction of the medulla and cervical cord after fitness exercises. *Stroke* 1989;20:292–294.

65. Taniguchi A, Wako K, et al. Wallenberg syndrome and vertebral artery dissection probably due to trivial trauma during golf exercise. *Rinsho Shinkeigaku* 1993;33: 338–340.

66. Sorensen B. Bow hunter's stroke. *Neurosurgery* 1978;2: 259–261.

67. Grinkler R, Guy C. Sprain of the cervical spine causing thrombosis of the anterior spinal artery. *JAMA* 1927;88: 1140–1142.

68. Suechting RL, French LA. Posterior inferior cerebellar artery syndrome following a fracture of the cervical vertebra. *J Neurosurg* 1955;12:187–189.

69. Schneider RC, Gosch HH, et al. Vascular insufficiency and differential distortion of the brain and cord caused by cervicomedullary football injuries. *J Neurosurg* 1970;33:363–375.

70. Marks RL, Freed MM. Non-penetrating injuries of the neck and cerebrovascular accident. *Arch Neurol* 1973; 28:412–414.
71. Nagler W. Vertebral artery obstruction by hyperextension of the neck: report of three cases. *Arch Phys Med Rehabil* 1973;54:237–240.
72. Tramo MJ, Hainline B, et al. Vertebral artery injury and cerebellar stroke while swimming: case report. *Stroke* 1985;16:1039–1042.
73. Ford FR. Syncope, vertigo and disturbances of vision resulting from intermittent obstruction of the vertebral arteries due to defect in the odontoid process and excessive mobility of the second cervical vertebra. *Bull Johns Hopkins Hosp* 1952;92:168–173.
74. Rogers L, Sweeney PJ. Stroke—a neurological complication of wrestling. *Am J Sports Med* 1979;7:352–354.
75. Hilton-Jones D, Warlow CP. Non-penetrating arterial trauma and cerebral infarction in the young. *Lancet* 1985;1:1435–1438.
76. Akhter J, Hyder S, et al. Cerebrovascular accident associated with anabolic steroid use in a young man. *Neurology* 1994;44:2405–2406.
77. Mochizuki RM, Richter KJ. Cardiomyopathy and cerebrovascular accident associated with anabolic-androgenic steroid use. *Phys Sports Med* 1988;16;109–114.
78. Jaillard AS, Hommel M, et al. Venous sinus thrombosis associated with androgens in a healthy young man. *Stroke* 1994;25:212–213.

Sports Neurology, Second Edition,
edited by Barry D. Jordan.
Lippincott–Raven Publishers, Philadelphia © 1998.

24

Abnormal Movement Disorders

A. J. Lees

*National Hospital for Neurology & Neurosurgery, Queen Square,
London WC1N 3BG, United Kingdom*

It might be imagined that the development of an abnormal movement disorder in a committed athlete would have early catastrophic effects on performance, but although this is often the case it is not inevitably so. Dyskinesias are often so task specific that although they may severely disrupt selective individual motor programs, those directly related to the sporting activity may be left unimpaired. For instance, I have looked after a patient who is a committed amateur golfer with a low handicap who has no problems at all putting the ball despite the presence of a devastatingly disabling writer's cramp. Ray Kennedy, the former English football player, was diagnosed as having Parkinson's disease at the age of 35, but retrospective video footage provided to me by British television clearly indicated that early signs of the disease were present in his arms while he was still playing at the highest level (1). This incredible occurrence may in fact have been related to the phenomenon of kinesia paradoxica in which patients with Parkinson's disease are able with the help of adrenaline surges to raise their motor response temporarily in emotionally charged situations. I have another patient with Parkinson's disease who despite moderately severe functional impairment involving his gait, posture, and balance is able to hang-glide efficiently, although there has been a concomitant marked deterioration in his skiing abilities.

Nevertheless, unexplained deterioration in sporting achievement may be the first sign of a neurodegenerative disorder and in retrospect may help to pinpoint the precise onset of the disorder (2). I have seen a number of patients with Parkinson's disease whose initial complaint was related to sporting pastimes. For example, a woman in her fifties complained that when playing tennis she began to have difficulty throwing the ball up to serve accurately and timing the shot; a golfer complained that over a period of 6 months he had lost a distance of about 50 yards on his drive, although his game on the green was unaffected. A keen swimmer began to note that he could no longer swim in a straight line and was continually veering to one side, tending to roll over during the strokes, and that after swimming about 200 m he would be unable to continue at all and would sink. On examination, he had early right-sided bradykinesia and rigidity. Fertl et al. (3) have retrospectively investigated the lifetime physical activity of 32 patients who had been diagnosed as having Parkinson's disease and compared them with a matched group of control subjects. They found that sporting activity prior to the onset of Parkinson's disease did not differ between the two groups. One of their patients, an accomplished downhill skier, noted that he was able to continue to ski downhill reasonably efficiently after the diagnosis had been made but that he had lost his ability to control balance at the end of the slope and now always fell when coming to a halt. At the time of diagnosis the patients were as physically active as the controls, but after diagnosis reduction of physical activity was greater in the parkinsonian group. Nevertheless, a significant proportion of the patients continued in their chosen sporting pastimes, although physically exhausting sports such as jogging or mountaineering were more likely to be abandoned. Some patients complained of stiffness and a fear of drowning during swimming and others of a devastating fatigue after walking or climbing short distances. Interestingly, cross-country skiing, a physical activity frequently adopted by the elderly to replace the more exhausting downhill skiing, was taken up by none of the patients but eight of the controls, raising the possibility that parkinsonians are less flexible in learning new motor plans.

Cumulative head trauma occurring in contact sports such as boxing (4), National Hunt steeplechasing (5), and occasionally in Association football (6) may result in damage to the basal ganglia and emergence of parkinsonian and dystonic syndromes. Athletes' cramps are an increasingly frequent cause of major morbidity in many professional sports, and an intriguing issue is whether Gilles de la Tourette syndrome may actually confer gifts with respect to sporting creativity. These highly selected aspects of the field of movement disorders in sport are discussed in some detail below.

PARKINSON'S SYNDROME IN BOXERS

Fragments of parkinsonism are a frequent and integral component of the punch drunk syndrome (7). In 1957 McDonald Critchley drew attention to a "striatal variety" as follows:

> Since the war one has been impressed with the greater frequency in civilian practice of types of punch drunkenness in which pallidal and striatal lesions are conspicuous. Here the clinical combination of a mask-like face, slurred monotonous speech, extrapyramidal rigidity, slowness of movement and tremors of the arms and head constitute a syndrome which superficially resembles a post-encephalitic Parkinsonian state.

Twenty-three of the 52 accounts of chronic traumatic encephalopathy before 1969 mention the presence of one or more of the cardinal signs of parkinsonism (8). In Roberts' own study of 250 randomly selected retired professional boxers, 13 of the 225 individuals he examined had a full-blown punch drunk syndrome and a further 24 had abnormal physical signs on examination, compat-

ible with previously described cases of chronic traumatic encephalopathy. Although parkinsonian signs were frequently described, the only case of a relatively pure parkinsonian syndrome was excluded from the analysis on the basis that this was an example of coincidental Parkinson's disease. This was a 57-year-old man who had fought more than 100 professional fights—mainly as a middleweight—who developed what sounded like a classical progressive Parkinson's syndrome with rest tremor at 47 years. However, memory deficits were detected early on, his speech was severely affected, and a left Babinski sign was present, diagnostic features that would probably exclude him from currently favored operational criteria for the clinical diagnosis of Parkinson's disease. In his monograph Roberts also observed that it was only in cases with prominent parkinsonian signs that progression of neurologic disabilities after stopping boxing were observed.

Very few examples of Parkinson's syndrome in boxers have subsequently been reported. Four of 15 pathologic cases reported by Corsellis et al. (9) had had a Parkinson's syndrome mentioned in their case records, and a Parkinson's dementia syndrome is also mentioned in some of the sparse earlier pathological reports (10–12). Two boxers with a Parkinson's syndrome and Babinski signs developing many years after their careers had finished have been reported (13, case 8; 14). Another report by Harvey and Newsom-Davis (15) described a 25-year-old professional middleweight who developed slurred speech and then started to shuffle mildly and complain of leg stiffness. Despite the onset of these mild signs he was able to win his last five professional contests before retiring and blamed his difficulties on an assault by the police! When examined 12 months after retirement at 25 he had depression, paranoia, and a symmetric bradykinetic-rigid syndrome with prominent speech and gait disturbance and a left extensor plantar. When reexamined neurologically 20 years later, he was easily distractible and depressed with a mild asymmetric bradykinetic rigid syndrome with marked speech and gait involvement; insignificant progression had occurred over two decades.

Undoubtedly the most famous example of Parkinson's syndrome caused by boxing is

Muhammad Ali, the former world heavyweight champion of the world, who continued to box into his late thirties. Three years before he retired mild slurring of speech was noted, and before the Holmes fight in 1980 he lost 38 pounds and was misdiagnosed by a private physician as having myxoedema and treated with thyroxine and benzamphetamine. Video review of this fight, in which Ali was a shadow of his former self, shows clear evidence of bradykinesia and hypomimia toward the end of the bout. Over the next 2 years incoordination of the legs, writing difficulties, and drooling of saliva were observed at medical examinations. Ali's neurologic condition is described by one of the neurologists who has examined him, Professor Stanley Fahn, in Thomas Hauser's biography of the fighter (16). In 1984 Ali was admitted to Columbia-Presbyterian Medical Center and was noted to have facial masking, reflex blepharospasm, a severe dysarthria, an asymmetric bradykinetic rigid syndrome with left-sided preponderance, and bilateral Babinski signs. His memory was intact and for short distances his gait was brisk. Neuroimaging revealed a cavum septum pellucidum and some brainstem damage. Fahn concluded that he had a posttraumatic Parkinson syndrome and he was begged not to state this to the media. Subsequently, Ali attributed his neurologic condition mainly to the injuries sustained in the third Frazier fight in Manila. Many of Ali's parkinsonian features are responsive to l-dopa (S. Fahn and A. Lieberman, personal communications) but his speech disturbance, which is disproportionately severe, is totally refractory to drug treatment. His neurologic condition has progressed relatively slowly over the past 10 years, although when opening the Atlanta Olympics he now had a marked rest tremor of the hand.

With the help of my colleagues in the Association of British Neurologists I have been able to examine seven professional boxers with a relatively pure Parkinson's syndrome. Five of these developed their symptoms at least 10 years after retiring from the ring and two as long as 30 years after. Although individual cases closely resembled patients with Parkinson's disease, a few differences in the clinical phenomenology can be detailed. Progression of the extrapyramidal syndrome once it has been established

is slow or nonexistent. Gratifying response to L-dopa therapy is relatively uncommon, and there is a disproportionate involvement of speech with rest tremor being less common than in Parkinson's disease. Four of the patients had a cavum septum pellucidum on neuroimaging, one or more Babinski signs were present in three, and early weakness in short-term verbal memory was also found in some of the patients. Magnetic resonance spectroscopy has been used to distinguish Parkinson's disease from some of the other multisystem degenerations such as strionigral degeneration and the Steele-Richardson-Olszewski syndrome (17). We have therefore carried out magnetic resonance spectroscopy on three of the boxers with Parkinson's syndrome, two of whom developed their symptoms decades after stopping fighting. Boxers, closely age-matched control subjects with idiopathic Parkinson's disease, and normal volunteers were scanned with a 1.5-tesla G.E. whole-body scanner. Proton density and T2-weighted coronal images of the brain were collected. A volume of interest between 4 and 6 mL was localized incorporating the putamen and globus pallidus. In the groups of patients this was performed in the basal ganglia subserving the clinically affected side. Spectroscopy was collected using a STEAM (stimulated echo acquisition mode) sequence. Parameters were repetition time 2.27 seconds and echo time of 200 msec. The spectra were line fitted using a commercial package called Sage provided by G E Medical Systems. Quantitation was achieved by using the fully relaxed water signal as an internal standard of reference. In marked contrast to the normal controls and patients with Parkinson's disease, all three boxers had a marked reduction in the N-acetyl aspartate creatinine ratio. It is known from pathologic studies that the putamen and globus pallidus may be damaged in the punch drunk syndrome, and these data therefore provide evidence that boxers with Parkinson's syndrome may have more extensive supranigral damage (18). They also provide further support for the view that the punch drunk syndrome may develop many years after the initiating head trauma.

Postmortem studies in dementia pugilistica have shown moderate to severe loss of the neuromelanine-containing cells, particularly in the ventrolateral tier of the pars compacta of the substantia nigra. In contrast to Parkinson's disease, however, Lewy bodies are rarely seen and neurofibrillary tangle formation is severe and invariable. Additional, often extensive, neuronal damage may be seen in the neocortex (especially the temporal lobe), the cerebellum, and other brainstem structures. The extensive neurofibrillary change and its distribution bear some similarity to the histopathologic findings reported in postencephalitic Parkinson's syndrome, Lytico-Bodig of Guam, and the Steele-Richardson-Olszewski syndrome (19). Roberts et al. (20) have also demonstrated the presence of numerous diffuse beta amyloid protein plaques in dementia pugilistica, linking it more closely to the pathology of Alzheimer's disease. In this regard it is of interest that there are sporadic cases in the literature of severe direct head trauma in young individuals being followed by a progressive Alzheimer dementia (21) and it is known that beta amyloid plaque formation can occur within a few days of severe closed head injury (22). There may therefore be a subgroup of constitutionally predisposed boxers in whom head trauma may be a triggering factor for the initiation of a neurodegenerative process. In the Parkinson's Disease Society Brain Tissue Bank in London there are a handful of patients' brains with histopathologic appearances compatible with chronic traumatic encephalopathy presenting with a pure Parkinson syndrome, although none of these are known to have been boxers.

ATHLETES' CRAMPS

The physical rigors of modern professional sport are now so great and the financial rewards so prodigious that it is scarcely surprising that sportsmen involved in games in which intricate and sustained dexterous activity is required may occasionally succumb to hand cramps. These are analogous to the well-recognized functional disturbances seen frequently in classical musicians and keyboard operators and writers' cramp of clerks, accountants, and students. However, they need to be clearly delineated from local musculoskeletal injuries, peripheral and cervical root

lesions, and incipient Parkinson's disease. Their cause is unknown but dilapidation of an ingrained motor program possibly occurring at the level of the basal ganglia has been proposed, and there are some authorities who consider them as a focal task-specific dystonia. Athletes' cramps have been most carefully detailed in professional golfers and darts players, but they may occur in a number of other sports. Task-specific essential tremors occurring in golfers, Olympic marksmen, and billiard players may also occur and Bill Werbeniuk, the Canadian snooker player, obtained tax relief for the alcohol required to damp down his essential tremor during major tournaments. As a sport becomes more high profile, gaining greater media coverage and perhaps more importantly revenue, the occurrence of cramps and tremors increasingly comes to light. Intriguingly, cramps seem restricted to the hands and have not yet been reported in soccer players. Michael Leach, former All-England Merit Crown Green bowling champion, was forced to quit competition bowls for 3 years because of "the twitch." He complained of a blockage between his brain and his hand and found the most successful therapy for solving the problem was a couple of drinks of alcohol before playing:

> I can't seem to play the wood I want to play, then frustration creeps in and I can't even release the bowl. My job as a solicitor is fairly pressurised, but I don't stammer in court, thankfully, so I can't really understand why it only happens in bowls.

Patsy Fagan, a professional snooker player, ran into difficulties shortly after reaching the 1978 world championship quarter finals when he suddenly found he was unable to play shots when using the rest and within a few weeks he dropped like a stone through the world rankings. Fagan reported that his difficulties occurred not just in competition but also in practice and that when requiring the rest or spider to complete a shot he was filled with terror. Attempting to use the rest, Fagan appeared to freeze and then would totally miscue. Fagan tried to cure the problem by playing left-handed and visiting hypnotists, psychiatrists, and behavioral therapists, all to no avail. Spin bowlers in cricket may also be affected; for a month in 1981 Phil Edmonds sent down an assortment of head-high full tosses and Fred Swarbrook, the

Derbyshire spin bowler, had such an acute problem including visualizing obstacles between him and the batsman that the county sent him—unsuccessfully—to a hypnotherapist. Perhaps the most famous example in recent years has been Roger Harper, the West Indian test off-spinner, whose bowling arm became so low and his deliveries so unpredictable that he lost his place in the team.

Most top-class professional golfers can recall at least one disastrous miss in competition that occurred as a direct result of an edgy, jerky shot. There are relatively few whose careers are threatened or ruined by what is known in the game as the "yips." Foster (23) has described the rise and fall of Ben Hogan, who, after being generally acclaimed as the greatest golfer of his generation, suddenly began to freeze at short putts and complained that he could not take the putter away from the ball because of spasm of his forearm and hand. The elegant stylist Sam Snead was another well-publicized victim who was able to continue in the sport only by first learning to putt the ball between his legs, and when this revolutionary technique was outlawed, he perfected the sidewinding technique, in which he would crouch feet together with the top of the putter supported in a reverse left-hand grip and the right-hand index finger extended and pushed down the grip of the putter with 18 inches or so separating the hand. He would then hit the ball outside the line of his right foot with a fluent swing. In the early 1980s Bernhard Langer's career was temporarily jeopardized by a severe attack of the "twitch:"

> It does not take an expert to see what is wrong. With the short putts I do not have a smooth action. I take the club away and there is a stop before I strike the ball.

Langer worked out that the main problem was tension in the forearm and shoulders and for a time used the cross-hand grip, with his left hand below the right and a very short back swing. Sam Torrance had this to say about his own yips:

> I feel faint standing over the ball. My hand starts shaking and it's an effort to take the club back. It seems like my right hand is taking over and jerking the ball off line and I haven't a clue how hard I am going to hit it.

McDaniel et al. (24) sent a 69-item questionnaire to 1050 professional and amateur golfers. Of the 42% who responded, 28% reported that they had suffered from the yips, which were described as jerks, tremors, or spasms affecting the hand, mainly during putting, but also during chipping. Both hands were involved in almost half the golfers and freezing was described in two-thirds. Sixty-eight percent reported a spontaneous remission; compensatory strategies were helpful in 52%, including cross-handed techniques, separating the hands on the putter grip, using a long putter, putting "side-saddle," changing the head position, and altering visual fixation. A quarter reported that activities other than golfing were also involved, including writing, playing a musical instrument, and playing billiards. Affected golfers also had a higher score on one item, obsessional thinking (e.g., "It's hard to concentrate because of unwanted thoughts or images that come into my mind and won't go away"). The mean age of the affected golfers was slightly greater than that of the unaffected ones (50 years, compared with 47 years). Sachdev (25) reviewed 20 Australian golfers with the yips and stated that the archetypal "victim" was a middle-aged man who had played competitive golf since his teens and developed a jerk, spasm, or freezing while putting or chipping. A number of golfers had particular difficulties fixing their gaze on the ball in a tournament. No specific psychopathology was found in the golfers with the yips compared with controls, but anxiety was felt to be important in exacerbating the problem. Cary Middlecoff attempted some years ago to provide a description for Henry Longhurst:

> A player with the putting yips is just somebody who temporarily at least is a real bad putter. He may have had a sound putting stroke and lost it, or he may have had a flaw in his stroke that finally caught up with him—like hooding the face of the putter going back. But it could be any one of a lot of things. Being too quick starting the backswing for instance, and getting quicker and jerkier as you go along.
>
> But I think that most bad puts are caused by indecision. The player doesn't fully make up his mind how he wants to stroke the putt so he changes his mind somewhere between the start of the backswing and the end of the forward swing. He decides that he ought to play for

more break, or for less break, so he changes his stroke pattern. Or maybe the thought hits him that he is about to hit the ball too hard, or too soft, so he slows down or speeds up his stroke. The result is a wavering, jerky, indecisive stroke. You must make up your mind in advance how you are going to stroke the ball and stick to your plan. When the mind wavers, the stroke wavers, and a wavering stroke won't do the job. Another danger to guard against during the stroke is becoming too anxious to see where the ball goes. Anxiety can, if you let it, make you raise your head before the ball is partway up the line to the cup.

In recent years large quantities of money have entered the sport of darts, which formerly was a leisure activity played in the public houses of the United Kingdom. The dart is probably the lightest missile used in competitive sport, weighing only a few grams, and because of this and the need for pinpoint accuracy, the effects of excessive anxiety can be particularly damaging. The main features of "dartitis" are a difficulty or inability to release the dart on certain throws and an accompanying self-consciousness. It is of some interest that professional rifle shooters may also experience similar problems of being unable to pull the trigger in competition. The dart throw becomes jerky or is pulled because of muscle tenseness and spasm in the hands and forearm. In an attempt to overcome the problem, the player shifts position frequently or uses auditory or visual cues to regain accuracy. Attacks are most likely to occur at times of important matches, but it may eventually make throwing difficult even in the privacy of a player's own home. As a generalization, dartitis sufferers tend to have an obsessive interest in the sport, considerable competence at the game, and a burning desire to win and improve their performance. Many increase their alcohol consumption during playing to allay anxiety. Factors predisposing to dartitis are an increased number of stressful life events in the year before onset, excessive anxiety, and an inward-looking, mildly obsessional personality.

A change of style or speed of throwing, the use of more proximal muscle groups in the arm with a new set of darts, and quiet, solitary practice may help to overcome the problem in 25%, and biofeedback and relaxation techniques may

also be of some help, The Crafty Cockney, Eric Bristow, tramped through the waiting rooms of psychologists, hypnotists, and masseurs in an unsuccessful attempt to solve his problem. Bristow began to find that increasingly frequently he would stand on the oche looking at his fully cocked dart, but being unable to release it and on occasions going off balance. Video analysis of Bristow's throwing technique showed a considerable change over his 10 years at the top, and at the Swedish Open Championship in 1987 the problem became so bad that he was obliged to employ a prompter to stand behind him encouraging him to let go of the darts. Bristow described his problem as follows:

> My mind says yes and my hand says no. I can't let go of the dart because my arm freezes and I lose balance.

Bristow finally managed to overcome the difficulty by improving his physical fitness and practicing for long periods every day.

GILLES DE LA TOURETTE SYNDROME AND THE QUESTION OF SPORTING CREATIVITY

Many ticqueurs give the impression of being particularly nimble and others are often described as being "nervy and wiry." Some appear to be particularly gifted with respect to music, and the distinguished English literary figure Samuel Johnson had multiple tics and obsessional behaviors. A number of accomplished professional sportsmen are known to have Gilles de la Tourette syndrome, including Jim Eisenreich, the Philadelphia Phillies baseball outfielder, and Abdul Rauff (née Chris Jackson), the Denver Nuggets guard. Witty, Ticcy Ray, one of Oliver Sacks' celebrated patients, excelled at table tennis because of his unexpected, startling improvisations. It is probable that Paul Gascoigne, the clown prince of English football, may have a mild form of the syndrome (26). Following a traumatic childhood incident in which Gascoigne witnessed the death of his best friend's young brother, he developed behavioral quirks. Keith Spraggan, Gascoigne's friend, described these in McGibbon's (1990) biography of Gascoigne:

He began to stutter more and more, and then he would blink all the time and make funny noises. He couldn't help it, he was just plain nervous.

At school, Gascoigne, in common with many aspiring soccer stars, showed interest in nothing except football and he developed an increasing number of nervous habits. Jeff Lambert, one of his sports teachers, described these as follows (27):

Paul developed a nervous swallow—a clearing of the throat which came out as a high-pitched squeak. He wouldn't be able to control it and some teachers would order him out of their classes because they thought he was taking the mickey, or trying to attract attention to himself by being stupid. But some muscular reaction forced the noise out, particularly when he was under pressure.

Ian Hamilton, in his book *Gazza Agonistes* (28), describes the first time he saw the young "Gazza" in action, playing for Newcastle United in 1987 in a team that included the Brazilian maestro Mirandinha. During the game Mirandinha on several occasions chastised Gascoigne for his play and Hamilton observed the following:

Gascoigne started to make strange spasmodic head movements and began muttering to himself. He kept licking his lips, flexing his jaw muscles, tucking his shirt in, pulling up his socks, and his face turned a more brilliant shade of pink. At the whistle though, as the teams were walking from the field, he was immediately at Mirandinha's side, chattering and joking, linking arms, the best of friends.

One of the Newcastle United scouts observed:

Gazza would get rid of one affliction, then another would start. When the barking stopped I'd say "You've got rid of the dog then Paul?". By then he had developed another nervous habit—a dry cough or something. I don't think he knew he was doing it. Other lads used to take the mickey and mimic him.

Before the England versus Czechoslovakia international game at Wembley stadium when much was expected of Gascoigne, Tony Dorigo, one of his teammates, recalled that he observed Gascoigne to be highly emotionally charged, nervy, tense, sweating, with a number of twitches. On New Years Day 1991, while playing for Tottenham Hotspur against Manchester United, Gascoigne was sent off the field of play for al-

legedly using foul language to the referee. At the press interview after the game he claimed, to guffaws of laughter from the press, that he had actually been swearing at himself and not at the referee. Around this time Gascoigne was described by the journalist Karl Miller as follows:

A highly charged spectacle on the field of play, fierce and comic, formidable and vulnerable, urchin-like and waif-like, a strong head and torso with comparatively frail-looking, breakable legs, strange eyed, pink faced, tense and upright, a priapic monolith in the Mediterranean sun.

Following his transfer to the Roman Club, Lazio, Gascoigne's comic indiscretions have continued to make headlines with his elfin pranks on teammates, his tongue protrusions during the national anthem, his inappropriate belching on Italian television, and his impulsive binge eating, self-destructive behavior, and compulsive orderliness. On the field of play, however, his outlandish inventiveness, histrionics, and capricious unpredictability continue to amuse and thrill the crowds. Even in Italy, where body language is an art form, Gazza's behavior is regarded with amusement and curiosity.

Whether those afflicted with Gilles de la Tourette syndrome have a particular inherent gift for sporting success or whether they are drawn to this field of human competitive activity because it helps them to sublimate emotional tension is unknown. It may be simply the only recourse left to individuals denied success in many other walks of life because of their social handicaps. Nevertheless, one cannot help but be struck by the frequency of sporting ability in a large number of children with tic disorders.

The tennis grunts of many professional players in the past few years also contain the germ of a tic. Although Monica Seles is the most celebrated exponent of this habit, it has grown to almost epidemic proportions, particularly on the female professional circuit. Each forceful shot is accompanied by a unique, stereotyped, emotionally charged, explosive vocalization that seems, as far as one can judge, to have a certain degree of irresistibility about it and with time it becomes an ingrained part of the playing ritual that is often distressing to opponents. The noise can be compared to the extempore vocalizations of some modern jazz players in that it reflects an outpouring of emotional and creative energy. Distinctive vocalizations associated with physical effort are also seen in other sports, including weight lifting, martial arts, and boxing.

CONCLUSIONS

The emergence of a progressive neurodegenerative disorder such as Parkinson's disease does not mean one should forgo an active lifestyle. Indeed, regular physical activity as part of a designed treatment program is advised, to maintain mobility and posture and to reduce stiffness. Physical activity may also provide mental stimulation, improve appetite and sleep, and reduce depression. Walking, bowling, swimming, and golf seem particularly suited to patients with Parkinson's disease and many continue exercise in health clubs. Young parkinsonians, who before the onset of their condition were involved in contact sports or team games, may have to make major adjustments as the restriction of fluent movement makes these activities increasingly difficult.

REFERENCES

1. Lees AJ. When did Ray Kennedy's Parkinson's disease begin? *Mov Disord* 1992;7:110–116.
2. Kasarskis EJ, Winslow M. When did Lou Gehrig's personal illness begin? *Neurology* 1989;39:1243–1245.
3. Fertl E, Doppelbauer A, Auff E. Physical activity and sports in patients suffering from Parkinson's disease in comparison with healthy seniors. *J Neural Transm (PD Sect.)*, 1993;5:157–161.
4. Critchley M. Medical aspects of boxing, particularly from a neurological point of view. *Br Med J* 1957;1:357–366.
5. Foster JB, Leiguarda R, Tilley PJB. Brain damage in National Hunt jockeys. *Lancet* 1976;1:981–982.
6. Anon. Brain damage in sport [Editorial]. *Lancet* 1976;1:401–402.
7. Martland HS. Punch drunk. *JAMA* 1928;91:1103–1107.
8. Roberts AJ. In: *Brain damage in boxers*. London; Pitman Medical Scientific Publications, 1969.
9. Corsellis JAN, Bruton CJ, Freeman-Brown D. The aftermath of boxing. *Psychol Med* 1973;3:270–273.
10. Brandenburg W, Hallervorden J. Dementia puglistica mit anatomischem Befund. *Virchows Arch Pathol Anatat Physiol Klin Med* 1954;325:680–709.
11. Grahmann H, Ule G. Beitrag zur Kenntnis der chronischen cerebralen Krankheitsbilder bei Boxern. *Psychiatr Neurol* 1957;134:251–283.
12. Constantinides J, Tissot R. Lésions neurofibrillaires d'Alzheimer generalisées sans plaques séniles. *Arch Suisses Neurol Neurochirug Psychiatr* 1967;100:117–130.
13. Mawdsley C, Ferguson FR. Neurological disease in boxers. *Lancet* 1963;2:795–801.
14. Friedman JH. Progressive parkinsonism in boxers. *South Med J* 1989;82:543–546.
15. Harvey PKP, Newsom-Davis J. Traumatic encephalopathy in a young boxer. *Lancet*, 1974;2:928–929.
16. Hauser T. *Muhammad Ali. His Life and Times.* New York: Simon & Schuster, 1991:489–492.
17. Davie CA, Wenning GK, Barker GJ, Tofts PS, Kendall BE, Quinn N, McDonald WI, Marsden CD, Miller DH. Differentiation of multiple system atrophy from idiopathic Parkinson's disease using proton magnetic resonance spectroscopy. *Ann Neurol* 1995;37:206–210.
18. Davie CA, Pirtosek Z, Barker GJ, Kingsley DP, Miller DH, Lees AJ. An MRS study of Parkinsonism related to boxing. *J Neurol Neurosurg Psychiatry* 1995;58:688–691.
19. Corsellis JAN. Boxing and the brain. *Br Med J* 1989; 298:105–109.
20. Roberts GW, Allsop D, Bruton C. The occult aftermath of boxing. *J Neurol Neurosurg Psychiatry* 1990;53:373–378.
21. Clinton J, Ambler MW, Roberts GW. Post-traumatic Alzheimer's disease; preponderance of a single plaque type. *Neuropathol Appl Neurobiol* 1991;17:69–74.
22. Roberts GW, Gentleman SM, Lynch A, Graham DI. Beta A4 amyloid protein deposition in brain after head trauma. *Lancet* 1991;338:1422–1423.
23. Foster J. Putting on the agony. *World Med* 1977;June 29:25–27.
24. McDaniel KD, Cummings JL, Shain S. The 'yips': a focal dystonia of golfers. *Neurology* 1989;39:192–195.
25. Sachdev P. Golfers' cramp. Clinical characteristics and evidence against it being an anxiety disorder. *Mov Disord* 1992;7:326–332.
26. Runciman D. Wazza Mazza wiz Gazza. *Modern Review,* Autumn edition 1991, 34.
27. McGibbon R. *Gazza—a biography.* London: Penguin, 1990.
28. Hamilton I. *Gazza Agonistes.* London; Granta, 1993.

Sports Neurology, Second Edition,
edited by Barry D. Jordan.
Lippincott–Raven Publishers, Philadelphia © 1998.

25

Multiple Sclerosis and Exercise

Brian R. Apatoff

Multiple Sclerosis Clinical Care and Research Center,
Department of Neurology & Neuroscience,
The New York Hospital-Cornell Medical Center, New York, New York 10021

CLINICAL FEATURES OF MULTIPLE SCLEROSIS

Multiple sclerosis (MS) is an inflammatory, demyelinating disorder of the central nervous system of presumed autoimmune etiology. It affects over 250,000 persons in the United States alone, affecting women more than men, and usually presenting early in life between the ages of 20 and 40. MS can have a highly variable clinical course with a broad spectrum of clinical severity. Typically there are acute attacks with focal neurologic deficits, including visual impairment, sensory disturbance, paralysis, motor incoordination, tremor, and gait disturbance (1). Magnetic resonance imaging (MRI) analysis of the brain and spinal cord usually demonstrates multiple areas of increased signal in the subcortical and periventricular white matter, representing old or active areas of demyelination. In addition to focal weakness, extreme generalized fatigue is a frequent complaint in MS that significantly limits activity. Depression is commonly experienced, and cognitive impairment is often seen with extensive white matter disease in MS. The condition also frequently affects normal bladder and bowel function, resulting in some combination of retention and/or incontinence. Symptoms of chronic pain can complicate the course of some patients (2,3).

NATURAL HISTORY AND TREATMENT OF MULTIPLE SCLEROSIS

While the pattern of disease activity can initially be characterized by a relapsing-remitting course, with acute exacerbations followed by variable improvement, at later stages there is often a chronic-progressive deterioration with increasing neurologic disability. Patients with a relapsing course that later evolves into a pattern of progressive disability are termed secondary progressive. This is to distinguish them from a smaller category, primary-progressive patients, who have an insidious onset of disease with an inexorable decline of function. In more "benign" forms of MS there can be infrequent attacks over decades with mild signs and symptoms and minimal disease on brain MRI. However, in more "malignant" forms of MS there can be rapid clinical progression over 1 to 5 years with severe neurologic disability and extensive white matter lesions evident on brain MRI. Moderately severe disability is noted in 10% of patients in 5 years, in 25% of patients within 10 years, and in 50% of patients within 18 years. The mean duration from disease onset to the need for unilateral assistance for walking is approximately 15 years (1).

The conventional treatment of MS has relied on immunosuppressive agents including corticosteroids, azathioprine, cyclophosphamide, and methotrexate, with only limited success in controlling disease (4,5) (Table 1). For acute relapses of moderate severity or rapidly progressive disease the recommended management initially is usually high-dose intravenous methylprednisolone (500 to 1000 mg QD for 3 to 7 days). Total lymphoid irradiation at lymphoablative doses has resulted in temporary benefits for chronic-progressive MS. Newer

TABLE 1. *Medications for multiple sclerosis*

Medication	Dosage	Indication, benefits
Immunosuppresive Therapy		
Prednisone	100 mg PO QD tapered over 20 to 30 days	Relapsing or progressive MS
Methylprednisolone	1000 mg IV QD for 3 to 5 days	Acute relapsing MS
Azathioprine	100–150 mg PO QD	Progressive MS
Methotrexate	7.5–25 mg PO or SC Q week	Progressive MS
Cyclophosphamide	Monthly cycles IV	Rapidly progressive MS
Cladribine	Monthly cycles IV-SC	Rapidly progressive MS
Immunomodulatory Therapy		
Interferon-beta 1a	6 mIU IM Q week	Relapsing-remitting MS
Interferon-beta 1b	8 mIU SC Q week	Relapsing-remitting MS
Gammaglobulin	0.2–0.4 mg/kg IV Q month	Relapsing-remitting MS
Copaxone	20 mg SC QD	Relapsing-remitting MS
Symptomatic Therapy		
Baclofen	5–20 mg PO TID to QID	Spasticity
Tizanidine	2–8 mg PO TID	Spasticity
Dantrolene	25–100 mg PO TID	Spasticity
Diazepam	2–5 mg PO BID	Spasticity
Amantadine	100 mg PO BID to TID	Fatigue
Pemoline	37.5 mg PO BID to TID	Fatigue
Methylphenidate	2.5 to 10 mg PO TID	Fatigue
Carbamazepine	200–400 mg PO TID	Pain, sensory disturbance
Phenytoin	100–300 mg PO QD	Pain, sensory disturbance
Clonazepam	1–2 mg PO TID	Pain, sensory disturbance
Amitriptyline (and other tricyclic analgesics)	25–150 mg PO QHS	Pain, sensory disturbance
Ibuprofen	400–600 mg PO QID	Pain, sensory disturbance
Morphine sulfate (and other narcotic analgesics)	10–30 mg PO TID	Pain, sensory disturbance

potent lympholytic drugs such as cladribine may also have benefits in slowing the rate of progression. Other immunomodulatory therapies such as interferon-beta have been shown to reduce attack frequency and brain lesions in milder relapsing-remitting forms of disease (5a). However, no standard therapy is curative or uniformly successful in controlling more severe forms of disease. The remainder of this chapter will focus on the role of exercise and symptomatic management in limiting the neurologic disability associated with MS.

EXERCISE TRAINING AND MULTIPLE SCLEROSIS

It is well documented that regular aerobic exercise in the general population results in substantial reduction in health risk, lowering blood pressure, reducing body fat, improving bone density, and extending life (6). In addition, the potential benefits of exercise training programs in reducing the neurologic disability related to MS and improving other parameters related to the quality of life have been established (7). For example, it was debated whether MS patients with moderate disability can exercise sufficiently to improve fitness without aggravating their underlying condition. For many years it was observed by patients and clinicians that infrequent vigorous physical activity could sometimes worsen many signs and symptoms of MS, and in some cases physical stress could be associated with an exacerbation of the MS. This raised the concern that exercise could be detrimental to the course of MS.

Clinical monitoring of disease progression in MS with the disability scales now in use in clinical trials is imperfect. The Expanded Disability Status Scale (EDSS) measures the disability in MS patients on the basis of the level of neurologic impairment; a score of 0 represents a normal neurologic examination and 10 represents death caused by MS (8). The EDSS is derived from ratings of individual functional systems (pyramidal, cerebellar, brainstem, sensory, bowel and bladder, visual cognitive) and degree of ambulatory impairment. Limitations of the EDSS include insensitivity to progression at certain stages and interrater variability. For example, there is lack of uniform representation across the grading scale, which is heavily weighted toward ambulatory function from scores 4 to 7.5. Research advances in neurologic rehabilitation, exercise physiology, and clinical outcomes analysis have demonstrated global benefits of physical therapy intervention in MS. Several carefully controlled studies have examined the effects of directed physical therapy and exercise training in MS. In one report by Petajan et al. (9), 46 moderately affected ambulatory MS patients were randomly assigned to exercise or nonexercise groups [mean expanded disability status scale (EDSS) of 3.8 and 2.9, respectively] and studied before and after 15 weeks of aerobic training (8). Aspects of physical fitness including maximal aerobic capacity, isometric strength, body fat composition, and blood lipids were measured with a variety of rating scales, as well as neurologic disability, activities of daily living, mood, and fatigue. Training consisted of three 40-minute sessions per week of combined arm and leg ergometry. With this modest regimen, the exercise group of MS patients had significant improvements in aerobic capacity, upper and lower extremity strength, body fat, and blood lipids. Mood and sense of well-being were favorably affected in the exercise group, as were some measures of fatigue. There was no significant change in the neurologic disability scale in the short period of time under study, except for improvement in bowel and bladder function (9). Presumably the exercise intervention promoted abdominal peristalsis and reduced the likelihood of obstipation. Thus with most objective and subjective measures, the exercise group experienced physical and psychologic improvements.

Kraft et al. (10,11) studied the effects of progressive resistive exercise training in eight MS patients, four with milder disease (EDSS 3.0) and four with more advanced disability (EDSS 6.0). After training sessions (knee and elbow flexors and extensors) over 3 months (45 minutes, three times weekly), both groups of patients had improve-

ments in ambulation and stair climbing functions. Formal quantitative measures of quadriceps, hamstrings, biceps, and triceps showed gains in strength in all groups. There were no adverse effects on clinical status attributable to the exercise program.

Svensson et al. (12) studied the benefits of endurance training in MS patients across a broad range of disability (EDSS 2 to 7), measuring repetitive knee and hip flexors over a 4- to 6-week period. The majority of patients showed increases in strength as well as improvements in subjective measures of fatigue, mood, and general health.

Although most persons with MS appear to tolerate exercise training and can experience global benefits of such activity, it is recommended that any exercise program be initiated under medical supervision (13). In normal individuals, regulation of blood pressure and circulation during physical and thermal stress is mediated by the autonomic nervous system. However, MS patients with more advanced disease may have abnormalities of autonomic cardiovascular function with significant increases in postural hypotension compared with controls and heart rate variation to deep respiration and Valsalva maneuvers (14,15). An attenuated pressor response to isometric exercise has been documented in persons with MS, such that normal blood pressure increases with sustained muscle contraction are not achieved (16). Dysfunction of cardiovascular regulation may be secondary to disseminated demyelinating lesions in brainstem autonomic nuclei or supramedullary spinal cord reflexes (14,16).

MANAGING SYMPTOMS IN MULTIPLE SCLEROSIS

As already outlined, a program of exercise can have global benefits for many parameters of physical and emotional well-being in MS patients. Certain limiting symptoms in MS may require specific strategies to maximize the therapeutic potential of exercise (16a). Any program of exercise should be discussed with a physician and the level of activity gradually increased only as tolerated.

Fatigue

Pathologic fatigue is a significant complaint for the majority of MS patients at some point in their condition and is often overwhelming and limiting, even in persons with otherwise minor or no focal neurologic disability (17–20). For many persons, small amounts of physical exertion tend to produce extreme fatigue, which is usually described as different from that experienced prior to the onset of their illness. Regular periods of rest and other attempts at energy conservation are only partially beneficial and may paradoxically increase the patient's physical limitations, because forced inactivity may promote muscular deconditioning and increase the level of exercise intolerance. Central nervous system stimulants such as amantadine, pemoline, or methylphenidate sometimes produce a modest improvement in symptoms. Other possible neuropsychiatric or medical contributors to fatigue in MS patients, such as depression, hypothyroidism, sleep disorder, or anemia, should be excluded. Certain antidepressants, including fluoxitine or bupropion, may benefit depression as well as help combat fatigue.

Weakness and Spasticity

Demyelination of the corticospinal tract in the brain and spinal cord can produce a variety of altered motor control, including weakness, slowness, and incoordination of movement and increased extensor tone, or spasticity. The leg "stiffness" or spastic gait typically seen in MS is an obvious impediment to normal ambulation and often requires circumabduction of the leg for forward movement, instead of a normal flexion stepping motion. Medication such as baclofen, tizanidine, dantrolene, or benzodiazepines, in combination with a daily program of stretching exercises, may help reduce the degree of spasticity (21). The antispasticity medication should be started at the lowest possible doses, even half a tablet (balcofen 5 mg, or tizanidine 2 mg, twice to three times a day), and increased gradually as tolerated. Clinical paresis may become more apparant at higher doses of drug as extensor tone in the lower extremities is reduced. Thus, medication must be carefully titrated for optimal response. The most common pattern of weakness in

the leg involves the hip flexion, thigh abduction, and foot dorsiflexion and eversion. Controlled studies support the concept that exercise can be beneficial for MS patients with focal weakness by increasing strength in paretic muscles and general aerobic capacity. Regular exercise should therefore be part of an ongoing treatment program even for persons with advanced disability. Patients with paraparesis can successfully use a stationary bicycle that is powered by a combination of arm levers and foot pedals, such as the Schwinn Aerodyne (which also has cooling fan blades on the flywheel), to provide both arm and leg exercise and range of motion (4). Even in a patient with complete paraplegia who is restricted to a wheelchair, regular use of an upper body ergometer preserves aerobic capacity and independence in daily activities such as transferring.

Heat Intolerance

Many patients with MS demonstrate an intolerance to minor elevations in body temperature. Excess environmental heat (e.g., warm, humid weather or taking a hot bath or shower) may greatly accentuate underlying symptoms. This appears to be a consequence of reduced axonal conduction in areas of marginal demyelination. Heat intolerance may be further aggravated by impaired thermal dissipation resulting from autonomic dysfunction, with resultant altered vasodilation and sweating. Heat-sensitive patients are advised to exercise with air-conditioning. Exercise outdoors should be planned for the coolest times of day; cooling helmets and vests can be obtained commercially.

Similarly, fever caused by infection can dramatically increase symptoms, with focal or generalized weakness and extreme fatigue. Patients must be instructed to monitor a fever and treat with vigorous hydration and antipyretics. Fever can also be an accompaniment of therapy with interferon-beta injections, and premedication with acetominophen is recommended for even low-grade fevers.

Gait Imbalance and Tremor

Demyelinating disease in the spinocerebellar pathways, or sometimes the dorsal proprioceptive pathways, can produce severe gait and truncal ataxia with limb dysmetria or tremor. Occasionally, flailing, choreiform movements of the arms can be most disabling. Even in the absence of significant focal weakness, many basic activities for some persons, such as standing, walking, feeding, and dressing, can no longer be performed independently. In cases in which gait imbalance or paraparesis impedes normal physical activity, a regular program of exercise can still be pursued in a properly equipped swimming pool (22). Such "aquatherapy" sessions are often sponsored by the local chapters of the National Multiple Sclerosis Society. In addition to providing buoyant body support for persons who otherwise have walking restrictions, the water provides a resistive element for dysmetric limb motion. Conductive thermal dissipation of heat in a properly cooled pool avoids the elevation in body temperature that makes exercise problematic for many MS patients and enables sustained aerobic exercise training.

MAINTENANCE OF GENERAL HEALTH MEASURES

Focal weakness in combination with spasticity, ataxia, pathologic fatigue, and heat intolerance typically leads to a progressive reduction in physical activity in persons with MS. However, a complication of reduced physical activity can be resultant deconditioning, which can further limit the patient's abilities to perform the activities of daily living (2,7). Simple activities such as walking, swimming, and using a stationary exercise bicycle, when performed on a regular schedule, may be of considerable value. Exercise should be performed in a cool environment whenever possible in patients who have heat-related declines in neurologic function. Swimming and water aerobics are particularly beneficial exercises in patients with limitations of balance or focal weakness, supporting and cooling the patient during activity.

For more severe disease with advanced disability, exercise with a physical and occupational therapist may be helpful in improving or maintaining neurologic function. The bracing of paretic portions of limbs, commonly an ankle–foot orthotic

for weakness of foot elevation, provides a significant benefit for gait stability (23,24). Patients should be evaluated by a rehabilitation specialist for the use of devices that provide support or balance assistance with walking (21). A cane or walker can reduce risk of falls and increase independent activity, thereby enabling patients to maintain a program of exercise.

Musculoskeletal complications can occur with weakness, spasticity, and reduced sensation in the legs, causing chronic hyperextension at the knee and damage of the posterior ligaments. This hyperextension injury may be reduced by the use of a knee brace (23). Similarly, an abnormal gait and posture resulting from weakness and imbalance may contribute to orthopedic problems in the hip or back with resultant pain and accelerated degenerative joint disease. Thus, complaints of localized musculoskeletal pain should be evaluated.

It is advisable for persons with MS to eat a balanced diet low in fat and high in bulk. Weight control is of increased concern because of reduced physical activity. Overweight patients are at increased risk of falls, which may result in serious injury. Although a variety of "special" diets are described for MS, there is no evidence to support claims of a specific benefit for the course of disease. Expensive nutritional and vitamin supplements are usually unnecessary and should be discussed with a physician. Rather, a simple generic multivitamin with iron used with a balanced diet and a calcium supplement (particularly in postmenopausal patients or patients taking corticosteroids) to reduce osteoporosis are normally adequate to promote good general health.

Acknowledgment

This work is supported by a generous grant from the Marc Haas and Helen Hotze Haas Foundation.

REFERENCES

1. Weinshenker BG. The natural history of multiple sclerosis. *Neurol Clin* 1995;13:119–146.
2. Ericsson RP, Lie MR, Wineinger MA. Rehabilitation in multiple sclerosis. *Mayo Clin Proc* 1989;64:818–828.
3. Frankel DI. Multiple sclerosis. In: Umphred DA, ed. *Neurologic rehabilitation*. St. Louis: Mosby–Year Book, 1990;545–557.

4. Taylor RS. Rehabilitation of persons with multiple sclerosis. In: Braddom RL, ed. *Physical medicine and rehabilitation.* Philadelphia: WB Saunders, 1995:1101–1112.

5. Weiner HL, Hohol MJ, Khoury SJ, Dawson DM, Hafler, DA. Therapy for multiple sclerosis. *Neurol Clin* 1995; 13:173–196.

5a. Rudick RA, Cohen JA, Weinstock-Guttman B, et al. Management of multiple sclerosis. *N Engl J Med* 1997; 337:1604–1611.

6. Kraft GH, de Lateur BJ. Exercise. *Phys Med Rehabil Clin North Am* 1994;5:243–392.

7. Delisa J, Hammond MC, Mikhulic MA, Miller RM. Multiple sclerosis. Part 1. Common physical disabilities and rehabilitation. *Am Fam Physician* 1985;32:157–163.

8. Kurtzke JF. Rating neurologic impairment in multiple sclerosis: an expanded disability status scale (EDSS). *Neurology* 1983;33:1444–1452.

9. Petajan JH, Gappamaier E, White AT, Spencer MK, Mino L, Hicks RW. Impact of aerobic training on fitness and quality of life in multiple sclerosis patients. *Ann Neurol* 1996;39:432–441.

10. Kraft GH, Alquist AD, de Lateur BJ. Effect of resistive exercise on physical function in multiple sclerosis. Consortium of MS Centers 1995 Meeting (abst).

11. Kraft GH, Alquist AD, de Lateur BJ. Effect of resistive exercise on strength in patients with multiple sclerosis. Consortium of MS Centers 1995 Meeting (abst).

12. Svensson B, Gerdle B, Elert J. Endurance training in patients with multiple sclerosis: five case studies. *Phys Ther* 1994;74:1017–1026.

13. Kosich D, Molk B, Feeney J. Cardiovascular testing and exercise prescription in multiple sclerosis patients. *J Neurol Rehabil* 1987;1:167–170.

14. Anema JR, Heijenbrok MW, Faes TJ, Heimans JJ, Lanting P, Polman CH. Cardiovascular autonomic function in multiple sclerosis. *J Neurol Sci* 1992;104:129–134.

15. Ponichtera-Mulcare JA. Exercise and multiple sclerosis. *Med Sci Sports Exerc* 1993;25:451–465.

16. Pepin EB, Hicks RW, Spencer MK, Tran ZV, Jackson CG. Pressor response to isometric exercise in patients with multiple sclerosis. *Med Sci Sports Exerc* 1996;28: 656–660.

16a. Stolp-Smith KA, Carter JL, Rohe DE, et al. Management of impairment, disability, and handicap due to multiple sclerosis. *Mayo Clin Proc* 1997;72: 1184–1196.

17. Freal JE, Kraft GH, Coryell JK. Symptomatic fatigue in multiple sclerosis. *Arch Phys Med Rehabil* 1984;65: 135–137.

18. Packer TL, Sauriol A, Brouwer B. Fatigue secondary to chronic illness: postpolio syndrome, chronic fatigue syndrome, and multiple sclerosis. *Arch Phys Med Rehabil* 1992;75:1122–1126.

19. Sandroni P, Walker C, Starr A. Fatigue in patients with multiple sclerosis: motor conduction and event-related potentials. *Arch Neurol* 1992;49:517–524.

20. Sharma KR, Kent-Braun J, Mynhier MA, Weiner MW, Miller RG. Evidence of an abnormal intramuscular component of fatigue in multiple sclerosis. *Muscle Nerve* 1995;18:1403–1411.

21. Smith CR, Scheinberg L. Symptomatic treatment and rehabilitation of patients with multiple sclerosis. In: Cook SD, ed. *Handbook of multiple sclerosis.* New York: Marcel Dekker, 1990:327–350.

22. Gehlsen G, Grigbsy S, Winant DM. Effects of an aquatic fitness program on the muscular strength and endurance of patients with multiple sclerosis. *Phys Ther* 1984;68: 653–657.

23. Schapiro RT, Laven L. Multiple sclerosis. In: Good DC, Couch JR, eds. *Handbook of neurorehabilitation.* New York: Marcel Dekker, 1995:551–583.

24. Schapiro RT. *Multiple sclerosis: a rehabilitation approach to management.* New York: Demos, 1991.

PART III

Sport-Specific Neurologic Injuries

Sports Neurology, Second Edition,
edited by Barry D. Jordan.
Lippincott–Raven Publishers, Philadelphia © 1998.

26

Auto Racing

Stephen E. Olvey

Department of Neurological Surgery, University of Miami School of Medicine,
1501 NW 9th Avenue, Miami, Florida 33136

BACKGROUND

Humans have raced in every mode of transportation available. Horses, canoes, chariots, clipper ships, and balloons all had their day. It is no surprise, then, that they would also race in automobiles. The first organized automobile race was a 79-mile run from Paris to Rouen, held on July 22, 1894. Since that time there have been automobile races of every description in practically every country. From the beginning, automobile racing was a dangerous pastime and, until recently was looked upon as more of a thrill show than a sport. Through the mid-1970s deaths in automobile racing were numerous. In fact, automobile racing was second only to flying homemade aircraft as the leading cause of death in sports (1).

In the early days of racing essentially no attention was paid to safety. Prize money was posted, and there were always enough entrants willing to risk their lives for it. Drivers were responsible for their own protection and almost nothing was done to protect the spectators. Initially races were run on public roads with no control over what might be in the way. Guardrails and safety crews were nonexistent. Nearly as many spectators as drivers were killed in the early days. In 1909 Carl Fisher, a man of great vision, built the Indianapolis Motor Speedway as a proving ground for the development of the automobile. He was also a promoter and expected to make a great deal of money. The first race was a balloon race; the 500-mile automobile race did not occur until 1911. In that race nine spectators and two drivers were killed; the event attracted over 80,000 spectators. The move to closed courses made automobile racing a big business. Today, motor sports enjoy the second highest attendance level of all sports. Drivers' salaries are in the millions of dollars and television ratings continue to climb.

Moving races to specially built tracks resulted in greater protection for spectators but did little to help drivers. Through the decades from 1911 to 1960 drivers were often killed instantly, dying mostly from massive head injuries or fatal burns. Helmets were cloth or leather until 1935, becoming metal in 1953 and then fiberglass during the 1960s (D. Davidson, U.S.A.C., personal communication, 1996). Helmets are now made of carbon fiber. Seat belts did not come into general use until the mid-1950s, with shoulder harnesses being introduced later that same decade. The delay in seat belt use was due to drivers initially faring better when they were thrown clear of the car and thus being reluctant to be restrained. The transition toward full restraint systems occurred during the late 1950s, when it became apparent that it was better to stay with the car.

Car construction in the deadlier decades featured front-engine cars with tubular steel frames. When a car crashed, most of the energy of the crash was transmitted directly to the driver. Cars involved in a fatal crash often showed little damage and could occasionally be repaired to race again at another event. Rear-engine cars evolved in Europe during the late 1950s and were introduced into the United States in 1961. By luck, not design, these cars were slightly safer because they basically exploded on impact, with each piece

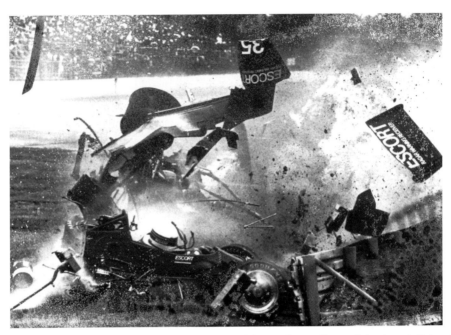

FIG. 1. Fragmentation of rear-engine racing car with driver safety cell remaining intact. Driver in this picture suffered minor concussion and fractured mandible. Speed on impact 180 mph (estimated).

that came apart expending energy (Fig. 1). The 1970s continued to see high fatality rates resulting from severe head injuries, largely because of a learning curve associated with aerodynamic principles and their application to vehicles traveling in excess of 200 mph on the ground. Materials also played an important role, especially with the introduction of carbon fiber as the principal material used in constructing the "tub" or safety cell in which the driver is restrained. The modern racing car now offers relatively good protection, considering that speeds have increased more than 20% in the past 15 years and both injury and death having decreased substantially (2,3). Several racing organizations have elected, for nostalgic and other reasons, to keep a more "stock" appearance to their vehicles. Tubular frames remain, and the engines are still in front of the driver. Injury and fatality rates in these series remain higher than in more modern forms of motor sport.

Modern racing cars can be divided into open- and closed-wheeled race cars. The simplest open-wheeled car is the Go-kart. Go-karts are raced throughout the world and provide a training ground for young, aspiring drivers. Several

world champions have learned the art of motor racing in Go-karts. These small cars can attain speeds of greater than 160 mph and offer virtually no driver protection. An infinite variety of other open-wheeled cars exist, culminating in the Indy and Formula 1 car. These are the fastest closed course vehicles, with top speeds in excess of 240 mph generating cornering forces greater than 5.5 Gs. Offshoots of open-wheeled race cars include drag race cars, 300-mph machines that travel only in a straight line, and off-road "buggies" that are used in desert and hill climb racing.

Closed-wheeled race cars are exemplified by the stock or "modified" car. The most popular form of motor sport in the United States today is NASCAR, which sanctions races using highly modified versions of common passenger cars. Several other varieties of closed-wheeled cars exist, including sports racing cars. These are modified versions of exotic passenger cars such as Jaguar, Ferrari, and Porsche. All types of cars are raced worldwide on and off the road, on any surface, and on ovals, road courses, and drag strips. There are sprint races and endurance races, rallies, and hill climbs. Some go for days;

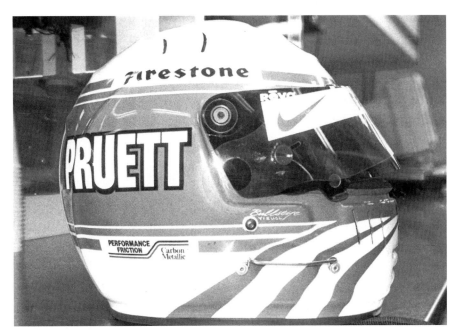

FIG. 2. Modern full face helmet, capable of 10 G impact without structural failure.

others last only a few seconds. They all have one thing in common: they are dangerous.

HEAD INJURY

CART is currently the only professional racing organization with accurate statistics on accident and injury rates for a defined period of time. Since 1981 head injuries have accounted for 29% of all injuries in CART (2,3). Three fatalities have occurred in that period, all due to severe head injury. Head injuries constitute over 90% of the neurologic injuries in this form of racing. It may be assumed that the same general percentages occur in other forms of motor sport. Both open and closed head injuries occur. Closed head injuries are by far the most common form of head injuries, and the majority of these are classified as mild brain injuries. All organized forms of racing require the use of an approved helmet. Today these are usually of the full-faced variety (Fig. 2). This type of helmet offers excellent protection from penetration and provides a substantial cushion to mitigate acceleration–deceleration injury. As a result, most head injuries are grade I concussions. The mechanism of such injury is either acceleration or deceleration as the helmet and head hit the inside of the cockpit or rotational as the car spins violently on its axis. Both mechanisms are identical to those found in boxing. The severity of the concussion is related to the amount of protection in the cockpit, the quality of the helmet, and the velocity of the crash. The most violent crashes result in diffuse axonal injuries as seen on the highway.

Mild brain injuries in motor sport constitute a higher percentage of all head injuries than in the general population. This is due to the use of high-quality helmets and the protection afforded by the required six-point safety harness. In the general population, mild head injury accounts for 60% to 80% of all head injuries (4). In automobile racing, mild head injury constitutes 95% of all head injuries. The incidence of serious sequelae of mild brain injury in auto racing has not been extensively studied. Subjectively, it appears that professional racing drivers have fared well after head injury. In the author's 25-year experience in CART, no driver has complained of postconcussion symptoms for more than 1 month after mild brain injury. Currently, because of the subjective impression that professional drivers do not suffer significantly from posttraumatic stress syndrome, a study is in progress evaluating 20 full-time professional drivers at the top of their sport. This experience seems to differ from that of the general population, in which an incidence of serious posttraumatic symptoms of as much as 40% of the injured population has been reported (4).

Severe closed head injuries in auto racing can run the gamut of head injuries but most often involve diffuse axonal injury secondary to shearing forces applied to the brain via the same mechanisms previously mentioned but of a greater magnitude. Diffuse axonal injury (DAI) is the term used to describe brain injury causing prolonged coma not due to a mass lesion or ischemic injury. Severe DAI is almost always due to vehicular injury and in the general population accounts for 16% of all severely head-injured patients (5). In auto racing, because of the factors mentioned previously, DAI accounts for less than 5% of all head injuries. Severe DAI results in shearing of small blood vessels and axons in the brain and the computed tomographic (CT) appearance of small, diffusely located punctate hemorrhages throughout the white matter. Recovery from DAI is rarely complete in the general population. Death occurs in 51% of the cases (5). In auto racing the results are better, most likely because the almost immediate medical attention given the injured driver at the scene leaves little or no chance for the driver to become hypoxic or hypotensive. Several examples of complete recovery from severe DAI have been documented, with some drivers able to return to competition. In CART racing since 1981 there have been four drivers with such severe injuries without other structural abnormalities, all of whom were able to return to competition. When DAI is associated with intracranial mass lesions or open head injury, the results are catastrophic. All four fatalities in CART since 1981 involved this type of combined injury.

A unique injury mechanism has been discovered in the General Motors Research and Development Center in Warren, Michigan. During a study of CART crashes it became apparent that drivers in crashes with very high G loads were surviving with relatively minor head injury.

These crashes often exceeded 60 G. It became clear that the driver's head in a CART crash fortuitously comes into contact with either the padded cockpit rim or the padded steering wheel when thrust forward on impact before reaching full excursion of the neck. The energy-absorbing nature of this padding mitigates the effect on the brain. In contrast, there have been two fatalities in another form of auto racing with lower G forces on impact due to basilar skull fractures as a result of the base of the skull being pulled away from the rest of the skull upon full head and neck excursion (Fig. 3). It appears that something needs to "catch" the head under controlled deceleration during impact to protect from devastating injury. These skull fractures were each associated with severe DAI.

Both epidural and subdural hematomas occur in auto racing but not to the extent that they do in passenger car crashes. This is obviously due to the wearing of suitable helmets. Intracranial hemorrhage related to contusion also occurs and accounts for most expanding intracranial lesions in auto racing. The head of the race car driver, even with a helmet on, is vulnerable to any number of objects coming into contact with it. Most notable are suspension parts, wheels, and tires. In addition to car parts, the head can make contact with support structures and retaining walls as well as the inside of the cockpit as mentioned. Any contact of sufficient magnitude can cause the head to decelerate, accelerate, or to rotate, causing injury. Penetration, however, is unusual and most frequently involves a rod or similar part of the suspension system. The most vulnerable part of the helmet for penetration is the visor area.

Case Report

The following is a case report of a diffuse axonal injury sustained in CART. The patient was a 28-year-old male racing driver who crashed while testing a car at the Indianapolis Motor Speedway. The crash was witnessed by track workers, who estimated that the car was traveling in excess of 220 mph when it went out of control and the right front of the car hit the second turn wall. The right front suspension was torn away, causing the wheel and tire assembly to make con-

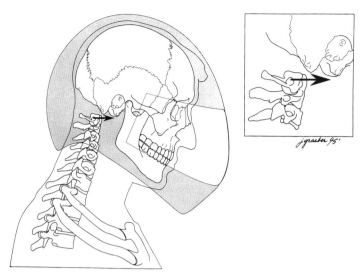

FIG. 3. Weight of helmet accentuates force of separation upon full excursion of unrestrained head causing basilar skull fracture.

tact with the driver's head and force it against the unpadded left side of the cockpit. At the scene the driver was unconscious, apneic, and given a Glasgow Coma Scale score of 4. He was intubated at the scene and transferred to the trauma center. Admitting CT scanning of the head showed punctate hemorrhages with nearly obliterated cisterns. Initial intracranial pressure was elevated and reached levels greater than 60, necessitating treatment with barbiturate coma, vasopressors, osmotherapy, and controlled hyperventilation. There were no expanding or mass lesions of the brain and no other associated injuries. The driver was comatose for approximately 3 weeks and then began a gradual awakening with complete neurologic recovery in 6 months after intense therapy. He continues to drive race cars without sequelae.

SPINAL INJURY

Since 1981, 20% of injuries in CART racing have been to the axial skeleton (6). During the decade 1981 through 1991, approximately 50 drivers have sustained injuries while driving Indy cars; nine involved the axial skeleton, three the cervical spine (6). Considering the forces involved in an auto racing crash, this seems remarkable.

Cervical Spine

The most frequent injury to the cervical spine in CART racing is a sprain or strain of the neck muscles on the left side. For years, drivers in races on oval tracks have worn a strap that attaches to the left side of the helmet and passes through the axilla to rejoin the helmet. This strap is used to combat the lateral G forces pulling the head and helmet to the right and making it difficult and tiring for the driver to hold the head upright. Lateral forces in modern oval track racing can exceed 5.5 G. In addition to the sprain or strain injury, this apparatus would also frequently cause paresthesias in the left arm occasionally lasting several days as a result of transient brachial plexus injury. Because of this type of injury, the use of these straps has declined; drivers now use a supporting pad to rest their head against during the race to keep it erect in the turns.

Fortunately, fractures of the cervical spine are rare. Direct frontal impact in an Indy car has rarely, if ever, produced a fracture of the cervical spine. A rear impact, however, frequently causes a flexion–extension type injury related to the whiplash effect aggravated by the weight of the helmet, which, with built-in radio, can be over 3 pounds. The extent of injury is related to the design and the amount of padding of the head rest coupled with the force of the crash. The most frequent fractures of the spine have been avulsions of the spinous processes and/or simple compression fractures of the cervical vertebral bodies (5). Disruption of the posterior ligaments also occurs. These injuries are fortunately rare. The most common type of crash that causes an injury to the spinal cord is a violent rollover. In this instance the driver's head is accelerated centrifugally out of the car, which, when coupled with either a forward or lateral flexion force, can produce serious injury to the cervical spine and spinal cord. Again, protection is offered by the roll bar, cockpit padding, and restraint system. In CART racing none of the cervical fractures sustained has resulted in a neurologic deficit. This enviable record, however, is not likely to remain intact, and an effort has been under way to develop a head and neck restraint system that will resist these disruptive forces. In other forms of auto racing the same mechanisms have, at times, resulted in spine injuries with deficits. At least one fatality has resulted from a hangman-type fracture when a stock car was hit broadside by another car, causing the driver's head and

neck to make contact with an ill-fitting shoulder strap and causing the driver literally to "hang" himself at the moment of impact. Proper fit of restraint mechanisms is vitally important.

In a drag racing accident a fracture dislocation of the lower cervical spine associated with quadriplegia occurred when a top fuel drag race car collided with a retaining wall and rolled over at the moment of impact. In spite of the fact that the roll bar kept the drivers' head from hitting the ground, a severe flexion-type injury occurred. A combination of forces applied to the head when the car hit the barrier and the resultant rollover caused a marked flexion–distraction deformity aggravated by the weight of the head with the helmet. A burst fracture of C-5 resulted. Forces involved in these types of high-speed crashes can generate an infinite number of combinations with marked potential for neurologic injury (5).

Dr. Robert Hubbard, from Michigan State University, has developed and tested the HANS device. This device tethers extreme movements of the driver's helmet and head with a stiff yoke and collar structure that is held to the torso by the existing shoulder straps (Fig. 4). The system

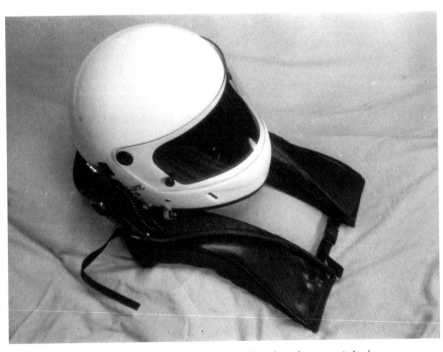

FIG. 4. HANS device. Tethered head and neck support device.

keeps the head and neck moving as one, with acceleration of the head in the event of an accident being controlled by tethers with inertia controlled release. When used properly, the HANS device will decrease neck loading as demonstrated by controlled tests in the General Motors and Wayne State University laboratories (Fig. 5). This system has been used with success in stock car racing as well as in sports racing cars. The drawbacks currently are the bulk of the system and the perceived lack of peripheral vision, although this has not proved to be an actual problem. This system is continually being refined and some form of inertia/tethering device will ultimately be in general use.

Thoracolumbar Spine

Injuries to the thoracolumbar spine are also relatively rare because the driver is so well restrained within the car. When an injury of this type does occur it is almost always associated with a frontal crash. The mechanism of injury is the result of the car striking a barrier or another car with sufficient force to cause the rear wheels to rise into the air and then come to rest on the ground, causing an axial load on the driver's buttocks and pelvis and consequently the thoracolumbar spine. Another mechanism of injury arises when the tub is shortened because of buckling of the bottom of the car as a consequence of a sudden

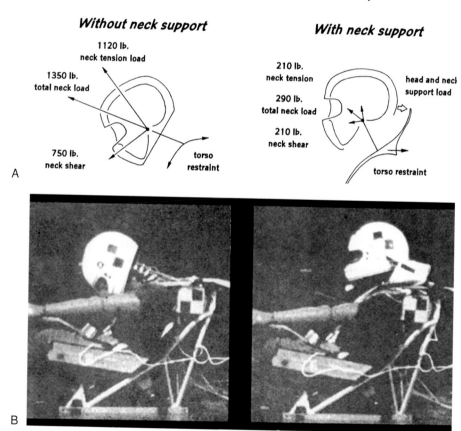

FIG. 5. (A) Crash test with and without HANS device demonstrating decreased neck loads with device. (B) Wayne State University tests showing decreased excursion of head and neck with HANS device in place (*right*) as compared with no HANS device (*left*).

stop against an object of some kind, producing an axial load on the driver's thoracolumbar spine. The driver in an Indy car is seated in a semiprone position and held there by the passive restraint systems previously mentioned. In this position the driver's spine is held in a slightly flexed position, forcing an aggravated flexion moment in the event of a frontal crash. As with cervical injuries, thoracolumbar injuries in CART since 1981 have not caused neurologic deficits, but obviously the potential is there.

Although precise data are not available for closed-wheeled racing, it appears that both cervical and thoracolumbar injuries are rare. In this form of racing the driver sits virtually upright. In 23 years of NASCAR racing there have reportedly been only three fractures of the cervical spine and no thoracolumbar fractures (6). Studies from General Motors Research have shown increasing neck loads in the event of a crash as the driver assumes a more reclined position (J. Melvin, General Motors, personal communications, 1982 to present). CART drivers compromise and sit in a 45° semireclined position, which, although causing higher neck loads in the event of a crash, makes the driver's head less exposed to flying objects and improves aerodynamic flow with greater comfort and performance.

PERIPHERAL NERVE INJURY

Peripheral nerve injuries have occurred with some regularity in auto racing. One type of injury has been previously mentioned and is due to compression of the brachial plexus by various straps used in an attempt to hold the driver's head upright on oval tracks to combat lateral G loads. Ulnar nerve palsies have also resulted from pressure against the ulnar nerve at the elbow because of poor driver seating positions and in-car protrusions. Compression injury to the sciatic nerve has resulted from an ill-fitting seat causing foot drop and pain. Also, the peroneal nerve has been involved through a similar mechanism. Obviously these types of injuries can be very dangerous. They are preventable by proper seating and the use of supports instead of straps to counter G loads.

PREVENTION OF NEUROLOGIC INJURY

Protecting the modern auto racing driver begins with the driver. Unlike the drivers in the barnstorming days of the past, modern racing drivers must be in excellent physical condition. Upper body strength and strong neck muscles are important. An accident in the Indy Lights series resulted in a comminuted fracture of C-5. As reported by his surgeon, the driver did not suffer a deficit because his neck musculature was extremely strong. Improved diets and aerobic training have reduced body fat in modern race drivers and improved their endurance. Reduced body fat enables one to better withstand the rigors of high ambient temperatures and to remain more focused during a prolonged event. Drivers' heart rates are known to exceed 85% of their maximum heart rates for the duration of a 3-hour event, with decreases in heart rate occurring only during pit stops and yellow caution periods (7). Fatigue often leads to inability to concentrate and therefore an increased likelihood of crashing. Enhanced endurance is therefore very important for driver safety.

Drivers are also responsible for their own personal protection, including an approved helmet and fire-resistant uniform with gloves, balaclava, socks, and shoes (Fig. 6). The driver also oversees the protection and comfort of the cockpit. This includes a six-point restraint system, padded steering wheel, and padded cockpit rim (Fig. 7). Padding must be an energy-absorbing foam such as Ensolite or other suitable product. Current restraint systems have a stretch factor of 15% to 20% on impact; therefore, energy-absorbing padding must extend to the steering wheel (5). The driver's helmet should make contact with the padded head rest when the driver is in a normal driving position. All sharp edges within reach of the driver's extremities should also be padded, rounded off, or removed altogether.

Crash study investigation in CART is ongoing; therefore, the cars are in a constant state of evolution. Currently, protection is afforded the

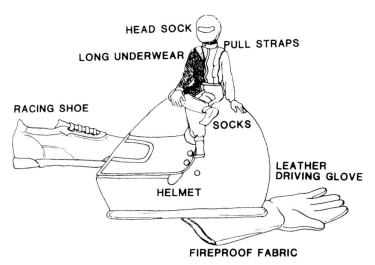

FIG. 6. Drivers' protective gear.

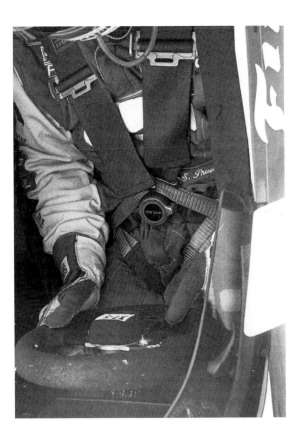

FIG. 7. Driver in car, showing restraint system and padding of cockpit rim and steering wheel.

driver by well-placed crushable structures; the side pods of the car and the nose cone are good examples. These structures absorb energy in the event of a crash and can deflect objects thrown about as a result of a crash. Strengthening of the tub and improvements in the location and anchoring of suspension parts have provided more energy-absorbing capabilities in an Indy car and lessened the chance of protrusion. The driver's feet have been placed behind a second bulkhead and the foot box area has been greatly strengthened. Finally, the driver is semireclined in the cockpit with the sides of the car reaching above the level of the shoulders. This arrangement makes it easier for the head to remain in the car in the event of impact or rollover and protects the driver from missiles generated by an accident (Fig. 8).

Attention to the race course is also of paramount importance. Armco barriers should be replaced by concrete wherever possible. Tire barriers are relatively inexpensive and provide excellent energy absorption when placed around stationary objects and at impact points. Sand traps also serve to retain an errant car and lessen the forces of impact. Any stationary objects that can be removed from the course should be removed. The surface itself should be as homogeneous as possible with no protrusions or leading edges from walls. Debris fencing should be of an approved type and placed substantially behind the frontal plane of any wall so that a driver's head is not likely to strike a post or support structure. All of these areas are under the jurisdiction of the sanctioning body and the insurer for the event. All arrangements in the interest of safety should be made a part of the sanction agreement.

The final line of defense against injury in auto racing is the rapid response of highly trained fire, safety, and medical personnel at the accident scene. The race track offers an excellent opportunity to utilize a complete emergency medical system (EMS). All events in CART are attended by two traveling physicians. One is an orthopedic surgeon, the other a critical care or trauma trained physician. Each doctor rides in one of the two safety trucks that are stationed

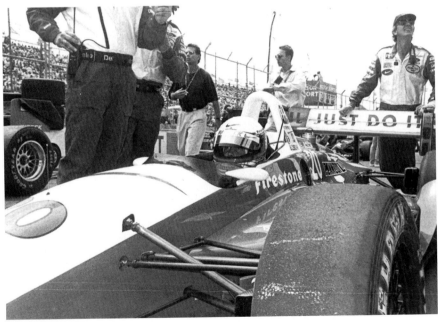

FIG. 8. Driver in car, revealing elevation of cockpit sides above shoulder level offering protection from debris and limited extrusion of body.

around the race course so as to be present at the scene of an accident within 60 seconds. Each truck also includes a paramedic and one or two firefighters. The same key individuals attend every race. Equipment on the trucks includes fire-suppressant materials, extrication tools, and emergency medical supplies. Items needed to perform any immediate lifesaving procedure are available. Both physicians are ATLS certified.

In the event of an accident, the physicians act as first responders and attend to the driver or drivers involved as soon as any fire is suppressed. Using trauma resuscitation protocols, it is immediately determined whether or not an airway is needed. This requires removal of the helmet. Two people are necessary: one to stabilize the cervical spine, the other to remove the helmet and its attachments. The only reason not to remove a helmet is that an object penetrates both the helmet and the head. In this case tools are available to cut out the face of the helmet, allowing easy access to the airway. Once the initial assessment is concluded and any immediate life-threatening problems are addressed, the driver's head, neck, and torso are immobilized on a custom-made short backboard and the driver is then carefully removed from the car. If extrication tools are needed to free the driver, it is the physician's responsibility to attend to the driver and ensure that further injury is prevented during the use of the extrication tools. Because carbon fiber splinters when cut, it is imperative that all parties protect their skin and eyes from flying pieces of carbon fiber debris. Once a controlled extrication of the driver has been completed, the driver is placed in a helicopter or ambulance under the care of the local medical authorities. Arrangements about the hospital to be used have been made prior to the event. One of the race physicians then accompanies the driver to the trauma center to act as liaison between the local medical personnel and the racing organization. In this way the entire operation is overseen by highly trained physicians with extensive experience in the recognition and treatment of racing injuries. Every effort is made to establish good rapport with the local medical authorities and to develop a good ongoing relationship. Close attention is given to the driver during hospitalization and

throughout rehabilitation and eventual return to work. Remarkably, with the exception of the three fatalities, in 20 years of CART racing, no driver has been so impaired from a crash as to be unable to return to competition.

Because we arrive at the scene so rapidly, some interesting observations have been made. In 1978 we first realized that all concussions of grade II or greater were associated with some period of apnea. This apneic period is directly proportional to the severity of the concussion. We are able, by virtue of early arrival on the scene, to assess and clear the airway immediately and ventilate the driver, if necessary. Usually a nasal pharyngeal airway is sufficient to stimulate respiration and provide a clear airway. We have also been impressed by the frequent occurrence of drivers, following a crash, removing themselves from the car, assessing the accident scene, and discussing the events with track workers, only to become obtunded and/or amnesic later. Normally these drivers develop only a grade I concussion and have a normal CT scan. It is imperative, however, that all drivers involved in a significant contact accident have the neck immobilized and undergo observation by trained personnel for at least 1 hour after the accident with thorough neurologic examination. CT scanning is always performed if there is documented loss of consciousness for any period or abnormal mental status for more than 5 minutes following the accident. Documented loss of consciousness also requires an overnight stay in the hospital in case of the rare development of a delayed, expanding, hemorrhagic contusion or clot.

RETURN TO COMPETITION FOLLOWING HEAD INJURY

Return to competition following head injury has been a much debated topic. Current practice has evolved from trial and error in sports such as boxing and football. In auto racing, until the mid-1970s, no one really paid any attention to a driver after mild brain injury. Drivers were left on their own regarding return to competition. The author knows of at least one instance in which a driver was knocked unconscious on

Friday night only to race again on Saturday and Sunday. On Monday he did not remember where he had been or how he had received a trophy. Currently, in CART the guidelines listed in Table 1 are used for return to competition.

"Second impact syndrome," described by Saunders and Harbaugh, is the rare occurrence of fatal cerebral swelling after a second brain injury in someone who is still symptomatic from the first injury. This possibility is of obvious concern in auto racing and must be vigorously guarded against.

For severe head injury and after prolonged hospitalization and rehabilitation, the following criteria must be met for return to competitive driving: The driver must have a normal neurologic examination performed by a certified neurosurgeon or neurologist and must have passed a full battery of neuropsychologic tests. There can be no seizures when seizure medication is not given and no residual lesion other than scarring on CT scan or magnetic resonance image. CART requires investigation at two institutions to eliminate any question of bias. After all of this, the driver must pass a strict performance test administered by the chief steward while observed by other licensed drivers. The driver who passes this test is then allowed to return to competition on a probationary basis. Using this format, CART has successfully integrated all of its severely head-injured drivers back into competition. One driver was unable to perform to his satisfaction in close racing situations and withdrew from further competition. Two other drivers have since retired from racing, leaving one driver still active and competitive.

A driver is allowed to return to competition after other neurologic injury when and if he or she can successfully perform the functions required to drive a racing car safely. This includes the ability to exit the car in a reasonable period of time in case of a fire or other reason for rapid evacuation. Prosthetic devices are allowed as long as they do not affect the safe operation of the vehicle and/or hamper the driver's performance. Braces have been used on the extremities to manage footdrop in a case of sciatic nerve injury, and special casts and shoes have been used to compensate for disabling injuries in a variety of circumstances. Racing drivers, by their nature, are extremely compliant with medical instructions and for the most part eager to return to competition as soon as it is safe to do so. Every effort is made to give a driver the opportunity to resume his or her career after injury. In auto racing, unlike most other sports, the previously injured

TABLE 1. *Guidelines for return to competition after head injury*

Injury	First concussion	Second concussion	Third concussion
Grade 1 (mild) No LOC <30 min PTA	May return to competition if asymptomatic for 1 week.	Return to competition in 2 weeks if asymptomatic at that time for 1 week.	Terminate season. May return to competition next season if asymptomatic.
Grade 2 (moderate) LOC <5 min PTA >30 min <24 h	Return to competition after asymptomatic for 1 week.	Minimum of 1 month. May return to competition then if asymptomatic for 1 week; consider terminating season.	Terminate season. May return to competition next season if asymptomatic.
Grade 3 (severe) LOC >5 min PTA > 24 h	Minimum of 1 month. May then return to competition if asymptomatic for 1 week.	Terminate season. May return to competition next season if asymptomatic.	

Adapted from Cantu RC, Micheli LJ. *American College of Sports Medicine's guidelines for the team physician.* Philadelphia: Lea & Febiger, 1991. In: National Athletic Trainers' Association Research & Education Foundation, Mild Brain Injury in Sports Summit Proceedings, Washington, DC, April 16–18, 1994, with permission.

driver is not the only one put at risk by the injury. Any lapse in performance not only may affect the injured racer but also could be catastrophic to other competitors or spectators.

Major strides have been made in the past decade in improving safety in auto racing. Today, in CART, a driver racing at speeds in excess of 200 mph has only a 1.2 times greater chance of being injured in a crash than an individual in a passenger car crashing in normal highway traffic at 50 mph (3). This relative safety is the result of the driver being adequately restrained in a safety cell or tub, surrounded by energy-absorbing material. The car is designed to break apart on impact, sparing the driver the brunt of the crash energy. Race courses have been improved with better barriers and safer runoff areas. Extremely rapid application of EMS at the scene has also improved outcomes, especially regarding head and spinal cord injury. What at one time was the second most dangerous sport in the world has now become relatively safe, with injuries on an annual basis no more frequent than those seen in professional football or hockey.

Acknowledgment

The author is indebted to his colleague Dr. Terry R. Trammell for the information regarding injury to the spine in auto racing.

REFERENCES

1. Metropolitan Life Insurance Company statistics.
2. Trammell TR, Olvey SE. Crash and injury statistics from Indy-Car racing 1985–1989. In: Association for the Advancement of Automotive Medicine, *Proceedings, 34th Annual Conference,* Scottsdale, AZ, Oct 1–3, 1990; 329–335. The Association, 1991.
3. Trammell TR, Olvey SE, Reed DB. Championship car racing accidents and injuries. *Physician Sports Med* 1986;14(5):114–120.
4. Ommaya AK, Salazar AM. A spectrum of mild brain injuries in sports. In: *Mild brain injury in sports summit proceedings,* National Athletic Trainers Association, Research and Education Foundation, Washington, DC, April 16–18, 1994;72–79.
5. Gennarelli, TA. Cerebral concussion and diffuse brain injuries. In: Cooper PR, ed. *Head injury,* 2nd ed. Baltimore: Williams & Wilkins, 1987:108–124.
6. Trammell TR. Motor sports. In: *Watkins, Robert's The spine in sports,* St. Louis: Mosby, 1995.
7. Lighthall JW, Pierce J, Olvey SE. A physiological profile of high performance race car drivers. In: Proceedings 1994 Motor Sports Engineering Conference, Society of Automotive Engineers, Dearborn, MI, Dec 5–8, 1994: 55–63.

Sports Neurology, Second Edition,
edited by Barry D. Jordan.
Lippincott–Raven Publishers, Philadelphia © 1998.

27

Ballet and Dance

Lyle J. Micheli, *Ruth Solomon, and †Peter G. Gerbino II

*Children's Hospital, Division of Sports Medicine, 319 Longwood Avenue,
Boston, Massachusetts 02115; *Department of Theater Arts, University of California, Santa Cruz,
California 95064; †Department of Orthopaedic Surgery, Division of Sports Medicine, Harvard
Medical School, Children's Hospital, 300 Longwood Avenue, Boston, Massachusetts 02115*

Typically, professional dancers, and even students who aspire to careers in dance, maintain that they must practice their art every day in order to meet its demands. Especially in large ballet companies this compulsion to dance may be reinforced by pressure from peers and management—by a nagging awareness that any hiatus from dance activity can have dire consequences in terms of status, performance opportunities, and even jobs lost. Hence, anything that threatens the dancer's ability to dance is anathema. It goes without saying that injuries tend to be right at the top of the dancer's list of such things.

Perhaps because injuries are associated with medicine, dancers have traditionally been distrustful of doctors. To see a doctor, they have often found, means to be told to take time off from all physical activity. This aversion to conventional medicine has probably been enhanced by the fact that dancers have traditionally been underinsured for their health needs. For one reason or another, at least until recently, many dancers have been more willing to seek the "quick fix," relatively inexpensive help for their medical problems available from chiropractors and other alternative-medicine practitioners than to see medical doctors. (There is good reason to believe that the better education available to both dancers and doctors through the emerging fields of dance medicine and dance science has begun to reverse this way of thinking.)

Unfortunately, the daily practice of movements that are both extreme and repetitive in their demands makes dancers far more susceptible to injury than the population at large. Unlike their fellow athletes in the contact sports, dancers seldom experience career-threatening traumatic injuries, but they do manifest a wide range of microtraumatic syndromes. The maxim in the field that "if you dance long enough, you will have injuries" is all too true.

Effective clinical management of dance injuries is, we have found, a five-step process. First, the problem must be understood by knowing the types of injuries that occur most frequently in this at-risk population, based on genetic makeup, body habitus, and the training demands of the discipline. These data provide clues to diagnosis and guidelines for prevention. Second, an accurate diagnosis must be made both generally (microtrauma, macrotrauma, or atrauma) and specifically. "Wastebasket" diagnoses rarely result in the rapid return of any athlete to full activity. Next, appropriate treatment is undertaken and monitored. To whatever extent possible, this should be done by a team approach, involving clinicians, therapists, the dance teacher or artistic director, and, when the patient is a child or adolescent, his or her parents. The fourth step is rehabilitation and return to dance, which requires planning that is specific to both the discipline and the patient. Finally, preventive measures must be taken to avoid recurrence.

EPIDEMIOLOGY

The epidemiology of neurologic injuries per se in dancers has yet to be written. In a practice such as ours, however, in which dancers are seen on a daily basis, one easily derives a clinical impression of which injuries are most common in this population of patients. We see that although dancers are susceptible to a wide range of neurologic problems, the largest concentration of injuries involves the low back, especially the lumbar spine. This finding is totally consistent with the research that is helping us understand the epidemiology of sports injuries in general. Spencer and Jackson (1), for example, reported that spine-related complaints constitute almost 10% of athletes' medical problems. Ferguson et al. (2) found that 75% of high-performance athletes have some sort of back pain. In the 142 top athletes in Sweden studied by Sward et al. (3), the incidence of low back pain ranged from 5% to 85%, depending on the sport. The demands of dance, with its extreme flexion of the spine and emphasis on hyperlordodis in movements to the rear, such as arabesque, suggest that it would lie toward the high end of the range (Fig. 1).

Lumbar Spine Injuries

Injuries to the lumbar spine usually result from either of two patterns of force generation: single-event, acute macrotrauma, or repetitive microtrauma with resulting "overuse" injury. Macrotrauma to the spine and back is most common in high-speed collision and aerobic sports; the current literature contains evidence of increased risk of spinal and thoracic macrotrauma in more than 20 different sports (4). Fortunately, such injuries are rarely encountered in dance, in which overuse injuries from repetitive microtrauma predominate (5).

One important caveat needs to be introduced immediately. The pattern of back injury in "older" dancers, broadly defined as postadolescent, tends to be quite different from that in the large number of serious child and adolescent participants who people this field. In the older dancer some significant degree of age-dependent segmental degeneration in the spine is to be expected. Hence, injury is commonly initiated in the anterior disc elements, producing discogenic pain and sciatica. Bone overgrowth at the facets may compromise the lateral recesses or neuroforamina, resulting in nerve encroachment and spinal stenosis. It is thus relatively easy for a minor twist or other sudden impact to result in nerve injury or irritation with associated swelling and pain. One of our studies involving subjects from the Division of Sports Medicine at Boston Children's Hospital can be referenced here to underscore this distinction. One hundred random cases of back pain encountered in athletic adolescents with a mean age of 15.8 years and range in age from 12 to 18 years were reviewed and compared with 100 adults seen in a back pain clinic in the period from 1989 to 1992. This group of adult subjects had a mean age of 31.9 years and range from 21 to 77 years. Sixty-two percent of the adolescents had derangements of their posterior elements associated with onset of back pain. Forty-seven of the 100 were ultimately shown to have spondylolysis stress fracture of the pars interarticularis. By contrast, 5% of adult subjects were found to have spondylolysis associated with low back pain. Conversely, discogenic back pain was the final diagnosis in 48 of the 100 subjects in the adult group, whereas only 11 of the 100 in the adolescent group had back pain attributable to disc abnormalities (6).

The differential diagnosis of back pain in dancers can be divided into four major categories: mechanical (including growth-related problems in the young dancer), discogenic, spondylolytic, and vertebral body fractures. Other causes of low back pain in the dancer are secondary to arthritic degeneration and spinal deformities.

Mechanical Low Back Pain

Mechanical back pain may be due to either acute or chronic musculotendinous or ligamentous injuries of the spine. Often this diagnosis is one of exclusion in the dancer, when careful physical examination has ruled out the other possible categories of injury. The only complaints of pain in this category may be of an aching back associated with prolonged standing or sitting or after dance training. Results of diagnostic techniques such as plain-film radiographs and bone scans are normal.

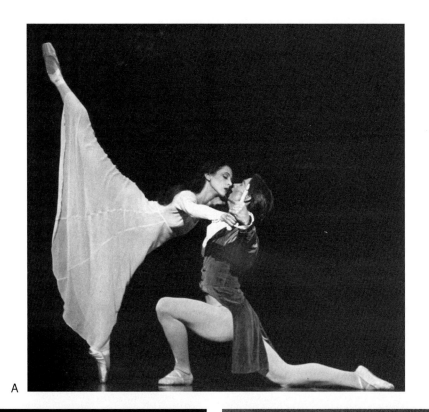

A

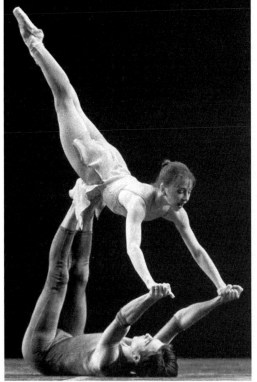

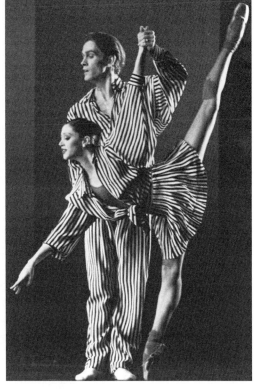

C

FIG. 1. Dance makes extreme demands on the spine, especially in movements involving leg extension to the rear. (Photographs by J. R. Phillips, courtesy of the Boston Ballet.)

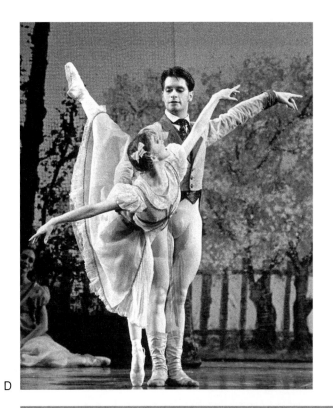

D

E

FIG. 1. *Continued.*

Mechanical and musculoskeletal problems such as postural lordosis and excessive tightness of the extensor musculature or weakness of the abdominals may be risk factors for this etiology. Poor technique can encourage all of these factors. Hyperlordosis is a special problem. Like any patient with chronic low back pain, the dancer must learn to limit the extension of the spine, specifically while dancing. However, the manner in which the dancer must do this is much more difficult. The average person involved in sitting or standing activities can usually learn to perform an effective pelvic tilt by using a combined action of the pelvic, gluteal, and abdominal muscles. The dancer has to rely primarily on the abdominal and paraspinal muscles, because the muscles in and below the pelvis are actively involved in dance technique. The frequently heard directive of the dance teacher to "pull up" into the chest is a reflection of this technical demand, which, it is hoped, results in good dance aesthetics as well as a safe position for the back.

Unfortunately, all too many dancers, particularly the younger ones, are hyperlordotic, which is noticeable when they perform *barre* or center floor work. This lordotic posture may reflect both anatomic malalignment and muscle–tendon imbalance and is almost always an acquired posture. True anatomic hyperlordosis is really quite rare, although individuals with certain genetic disorders such as chondroplasia or cleidocranial dysostosis appear to have an increased incidence of anatomic hyperlordosis. Much more frequently the hyperlordosis of the young dancer is due to a combination of muscle imbalance with relatively weak abdominals and relatively tight lumbodorsal fascia and poor technique, especially attempting to increase "turnout" at the hip by swaying the back.

Increased lordosis at the lumbopelvic junction is associated with flexion at the hip joints and resultant increased external rotation. This "trick" of swaying the back in order to increase turnout at the hips can be observed in many young dancers, but it must never be allowed as it not only interferes with the development of good technique but also increases the risk of back injury.

In addition, mechanical back pain may represent a transient "overgrowth" syndrome. The bony elements outstrip the ligaments and tendons during the second growth spurt, and this results in a combination of tight lumbodorsal fascia and hamstrings posteriorly, weak abdominal muscles anteriorly, and a posterior decompensation of the torso over the pelvis. Some of these children, usually boys, compensate for this structural imbalance by developing a mild roundback posture in an attempt to rebalance the torso forward over the pelvis and can develop wedging of the vertebral bodies at the apex of the compensating kyphosis. In these cases, proper treatment consists of flexibility exercises for the tight lumbodorsal fascia and hamstrings and anterior abdominal muscle strengthening. Antilordotic bracing may also be required. The back pain experienced by these patients must not be attributed to the roundback posture and treatment limited to dorsal extension exercises.

A particular instance of the interaction between technique, muscle strength, and postural alignment must be mentioned. The lifting technique of many male dancers is often unsafe, with the lift both initiated and executed with a lordotic back. Too often, the young male dancer gets into a pattern of lifting with a swayed back (Fig. 2). Choreography may demand that he be leaning forward or turning while lifting, which contributes to this habit. This pattern is typically not corrected as he advances professionally. We have been pleased with the results of a total body weight training program for a number of our dancers in the Boston Ballet. Improving the strength not only of the upper body but also of the abdominal and torso muscles has resulted in a significant improvement in body posture while lifting and has helped to minimize this swaybacked tendency, which is not only dangerous but also aesthetically displeasing.

Muscle and tendon macrotraumas in the form of strains are not infrequent occurrences in dancers. Many, if not most, of these injuries never come to the attention of a medical provider, as the dancer resolves his or her symptoms unaided within 4 to 6 weeks. Soft tissue scarring and shortening may occur, making recovery difficult and requiring physical therapy to regain flexibility. Perhaps the most important point regarding low

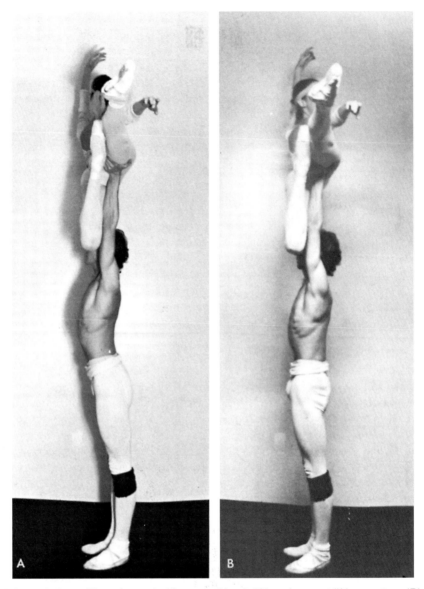

FIG. 2. A dance lift performed with swayed back (**A**) and correct lifting posture (**B**).

back strain is that it becomes chronic far less frequently in children than adults and heals far more readily. The diagnosis of back strain in a young dancer should be suspect unless an exact date and mechanism of injury are known. Back pain that does not resolve should not be diagnosed as "chronic mechanical low back pain" unless all other diagnoses have been ruled out (4).

Discogenic Back Pain

Discogenic back pain is rare in the prepubescent child, but the incidence in athletically active adolescents may be higher than in less active youths. A study carried out by the Mayo Clinic demonstrated increased disc disease with resultant back pain and sciatica in the adolescent age group in correlation with increased participation in sports (7). Activities such as dance that involve axial compression and flexion are typically associated with this injury. Hence, it must always be included in the differential diagnosis. The introduction of magnetic resonance imaging (MRI) has greatly aided in the early diagnosis of this condition.

The clinical presentation of discogenic back pain is often quite different in younger dancers from that in adults. Pain is not always the chief complaint; back stiffness, abnormal gait, or loss of hamstring flexibility may be more prominent. On examination, dramatic tightness of the lumbodorsal fascia and hamstrings is frequently found, often with an associated reactive lumbar or thoracolumbar scoliosis. A positive straight leg raising test or Lasègue's sign may reflect sciatic irritation. Asymmetric hamstring tightness may sometimes be the only warning of disc herniation. Loss of reflexes or muscle wasting is unusual.

Lumbar spine films are usually unremarkable initially, although they may occasionally show decreased disc space or an irregularity of the vertebral end plates at the level of involvement. Computed tomography or magnetic resonance imaging is usually diagnostic. The absence of radiation may make MRI the examination of choice in this age group.

Younger dancers and athletes with back pain related to disc deterioration may harbor genetic predispositions to disc disorder. A number of patients who came to our clinics with discogenic pain and sciatica showed evidence of multilevel disease, indicating a possible early familial tendency. A possible anatomic predisposition to adolescent disc disease has also been suggested, with a clover-shaped spinal canal and short pedicle increasing the chances of symptomatic disc protrusion (8).

Conservative treatment with bed rest, nonsteroidals, and progressive mobilization is recommended initially. Bracing therapy and exercise have been effective (9); we have found bracing to be far more beneficial than use of a soft lumbar support. If bracing, antiinflammatories, and physical therapy are unsuccessful at 12 weeks, epidural corticosteroids may be employed.

One study suggests that early surgical herniated nucleus pulposus (HNP) excision is required to prevent long-term back problems in children and adolescents (7). Our data on using the Boston brace are still being compiled, but our clinical impression is that most of these dancers have resolution of their back and leg pain without surgery. Repeated MRI at 1 year has shown complete resolution of the HNP in one patient (Fig. 3).

With the exception of bracing instead of corset use, we follow the discogenic back pain algorithm as described by the Pennsylvania Hospital group (10), modified by the special circumstances of the young dancer or athlete. Once cauda equina syndrome is ruled out, nonoperative therapy is all that is required for the majority of dancers with discogenic back pain. There may be a high incidence of continued back complaints in these patients as adults, but the effect of continuing dance or athletic participation on the natural history is not known (7).

Sciatica can, of course, be present with any discogenic condition. Sammarco (11,12) has observed that dancers (like gymnasts) may be at additional risk for sciatica because their habitual lack of adipose tissue exposes the sciatic nerve to traumatic injury when the buttocks strike the floor in splitlike movements. Also, a chronic sciatic neuritis might result from the repetitive practice of extreme low back and hamstring stretches or from imperfect technique in landing jumps (12). In addition to following a normal treatment regimen consisting of antiinflammatory medication, hot packs, and gentle stretching exercises, dancers with sciatic neuritis should reduce the number of classes they take during the 6 to 8 weeks that may be required for convalescence. A water *barre* can be helpful at this time as a relatively safe means of maintaining adequate conditioning.

Because the sciatic nerve passes under or sometimes through the tissues of the piriformis muscle, spasming or hypertrophy of that muscle may cause nerve entrapment, resulting in pain that mimics sciatica or other possible symptoms of disc herniation. The redundancy of internal and external hip rotation utilized by dancers in the practice of all dance techniques makes them particularly susceptible to chronic strain and/or spasming of the piriformis, one of the external

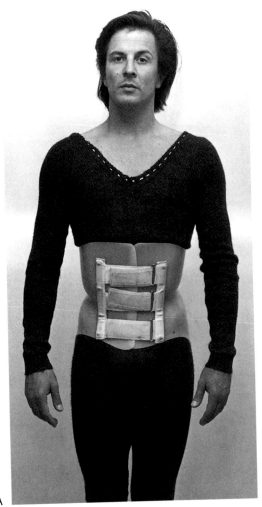
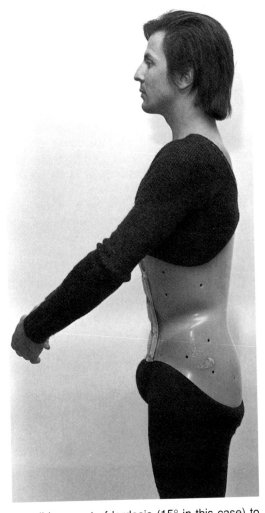

A   B

FIG. 3. The Boston brace can be constructed with a mild amount of lordosis (15° in this case) to minimize stresses on the discs, as in the treatment of disc herniation.

rotators of the hip. The dancer presents with deep posterior hip (gluteal) pain, and there may be sciatic radiation. Physical examination elicits pain on internal or external hip rotation against resistance. Positive straight leg raising and Lasègue's sign may not be present. Treatment consists of stretching and strengthening the external rotators of the hip, antiinflammatories, and physical therapy modalities including ultrasonography.

Spondylolytic Back Pain

Spondylolysis as a cause of back pain in dancers (and athletes) today appears to be increasing in frequency; its incidence in dancers is definitely greater than in the general population, perhaps equivalent to that found in gymnasts (13). Spondylolysis occurs only in the bipedal human; a study carried out in a group of institutionalized patients who never walked showed that risk of spondylolysis was almost zero (14). There do appear to be genetic risk factors, however. An association of spondylolysis with spina bifida occulta in 20% of young athletes has been found in previous studies (8).

Most authors now feel that spondylolysis and prespondylolytic stress reaction are overuse injuries (15–17). The mechanism of injury is repetitive microtrauma resulting from extreme flexion, extension, and rotation of the spine. This may result in damage to all of the posterior elements of the lumbar spine, including the pars interarticularis, facets, pedicles, lamina, and spinous processes. However, the pars is the most common site of injury (Fig. 4). Studies have suggested that hyperextension, in particular, results in shear stress at the pars, with eventual stress fracture (17).

The dancer is at first symptomatic only during certain maneuvers. The pain often becomes progressively more severe with daily routine activities or even at rest. It is typically relieved by supine positioning or by simply reducing the activity level. Occasionally, a single macrotraumatic event may result in acute onset of pain.

Physical examination again often reveals a hyperlordotic posture, with a painless limitation of motion in the lumbar spine on forward flexion

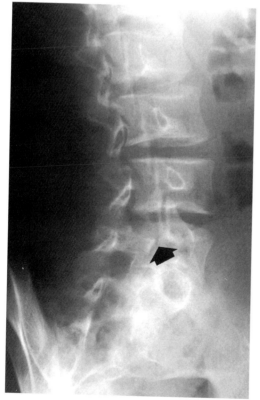

FIG. 4. Spondylolysis; stress fracture of the pars interarticularis as seen on oblique radiograph.

but pain with provocative hyperextension. A positive finding with the hyperextension test is usually indicative of posterior element damage. The dancer, standing on one leg and then the other, will elicit pain while hyperextending the back. The pain is often exaggerated on the ipsilateral side of the pathologic defect during this maneuver. Tight hamstrings and loss of flexibility may accompany these findings.

The diagnosis of *early* spondylolysis cannot be made with plain radiographs, even including obliques, because the pars has not yet fractured (Fig. 5A). Instead, studies from Children's Hospital in Boston and elsewhere suggest that single photon emission computed tomography (SPECT) bone scans are necessary to demonstrate these early lesions (Fig. 5B) (18–22). We recommend initial anteroposterior lateral and oblique radiographs in young athletes suspected of spondylolysis and with symptoms that have persisted longer than 3 weeks. If these are negative and there is no clinical evidence of herniated disc, we proceed to a SPECT bone scan, especially if repetitive hyperextension is involved, as in dance, and hyperextension testing exacerbates symptoms.

Spondylolysis in the young dancer is not considered an incidental finding as it might be for an adult. It is a pars interarticularis stress fracture and treated with bracing and physical therapy until healed or asymptomatic. This may take up to 9 months. The device used for bracing is the Boston overlapping brace with zero degrees of lordosis (Fig. 6) (8,9). Prespondylolytic pars stress reaction is treated the same way. Either may require repeated SPECT to confirm healing (8,9,23–26).

Occasionally, sciatica may be associated with spondylolysis. This may be due to compression of the L-5 nerve root by hyperplasia of the synovial and fibrous tissue at the site of the pseudoathrosis or associated disc disease. MRI can be useful for differentiation in these cases. Eighty-five percent of lesions are at L-5, and almost all the rest are at L-4.

It is essential to make the diagnosis of spondylolysis and initiate protective treatment as early as possible, before frank fracture or spondylolisthesis has occurred. There is an un-

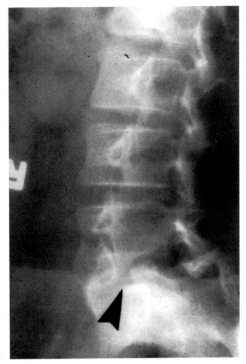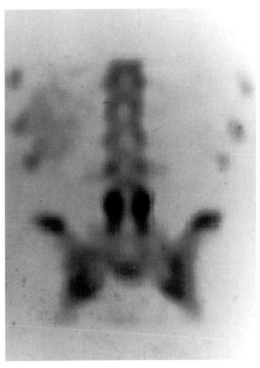

A   B

FIG. 5. **A:** Oblique radiograph showing obvious L-5 spondylolysis. When the fracture is this apparent it is probably of long standing. **B:** SPECT bone scanning (showing L-4 spondylolysis) is the diagnostic tool of choice for detecting this injury.

fortunate tendency with this lesion, perhaps a holdover from the time when this entity was thought of as a developmental defect and not recognized as a stress fracture, to withhold treatment unless lysis is evident on plain radiographs. No clinician, of course, would use such an approach with a tibial stress fracture, and to use it with stress fracture of the pars, which has an even greater potential for complete fracture and subsequent nonunion, is unacceptable. Treatment of spondylolisthesis is similar to that already described, with antilordotic bracing and hamstring stretching. Union may occur occasionally in grade I spondylolisthesis, but more commonly the goal is less to attain union or reduction than to return the dancer to full painless activity. If symptoms persist or increased slippage occurs, repair of the pars defect or fusion may be considered (27,28) All dancers with this condition are permitted to perform in the brace if symptoms have been relieved.

Return to dancing is entirely based on resolution of symptoms. If pain resumes when the brace is removed, the dancer is instructed to perform in the brace. If pain persists in the brace, dance activities are stopped until they can be resumed painlessly. The dancer with unilateral spondylolysis despite adequate bracing may return to full performance out of the brace when symptoms have resolved. In this case efforts are made to ensure that the contralateral pars does not fracture (8,9,29).

Both the prevention and rehabilitation of low back pain rest primarily on strict adherence to a systematic and balanced program of stretching and strengthening exercises. For stretching, the proprioceptive neuromuscular facilitation (PNF) technique is recommended. PNF stretching of the hamstrings and lumbodorsal fascia while the pelvis is stabilized can be extremely useful. With this technique the dancer might place one leg on the ballet *barre* and contract the quadriceps and

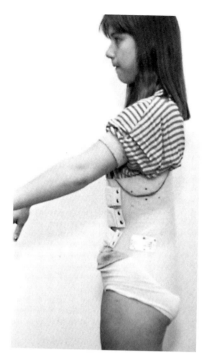

FIG. 6. The Boston brace antilordotic version (0° of lordosis) is used to treat posterior element conditions such as spondylolysis or facet arthrosis.

hamstrings strongly for 8 to 10 seconds, then release the contraction and slowly bend forward over the leg, stretching for another 8 to 10 seconds. During this stretch the supporting leg should first be in parallel position. Then the stretch should be repeated with the supporting leg turned out. (Dancers tend to do these stretches only turned out and need to be instructed carefully.) The PNF stretching technique can also be employed while lying supine on the floor, particularly with a young dancer who is very tight. It is important that the dorsal spine be protected while stretching the lumbar spine. This is accomplished by crossing the arms behind the back and maintaining an adducted posture of the scapula while forward bending stretches are being performed.

It is also important to stretch the lateral lumbodorsal fascia and to include stretching of the head and neck elements. In addition, stretching of the anterior hip along with the spinal elements

should be emphasized, as hip flexion contractures are often seen in combination with hyperlordosis of the low back.

A program of abdominal and pelvic strengthening exercises must be included in any rehabilitation regimen for the low back. We recommend a program of pelvic tilts, performed in both the standing and supine positions. We have found that, in general, careful instruction by a physical therapist is required to ensure that these exercises are done properly. Often several sessions are required. Initially, we use single leg lifts done slowly in the supine position while the opposite leg is flexed up. Three sets of 10 repetitions each are performed. This usually precedes the use of any type of situp exercise, because at first the injured dancer may not be able to tolerate the full torso-lifting technique. When we are able to go to a situp program, this is once again done in a slow fashion, with the knees and hips flexed at 90° and the scapula maintained in the adducted position.

In the later stages of the rehabilitation program weight training with a universal gym or free weights should be added. Vertical and horizontal rowing exercises are useful for strengthening the upper portions of the dorsal spine, as are latissimus pulls.

An important component of our rehabilitation program for low back injury is early use of swimming. This seems to be well tolerated, can be performed often in a functional and painless fashion, and is useful for synchronizing activity of the low back and pelvic musculature. As in the rehabilitation of any athletic injury, slow progression of training done in a painless fashion is important if the body is to return to full function (30).

Vertebral Body Fractures

Vertebral body microfracture at the anterior margin is a fourth cause of low back pain in the dancer. These fractures appear to be the result of microtrauma, usually from repetitive flexion, which injures the anterior portions of the vertebral endplates and can lead to frank wedging and Schmorl's node formation. The most frequent site of involvement is at the thoracolumbar junction, typically in one or two vertebral levels but occasionally involving three or more. These lesions have been referred to as "atypical Scheuermann's disease" (31). Often this occurs in gymnasts who begin their training before the age of 5 (30), so the crossover to young dancers is to be expected. Sorenson (32) characterized "classical Scheuermann's" as wedging of at least three consecutive thoracic vertebrae with Schmorl's node formation and a structural round back. Some cases that meet the criteria of true thoracic Scheuermann's disease may actually be the result of severe lumbar extension contracture with excessive flexion demands transferred to the thoracic spine and resultant anterior vertebral plate fracture with secondary bony deformation of the vertebra (30). In addition to dance, sports in which this type of injury is seen include rowing, gymnastics, tennis, and diving.

A sagittal "flatback" alignment of the spine with lumbar hypolordosis and thoracic hypokyphosis, such as is frequently seen in fully mature ballerinas, appears to increase the susceptibility to atypical Scheuermann's at the thoracolumbar junction (33). Tight lumbodorsal fascia, causing forward flexion to occur in the dorsal spine rather than in the lower lumbar spine, may also be a factor. Plain radiographs are usually sufficient for the diagnosis of this injury. Treatment consists of hyperextension bracing (15° to 30°), strengthening, and stretching with emphasis on the hamstrings. Here, McKenzie-type extension exercises are stressed (34). If diagnosed early, these dancers become asymptomatic in 4 to 6 weeks and can gradually return to full activity over 3 to 6 months (35). Strengthening in these dancers should follow guidelines described elsewhere (36–39). Without better epidemiologic data, prevention guidelines are theoretical. Observing dancers with increased or decreased lumbar lordosis and stressing flexibility and perilumbar strengthening may help.

To this point our discussion of stress fractures and fractures has focused on the pars interarticularis, which is clearly one of the most vulnerable components of the spinal column. It should be noted, however, that the pedicles are not immune to such injuries in dancers. At least two factors can explain the relatively low rate of fracture through the pedicles compared with the incidence of fracture through the pars interarticularis

(40). First, the pedicle is mechanically stronger than the pars interarticularis (41–43). Second, the anatomy and biomechanics of the lumbar spine serve to concentrate shear stress at the pars interarticularis selectively (30,43). Krenz and Troup (44) demonstrated anatomically that the thickest area of the pars interarticularis is anterolateral and the narrowest region is posteromedial, where stress fracture begins. They concluded that shear stress on the articular processes accounted for this selective cortical thickening. Abel (45) showed that spondylotic defects begin at the inferior margin of the pedicle, which is under the highest concentration of stress, and are then propagated obliquely across the pars interarticularis as the forces increase.

In an earlier paper we reported on our experience with the diagnosis and treatment of stress fractures of both pedicles of the second lumbar vertebra in a young ballet dancer, and her case can be used to summarize much of what we have said here (46). This 18-year-old woman, who had trained to be a ballet dancer for 10 years, had the gradual onset of pain in the middle and lower parts of the back over a period of several months. The pain began 1 month after she increased her daily training from 3 hours to 6 hours. She recalled no incident of acute injury, there was no history of pain in the back, and she had not sustained any prior stress fractures. Coughing, prolonged sitting, arising from a chair, and certain dance maneuvers, including *jeté,* forward bending of the lumbar spine, and hyperextension of the lumbar spine when being lifted, all made the pain worse. The pain did not radiate.

A night's rest decreased the pain enough for the patient to train for 6 hours a day for 3 months after the onset of symptoms (a good example of dancers' ability to "live with pain"). The discomfort recurred daily; it was exacerbated by movements that involved flexion and extension of the lumbar spine but not those involving rotation. The menses were normal, and the patient's diet was well balanced nutritionally.

Physical examination revealed pain on hyperextension of the lumbar spine. There was no evidence of scoliosis or spasm of the paravertebral muscles. The findings on neurologic examination were negative, and the findings on antero-

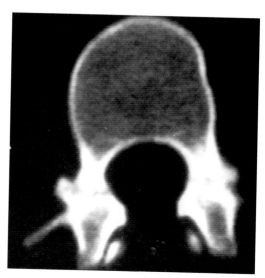

FIG. 7. This computed axial tomographic section shows bilateral stress fracture of the pedicle of the second lumbar vertebra.

hyperextension test was negative, and there were no abnormal neurologic findings.

A plain lateral radiograph showed a lucent defect of the pedicles of the second lumbar vertebra with surrounding sclerosis (Fig. 8). These abnormalities could not be identified on the anteroposterior or oblique radiographs. Computed axial tomographic sections showed persistent nonunion of both pedicles of the second lumbar vertebra, a finding similar to that seen 3 years previously. A bone scan showed a focal area of increased uptake that involved the right side of the fourth lumbar vertebra but not the area in question, the second lumbar vertebra.

The patient was managed with a program of exercise that included pelvic tilting, stretching of the thoracolumbar fascia, and strengthening of the

posterior, lateral, and oblique radiographs of the lumbar spine were normal. Because of the persistence of pain, computed axial tomographic sections of the lumbar vertebrae were made 3 months after the initial visit. One section showed bilateral fracture of the pedicle of the second lumbar vertebra (Fig. 7).

The initial treatment consisted of modification of the patient's dance technique to avoid painful maneuvers, taping the torso and back, exercises to strengthen the abdominal muscles, and pelvic tilt exercises. The patient was able to dance without limitation or pain 3 months after the initial diagnosis was made.

The patient became a professional ballet dancer and remained asymptomatic for 2 ½ years. Then, during a particularly strenuous rehearsal, she had an onset of pain that was similar to the first episode. The pain increased to the point that she could no longer dance effectively.

Clinical examination revealed no spasm of the paravertebral muscles or scoliosis. Forward flexion of the lumbar spine was limited by pain, and returning to an upright posture from a position in which the lumbar spine was flexed caused sharp pain in the midline of the lumbar area. This pain did not radiate to the lower limbs. The result of a

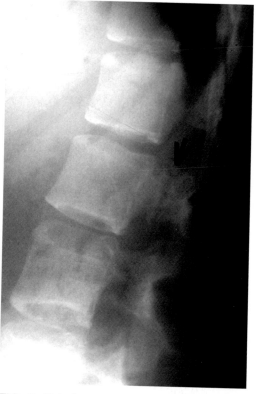

FIG. 8. This lateral radiograph of the lumbar spine demonstrates a radiolucent area at the site of the stress fracture of the pedicles. There is sclerosis of the bone on both sides of the radiolucent area.

gluteal muscles. She wore a Boston brace constructed to keep the spine in 0° of lordosis. It was suggested that she wear the brace full time, but in fact she wore it only at night for 2 months. The pain decreased to the point that she was able to perform her daily activities and exercises comfortably, but she did not dance during this period. She resumed dancing when she stopped wearing the brace but avoided specific movements that exacerbated the pain. She remained free of pain 1 year later and continued the exercise program for strengthening and stretching the abdominal and lumbar paravertebral muscles (46).

Lumbar Spondylosis

One additional source of low back pain resulting from repetitive microtrauma deserves mention: arthritic degeneration. In the adult, the facet joints would be the most likely source (facet degenerative arthritis as a result of microtrauma has not been reported in children). "Facet syndrome" has been described and may be another hyperextension overuse injury (47). This condition is not uncommon in the older dancer, in whom many years of stress on the facet joints due to excessive hyperextension may have caused degenerative changes, including erosion of the cartilage surface and joint space narrowing with osteophyte formation at the edges of the joints (Fig. 9). Progressive stenosis ensues. The pain may be localized or may radiate down the lower extremity because of irritation of the nerve root adjacent to the facet (48). Treatment consists of rest, antiinflammatories, and antilordotic exercises. If pain persists, immobilization with an antilordotic brace should be considered.

Spinal Deformities

A less common source of back pain in the dancer may be a transitional vertebra at the lumbosacral junction, with painful pseudoarthrosis at the sacroiliac junction (4). The types most predisposed to pseudoarthrosis formation are those with an enlarged transverse process or laterally fused mass. The mass may make direct contact with the iliac wing or sacrum, leading to degenerative changes and pain with movement (49). Originally described by Bertolotti (50), this is a well-known source of low back pain (49,51). Bracing, rest, and antiinflammatories can frequently reduce the pain, but the process is progressive and may persist. Corticosteroid injections to the pseudoarthrosis have been used with some success, but definitive treatment may require fusion or, more recently, resection of the bone impingement (51). Once symptoms have resolved, there are no contraindications to gradual return to full activity. If an impinging transitional vertebra is found incidentally on radiographs, the patient can be forewarned of the predisposition.

Sacroiliac and coccygeal pains are unlikely to result from repetitive microtrauma, although one report exists of sacroiliac stress fracture (52). If there has been no macrotrauma, one of the atraumatic arthritides should be suspected in these areas.

One further condition, idiopathic adolescent scoliosis, should be noted. It occurs in 10% to 16% of the general population (53–55) but has been reported to have a higher rate of occurrence in dancers (56). The diagnosis and treatment of this condition are well described elsewhere (57,58). Dancers with curves requiring bracing (those beyond 20° to 25°) may still participate in a complete program of dance training, particularly with regimens incorporating a maximum of 18 hours per day of bracing.

CERVICAL SPINE INJURIES

We have said virtually nothing to this point about the cervical spine because dancers, with only one notable exception, do not seem to be unusually vulnerable to injury in that region. The exception results from the practice of "spotting," a technique used especially by ballet dancers to ward off vertigo when performing a series of rapid turns such as *pirouettes* or *fouettés*. When spotting, the dancer fixes his or her gaze for as long as possible on some distant object while rotating the body through a full 360° turn, then suddenly rotates the head in the direction of the turn to reestablish visual contact with the object. Endless repetitions of this maneuver can cause cervical radiculitis, characterized by neuralgia that may travel from the neck to the fingers with resulting

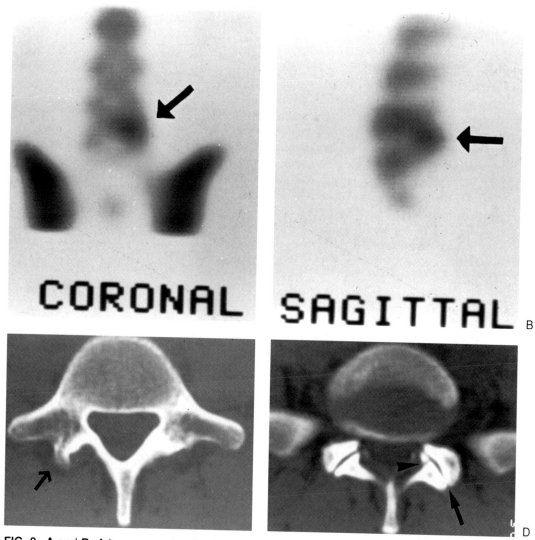

FIG. 9. A and **B:** A bone scan showing increased activity of the posterior elements of the left L4-5 region in a 36-year-old ballet dancer who developed left lumbar back pain following a vigorous summer program. **C:** CT scan of the same area, demonstrating left L4-5 facet arthrosis, with osteophyte and fracture of the inferior L-4 facet. **D:** CT scan of a 32-year-old ballet dancer who had intermittent low back pain radiating to the back of her left leg associated with leg extension movements. It reveals arthrosis of the L5-S1 facet joints.

hypesthesia, paresthesia, and loss of normal muscle reflexes. Treatment requires rest with immobilization of the neck using a soft collar, antiinflammatory medication, and the local application of moist heat. In extreme cases, where symptoms are severe and do not respond to this initial treatment, disc herniation must be suspected. The use of MRI for further diagnosis is then indicated (59,60).

PERIPHERAL NERVE INJURIES

Femoral neuritis results from traction or stretch of the femoral nerve and has been reported by both Sammarco and Miller (12,60,61). The patient presents with weakness in the thigh, usually demonstrated in movements that require simultaneous hip extension and knee flexion, such as the "Horton hinge" (Fig. 10). Electromyography may be helpful in the diagnosis of this injury. Treatment includes antiinflammatories and avoiding movements that cause traction of the femoral nerve.

Peroneal neuritis presents with hypesthesia and paresthesia in the forefoot between the first and second phalanges, with tenderness over the nerve at midfoot. The etiology may be external trauma causing damage to the nerve. Another rare source of peroneal nerve irritation is the pressure from tight ribbons and elastic used to secure pointe shoes (62).

Trauma at the ankle may result in sural neuropathy, causing pain and Tinel's sign in the lateral forefoot. Modern dance, done in bare feet, makes the dancer more vulnerable to lateral foot pressure against the floor with unusual maneuvers. Padding and changes in choreography to remove pressure from the subcutaneous sural nerve usually cause this condition to subside over time (62).

In modern dance, sitting on the feet with pressure on the dorsum of the foot against the floor can cause dorsal cutaneous neuritis. Tinel's sign and paresthesia between first and second phalanges are usually apparent upon examination (63).

Interdigital neuromas occur often in the general population but are particularly problematic

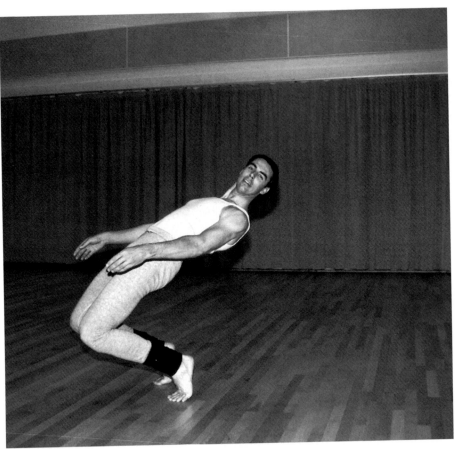

FIG. 10. A typical modern dance movement (the "Horton hinge"), requiring simultaneous hip extension and knee flexion. The resulting traction of the femoral nerve can cause neuritis. (Photograph by B. Berryhill.)

in dancers because of the persistent weight bearing on the metatarsal heads required by most forms of dance. The most frequently affected area of irritation is between the third and fourth metatarsal heads. Nerve entrapment, fibrosis, and thickening create sharp, shooting, "electric shock" pain. Conservative treatment using metatarsal pads to raise the heads and relieve pressure on the nerve is sometimes effective. If pain persists, corticosteroid injection may be helpful. Surgical excision of the neuroma is recommended when the preceding measures are not successful (64).

In conclusion, peripheral nerve conditions can interfere with training and performing to a great extent and thus seriously affect the degree to which a dancer can participate fully in his or her art form.

DISCUSSION

This overview of neurologic injuries in dancers is somewhat reductionistic in that it tends to treat all dancers alike. In reality, of course, dancers come in many varieties: they are male and female, professional and novice, relatively old and relatively young, and so on. Also, they practice different types of dance—most essentially ballet, modern, jazz, and aerobics—and, as has been well demonstrated in the literature by now, each of these subgenres makes unique demands on the body (65). In an earlier study we were even able to suggest that the various techniques employed by modern dancers produce different patterns of injury (66). All of these distinctions complicate the problems involved in dealing efficiently with dance injuries.

Nonetheless, the fact remains that dancers as patients do share with one another certain needs that are less pressing in the general population of patients. As these needs are similar to those experienced by athletes, a much larger base of patients in any medical practice, the tendency has been to encourage dancers to seek medical assistance in the same places, from the same doctors, as do athletes (67). For example, most of the dancers who come to us at Children's Hospital, Boston, are seen initially in our Sports Medicine Clinic.

As a result of this development, a relatively new medical specialist, the sports dance medicine doctor, has come into being. These individuals are emphasizing the prevention of injury in active children and adults as never before and are creating a more active role for the patient in the management of his or her own injury. Where patients were once required to immobilize injured body parts, they are now often encouraged to use stretching and strengthening exercises for both curative and rehabilitative purposes. Thus, by addressing the needs of our most active patients we move forward in ways that will eventually benefit all.

REFERENCES

1. Spencer GW, Jackson DW. Back injuries in the athlete. *Clin Sports Med* 1983;2:191–216.
2. Ferguson RJ, McMaster JH, Stanitski CL. Low back pain in college football linemen. *Am J Sports Med* 1974; 2(2):63–69.
3. Sward I, Hellstrom M, Jacobsson B, Hyman R, Peterson L. Disc degeneration and associated abnormalities of the spine in elite gymnasts: a magnetic resonance imaging study. *Spine* 1991;16:437–443.
4. Gerbino PG, Micheli LJ. Back injuries in the young athlete. *Clin Sports Med* 1995;14:571–589.
5. Solomon R, Micheli L. Concepts in the prevention of dance injuries: a survey and analysis. In: Shell CG, ed. *The 1984 Olympic scientific congress proceedings,* vol 8: *The dancer as athlete.* Champaign, IL: Human Kinetics Publishers, 1986:201–212.
6. Micheli LJ, Wood R. Back pain in young athletes. *Arch Pediatr Adolesc Med* 1995;149:15–18.
7. DeOrio JK, Bianco AJ. Lumbar disc excision in children and adolescents. *J Bone Joint Surg Am* 1982; 64A: 991–995.
8. Steiner ME, Micheli LJ. The use of a modified Boston brace to treat symptomatic spondylolysis. *Orthop Trans* 1983;7(1):20.
9. Micheli LJ, Hall JE, Miller ME. Use of modified Boston brace for back injuries in athletes. *Am J Sports Med* 1980;8:351–356.
10. Wisneski RJ, Rothman RH. The Pennsylvania Plan II: an algorithm for the management of lumbar degenerative disc disease. *Instruc Course Lect* 1985;34:17–36.
11. Sammarco GJ. The dancer's hip. *Clin Sports Med* 1983; 2:485–498.
12. Sammarco GJ. The hip in dancers. *Med Prob Perf Artists* 1987;2(1):5–14.
13. Jackson DW, Wiltse LL, Cirincione RJ. Spondylolysis in the female gymnast. *Clin Orthop* 1976;117:68–73.
14. Rosenberg NJU, Bargar WL, Feiedman B. The incidence of spondylolysis and spondylolisthesis in nonambulatory patients. *Spine* 1981;6:35.
15. Troup JDG. Mechanical factors in spondylolisthesis and spondylolysis. *Clin Orthop* 1976;149:59–67.

16. Weir MR, Smith DS. Stress reaction of the pars inter-articularis leading to spondylolysis. A cause of adolescent low back pain. *J Adolesc Health Care* 1989; 10: 573–577.

17. Weiss GB. Stresses at the lumbosacral junction. *Orthop Clin North Am* 1975;6:83–91.

18. Bellah RD, Summerville DA, Treves ST, et al. Low-back pain in adolescent athletes: detection of stress injury to the pars interarticularis with SPECT. *Radiology* 1991;180:509–512.

19. Collier BD, Johnson RP, Carrera GF, et al. Painful spondylolysis or spondylolisthesis studied by radiography and single photon emission computed tomography. *Radiology* 1985;154:207–211.

20. Papanicolaou N, Wilkinson RH, Emans JB, et al. Bone scintigraphy and radiography in young athletes with low back pain. *AJR* 1985;145:1039–1044.

21. Pennell RG, Maurer AH, Bonakdarpour A. Stress injuries of the pars interarticularis: radiologic classification and indications for scintigraphy. *AJR* 1985; 145: 763–766.

22. Rosen PR, Micheli LJ, Treves S. Early scintigraphic diagnosis of bone stress and fractures in athletic adolescents. *Pediatrics* 1982;70(1):11–15.

23. Micheli LJ. Sports following spinal surgery in the young athlete. *Clin Orthop* 1985;198:152–157.

24. Micheli LJ. The spine and chest wall. In: Johnson RL, Lombardo J, eds. *Current review of sports medicine.* Philadelphia: Current Medicine, 1994:1–16.

25. Micheli LJ, Allison G. Lumbar spine injury in young athletes. In Proceedings of sports neurology symposium at the 1992 annual meeting of the American College of Sports Medicine. *Med Sci Sports Exerc,* in press.

26. Micheli LJ, Micheli ER. Back injuries in dancers. In: Shell CG, ed. *The 1984 Olympic scientific congress proceedings,* Vol 8: *The dancer as athlete.* Champaign, IL: Human Kinetics Publishers, 1986:91–94.

27. Hardcastle PH. Repair of spondylolysis in young fast bowlers. *J Bone Joint Surg Br* 1993;75B:398–402.

28. Stinson JT. Spondylolysis and spondylolisthesis in the athlete. *Clin Sports Med* 1993;12:517–528.

29. Blanda J, Bethem D, Moats W, et al. Defects of pars interarticularis in athletes: a protocol for nonoperative treatment. *J Spinal Disord* 1993;6:406–411.

30. Micheli LJ. Low back pain in the adolescent: differential diagnosis. *Am J Sports Med* 1979;7:362–364.

31. Hensinger RN. Back pain and vertebral changes stimulating Scheuermann's disease. *Orthop Trans* 1982;6:1.

32. Sorenson HK. *Scheuerman's juvenile kyphosis.* Copenhagen: Junksgaard, 1974.

33. Blumenthal SL, Roach J, Herring JA, et al. Lumbar Scheuermann's: a clinical series and classification. *Spine* 1987;12:929–932.

34. McKenzie RA. *The lumbar spine: mechanical diagnosis and therapy.* Lower Hutt, New Zealand: Spinal Publications, 1981.

35. Yancey RA, Micheli LJ. Thoracolumbar spine injuries in pediatric sports. In: Stanitski CL, DeLee JC, Drez D Jr., eds. *Pediatric and adolescent sports medicine (Orthopaedic sports medicine: principles and practices,* vol 3). Philadelphia. WB Saunders, 1994:162–174.

36. Maffulli N, King JB, Helms P. Training in elite young athletes (the training of young athletes [TOYA] study): injuries, flexibility and isometric strength. *Br J Sports Med* 1994;28(2):120–136.

37. Micheli LJ. Physiological and orthopedic considerations for strengthening the prepubescent athlete. *Natl Strength Conditioning Assoc J* 1985;7(6):26–27.

38. Sewall L, Micheli LJ. Strength training for children. *J Pediatr Orthop* 1986;6(2):143–146.

39. Webb DR. Strength training in children and adolescents. *Pediatr Clin North Am* 1990;37:1187–1210.

40. Cyron BM, Hutton WC. The fatigue strength of the lumbar neural arch in spondylolysis. *J Bone Joint Surg Br* 1978;60B:234–238.

41. Grogan JP, Hemminghytt S, Williams AL, Carrera GF, Haughton VM. Spondylolysis studied by computed tomography. *Radiology* 1982;145:737–742.

42. Hollinshead WH. *Anatomy for surgeons,* Vol 3. *The back and limbs.* 2nd ed. New York: Harper & Row, 1969: 82–122.

43. Lamy C, Bazergui A, Kraus H, Farfan HF. The strength of the neural arch and the etiology of spondylolysis. *Orthop Clin North Am* 1975;6:215–231.

44. Krenz J, Troup JDG. The structure of the pars interarticularis of the lower vertebrae and its relation to the etiology of spondylolysis. With a report of a healing fracture in the neural arch of the fourth lumbar vertebra. *J Bone Joint Surg Br* 1973;55B:735–741.

45. Abel MS. The radiology of low back pain associated with posterior element lesions of the lumbar spine. *CRC Crit Rev Diagn Imaging* 1984;20:311–352.

46. Ireland ML, Micheli LJ. Bilateral stress fracture of the lumbar pedicles in a ballet dancer: a case report. *J Bone Joint Surg AM* 1987;67A:140–142.

47. Hochschuler SH. *The spine sports.* Philadelphia: Hanley and Belfus, 1990.

48. Trepman E, Walaszek A, Micheli LJ. Spinal problems in the dancer. In: Solomon R, Minton SC, Solomon J, eds. *Preventing dance injuries: an interdisciplinarv perspective.* Reston, VA: American Alliance for Health, Physical Education, Recreation, and Dance, 1990: 103–131.

49. Mann DC, Keene JS, Drummond DS. Unusual causes of back pain in athletes. *J Spinal Disord* 1991;4:337–343.

50. Bertolotti M. Contributo alla conoscenza dei vizi di differenzazione regionale del rachide con speciale riguardo alla assimilazione sacrale della v lombare. *Radiol Med* 1917;4(5–6):113–144.

51. Santavirta S, Tallroth K, Ylinen P, et al. Surgical treatment of Bertolotti's syndrome: follow-up of sixteen patients. *Arch Orthop Trauma Surg* 1993;112(2):82–87.

52. Marymount JV, Lynch MA, Henning CE. Exercise-related stress reaction of the sacroiliac joint: an unusual cause of low back pain in athletes. *Am J Sports Med* 1986;14:320–323.

53. Brooks HL, Azen SP, Gerberg E, Brooks R, Chan L. Scoliosis: a prospective epidemiological study. *J Bone Joint Surg Am* 1975;57A:968–972.

54. Bunnell WP. The natural history of idiopathic scoliosis. *Clin Orthop Relat Res* 1988;229:20–25.

55. Edmonson AS. Scoliosis. In: Crenshaw AH, ed. *Campbell's operative orthopaedics,* 7th ed, vol 4. St. Louis: CV Mosby, 1987:3167–3236.

56. Warren MP, Brooks-Gunn J, Hamilton LH, Warren LF, Hamilton WG. Scoliosis and fractures in young ballet dancers: relation to delayed menarche and secondary amenorrhea. *N Engl J Med* 1986;314:1348–1353.

57. Lonstein JE. Natural history and school screening for scoliosis. *Orthop Clin North Am* 1988;19(2):227–238.

58. Winter RB. Spinal problems in pediatric orthopaedics. In: Morrissy RT, ed. *Lovell and Winter's pediatric orthopaedics,* 3rd ed., vol 2. Philadelphia: WB Saunders, 1990:625–702.
59. Hamilton WG. Ballet and your body: an orthopedists view: cervical and thoracic injuries. *Dancemagazine* 1978;52(11):48–49.
60. Sammarco GJ. Neurapraxia of the femoral nerve in a modern dancer. *Am J Sports Med* 1991;19:413–414.
61. Miller EH, Benedict FE. Stretch of a femoral nerve in a dancer: a case report. *J Bone Joint Surg Am* 1985; 67A:315–317.
62. Sammarco GJ, Miller EH. Forefoot conditions in dancers: part II. *Foot-Ankle* 1982;3(2):93–98.
63. Sammarco GJ. The foot and ankle in classical ballet and modern dance. In: Jahss M, ed. *Disorders of the foot.* Philadelphia: WB Saunders, 1982:1626–1659.
64. Sammarco GJ. Dance injuries. In: Nicholas JA, Hershman EB, eds. *The lower extremity and spine in sports medicine.* St. Louis: CV Mosby, 1986:1406–1439.
65. Schafle M, Requa RK, Garrick JG. A comparison of patterns of injury in ballet, modern, and aerobic dance. In: Solomon R, Minton SC, Solomon J, eds. *Preventing dance injuries; an interdisciplinary perspective.* Reston, VA: American Alliance for Health, Physical Education, Recreation, and Dance, 1990:1–14.
66. Solomon R, Micheli LJ. Technique as a consideration in modern dance injuries. *Phys Sports Med* 1986; 14(8):83–92.
67. Ryan AJ. Finding the right physician. In: Solomon R, Minton SC, Solomon J, eds. *Preventing dance injuries: an interdisciplinary perspective.* Reston, VA: American Alliance for Health, Physical Education, Recreation, and Dance, 1990:305–309.

Sports Neurology, Second Edition,
edited by Barry D. Jordan.
Lippincott–Raven Publishers, Philadelphia © 1998.

28

Boxing

Barry D. Jordan

Neurobehavior Program, Reed Neurological Research Center,
UCLA School of Medicine, 710 Westwood Plaza, Los Angeles, California 90095-1769

Permanent and irreversible neurologic dysfunction is the primary medical concern of boxing. The proper analysis of neurologic injuries in boxing requires differentiation between acute and chronic traumatic brain injury as well as between amateur and professional boxing. Acute traumatic brain injury (ATBI) among boxers have a different pathophysiologic mechanism and clinical presentation than the chronic traumatic brain injury (CTBI) that is encountered primarily among retired boxers. Amateur boxing differs from professional boxing in several aspects (Table 1). This chapter discusses acute and chronic neurologic injuries commonly seen among amateur and professional boxers and describes their evaluation, treatment, and prevention.

ACUTE TRAUMATIC BRAIN INJURY

Epidemiology

Studies analyzing the frequency of ATBI in amateur boxing indicate that permanent and irreversible neurologic dysfunction rarely occurs. Blonstein and Clarke (1) assessed boxing injuries in amateur boxers over a 7-month period and found that only 29 boxers (0.58%) were severely concussed or knocked out more than once. Twenty-three boxers were knocked out twice, and six were severely concussed once. Injury reports of 1981 and 1982 USA National Amateur Boxing championships noted that 48 of 547 bouts (8.7%) were stopped because of knockouts or blows to the head (2). This yielded a rate of 4.38 head injuries per 100 personal exposures. The in-

vestigators in this study concluded that this rate reflected a "strict and conscientious over-call or sensitivity to ongoing safety in the ring" (2). Larson et al. (3) reported acute head injuries in the 1950 and 1951 Swedish junior championships and the 1951 Swedish championships and found that 35 of 75 boxers were knocked down: 14 of these were knockouts. Jordan et al. (4) reviewed all boxing injuries sustained by amateur boxers at the United States Olympic Training Center (USOTC) during a 10-year period. Among the total of 477 injuries, only 29 (6.5%) were brain injuries. Although the severity was difficult to ascertain, 26 out of 28 concussions were described as being mild. This lower injury rate was probably a reflection of a low injury rate associated with sparring and training. In another survey of amateur boxers in Denmark, 5.7% to 7.8% of boxing competitions resulted in a knockout (KO) and 0.8% to 5.4% of the bouts were terminated because the referee stopped the contest secondary to head blows (RSCH) (5).

Two studies of acute boxing injuries among U.S. military personnel have been conducted (6,7). Welch et al. (6) conducted a survey of boxing injuries that occurred during an institutional boxing program at the U.S. Military Academy (USMA) in West Point, New York, over a 2-year period. Although approximately 2100 cadets received boxing instruction, only 22 cases of blunt head trauma were reported, none of which resulted in neurologic deficits. In another study, assessing amateur boxing injures among military personnel, Enzenauer et al. (7) retrospectively reviewed all hospitalizations for boxing-related

TABLE 1. *Amateur versus professional boxing*

Aspect	Amateur	Professional
Regulatory agency	One national regulatory agency (USA Boxing Inc.)	Multiple state or local commissions; also the Association of Boxing Commissions (ABC) that was empowered by the Professional Boxing Safety Act
Headgear	Yes	No
Rounds	Three 3-minute rounds or Five 2-minute rounds	Four to twelve 3-minute rounds
Gloves	8–12 oz.	8–10 oz.

injuries in U.S. Army hospitals for a 6-year period from 1980 through 1985. During this period of observation, there were 401 admissions for boxing-related injuries. Among these injuries, head injuries comprised 68% of all injuries. However, the exact number of brain injuries within this group is indeterminate because all head injuries were broadly lumped together.

McCown (8), in a medical and statistical report of injuries among professional boxers in New York State from 1952 to 1958, observed 325 knockouts and 789 technical knockouts among 11,173 participants. Of the 325 boxers with knockouts, 10 required hospitalization. Jordan and Campbell (9) reviewed all acute boxing injuries among professional boxers in New York State from August 1982 through July 1984. During this 2-year period there were 3110 rounds fought and 376 injuries, of which 262 were head injuries. This yielded a frequency of 0.8 head injuries per 10 rounds fought and 2.9 head injuries per 10 boxers. Rarely did head injuries result in permanent neurologic dysfunction. Four boxers required immediate neurologic evaluation at a hospital after their fights. In a survey of a representative sample of active professional boxers in New York State, the prevalence of a self-reported TKO or KO was 42% (143 boxers) (10). Also observed in New York State was a tendency for TKOs or KOs to occur in the earlier rounds. In one year, 122 of 189 bouts (65%) resulted in a TKO or KO and 80% of these occurred within the first three rounds (11).

Fatalities in the ring are uncommon in both amateur and professional boxing. Worldwide figures indicate that from 1945 through 1979 there

were 335 deaths in amateur and professional boxing (12). This is approximately between 9 and 10 deaths per year. In New York State there were seven deaths among professional boxers during the 7-year period of 1945 through 1952, yielding an average of one death per year; however, in the subsequent 7 years, no fatalities were noted (5). Fatalities occur less frequently among amateur boxers than professionals. Among 645 boxing fatalities reported between 1918 and June 1983, 190, or approximately one-third, were among amateurs (13). Among military personnel who boxed worldwide during a 6-year period only one death was reported (7).

Well-documented risk factors for ATBI in boxing derived from large well-defined boxing populations are limited. Welch et al. (6) observed that acute injury rates tended to be higher during competition than during sparring. However, the absolute number of acute boxing injuries tended to be higher during sparring instruction (6). This finding was a reflection of more exposure to sparring and instruction than to competition. Although risk factors for ATBI are poorly delineated, several clinical situations may predispose a boxer to an increased risk of acute neurologic injury. The poorly conditioned athlete who does not adequately train prior to a competition is at increased risk of injury. Any boxer who enters the ring needs to be well conditioned and strong. Accordingly, any medical condition (e.g., flu, fever, malaise) can have detrimental effects on a boxer's performance. Another important but often neglected factor that may increase a boxer's risk of acute injury in the ring is rapid and extreme weight loss prior to a boxing competition. Boxers who lose several pounds within 24 hours of a bout are at increased risk of injury because these boxers tend to be dehydrated. Dehydration before a competition can reduce alertness and reaction time, thus making a boxer more susceptible to the offensive attack of the opponent. Whether dehydration physiologically increased the risk of a concussion has not been scientifically demonstrated.

Clinical Presentation

The knockout in boxing is synonymous with a cerebral concussion and is the most common acute neurologic injury in boxing. The knockout can vary in severity and can be classified in four categories (1). Type 1 is the mildest form and is classically known as being "out on one's feet." The boxer is usually unable to defend himself and is dazed to the extent that he staggers around the ring or rests on the ropes. Type 2 is the mild knockout in which the boxer is knocked down and cannot rise before the count of 10 but does not experience loss of consciousness. Types 3 and 4 are moderate and severe knockouts, respectively. The boxer who suffers a type 3 knockout is rendered unconscious but recovers quickly. The type 4 knockout is similar to type 3 except that the period of unconsciousness is longer.

Sercl and Jaros (14) analyzed the acute neurologic findings in 427 boxers involved in 1165 matches. Three hundred thirty-six (79%) boxers had clinical abnormalities that resolved within several minutes and 91 (21%) had neurologic symptoms lasting up to 24 hours. The most common clinical finding was derangement of muscular tone (380 cases), followed by cerebellar and vestibular signs (319 cases) and pyramidal symptoms (253 cases). Other findings included unconsciousness (112 cases), extrapyramidal signs (191 cases), and general muscular weakness (142 cases). Cranial nerve lesions were exceedingly rare (7 cases).

Amnesia is not an infrequent consequence of acute brain injury in boxing. Characteristic of many knockouts seems to be an amnestic period with confusion (3), but amnesia can occur without a knockout and should be regarded as evidence of serious injury (15). Blonstein and Clarke (1) described a boxer who won a decision but was amnesic for the entire fight despite not being knocked out. Both retrograde and anterograde amnesia have been described in boxing (16).

A boxer may also experience neurologic symptoms after a bout. Critchley (16) described this as the "groggy state," which can be synonymous with the postconcussion syndrome. Usually a boxer experiences transient nonspecific symptoms such as headache, dizziness, imbalance, irritability, fatigue, poor memory, and dysarthria that usually passes, and he returns to his status quo. Nevertheless, Critchley (16) suggested that accumulation of groggy states may predispose a boxer to the "punch drunk" state.

More recently, the second impact syndrome (SIS) has been described in boxers (17). The SIS represents an exaggerated, commonly fatal response to a second concussion while an athlete is symptomatic from an earlier concussion. In boxing, the SIS may occur in a tournament setting where a boxer competes more than once over a selected time period (typically a few days to a week), or it can occur less frequently within a given bout associated with multiple concussive blows (17). The pathophysiologic mechanism of SIS appears to loss of vasomotor autoregulation leading to massive brain swelling and malignant edema (see chapter 17).

Pathology

The concussion represents the most common ATBI encountered in boxing and typically is not associated with any gross pathologic changes. Microscopically, animal studies suggest that chromatrolysis can occur after concussion (18). However, when extrapolating to humans, the severity of the head trauma experienced by the experimental animals in these investigations may be more significant than what is typically encountered in boxing. In human studies, Oppenheimer (19) observed microscopic changes such as axonal retraction balls and myelin destruction in the setting of microglial clusters after a concussion. However, the contribution of anoxia to these neuropathologic changes was difficult to assess. Accordingly, whether the uncomplicated concussion in boxing (i.e., without anoxia or reduced cerebral perfusion) results in structural damage remains to be determined.

Although uncommon, acute pathologic lesions such as diffuse axonal injury, subdural hematoma, epidural hematoma, cerebral contusion, intracerebral hemorrhage, injury to the carotid, and subarachnoid hemorrhage may be encountered in boxers (20,21). For a detailed discussion on traumatic brain injury in sport see Chapter 17.

Pathophysiology

The concussive properties of a boxer's punch are related to the manner in which the punch is delivered and how the mechanical forces are transferred and absorbed through the intracranial cavity. Blows thrown from the shoulder, such as the roundhouse or the hook, tend to deliver more force than the straightforward jab. The force transmitted by a punch is directly proportional to the mass of the glove and the velocity of the swing and is inversely proportional to the total mass opposing the punch (22).

The essential feature of a concussive force is that it is sufficient to accelerate the skull. Rotational (angular) acceleration, linear (translational) acceleration, and impact deceleration can all play a role in the development of acute cerebral injury (20). Angular acceleration occurs when a punch causes a rotational movement of the skull that can potentially stretch and tear cerebral blood vessels. Subdural hematomas typically result from tearing of the bridging veins secondary to rotational acceleration. Rotational acceleration is also responsible for diffuse axonal injury. Linear acceleration occurs with blows directly to the face that propel the skull in an anterior-to-posterior direction. Linear acceleration may result in gliding contusions.

CHRONIC TRAUMATIC BRAIN INJURY

CTBI, also known as dementia pugilistica, chronic traumatic encephalopathy, chronic neurologic injury, or the "punch drunk" syndrome, represents the long-term cumulative neurologic consequences of repetitive concussive and subconcussive blows to the head. Traditionally, this syndrome has been described primarily in boxers; however, it may be anticipated in other sports such as American football, ice hockey, and perhaps soccer. This syndrome was first described in the medical literature by Martland (23) in 1928 when he described a 38-year-old retired boxer with advanced parkinsonism, ataxia, pyramidal tract dysfunction, and behavioral changes.

Epidemiology

Roberts (24) conducted a comprehensive study of the epidemiologic aspect of CTBI. He randomly sampled 250 of 16,781 ex-professional boxers who were licensed by the British Board of Control for at least 3 years from 1929 through 1955. Among the 250 boxers, 224 were examined and 26 were excluded on the basis of either death, emigration, or refusal. Thirty-seven boxers (17%) had clinical evidence of central nervous system lesions attributable to boxing. Roberts concluded that the prevalence of lesions increased when exposure to boxing increased. Putative and established risk factors for CTBI are presented in Table 2. Documented risk factors for CTBI in boxing include later retirement (i.e., over 28 years of age), increased duration of career (i.e., more than 10 years), and a greater number of bouts (i.e., more than 150 bouts) (24). Clinical studies suggest that risk factors for the development of CTBI include poor performance (i.e., second- or third-rate boxers), boxing style (i.e., being a slugger, rather than a scientific, intelligent boxer), boxers who are notorious for their ability to "take" a punch, and being a professional boxer as opposed to amateur (25). The age at examination also influenced the prevalence of CTBI. Boxers who were examined after

TABLE 2. *Putative and documented risk factors for chronic traumatic brain injury*

Total number of fights
Number of knockouts experienced
Number of losses
Duration of boxing career
Fight frequency
Age of retirement from boxing
Sparring exposure
Poor performance or skills

the age of 50 had a higher prevalence of CTBI than those examined before that age of 50 (24). A more recent study implies that increasing sparring exposure may increase the risk of neurocognitive decline among professional boxers (26). A history of a technical knockout (TKO) or knockout (KO) has also been reported to be associated with an abnormal computed tomographic (CT) scan of the brain (10). In addition, progressive changes on CT scans been noted in boxers who lose more than 10 bouts (27).

Clinical Presentation

In a comprehensive review of the neuropsychiatric aspects of boxing, Mendez (28) classified the clinical manifestations of CTBI into motor, cognitive, and psychiatric symptoms. Early signs of CTBI may include dysarthria, mild incoordination, tremor, and decreased complex attention. Psychiatric symptoms may include emotional lability and other mild behavioral disturbances such as euphoria or hypomania and increased irritability. Although it has been observed that the initial manifestations of CTBI are predominantly psychiatric or behavioral in nature (29), it is the experience of the author that the behavioral and personality disturbances may be difficult to as-

sess early in the disease. This is particularly the case when the examiner lacks knowledge of the boxer's premorbid personality. The second or moderate stage of CTBI is characterized by a progression of the motor, cognitive, and/or behavioral symptoms (28). Motorically, boxers exhibit signs of parkinsonism and/or progressive difficulty in coordination and ambulation. Cognitive deficits include mild deficits in memory, attention, and executive function. Psychiatric manifestations may include inappropriate behavior, morbid jealousy, paranoia, and violent outbursts. The third or severe stage of CTBI is often referred to as dementia pugilistica (28). During this phase of the disorder, the boxer exhibits significant motor dysfunction characterized by prominent pyramidal, extrapyramidal, and/or cerebellar symptoms. Cognitive dysfunction as evidenced by amnesia, executive–frontal lobe dysfunction, and psychomotor retardation may be observed. Behaviorally, boxers may exhibit disinhibition, violent outbursts, hypersexuality, and psychosis (28).

Clinical criteria for CTBI in boxing are presented in Table 3 (30). Because chronic neurologic impairment in boxing is not temporally related to the effects of a single blow to the head, the diagnosis of CTBI can be problematic. Accordingly, if a boxer exhibits neurologic dys-

TABLE 3. *Clinical criteria of chronic traumatic brain injury (CTBI)*

	Definition	Clinical examples
Probable	Any neurologic process characterized by two or more of the following conditions: dementia, cerebellar dysfunction, pyramidal tract disease, or extrapyramidal disease. Clinically distinguishable from any known disease process and consistent with the clinical description of CTBI.	Dementia and extrapyramidal dysfunction suggestive of parkinsonism with associated cerebellar dysfunction that is inconsistent with parkinsonism.
Possible	Any neurologic process that is consistent with the clinical description of CTBI but can be potentially explained by other known neurologic disease.	Alzheimer's disease and other primary dementia; Parkinson's disease; primary cerebellar degeneration; Wernicke-Korsakoff's.
Improbable	Any neurologic process that is inconsistent with clinical description of CTBI and can be explained by a pathophysiologic process unrelated to trauma.	Cerebrovascular disease; multiple sclerosis; brain neoplasm; inherited neurologic disorders.

TABLE 4. *Chronic Brain Injury (CBI) scale (31)*

Motor	
Normal	0
Mild incoordination, dysarthria, parkinsonism, gait disturbance, or pyramidal signs	1
Moderate incoordination, dysarthria, parkinsonism, gait disturbance, or pyramidal signs	2
Severe incoordination, dysarthria, parkinsonism, gait disturbance, or pyramidal signs	3
Cognitive	
Normal or MMSE[a] = 28–30	0
Mild deficits in mental speed, memory, attention, executive function, language or visuospatial function, or MMSE = 20–27	1
Moderate deficits in mental speed, memory, attention, executive function, language or visuospatial function, or MMSE = 10–19	2
Severe deficits in mental speed, memory, attention, executive function, language or visuospatial function, or MMSE ≤ 9	3
Behavioral	
Normal	0
Mild agitation or aggression, delusions, hallucinations, dysphoria, anxiety, euphoria, apathy, disinhibition, irritability or lability, or aberrant motor behavior	1
Moderate agitation or aggression, delusions, hallucinations, dysphoria, anxiety, euphoria, apathy, disinhibition, irritability or lability, or aberrant motor behavior	2
Severe agitation or aggression, delusions, hallucinations, dysphoria, anxiety, euphoria, apathy, disinhibition, irritability or lability, or aberrant motor behavior	3
Total CBI score (range 0–9)	____

[a] MMSE, Mini-Mental State Examination.

function in later life, it must be determined whether the neurologic deficits are attributable to boxing. The likelihood of CTBI being attributable to boxing can be classified as probable, possible, or improbable (30).

A chronic brain injury (CBI) scale has been devised to assess the severity of CTBI in boxing (31). This 10-point grading scale classifies the neurologic symptoms into motor, cognitive, and behavioral aspects (Table 4). A boxer who exhibits a totally normal neurologic examination will score zero. Mild CTBI is represented by a score of 1 or 2. Boxers scoring in the mild range may demonstrate mild balance problems (i.e., an abnormally sharpened Romberg), mild incoordination, mild dysarthria, and/or mild deficits in memory and attention. Boxers with more significant neurologic impairment are classified as moderate (CBI score of 3 or 4) or severe (CBI score greater than 4).

Pathology

Corsellis et al. (32,33) described four types of central nervous system changes among 15 ex-boxers: septal and hypothalamic anomalies, cerebellar changes, degeneration of the substantia nigra, and regional occurrence of Alzheimer's

neurofibrillary tangles (NFTs). Twelve cases demonstrated a fenestrated septal cavum, and frequently the floor of the hypothalamus appeared to be stretched while the fornix and mammillary bodies were atrophied. The cerebellum was notable for scarring of the folia in the region of the cerebellar tonsils, and there was a reduction in the number of Purkinje cells on the inferior surface of the cerebellum. Neurofibrillary tangles primarily involved parts of the hippocampus and the medial temporal gray matter. The neurofibrillary changes in the limbic gray matter were not accompanied by senile plaques. The substantia nigra tended to lack pigment, and nerve cells became gliosed.

Roberts et al. (34), utilizing immunocytochemical methods and an antibody raised to the beta-protein present in Alzheimer's disease (AD) plaques, found that retired boxers with dementia pugilistica and substantial neurofibrillary tangles showed evidence of extensive beta-protein immunoreactive deposits (plaques). These "diffuse" plaques were not visible with Congo red or standard silver stains. Because the degree of beta-protein deposition was comparable to that seen in AD, it was postulated that in dementia pugilistica the pathogenic mechanism of tangle and plaque formation may be similar to that of

AD. Support of this hypothesis was provided by Tokuda et al. (35) when these investigators demonstrated tau immunoreactive NFTs and beta-protein immunoreactive senile plaques in boxers exhibiting dementia.

Another important neuropathologic observation has been the presence of ubiquitin in the neurofibrillary tangles in the brains of boxers with dementia and patients with AD (36). Ubiquitin, which has been identified as a component of neurofibrillary tangles in AD, is thought to be a protein involved in the ATP-dependent non-lysosomal degradation of abnormal proteins. It has been speculated that dementia may result from the dysfunction of cells bearing ubiquitin tangles. Among 16 boxers studied in this investigation, 11 exhibited dementia. Among the 11 boxers with dementia, 9 had evidence of ubiquitin immunoreactivity in the NFTs. None of the five boxers without dementia demonstrated staining of the neurofibrillary tangles with anti-ubiquitin.

Uhl et al. (37) also presented evidence documenting similarities between CTBI and AD. These investigators conducted a pathologic and neurochemical examination of the brain of a 52-year-old former boxer with well-documented dementia pugilistica. In addition to documenting NFTs in the cortex and the nucleus basalis of Meynert (nbM), they noted a significant reduction of choline acetyltransferase activity in the nbM and in several regions of the cerebral cortex. These findings are similar to those noted in AD.

Although there are several similarities between AD and DP, Hof et al. (38) reported that a more circumscribed population of cortical pyramidal neurons might be affected in CTBI than in AD. In CTBI the NFTs are concentrated primarily in the superficial layers (II and III) of the neocortex, whereas in AD the NFTs are distributed in the superficial and deep layers with a predominance in the deeper layers. In the hippocampus, the distributions of NFTs in AD and CTBI are similar.

Pathophysiology

The pathophysiology of CTBI is unknown; however, one can develop hypotheses that might explain the pathologic substrates for the clinical findings in boxers suffering from CTBI. The parkinsonian syndrome and ataxia–dysequilibrium are related to changes in the substantia nigra and the cerebellum, respectively, whereas the cognitive and memory deficits could possibly be explained on the basis of the changes noted in the hippocampus, mammillary bodies, and fornix. Frontal lobe damage may contribute to the personality or behavioral changes encountered in CTBI, as well as attention and memory function.

It has been hypothesized by Martland (23) that this syndrome is secondary to single or repeated head blows resulting in multiple petechial hemorrhages in the deeper portions of the cerebrum that are later replaced by gliosis or a progressive degenerative lesion. Alternatively, it can be theorized that in order to develop clinical symptoms of CTBI, a critical number or percentage of functional neurons must be damaged or experience cell death. Conceivably, a boxer who terminates a boxing career and has experienced some neuronal loss does not exhibit clinical symptoms consistent with CTBI because he has a critical number or percentage of functional neurons. However, as he experiences normal or accelerated neuronal dropout associated with aging, he may develop clinical signs of CTBI because he has less than the critical threshold level of functioning neurons. This theory would explain why CTBI appears to progress after the termination of a boxing career and the cessation of cerebral trauma.

Any account of the pathophysiology of CTBI would have to consider the pathologic role of abnormal amyloid deposition and central cholinergic system dysfunction. It has been speculated that potential blows to the head could conceivably produce local changes in the blood–brain barrier (BBB) that may enable the deposition of beta amyloid in the injured areas (39). Alternatively, cerebral concussion may damage the BBB, thus allowing the extravasation of serum proteins that may serve as antigenic initiators of a secondary immune response that attenuate normal CNS function (40). The role of the cholinergic system in the pathogenesis of CTBI remains to be determined. Animal studies indicate that concussive head injury has a profound effect on central cholinergic neurons (41). Furthermore, the cholinergic system has been implicated in the pathophysiology of AD and is probably involved in the physiologic basis of learning and memory (42). Accordingly, any theory of the pathogenesis of CTBI must delineate the interactions between head trauma, amyloid deposition, central cholinergic function, and cognitive impairment.

In addition to the foregoing factors, the potential role of apolipoprotein E (APOE) e4 allele in the development of CTBI needs to be explored. Evidence suggests that the presence of APOEe4 allele may promote the deposition of cerebral amyloid in individuals experiencing traumatic brain injury (43). Mayeaux et al. (44) noted a 10-fold synergistic increased risk of AD in individuals with traumatic brain injury and the presence of APOE e4, whereas an addictive increased risk of AD in patients with head trauma and APOE e4 was observed by Katzman et al. (45). Based on our observation of extensive parenchymal cerebral amyloid deposition and cerebral amyloid angiopathy in a demented boxer who harbored an APOE e4 allele (46), we conducted a study to determine whether APOE e4 is associated with CTBI (31). In an analysis of 30 active and retired boxers, we found that APOE e4 was associated with an increased severity of CTBI in high-exposure boxers (i.e., boxers with more than 12 professional bouts). This finding suggests that there may be a genetic predisposition to the untoward effects of a long boxing career (31).

CERVICAL SPINE INJURIES

Cervical spine injuries are rare in boxing. Strano and Marias (47) reported a fracture in the anterior arch of the atlas in a 27-year-old amateur boxer who presented with persistent occipital headaches. Although the exact mechanism of this fracture was uncertain, the investigators speculated that a direct blow to the head with the neck hyperextended (when the odontoid lies against the anterior arch of the atlas) may deliver sufficient force to fracture the anterior arch of the atlas. Kewalramani and Krauss (48) reported a case of quadriplegia secondary to a C-6 vertebral body fracture in a boxer but did not comment on

the mechanism or circumstances of the injury. Jordan et al. (49) encountered a stable unilateral fracture of the lamina of C-3 in a professional boxer who struck his neck on the bottom rope of the ring while falling to the canvas. A recent personal observation has been the onset of a cervical radiculopathy in two amateur boxers. One boxer had a previous history of a cervical disc herniation and the other had onset of radicular symptoms without a prior history of cervical dysfunction.

NEUROLOGIC EVALUATION OF THE BOXER

The proper evaluation of the boxer should at a minimum include a complete neurologic examination (Table 5). Whether auxiliary neurodiagnostic tests are utilized depends on the clinical judgment of the examining physician or the rules of the governing boxing organization.

Neurologic Examination

The neurologic examination can be separated into three distinct phases that require variable techniques in assessment; these include the prefight, intrafight, and postfight examinations.

The prefight neurologic examination should be comprehensive and establish a neurologic baseline for future comparisons (i.e., with the intrafight and postfight examinations). Ideally, the physician conducting the prefight examination should be present at ringside during the bout. Included in the prefight examination of the boxer is a detailed history that inquires about past knockouts, medical suspensions, neurologic symptoms and disorders, and prior episodes of unconsciousness outside the ring. The neurologic examination should test

TABLE 5. *Neurologic evaluation of the boxer*

Neurologic examination
  Prefight
  Intrafight
  Postfight
Neurodiagnostic testing
  Electroencephalogram (EEG)
  Computed tomographic (CT) scan
  Magnetic resonance imaging (MRI) scan

higher integrative function, cranial nerves, sensory function, motor strength, coordination, and reflexes. The mental status examination should be simple to accommodate the boxer's educational level and should be in the boxer's primary language. Any boxer exhibiting an abnormal prefight neurologic examination should undergo further neurologic evaluation before continuing his boxing career.

The ringside neurologic examination of the boxer during the fight is mainly observational. It is intended to identify boxers who are neurologically injured or those predisposed to being neurologically injured. Early in a fight, the ringside physician should familiarize himself or herself with the boxing style of both fighters. During the fight, the physician should be alerted to signs of deteriorating motor control or signs of decreased activity. These signs can be indicative of existing or impending brain injury. Evidence of deteriorating motor control includes wobbly knees, unsteady gait, loss of head control, excessive leaning against the ropes, and wild, uncontrolled punches. Signs of decreased activity include slowed reflexes, no avoidance of punches, and no active offensive or defensive maneuvers. Between rounds the physician should observe how the boxer walks back to his corner, his ability to find his corner, his interaction with his corner attendants, and his posture while sitting in the corner. If the ringside physician is required to perform a neurologic examination of a boxer between rounds, it should be conducted expeditiously. Because the ringside physician has been observing the boxer's motor coordination and control during the round, assessment between rounds should be primarily directed toward establishing a normal mental status. The mental status examination should be simple, understandable, and in the native language of the boxer. It should test orientation, alertness, and comprehension. If the boxer does not exhibit a clear and alert sensorium, the fight should be terminated.

At the conclusion of a bout, a modified neurologic examination should be conducted on any boxer suspected of sustaining neurologic injury. All boxers experiencing an excessive number of head blows, regardless of whether they won or lost the fight, should be included in this group. The postfight neurologic examination should also be conducted on any boxer who has neurologic complaints. The boxer who sustains a head injury with rapid recovery, together with his manager or coach, should be informed about recurrent neurologic symptoms that could represent ongoing neurologic injury and be instructed to notify a physician in case these appear.

Neuropsychologic Testing

Neuropsychologic testing can serve as an important adjunct in the evaluation of the boxer and has been employed to assess CTBI in retired boxers and to evaluate cognitive functioning in active amateur and professional boxers. However, the utilization of neuropsychologic testing in boxing is associated with methodologic concerns (50). First, normative data for boxers are essentially nonexistent. Accordingly, comparing neuropsychologic test scores with normative scores of individuals who are distinctly different is inappropriate. Another methodologic consideration is the selection of proper control groups. For example, Thomassen et al. (51) conducted a case-control study comparing 53 former champion amateur boxers with 53 former soccer players. Although subtle differences in neuropsychologic testing were noted between the groups, the significance of these findings should be interpreted with caution because the soccer players differed from boxers in background variables such as age, schooling, and exposure to head trauma unrelated to their respective sporting activities. Furthermore, soccer players may also be vulnerable to the cumulative effects of head trauma from concussion and/or heading of the ball (see Chapter 38). Accordingly, the selection of soccer players in this investigation may be inappropriate. A third methodologic concern in the utilization of neuropsychologic testing in boxers is the screening for comorbidities that may influence neurologic functioning (50).

Several investigations have utilized neuropsychologic testing in the evaluation of active and retired boxers (24,26,51–65). In general, it appears that amateur boxing is associated with less neuropsychologic impairment than professional boxing. According to Butler (66), a review of 10 studies assessing 289 amateur boxers found that amateur boxers did not exhibit any significant signs of neuropsychologic dysfunction. This review did suggest that a long amateur career might reduce fine motor movements, but it was felt these findings were within the normal range and did not represent central neuropsychologic functioning. Among professional boxers the profiles of neuropsychologic function are consistent with those encountered in CTBI. These include variable impairment in memory, information processing speed, finger-tapping speed, complex attentional attacks, sequencing abilities, and frontal–executive function (28).

Electroencephalogram

The electroencephalogram (EEG) is a commonly utilized neurodiagnostic test in the evaluation of boxers. Although the EEG is not a required screening test in amateur boxing, it is employed by several professional boxing commissions. Compared with nonfunctional neuroimaging (i.e., CT or MRI), the EEG has the advantage of being able to assess physiologic function when the CT or MRI can assess only anatomic lesions independent of function. Accordingly, the EEG should not be substituted for CT or MRI or vice versa. The EEG should be utilized to complement neuroimaging in the evaluation of a boxer. Any boxer who exhibits an abnormal EEG should not be allowed to participate in the sport of boxing. Although the EEG is a useful preparticipation screening test, its role in distinguishing chronic brain injury is less clearly delineated. Selected investigations utilizing EEG are cited in the following.

Kaplan and Browder (68) preformed 1400 EEGs on 1043 professional fighters and correlated the brain wave patterns with clinical and ringside observations, cinematography, and performance data. It was concluded that boxers with low ratings had a statistically significant greater percentage of disorganized EEGs compared with high-rated boxers. No statistically significant correlation was noted with age, number of fights, type of fighter, weight division, win–loss record, or number of knockouts. Forty of these boxers had repeat EEGs performed within 10 minutes of losing a fight (either by TKO or decision), and the EEGs did not demonstrate any changes from the prefight tracings. In the same study, 197 of the 1043 fighters evaluated underwent one to six repeated EEGs spanning a period of up to 4 years. Forty-eight records demonstrated changes in the brain wave pattern from previous tracings. These changes usually took the form of increased slow-wave activity with the development of paroxysmal dysrhythmia, improvement of alpha-wave activity, less paroxysmal dysrhythmia, or less slow-wave activity. The number of boxers exhibiting each of these changes was not mentioned.

Busse and Silverman (69) performed 30 EEGs on 24 professional boxers and found dysrhythmic patterns in 9 (37.5%); this was statistically higher than that reported in control groups. Although these investigators lacked background information on the careers of these boxers, they concluded that boxers who had been knocked out showed more severe disturbances that those who had not.

Roberts (24) performed 168 EEGs on retired professional boxers and found no significant difference between cases clinically diagnosed as having CTBI and normal ex-boxers without CTBI. Roberts concluded that it was unwise to use a single EEG to support the diagnosis of CTBI. Similarly, Thomassen et al. (51) compared the EEG patterns of 53 former amateur boxers with those of 53 former soccer players and noted no differences between the two groups.

In a review of 1190 consecutive EEG reports among a representative sample of active professional boxers in New York State, 6% (67 tracings among 45 boxers) were interpreted as abnormal or borderline (67). The most common abnormality (23 cases) was focal slowing localized to the frontal and/or temporal lobes. Other types of abnormalities included diffuse slowing (eight cases) and paroxysmal dysfunction (six cases). When compared with boxers with normal tracings, boxers with abnormal EEGs tended to be older (more than 30 years of age). This increased association between older age and exhibiting an abnormal EEG may reflect longer exposure to boxing and/or an increased susceptibility of the older boxer to the trauma associated with boxing.

This clinical observation provides data to support the concerns about older boxers participating in the sport.

Computed Tomography

Several clinical investigations have utilized CT scanning to evaluate neurologic injury in boxers (10,27,51,53,59,70–73). However, the majority of these studies have utilized small sample populations.

Casson et al. (70) performed detailed neurologic examinations, EEGs, and CT scans on ten active professional boxers aged 20 to 31 years shortly after they had been knocked out. Although no subdural or intracerebral hematomas were noted, cerebral atrophy was noted in five boxers. Of the five abnormal scans, three demonstrated generalized cerebral atrophy and two demonstrated ventricular dilation. One of these boxers had a cavum septum pellucidum. Among the five boxers with atrophy, all had a normal neurologic examination and one had an abnormal EEG characterized by increased theta waves anteriorly. According to the investigators of this study, the more proficient fighters and the fighters with the most bouts were more apt to have cerebral atrophy. The findings of this study must be interpreted with caution. First, ten boxers is too limited a sample size to extrapolate accurate information regarding the general boxing population. Furthermore, the significance of cerebral atrophy is difficult to determine because there was no documentation that these boxers had previously normal CT scans. In the absence of focal abnormalities on CT scans that can be temporally related to boxing events, a CT scan must document a change to provide sufficient evidence that the findings are secondary to boxing.

Kaste et al. (53) performed CT scans on six professional and eight amateur boxers together with neurologic examinations, psychologic testing, and EEG testing. Three of the six professionals and one of the eight amateurs had evidence of cerebral atrophy. Cavum septum pellucidum was noted in two professionals and one amateur. Of the four professionals whose CT scans demonstrated atrophy or cavum septum pellucidum (or both), one had an abnormal neurologic examination, one had an abnormal EEG, and two had abnormal psychologic tests. The one amateur with an abnormal CT scan also had an abnormal EEG. The investigators in this study concluded that, despite modern medical control of boxing, chronic brain injuries do occur.

Sironi et al. (71) evaluated ten professional boxers with CT scanning, EEG testing, and neurologic evaluation. Although the neurologic examination was normal in all ten boxers, four cases had borderline cerebral atrophy and two exhibited definite cerebral atrophy. The CT abnormalities in this study correlated with the frequency of knockouts and were independent of the number of years or matches fought.

Ross et al. (72), in a larger study, evaluated the neurologic status of 40 former boxers. A statistically significant relationship was found between cerebral atrophy on CT scans and the number of bouts fought but not the number of knockouts or technical knockouts. Furthermore, abnormalities on neurologic examination did not correlate significantly with the number of bouts.

Casson et al. (59) evaluated 13 former boxers, 2 active professional boxers, and 3 active amateur boxers for evidence of brain damage utilizing the neurologic examination, EEG, CT scan, and neuropsychologic testing. Thirteen of the 15 former and active professional fighters (87%) had abnormal results on at least two of four tests, whereas the 3 amateur boxers had normal neurologic examinations, EEGs, and CT scans. Eight boxers had an abnormal CT scan demonstrating atrophy, and a cavum septum pellucidum was noted in three of these eight. Six of the eight boxers with more than 20 professional bouts had abnormal CT scans. Boxers with abnormal CT scans were also noted to have more impairment on neuropsychologic testing than those with normal CT scans.

The above mentioned CT investigations of boxers failed to utilize a representative sample of boxers and are limited by small sample size. To address this issue, we analyzed CT scans in a representative sample of 338 active professionals in New York (10). Twenty-five boxers (7%) exhibited abnormal CT scans. The most common CT abnormality was brain atrophy (22 cases). Focal lesions of low attenuation consistent with post-traumatic encephalomalacia were noted in only three boxers. There was an association between exhibiting an abnormal CT scan and a previous history of a technical knockout or a knockout. Among the 338 boxers, a cavum septum pellucidum (CSP) was noted in 45 boxers (13%). The presence of CSP correlated with cerebral atrophy on CT. The presence of a CSP on CT in boxers probably represents an acquired condition because it has been observed to develop in boxers (27).

Magnetic Resonance Imaging

MRI appears to be more sensitive than CT in the detection of traumatic brain injury in boxers (73). The MRI can detect white matter changes, cerebral contusions, and small subdural hematomas that may be missed on CT. Despite the advantage of MRI over CT, the utilization of MRI in the evaluation of boxers has been limited. Levin et al. (50), in an MRI evaluation of young boxers, failed to observe any evidence of cognitive deterioration or abnormalities. Similarly, Jordan and Zimmerman (74) failed to document any abnormalities on MRI scanning and neurologic examination in nine amateur boxers who were medically suspended secondary to a knockout or excessive head blows. Davie et al. (75) utilized magnetic resonance spectroscopy (MRS) to evaluate boxers with parkinsonism (see Chapter 24).

Single Photon Emission Computed Tomography

Single photon emission computed tomography (SPECT) assesses cerebral perfusion and may serve as an extremely sensitive indicator of cerebral dysfunction. To date, SPECT has been utilized to evaluate amateur and professional boxers (76,77). Kemp et al (76) performed SPECT scans on 34 amateur boxers and 34 controls and reported the frequency of abnormal scans among the amateur boxers to be 41% compared with 14% of the controls. Dane et al. (77) found SPECT to be more sensitive than CT, MRI, EEG, or neurologic examination in the detection of brain dysfunction in a referred population of professional boxers. As one might expect, frontal and temporal hypoperfusions were the most frequent abnormalities observed on SPECT.

TREATMENT OF NEUROLOGIC INJURY

Acute Traumatic Brain Injury

The treatment of ATBI in boxing is dependent on whether a structural lesion of the central nervous system (e.g, subdural hematoma, brain contusion, or epidural hematoma) is suspected (Table 6). A structural lesion should be suspected in any boxer experiencing prolonged loss of consciousness (greater than 1 to 2 minutes), relapsing unconsciousness after a period of lucidness, seizures, or focal neurologic deficits. If a structural lesion is suspected, immediate medical care should be instituted at ringside and the boxer should be prepared for transport to a medical facility close to the arena. Ideally, an ambulance should be present at all boxing matches to ensure prompt emergency transportation, and the medical facility should have emergency neuroradiologic and neurosurgical services readily available. Furthermore, the ringside physician should accompany

---

TABLE 6. *Treatment of neurologic injury*

Acute brain injury
  Nonstructural lesion: Temporary medical suspension from contact boxing for at least 1 month with a neurologic evaluation before reinstatement.
  Structural lesion: Intravenous mannitol and hyperventilation if associated with herniation: immediate transfer to hospital; permanent medical suspension from boxing.
Chronic brain injury
  Parkinsonism: Levodopa–carbidopa (Sinemet) (?)
  Posttraumatic amnesia and/or dementia: Cholinergic drugs (?) (e.g., Tacrine, Donepezil)
  Psychiatric disturbances: Antidepressants or tranquilizers (?)
Cervical spine injury
  Immediate immobilization of the cervical spine and transfer to the hospital; cardiopulmonary resuscitation initiated at ringside if indicated.

the boxer in the ambulance to continue emergency medical care initiated at ringside and to convey the history to the receiving physicians. Whether surgical or medical treatment is needed for traumatic intracranial lesions is dependent on the type of injury (see Chapter 17). Any boxer who acquires a structural lesion should be permanently suspended from boxing and contact sports, regardless of the level of recovery.

ATBI in boxing that is not associated with a structural lesion of the central nervous system usually do not require immediate neurologic care but nonetheless should be fully evaluated before contact boxing (i.e., sparring or actual competition) is continued. Any boxer experiencing significant or excessive head blows during a boxing match or who has a fight terminated secondary to being knocked out or sustaining multiple head blows should automatically be considered to have an ATBI. Furthermore, any boxer, regardless of whether he won or lost the fight, should also be considered to have ATBI if he experiences substantial head trauma as determined by the clinical judgment of the ringside physician. Therefore, it is vital that the ringside physician be experienced and well trained in boxing medicine.

All boxers with acute nonstructural injury to the central nervous system (e.g., concussion or posttraumatic amnesia) should be medically suspended and undergo a mandatory rest period from contact boxing (i.e., sparring, exhibitions, or competitive bouts). Although the duration of the medical suspension and rest period depends on the severity of the neurologic injury, the minimum time should be 1 month. Medical reinstatement should be conditional on the athlete's fulfillment of the mandatory rest requirement and a normal neurologic evaluation. The neurologic evaluation, at minimum, should include a neurologic examination. Whether further neurodiagnostic procedures are utilized is at the discretion of the ringside physician or the regulations and rules of the governing or sanctioning body. For example, in New York State, professional boxers who receive a TKO or a KO are required to have a CT scan and an EEG in addition to the neurologic examination on medical reinstatement (78). An abnormal CT scan, EEG, or neurologic examination precludes reinstatement.

Chronic Traumatic Brain Injury

At present, the treatment of CTBI is largely empirical and theoretical (see Table 6). Boxers exhibiting parkinsonism that interferes with daily functioning should be empirically treated with levodopa–carbidopa (Sinemet) or other antiparkinsonism medications. The treatment of dementia associated with CTBI is speculative. Goldberg et al. (79) observed an improvement in verbal memory but not visual memory in a non-boxer experiencing posttraumatic amnesia treated with physostigmine and lecithin. Whether antidepressants or tranquilizers are effective in the treatment of psychiatric disorders associated with CTBI is unknown. An active boxer who displays progressive characteristics of CTBI should be medically suspended from boxing.

Cervical Spine Injury

Acute cervical spine injuries should be managed cautiously and expeditiously (see Table 6). If a cervical spine injury is suspected, the neck should be immobilized immediately with a cervical collar or spineboard. In the situation in which respirations have ceased, an airway should be established and ventilation initiated. The boxer should then be transported by ambulance to the hospital, where appropriate radiologic studies can be conducted. The treatment and further management of cervical spine injuries are dependent on the type and severity of the injury (see Chapter 11).

PREVENTION OF NEUROLOGIC INJURY

Boxing is an inherently dangerous sport and the prevention of neurologic injury is of primary importance. Increasing medical safety in boxing requires active participation by the ringside physician, boxing regulatory agencies, trainer, promoter or matchmaker, and the boxer himself (80).

The role of the ringside physician in providing safety in the ring cannot be overemphasized. Theoretically, a physician should be in attendance at all boxing matches. In certain jurisdictions the ringside physician has the authority to

TABLE 7. *Health and safety issues of the Professional Boxing Safety Act (82)*

A physical examination must be performed certifying whether a boxer is fit to fight.
An ambulance or medical personnel with appropriate resuscitation equipment must be present at ringside.
A physician must be present at ringside.
Each boxer must have health insurance to provide medical coverage for any injuries sustained in a match.
No boxing match can be held in a state that does not have a boxing commission.
Each boxer must be registered with a boxing commission and will be issued an identification card.
No boxer will be permitted to box while under suspension from any boxing commission.
A central registry of boxers is to be maintained that contains information on current suspensions and results of boxing matches.

enter the ring during the progress of a bout or between rounds and can terminate any boxing bout to prevent severe physical injury. On a nationwide basis, however, most ringside physicians do not have the authority to terminate a professional fight. In addition, any physician at ringside should be equipped with the necessary emergency equipment to administer first aid to any injured boxer.

In amateur boxing, USA boxing serves as the national regulatory agency and governs all amateur boxing within the United States. USA boxing provides many functions that protect the health and safety of the amateur boxer. Their functions include the assignment of ringside physicians, prebout physical examinations, postbout medical evaluation and treatment of injuries, and the training of referees (81).

On the administrative level, professional boxing has lacked a national regulatory agency to enforce uniform medical standards. Traditionally, state or local agencies have governed professional boxing in their respective areas, often lacking the proper communication channels for medical surveillance of boxers and reciprocal enforcement of medical suspensions. However, legislation entitled the Professional Boxing Safety Act has been implemented and represents the first attempt to regulate boxing on a national level (82). The purpose of the Professional Boxing Safety Act is to expand the system of safety precautions that protects the welfare of professional boxers and assist state boxing commissions to provide proper oversight for the professional boxing industry in the United States. Health and safety requirements established by the Professional Boxing Safety Act are listed in Table 7. The Professional Boxing Safety Act also recognizes the Association of Boxing Commissions as a distinct entity to assist in protecting the health and safety of the professional boxer. The ABC represents a volunteer organization of the boxing commissions within the United States.

CONCLUSION

Boxing is an inherently dangerous sport with particular risk to the nervous system. Banning boxing would curtail boxing but would not halt it, and "bootleg" boxing would resurface. If boxing submerged underground, where there would be no medical or legal supervision, the magnitude of neurologic injury would escalate. Accordingly, increasing medical safety represents the most practical approach to boxing in today's society.

REFERENCES

1. Blonstein JL, Clarke E. Further observations on the medical aspects of amateur. *Br Med J* 1957;1:362–364.
2. Estwanik JJ, Boitano M, Ari N. Amateur boxing injuries at the 1981 and 1982 USA/ABF national championships. *Phys Sports Med* 1984;12:123–128.
3. Larson LW, Melin KA, Nordstrom-Ohrberg G, et al. Acute head injuries in boxers. *Acta Pyschiatr Neurol Scand* 1954;95(Suppl):1–42.
4. Jordan BD, Voy RO, Stone J. Amateur boxing injuries at the United States Olympic Training Center. *Phys Sports Med* 1990;18(2):80–90.
5. Schmidt-Olsen S, Jensen SK, Mortensen V. Amateur boxing in Denmark: the effect of some preventive measures. *Am J Sports Med* 1990;18:98–100.
6. Welch MJ, Sitler M, Kroeten H. Boxing injuries from an instructional program. *Phys Sports Med* 1986; 14(9):81–89.
7. Enzenauer RW, Montrey JS, Enzenauer RJ, et al. Boxing related injuries in the US Army, 1980 through 1985. *JAMA* 1989;261:1463–1466.
8. McCown LA. Boxing Injuries. *Am J Surg* 1959; 98: 509–516.
9. Jordan BD, Campbell E. Acute boxing injuries among professional boxers in New York State: a two-year survey. *Phys Sports Med* 1988;16:87–91.

10. Jordan BD, Jahre C, Hauser WA et al. CT of 338 actve professional boxers. *Radiology* 1992;185:509–512.

11. Jordan BD. Professional boxing: experience of the New York State Athletic Commission. In: Cantu RC, ed. *Boxing and medicine.* Champaign, IL: Human Kinetics, 1995:177–185.

12. Moore M. The challenge of boxing: bringing safety into the ring. *Phys Sports Med* 1980;8:101–105.

13. Ryan AJ. Eliminate boxing gloves. *Phys Sports Med* 1983;11:49.

14. Sercl M, Jaros O. The mechanisms of cerebral concussion in boxing and their consequences. *Work Neurol* 1962;3:351–357.

15. McCunney RJ, Russo PK. Brain injuries in boxers. *Phys Sports Med* 1984;12:53–67.

16. Critchley M. Medical aspects of boxing, particularly from a neurological standpoint. *Br Med J* 1957; 1:357–362.

17. Cantu RC, Voy R. Second impact syndrome: a risk in any sport. *Phys Sports Med* 1995;23.

18. Windle WF, Groat RA. Disappearance of nerve cells after concussion. *Anat Rec* 1945;93:201–209.

19. Oppenheimer DR. Microscopic lesions in the brain following injury. *J Neurol Neurosurg Psychiatry* 1968; 31:299–306.

20. Lampert PW, Hardman JM. Morphological changes in brains of boxers. *JAMA* 1984;251:2676–2679.

21. Unterharnscheidt F. About boxing: review of historical and medical aspects. *Tex Rep Biol Med* 1970; 28:421–495.

22. Parkinson D. The biomechanics of concussion. *Clin Neurosurg* 1982;29:131–145.

23. Martland HAS. Punch drunk. *JAMA* 1928; 91: 1103–1107.

24. Roberts AH. *Brain damage in boxers.* London: Pitman Publishing, 1969.

25. Critchley M. Medical aspects of boxing, particularly from a neurological standpoint. *Br Med J* 1957; 1:357–362.

26. Jordan BD, Matser E, Zimmerman RD, et al. Sparring and cognitive function in professional boxers. *Physician Sports Med* 1996;24(5):87–98.

27. Jordan BD, Jahre C, Hauser WA. Serial computed tomography in professional boxers. *J Neuroimaging* 1992;2:181–185.

28. Mendez MF. The neuropsychiatric aspects of boxing. *Int J Psychiatry* 1995;25:249–262.

29. LaCava G. Boxer's encephalopathy. *J Sports Med Physical Fitness* 1963;87–92.

30. Jordan BD. Epidemiology of brain injury in boxing. In Jordan BD, ed. *Medical aspects of boxing.* Boca Raton, FL: CRC Press, 1993:147–168.

31. Jordan BD, Relkin NR, Ravdin LD, et al. Apolipoprotein E e4 associated with chronic traumatic brain injury in boxing. *JAMA* 1997;278:136–140.

32. Corsellis JAN, Bruton CJ, Freeman-Browne C. The aftermath of boxing. *Psychol Med* 1973;3:270–303.

33. Corsellis JAN. Posttraumatic dementia in Alzheimer's disease. In: Jatzman R, Terry RD, Bick K, eds. *Senile dementia and related disorders.* New York: Raven Press, 1978:125–133.

34. Roberts GW, Allsop D, Bruton C. The occult aftermath of boxing. *J Neurol Neurosurg Psychiatry* 1990; 53:373–378.

35. Tokuda T, Ikeda S, Yanugesa N, et al. Re-examination of ex-boxers brain using immunohistochemistry with antibodies to amyloid beta protein and tau protein. *Acta Neuropathol* 1991;82:280–285.

36. Dale GE, Leigh PN, Luthert P, et al. *J Neurol Neurosurg Psychiatry* 1991;54:116–118.

37. Uhl GR, McKinney M, Hedreen JC, et al. Dementia pugilistic: loss of basal forebrain cholinergic neurons and cortical cholinergic markers. *Ann Neurol* 1982; 12:99.

38. Hof PR, Bouras C, Buee L, et al. Differential distribution of neurofibrillary tangles in the cerebral cortex of dementia pugilistic and Alzheimer's disease cases. *Acta Neuropathol* 1992;85:23–30.

39. Merz B. Is boxing a risk factor for Alzheimer's? *JAMA* 1989;261:2597–2598.

40. Mortimer JA, French LR, Hutton JT, et al. Head injury as a risk factor for Alzheimer's disease. *Neurology* 1985;35:264–267.

41. Saija A, Hayes RL, Lyeth BG, et al. The effects of concussive head injury on central cholinergic neurons. *Brain Res* 1988;452:303–311.

42. Smith CM, Swash M. Possible biochemical basis of memory disorder in Alzheimer's disease. *Neurology* 1978;3:471–473.

43. Nicoll JAR, Roberts GW, Graham DI. Apolipoprotein Ee4 allele is associated with deposition of amyloid beta protein following head injury. *Na Med* 1995;1:135–137.

44. Mayeaux R, Ottoman R, Maestre G, et al. Synergistic effects of traumatic head injury and apolipoprotein e4 in patients with Alzheimer's disease. *Neurology* 1995; 45:555–557.

45. Katzman R, Galosko DR, Saitoh T, et al. Apolipoprotein e4 and head trauma: synergistic or additive risks? *Neurology* 1996;46:889–892.

46. Jordan BD, Kanick AB, Horwich MS, et al. Apolipoprotein Ee4 and fatal cerebral amyloid angiopathy associated with dementia pugilistica. *Ann Neurol* 1995;38:698–699.

47. Strano SD, Marias AD. Cervical spine fracture in a boxer—a rare but important sporting injury: a case report. *S Afr Med J* 1983;63:328–330.

48. Kewairamani LS, Krauss JF. Cervical spine injuries resulting from collision sports. *Int Med Soc Paraplegia* 1981;19:303–312.

49. Jordan BD, Zimmerman RD, Devinsky O, et al. Brain contusion and cervical fracture in a professional boxer. *Phys Sports Med* 1988;16:85–88.

50. Levin HAS, Jordan BD. Neuropsychological assessment of brain injury in boxing. In: Jordan BD, ed. *Medical aspects of boxing.* Boca Raton, FL: CRC Press, 1993: 197–206.

51. Thomassen A, Juul-Jensen P, Olivarius B, et al. Neurological electroencephalographic and neuropsychological examination of 53 former amateur boxers. *Acta Neurol Scand* 1979;60:352–362.

52. Brooks N, Krysshik G, Wilson L, et al. A neuropsychological study of active amateur boxers. *J Neurol Neurosurg Psychiatry* 1987;50:997–1000.

53. Kaste M, Vilkki J, Sainio K, et al. Is chronic brain damage in boxing a hazard of the past? *Lancet* 1982; 2:1186–1188.

54. Ross RJ, Casson IR, Siegel O, et al. Boxing injuries: neurologic, radiologic and neuropsychologic evaluation. *Clin Sports Med* 1987;6:41–51.

55. Heilbronner RL, Henry GK, Carson-Brewer M. Neuropsychologic test performance in amateur boxers. *Am J Sports Med* 1991;19:376–379.

56. Levin HAS, Lippold SC, Goldman A, et al. Neurobehavioral functioning and magnetic resonance imaging findings in young boxers. *J Neurosurg* 1987; 67:657–667.

57. Drew RH, Templer DI, Schuyler BA, et al. Neuropsychological deficits in active licensed professional boxers. *J Clin Psychol* 1986;42:520–525.

58. Butler RJ, Forsythe WI, Beverly DW, et al. A prospective controlled investigation of the cognitive effects of amateur boxing. *J Neurol Neurosurg Psychiatry* 1993;56:1055–1061.

59. Casson IR, Siegel O, Sham R, et al. Brain damage in modern boxers. *JAMA* 1984;251:2663–2667.

60. McLatchie G, Brooks N, Gailbraith S, et al. Clinical neurological examination, neuropsychology, electroencephalography, and computed tomographic head scanning in active amateur boxers. *J Neurol Neurosurg Psychiatry* 1987;50:96–99.

61. Stewart WF, Gordon B, Selnes O, et al. Prospective study of central nervous system function in amateur boxers in the United States. *Am J Epidemiol* 1994; 139:573–88.

62. Johnson J. Organic psychosyndromes due to boxing. *Br J Psychiatry* 1969;115:45–53.

63. Jordan BD, Matser JT, Zimmerman RD, et al. Sparring and cognitive function in professional boxers. *Phys Sports Med* 1996;24(5):87–98.

64. Murelius O, Haglund Y. Does Swedish amateur boxing lead to chronic brain damage? A retrospective neuropsychological study. *Acta Neurol Scand* 1991;83:9–13.

65. Haglund Y, Eriksson E. Does amateur boxing lead to chronic brain damage? A review of some recent investigations. *Am J Sports Med* 1993;21:97–109.

66. Butler RJ. Neuropsychological investigation of amateur boxers. *Br J Sports Med* 1994;28:187–190.

67. Brookler KH, Itil T, Jordan BD. Electrophysiologic testing in boxers. In: Jordan BD, ed. *Medical aspects* of boxing. Boca Raton, FL: CRC Press, 1993;207–214.

68. Kaplan HA, Browder J. Observations on the clinical and brain wave patterns of professional boxers. *JAMA* 1954;156:1138–1144.

69. Busse EW, Silverman AJ. Electroencephalographic changes in professional boxers. *JAMA* 1952; 149: 1522–1525.

70. Casson IR, Sham R, Campbell EA, et al. Neurological and CT evaluation of knocked-out boxers. *J Neurol Neurosurg Psychiatry* 1982;45:170–174.

71. Sironi VA, Scotti G, Ravagnati L, et al. CT scan and EEG findings in professional pugilists: early detection of cerebral atrophy in young boxers. *J Neurosurg Sci* 1982;26:165–168.

72. Ross RJ, Cole M, Thompson JS, et al. Boxers—computed tomography, EEG, and neurosurgical evaluation. *JAMA* 1983;249:211–213.

73. Jordan BD, Zimmerman RD. Computed tomography and magnetic resonance imaging comparisons in boxers. *JAMA* 1990;263:1670–1674.

74. Jordan BD, Zimmerman RD. Magnetic resonance imaging in amateur boxers. *Arch Neurol* 1988;45:1207–1208.

75. Davie CA, Pirtosek Z, Barker GJ, et al. Magnetic resonance spectroscopic study of parkinsonism related to boxing. *J Neurol Neurosurg Psychiatry* 1995; 58:688–691.

76. Kemp PM, Houston AS, Macleod MA, et al. Cerebral perfusion and psychometric testing in military amateur boxers and controls. *J Neurol Neurosurg Psychiatry* 1995;59:368–374.

77. Dane SD, Jordan BD, Rowen, et al. SPECT scanning in professional boxers, in preparation.

78. New York State Department of State. Laws and rules regulating boxing and wrestling matches, 1984.

79. Golberg E, Gerstman LJ, Mattis S, et al. Effects of cholinergic treatment on posttraumatic anterograde amnesia. *Arch Neurol* 1982;39:581.

80. Jordan BD. Increasing medical safety in boxing. In: Jordan BD, ed. *Medical aspects of boxing.* Boca Raton, FL: CRC Press 1993:17–21.

81. USA Boxing. Rules and Regulations.

82. Professional Boxing Safety Act of 1996 (HR 4167). Public Law 104-272. 104th Congress.

Sports Neurology, Second Edition,
edited by Barry D. Jordan.
Lippincott–Raven Publishers, Philadelphia © 1998.

29

Cycling

Carl Heise

Department of Neurology, Hospital for Special Surgery,
535 East 70th Street, New York, New York 10021

Bicycling has become increasingly popular in this country as a recreational activity, form of aerobic exercise, competitive sport spanning many age groups, and energy-saving means of transportation. The latter two, however, are much less prevalent than in some European and Asian countries, most likely for a variety of cultural and geographic reasons. These include Americans' love affair with the automobile, large distances and suburban sprawl, automobile and truck traffic, and limited designated bicycle lanes and paths.

In the United States, recreational cycling far surpasses competitive cycling in terms of sheer numbers. The United States Cycling Federation (USCF) estimates that there are about 70,000 licensees for racing competition, which is split almost evenly between on-road and off-road races (H. Monaghan, USCF, personal communication). Estimates of total users reached about 85 million in 1989 (1). The discrepancy is much less pronounced in many European countries in which cycling is the second most popular sport after soccer. For example, in Italy the organization of cycling rivals that of baseball in the United States, with multiple associations at the amateur level that organize competitions for people ranging from children through the elderly. This does not include the national federation, which governs the professionals, as well as the so-called dilettantes or younger cyclists who are eligible for the Olympics and supply the professional ranks.

In spite of the popularity of cycling, it is not well appreciated that it is a hazardous activity. The literature provides ample and interesting statistics in terms of recreational cycling, but information regarding injuries incurred during races is limited and the USCF does not maintain statistics. The insurance carrier for the USCF estimates that there are on average 50 head injuries per season, but the type and severity are not known (Insurance carrier, USCF, personal communication). There were apparently two cervical spine injuries resulting in paralysis during the past season, and the insurance carrier estimates an average of one case per year over the past several years. One of the spine injuries occurred in an off-road race and the other in a road race.

In spite of the higher speeds involved, racing would seem to be a safer activity than pure recreational cycling, and a representative of the cycling federation confirmed that the majority of racers are injured during training (H. Monaghan, USCF, personal communication). There are probably several reasons for the relative safety of racing and these will be only touched on here.

Races are generally held in areas or on roads that have been closed to vehicular traffic, so there are fewer possibilities for chance encounters with cars and other obstacles (pedestrians, animals, other recreational cyclists, and the like). The racers are generally all more focused and alert, because of the circumstances, and thus less prone to the falls and collisions resulting from inattentiveness to which recreational cyclists are prone. The racers are all traveling in the same direction, and any falls that do occur tend to be lateral and not head-on collisions (this is not always the case in races from one location to another).

Probably the most important difference is that racers are required to wear helmets (see later). In Europe, however, not all professionals are required to wear helmets and they are certainly frowned upon for training, and this may explain the greater number of injuries noted in training both here and abroad.

Because of the racing position with head forward, the attachment of the feet to the pedals, and the hands gripping the handlebars, the head is a common point of impact, along with the shoulder. The design of the modern racing bicycle sacrifices stability, and even minimal contact of the front wheel with a stable rear wheel or irregularity in the road surface results in the rider being pitched suddenly and violently to the pavement. As a rule, there is no time to alter course or break one's fall.

The traditional bicycle shoe was attached to the pedal by a plate nailed to the shoe bottom with a groove that adapted to the frame of the pedal as well as a strap surrounding the shoe. This increased the power and efficiency of the pedal stroke on the crank. Newer pedal designs and shoe attachments allow easier and safer egress from the pedal, but, as with the older system, this requires a significant amount of force, as in a fall.

TYPES OF COMPETITION

In the United States, cycling competitions may be divided into on-road and off-road races, whereas in Europe road racing predominates. According to the USCF, the two types are approximately evenly split in enrollment. The number includes collegians and professionals.

Their versatility and ease of use have contributed to the rising popularity of off-road bicycles or so-called mountain bikes and the development of their own genre of competition with climbs, descents, and so forth. Actually, the Europeans had their own brand of off-road cycling known as cycle-cross using modified road bikes. This takes place during the winter months and serves as a means of maintaining conditioning. It involves running while carrying the bicycle on the shoulder, jumping small obstacles, and pedaling in mud.

Road races in this country are similar in type to those in Europe. The principal types include the stage race, the time trial or chronometer, and the races that take place from one town or location to another. In addition, for logistic reasons, there are circuits or "circle" races in which multiple laps are run around a course on local roads or city streets closed to traffic. These are the most common types of race among amateurs, because the races are shorter and multiple races may be conducted in the course of a day for different age groups.

Stage races range in length and duration from a few days to 3 weeks as in the Tour de France and Giro d' Italia, which are the two most famous road races in Europe. Time trials are also of varying lengths, but the racers race separately, leaving the starting line every minute or two and competing against the clock. These races are extremely intense and the cyclists must sustain their maximum velocity throughout without any rest or break in effort and without being able to "draft" other racers.

The races in line or from one place to another are generally longer and with more demanding terrain than the individual stages in a stage race and some are referred to as "classic," such as the Milano–Sanremo, Paris–Roubaix, and Liegi–Bastone–Liegi races. Although it is not readily apparent to the observer, cycle racing is extremely tactical as well as a curious blend of team and individual sport. Generally each team has a captain, who is the strongest of the group and the most likely to win. The main function of the others is to help the captain to win. This may take the form of supplying water bottles, furnishing a fresh tire in case of a flat or even a bicycle, and most commonly helping to break the wind or pulling the captain up to the main group in case of a fall or "pit stop." If the captain is primarily a sprinter, the team will allow the captain to draft until just the right moment during a final sprint.

Racers differ in individual physiognomy and athletic characteristics, some being considered climbers, others sprinters, and others especially suited to sustained velocity as in time trials. Those who excel in stage races are considered the most "complete" and need to combine all of the foregoing characteristics as well as have remarkable recuperative powers in order to compete on a high level for three straight weeks.

MECHANISMS OF INJURY

Injuries to racers tend to occur more frequently during training, especially during unofficial outings involving large numbers of cyclists. Although helmets are required in all amateur races, this is not universally true of the professionals, and helmets are shunned during training, particularly in Europe.

The most spectacular falls and injuries occur during high-speed, crowded, group sprints in which there are sudden changes in direction, similar to "cracking the whip" on ice, with bicycles or riders touching and causing a chain reaction type of fall. In the European amateur races, there may be sprints along town streets that have not been cleared of cars, and the front racers may graze automobiles while attempting to "brush off" those who are behind with an obstructed view. In criteriums, besides the sprints, falls tend to occur at corners and changes in caliber of the roadway, both of which produce sudden changes in velocity. These may be minor for the front runners but are magnified manyfold as they are transmitted back in the group, where those in the middle and rear may come to a complete halt and then be forced to sprint at top speed to reach the group once again.

In linear races with descents, sometimes fatal falls may occur with a variety of causes if the racers exit the road from high precipices. An error in judgment of velocity, a sudden blowout, hitting an unexpected patch of water or sand, or swerving to avoid another cyclist may all result in disaster at high speeds.

In spite of relatively frequent falls in races, injuries other than abrasions, contusions, and fractures are rare. Although not well publicized in Europe, there are generally one or two serious or fatal injuries per year. In any event, the serious or fatal injuries to racers do not differ substantially in nature from those to recreational cyclists, other than being much less common and not involving automobiles. The overwhelming majority of serious and fatal injuries involve the nervous system, and these are the subject of the bulk of this chapter.

NEUROLOGIC INJURY IN CYCLING

The principal types of neurologic injury related to bicycles may be divided into those that are acute and traumatic and those that are chronic and compressive in nature. The former generally involve the central nervous system (CNS), consisting of head (brain) injuries and less frequently spinal cord injuries. The latter are related to sites of prolonged contact between the cyclist and the bicycle, most notably the hands and the perineum, and involve the peripheral nervous system. The most frequently compressed nerves are the ulnar and pudendal nerves, but involvement of the median, sciatic, and posterior cutaneous nerves of the thigh has been reported (2–4).

Head Trauma

According to various sources, upward of 1300 bicycle-related deaths occur in the United States each year, and the vast majority are due to head injury (1,5,6). In 1985, cycling injuries resulted in approximately 574,000 emergency room visits, with similar numbers for 1982 (1,7). Many of these were related to head injuries.

A 2-year study of head injuries in children revealed that the single most common cause was a fall from a bicycle, producing 12% of all the head injuries (8). In a 1-year sample of bicycle-related admissions to three major hospitals in Calgary, Alberta, 73 or 67% of the injuries were related to craniocerebral trauma and none of the riders were wearing helmets. One-fifth suffered a skull fracture and five developed subdural hematomas (SDHs), four of which were fatal. There were three cervical spine injuries, two with neurologic deficit, although the type was not specified. Notable was the fact that although only a minority were due to encounters with automobiles, these produced all the fatalities. Bicycle accidents not involving a car were the most common cause of brain injuries sustained in recreational activities. These involved falls from the bicycle after impact with another object or loss of control. The authors remarked that even though 88% of the brain injuries were mild, there is an increasing body of literature indicating significant morbidity (in terms of physical, mental, and behavioral changes), even with "mild" head trauma (1,7,8, and Neuro Alert).

Friede et al. (7) found that 63.4% of all bicycle-related deaths in 1980 were in those younger than 20 years of age (5). Collisions with automobiles, which produced 27% of the injuries, were six times more likely to result in hospital admission. Ninety-five percent of the fatalities of children related to bicycling injuries involved automobiles. They also commented on helmets, citing data from an evaluation (9). Of 24 helmets evaluated, only 10 provided adequate deceleration (less than 300 G) from a 5-foot impact height and only 6 were protective from 6 feet. The seated cyclist's head is either slightly higher or lower than their height, depending on trunk position and type of handlebars. The traditional helmet in Europe did not pass even a 6-inch drop height (5).

Sachs et al. (10) reviewed mortality data from the National Center for Health Statistics and morbidity data from the Consumer Product Safety Commision's National Electronic Injury Surveillance System from 1984 to 1988. They found 2985 head injury deaths related to cycling and 905,752 head injuries (32% of all persons treated in an emergency room with cycling injuries). The deaths related to head injury represented 62% of all cycling deaths. Forty-one percent of the deaths and 76% of the injuries were sustained by children younger than 15 years. Of the deaths caused by head injury, 87% were due to bicycle–car collisions. The authors cited Weiss and *Consumer Reports* in estimating helmet use as 10% overall and only 2% in youngsters (11).

Thompson et al. (1) looked at the effectiveness of helmets in a case-control study in the Seattle area. They found that only 7% of the head-injured cyclists were wearing helmets, compared with about 24% of cyclists with other types of injuries in the control group. Of the 99 with serious brain injury, only 4% wore helmets. They estimated an 85% decrease in the risk of head injury and 88% decrease in the risk of brain injury with helmet use (4). This corresponds closely to the estimates of Sacks et al.

In an autopsy review of all bicycle-related deaths in the Miami metropolitan area, Fife et al found that in 86%, the head and the neck were the most seriously injured area. None of the fatalities were wearing helmets and all were involved in encounters with automobiles (12).

Types of Head Injury

The majority of articles concerning head injury (HI) in bicycling do not look closely at the specific types of head or brain injury, generally grouping them according to severity into mild, moderate, and serious. One may reasonably assume that they are similar in type and mechanism to those sustained in other sports, particularly those in which the head is one of the initial points of impact.

Weiss, in *Clinics in Sports Medicine* (6), states that fatal head trauma in cyclists is nearly always caused by intracranial hemorrhage, such as epidural hematomas associated with skull fractures and subdural hematomas (SDH).

Thompson et al. (1) found that 42% of their patients had concussions or worse. Almost 70% were considered mild or minor, with the remainder related to contusions, lacerations, or SDH's. Subdural hematomas were associated with a poor prognosis, with 80% fatality rate in one study (although of limited number). (9).

The autopsy review by Fife et al. (10) of fatally injured cyclists in Dade County found contusions to be the most common serious brain injuries (90 cases) and often associated with hemorrhage or laceration. They found an association between skull fractures and brain injury. Ninety-two percent of the patients with skull fractures had associated brain injuries, even with linear, nondisplaced fractures. Of cases with fatal head and neck injuries, 74% had head injuries alone, 20% had both, and only 6% had isolated cervical injuries. Although there has been some concern regarding helmet use contributing to cervical injuries, given the preponderance of head injuries, it would seem clear that the relative benefits far outweigh the risks.

In spite of evidence supporting the use of bicycle helmets (1,10), Weiss (6) cited several community-based campaigns to increase helmet use that produced only modest (at best) gains in actual usage. Interestingly, although it has been advocated by various groups and in several articles, Weiss pointed out that separation of bicycles and motor vehicles may not provide an easy remedy to cycling injuries. He stated that although a high percentage of motor vehicle–bicycle collisions are fatal, they are not the major cause of fatality or injury. Most morbidity and mortality are related to collisions with road hazards and irregularities in the road surface. In fact, he cited data from the League of American Wheelmen that indicate a 2.6% greater risk of injury on bicycle paths compared with roads. This is thought to be due to use by multiple types of vehicles and modes of locomotion, most with much lower velocity than the bicycle.

In summary, bicycle-related head injuries are an underrecognized major cause of mortality and morbidity. Head injuries occur most frequently in children and adolescents and are generally related to nonuse of helmets.

Spine Injuries

Possibly because of the predominance of head injuries, literature on bicycle-related injuries to the spine is lacking, except for mention in a few articles on head injuries. A 2-year British survey of admissions to a spinal cord center found that up to 50% were road or motor vehicle related, with only 3% involving bicycles. Bicycles were a less common cause than diving, gymnastics, and skiing.

In assessing the effectiveness of helmets in 235 cyclists with head injuries, Thompson et al. (1) found four with cervical spine fractures, all without paralysis. Three of the four also had associated head injuries, but the fourth, who was wearing a helmet, did not.

In the Dade County study (10), one of the two fatalities related to extended mirrors on pickup trucks had a fracture of C-1 and the skull, with severance of the brainstem. Friede et al. (7), who lumped skull and spine fractures together, found 6 of the latter out of 573 injuries.

In a 1-year study of bicycle injuries in Calgary, Guichon et al. (9) found 3 cervical injuries, two with neurologic deficits, out of 107 patients, but did not clarify the type.

In the Dade County experience of fatal injuries (10), the head and neck were the most severely involved in 86% of 173 cyclists, but 75% of injuries involved the head alone and only about 6% the spine alone. However, three of their cases with dislocation of skull on C-1 and brainstem injury were classified as head (brain) injuries. The authors commented on spine fractures but did not talk about spinal cord injuries or other neurologic injuries, in spite of autopsy studies. They found that spine fractures were second only to skull fractures in frequency and that cervical fractures alone were third. The most frequently fractured site was C-1, with a progressive reduction in frequency farther down the spine.

Fife et al. (10) did say that because spinal cord injuries above C-5 (because of respiratory compromise) involve significantly higher mortality than those below, their data may have been skewed toward an excess of C-1 and C-2 fractures, as they looked only at fatalities. Although it was not stated, one can presume that all the cases with spine injury alone and a percentage of those with both head and spine injuries were related to upper cervical spinal cord injury with respiratory or ventilatory insufficiency, because this is the most mobile portion of the spine and the most common site of cord injury (13).

The Peripheral Nervous System: "Nontraumatic" Injury to Peripheral Nerves

Compression injury to peripheral nerves also occurs in cycling, tending to be chronic and repetitive, although at times acute. These nerve injuries are common although less important in terms of severity than those of the central nervous system. They occur at the principal points of contact between the cyclist and the cycle. Thus the most common sites are the hands and perineum, with the feet a distant third.

Of the problems that arise from contact with the bicycle seat, pudendal neuropathy and impotence are the principal neuropathic ones. It is during its passage along the sides of the perineum, or beneath the symphysis for the terminal branch, that the nerve may become compressed and give rise to symptoms. Weiss (14) looked at the frequency and severity of symptoms in 113 of 132 cyclists engaged in a 500-mile, 8-day tour. He found that

45% developed some degree of perineal numbness and that in 10% it was of significant severity, causing 2% to discontinue riding temporarily.

In another review of bicycling injuries, the same author stated that up to 50% of cyclists on long-distance rides complain of numbness and in those cyclists it is a frequent symptom. The symptoms consist of paresthesias and/or hypesthesias of the scrotum or penile shaft (15,16). Weiss, as did Bond (17) in a 1975 report, attributed the penile numbness to a temporary ischemic insult to the dorsal nerve of the penis, which is compressed by the bicycle seat as it passes beneath the symphysis pubis.

Weiss further stated that the genital branch of the genitofemoral nerve may be involved, particularly with symptoms of scrotal anesthesia. He did not specify whether the scrotal numbness was anterior or posterior, but because the majority of the scrotum is supplied by branches of the perineal division of the pudendal nerve and cluneal branches of the posterior cutaneous nerve of the thigh (18), it appears more likely that the sensory loss was due to compression of one or both of the nerves as they pass through the perineum. Generally, the anterosuperior portion of the scrotum is supplied by the ilioinguinal and genitofemoral nerves. Although possible, because of the prolonged flexion of the trunk on the thigh at the hip associated with the "down" position in racing, it seems much less susceptible to pressure than the nerves compressed by the cyclist's weight.

Weiss included impotence as a second neuropathic problem in cycling and commented that it is probably underreported, given the nature of the male psyche. Solomon and Cappa (19) reported the case of a physician with a transient sensation of tightness of the glans penis associated with use of a stationary bicycle. He later developed impotence, which resolved 1 month after cessation of cycling exercise. They attributed the patient's impotence to perineal nerve pressure. They went on to say that perineal trauma is not even considered as a cause of impotence in several large reviews, although documented with pelvic fractures and use of a perineal post in hip surgery and fractures; instead, vascular causes are more widely incriminated.

Goodson (15) reported an individual who developed penile numbness, without impotence, shortly after completing a 2-day, 180-mile bike ride. His symptoms resolved slowly over the course of a month, with decreased mileage. This was attributed to compression of the terminal sensory branch of the pudendal nerve (dorsal nerve of the penis).

Weiss (20) also cited a report by Desai and Gingell (21) of a young man with impotence immediately after a 2-day, 135-mile bicycle race. This persisted for several months. They did not mention associated neuropathic symptoms, but electrophysiologic study demonstrated an abnormal response for the dorsal nerve of the penis. They attributed this to a "reversible ischemic neuropathy" of the dorsal nerve of the penis and cavernous nerves of the penis (vasomotor = perineal) secondary to compression between the pubic bone and the bicycle seat.

Probably the best known compressive neuropathy related to cycling is that of the ulnar nerve in the hand, also known as "handlebar neuropathy" (14,22–25). Inexperienced cyclists tend not to vary their hand position as often as recommended [Wilmanth and Nelson, in Richmond's chapter on handlebar problems, suggest every 3 to 4 minutes (26)] and also seem to spend an excessive amount of time in the "down" position. In general, the hand position should be varied every 5 minutes, but this depends on the terrain and type of cycling and may be problematic at times.

The onset of ulnar neuropathy in cyclists may be relatively acute, after an unaccustomed long ride; subacute, after a multistage ride; or chronic, with progression of symptoms. Like carpal tunnel syndrome (CTS), it usually presents with sensory symptoms (hypesthesia or paresthesias).

Burke (22) stated that cyclist usually notice numbness or weakness in the hand, with or without loss of coordination. This classically involves sensation to the volar aspect of the last 1½ digits (fourth and fifth), as well as the dorsal tips and distal, ulnar aspect of the palm. It also involves the intrinsic muscles of the hand. If the effect is significant, the cyclist may begin to notice atrophy of the first dorsal interosseus muscle and even a claw hand deformity.

In the survey by Kulund and Brubaker (23) of 89 of the 1200 cyclists participating in the BikeCentennial Tour, 32 (35%) developed hand numbness. Two riders had numbness only in the index finger and seven had numbness in both a median and ulnar nerve distribution. The majority had bilateral symptoms. They also found that the symptoms, once present, tended to persist. Several developed difficulty with abduction and adduction of the fingers or poor pinch, which likewise did not improve with continuation of the activity.

Noth et al. (24) described neurophysiologic testing in four cyclists with ulnar neuropathy (see later). Three of the four had sensory symptoms and later developed weakness after long tours. The fourth had only ulnar sensory symptoms. The paresis in the first three persisted for several months.

Hankey and Gubbay (25) studied two patients with isolated hand weakness and no sensory symptoms (bilateral in one and unilateral in the other). They diagnosed a neuropathy of the deep palmar branch of the ulnar nerve.

Eckman et al. (27) described three patients with ulnar neuropathies after extended periods of cycling. One man cycled across the country at 100 miles a day for a month and had bilateral weakness and wasting of intrinsic hand muscles (ulnar) without sensory symptoms. The other two had evidence of involvement of both the sensory and motor branches of the ulnar nerve.

Weiss (14) surveyed 113 of 132 participants in an 8-day, 500-mile bicycle tour and found that palm numbness occurred to some extent in 32% of riders, was severe in about 10%, and was less frequent than perineal numbness (45%). Although commonly described in the literature, it did not require cessation of the tour, although follow-up was lacking. Two-thirds of their cyclists with hand numbness had ulnar symptoms and about a third had numbness of the entire hand (median and ulnar).

Richmond (26) cited two neurophysiologic studies of long-distance cyclists, one of which compared sensory distal latencies of the ulnar nerve in 15 cyclists and 10 control subjects. The study found prolonged sensory latencies in all the cyclists. However, in another study of 20 cyclists,

9 of whom had transient symptoms, both motor and sensory nerve conductions were normal.

On the basis of Hoyt's experience with 117 cases of "cyclist's palsy," all of whom resumed cycling with resolution of symptoms, Richmond suggested neurophysiologic testing only in cases that do not improve appropriately with corrective measures or in whom the diagnosis is less than clear. I would also add those with significant weakness or atrophy.

Although the prognosis appears good, cyclists would do well to become aware of the potential for nerve injury and to heed early, more minor, sensory symptoms with the hope of circumventing potentially disabling weakness and a lengthy recovery. However, it is worth noting that in some cases the weakness was insidious.

Possibly because the transverse carpal ligament provides a more resistant roof to the carpal tunnel, or possibly because of hand positioning, carpal tunnel syndrome is much less commonly reported. Kulund and Brubaker found 9 of 32 cyclists with numbness of the entire hand or index only (7 and 2, respectively). Braithwaite (4) reported bilateral CTS in a cyclist.

Weiss (14) found that one-third of cyclists reporting hand paresthesias had symptoms in the entire hand, suggesting either combined median and ulnar involvement or, more likely, CTS, because the latter is well known to produce more diffuse symptoms.

Weiss (14) found neck and shoulder pain to be a fairly frequent complaint (about 20%), but this was generally limited to the area of the trapezius muscle and was not radicular (95%). About 5% also complained of numbness in that area, however, suggesting possible midcervical nerve root impingement or irritation. Richmond (26), related the neck pain to hyperextension of the cervical spine, particularly in cyclists pedaling in the down position (racers, neophytes) or with poorly fitting frames or attachments. This occurs with overreaching if the bicycle is too long, the seat too far back, or the stem to the handlebar too long.

Also reported by Weiss (14), as well as Kulund and Brubaker (23), has been numbness of the plantar aspect of the foot. This was noted in eight (7%) of those studied by the former and consisted of pain or paresthesias in the bottom of the foot.

On the BikeCentennial Tour this was infrequent, being noted in only two women with numbness of the great toe and one man with numbness of the "ball" of the foot. Another had dorsal forefoot numbness.

Without more details or neurophysiologic studies, it is difficult to determine the exact cause of the preceding symptoms. However, the distribution of symptoms suggests pedal pressure on the plantar nerves or on the digital branch of the medial plantar nerve (great toe numbness). The dorsal numbness suggests shoe pressure on the medial or intermediate branches of the superficial peroneal nerve.

Other isolated reports have noted the association of cycling with sciatic neuropathy resulting from pressure on the buttock (28), as well as a neuropathy of the posterior cutaneous nerve of the thigh (29).

REFERENCES

1. Thompson RS, et al. A case-control study of the effectiveness of bicycle helmets. *N Engl J Med* 1989;320:1361–1367.
2. Stewart JD, et al. Sciatic neuropathies. *Br Med J* 1983;287:1108–1109.
3. Arnoldussen WJ, Korten JJ. Pressure neuropathy of the posterior femoral cutaneous nerve. *Clin Neurol Neurosurg* 1980;82:57–60.
4. Braithwaite IJ. Bilateral median nerve palsy in a cyclist. *Br J Sports Med* 1992;26(1):27–28.
5. Division of Injury Epidemiology and Control, Center for Environmental Health, Centers for Disease Control. Bicycle-related injuries: data from the National Electronic Injury Surveillance System. *JAMA* 1987;257:3334–3337.
6. Weiss B. Bicycle-related head injuries. *Clin Sports Med* 1994;13(1):99.
7. Friede AM, et al. The epidemiology of injuries to bicycle riders. *Pediatr Clin North Am* 1985;32:141–151.
8. Ivan LP, et al. Head injuries in childhood: a 2-year survey. *Can Med Assoc J* 1983;128:281–284.
9. Guichon DM, Myles ST. Bicycle injuries: one-year sample in Calgary. *J Trauma* 1975;15:504–506.
10. Sachs JJ, et al. Bicycle-associated head injuries and deaths in the US from 1984–1988. *JAMA* 1991;266:3016–3018.
11. Fife D, et al. *J Trauma* 1983;23:745–755.
12. Rimel RW, et al. Disability caused by minor head injury. *Neurosurgery* 1981;9:221–228.
13. Chiles BW, Cooper PR. Acute spinal injury. *N Engl J Med* 1996;514–520.
14. Weiss BD. Nontraumatic injuries in amateur long distance bicyclists. *Am J Sports Med* 1985;13:187–192.
15. Goodson JD. Pudendal neuritis from biking. *N Engl J Med* 1981;304:365.
16. Mellion MB. Common cycling injuries: management and prevention. *Sports Med* 1991;11:52–70.
17. Bond RE. Distance cycling may cause ischemic neuropathy of penis. *Sports Med* 1975;3:54–56.
18. Stewart JD. *Focal peripheral neuropathies*, 2nd ed. Amsterdam: Elsevier, 1993:197–225.
19. Solomon S, Cappa KG. Impotence and bicycling. *Postgrad Med* 1987;81:99–102.
20. Weiss BD. Clinical syndromes associated with bicycle seats. *Clin Sports Med* 1994;13:175–186.
21. Desai K, Gingell JC. Hazards of long distance cycling. *Br Med J* 1989;298:1072–1073.
22. Burke ER. Ulnar neuropathy in bicyclists. *Physician Sports Med* 1981;9(4):53–56.
23. Kulund DN, Brubaker CE. Injuries in the BikeCentennial tour. *Physician Sports Med* 1978;6:74–78.
24. Noth J, Dietz V, Mauritz KH. Cyclist's palsy: neurologic and EMG study in four cases with distal ulnar nerve lesions. *J Neurol Sci* 1980;47:111–116.
25. Hankey Graeme J, Gubbay, Sasson S. Compressive mononeuropathy of the deep palmar branch of the ulnar nerve in cyclists. *J Neurol Neurosurg Psychiatry* 1988;51:1588–1590.
26. Richmond DR. Handlebar problems in Bicycling. *Clin. Sports Med.* 1994;13:165–173.
27. Eckman PB, Perlstein G, Altrocchi PH. Ulnar neuropathy in bicycle riders. *Arch Neurol* 1975;32:130–131.
28. Haig AJ. Pedal Pusher's palsy. *N Engl J Med* 1989;320:63.
29. Arnoldussen, WJ, Korten JJ. Pressure neuropathy of the posterior femoral cutaneous nerve. *Clin Neurol Neurosurg* 1980;82:57–60.

Sports Neurology, Second Edition,
edited by Barry D. Jordan.
Lippincott–Raven Publishers, Philadelphia © 1998.

30

Diving

Charles H. Tator

Division of Neurosurgery, The Toronto Hospital, 399 Bathurst Street, Toronto, Ontario M5T 2S8, Canada

Aquatic injuries are the leading cause of catastrophic injury related to sports and recreation (1). Sports and recreational injuries account for a significant proportion of all neurotrauma. Indeed, in some geographic areas sports and recreation rank after motor vehicle accidents as the second most frequent cause of acute spinal cord injury (2,3). In many countries, diving is the most common sport or recreation leading to spinal cord injury (2,4). In some series up to 75% of spinal cord injuries related to recreational activities were due to diving (5). The serious nature of aquatic injuries is underlined by the fact that these injuries often cause major neurologic deficits, often occur in young people in whom the disability can last the lifetime of the victim, and cost society enormous amounts of money for medical services and lost earnings. Of great importance is the fact that almost all aquatic injuries are preventable (1), and thus knowledge of the epidemiology of these injuries can be the first step to prevention. This chapter reviews in detail the findings of several studies of aquatic injuries conducted by the author and also provides an overview of the important findings of other investigators. Excluded are scuba-diving injuries, which are discussed in detail in another chapter.

EPIDEMIOLOGY

In a study of patients with acute spinal cord injuries admitted to two Toronto hospitals from 1948 to 1973, we found that 15% of the 358 cases were due to accidents related to sports and recreation (6). Diving accounted for 38 or 10.6% of the total number of cases, and indeed diving was the most common cause of spinal cord injury sustained during sports and recreational activities (7). All other types of sports and recreational activity, including football, hockey, and soccer, were much lower in frequency as causes. The median age of the 38 divers was 21 years, compared with an average age of 34 years for other patients with spinal cord injury. There were 32 males and 6 females.

To study specifically the issue of spinal cord injury related to diving, the author created a Task Force on Spinal Injuries, which prospectively studied the incidence and circumstances of spinal cord injuries in Ontario, Canada during the calendar year, 1979 (8). The data were collected with questionnaires sent to all neurosurgeons, orthopedic surgeons, and physical and rehabilitation medicine specialists. During 1979, there were 54 Ontario residents who sustained a spinal injury in diving or other aquatic activities, 51 males (94.4%) and 3 females (5.6%). The median age was 22, with a range of 12 to 49 years. Almost 39% of patients were in the 11- to 20-year-old group, and more than 80% were 30 years old or younger. Diving was the cause of the spinal cord injury in 92% of cases. Kite skiing, water skiing, and being pushed into water made up the remainder. The locations of the accidents included the following: private swimming areas, 72.5%; public swimming areas, 21.6%; and camps, 5.9%. Swimming pools were the site of 45% of the injuries, and 55% occurred in lakes, rivers or quarries. Alcohol consumption was known to be a factor in 16 patients, and alcohol or drugs were suspected in 14 others. Late evening and night were the most common times of the day for these injuries.

In 1986, our center conducted the first comprehensive study of all catastrophic sports and recreation injuries in a given geographic region (1). The entire Province of Ontario, comprising approximately one-quarter of the land mass and one-third of the population of Canada, was surveyed prospectively for the incidence and causes of all sports and recreation injuries of all types occurring in the calendar year 1986. Catastrophic injury was defined as an injury causing actual or potential long-term or permanent injury or death and included all brain and spinal cord injuries beyond simple concussions or spinal strains. A total of 530 cases were identified, including 87 fatalities in the Province of Ontario (approximately 8 million population). The study was conducted by sending quarterly questionnaires to 4000 selected members of the Ontario Medical Association, including specialists who commonly treat trauma patients such as emergency physicians, neurosurgeons, and orthopedic surgeons. Aquatic activities were the leading category (104 cases) and accounted for 19.8% of the injuries. Seventy-three cases (13.8%) were due to miscellaneous water sports and 32 cases (6.0%) to diving. More than half the deaths (51.6%) were due to water sports, with fishing being the leading aquatic activity (21 cases) causing fatality. Other aquatic fatalities occurred in boating (15 cases), swimming (4 cases), scuba diving (3 cases), and wind surfing (2 cases). Males constituted more than 80% of all injured victims, and almost 75% of all victims were 30 years of age or less.

The large number of fatalities in boating and fishing was explained in part by lack of life preservers. Alcohol consumption was a factor in 40% of the deaths (when this information was available). Also, a significant number of deaths occurred in cold weather months, indicating that hypothermia was a factor (1). Alcohol has been a prominent factor in several other series of diving injuries (9–11). For example, Bailes et al. (9) documented the use of alcohol in 97 (44.7%) of 220 patients with injuries of the cervical spine sustained in diving.

Kurtzke (4) compared the incidence of diving as a cause of spinal cord injury among various countries and found that the percentages of all cord injuries related to diving were 2.2% in South Africa, 4.4% in Austria, 5.3% in the United States, 6.2% in England, 8.0% in Norway, and 8.3% and 14.0% in two different regions of Australia. It is of interest that in England, the proportion of diving injuries in relation to the total number of sports-related injuries has remained constant from the 1950s to the 1980s (12). There are significant differences in the circumstances of the injuries in specific locations. In the Los Angeles area, for example, the ocean was the site of the injuries in 40% and swimming pools in 29% (13), and in Maryland, body surfing has been a frequent cause of cervical spine injury (14).

It should be noted that head and spinal cord injuries are extremely rare in competitive divers who have received training in diving techniques and that almost all diving injuries have occurred in noncompetitive, unsupervised aquatic activities. Similarly, there have been very few diving injuries in pools or natural swimming areas under direct supervision of trained personnel, such as swimming pools in schools.

CLINICAL FEATURES
OF DIVING INJURIES

In our study of diving injuries from 1948 to 1973 (7) the most common vertebral level of injury was C5-6 (39%) with the next most frequent levels being C4-5 (24%), C-5 (16%), C-6 (8%), C6-7 (8%), C7-T1 (3%), and T-12 (3%). The most common type of injury to the vertebral column was a posterior fracture–dislocation in 37%, with other common types being anterior fracture-dislocation (24%), compression fracture (18%), and burst fracture (8%). In a series reported by Bailes et al. (9) in which computed tomographic (CT) scanning was frequently performed, burst-type fractures were identified in 51.8% of patients. The seriousness of these injuries is emphasized by the finding that 25 of 38 patients had complete neurologic injuries with no voluntary motor function and no appreciation of sensation below the level of injury, which was in the cervical region in all 25 cases (7). Three patients died within 12 months of injury. Our 1979 study (8) also showed that C5-6 was the most common level of injury in the 54 cases. In 33 there was injury to the spinal cord, 8 cases had root injury only, and in the remaining 13 there was a fracture or dislocation of the spinal column without spinal cord or root injury. Twenty of the 33 cord injuries were complete, and 2 of the patients died within 12 months.

The biomechanics of diving injuries usually involve the top of the head striking the bottom of the natural body of water or swimming pool or rarely another swimmer or a submerged object. The cervical spine suffers compression between the immobilized, decelerated head and the weight of the after-coming body. The compression load on the cervical spine is transmitted axially and results in fracture-dislocation, either anterior or posterior, or burst fractures of the vertebral bodies. As already noted, most injuries occur at the midcervical region, although there have also been injuries more cephalad or caudal. High cervical injuries with major cord compression are not common, perhaps because they cause apnea and drowning. Indeed, the incidence of spinal injuries in diving may be even higher than reported, because some drowning victims may have harbored undetected spinal cord injuries (10,15). The biomechanical reasons for the predilection for the midcervical region may be related to the increased range of motion at this level.

Major head injuries or other associated injuries in diving are surprisingly rare. For example, Bailes et al. (9) analyzed 220 patients with neck fractures sustained in diving and found no intracranial mass lesions or systemic injuries, although 36.8% of patients sustained a loss of consciousness for more than 5 minutes. Nine patients (4.1%) in this series were near-drowning victims and had water aspiration pneumonia.

MANAGEMENT

Details of the management of the acute neurologic injuries accompanying diving and other aquatic activities are beyond the scope of this chapter. Emergency management of acute cervical spinal cord injury is given in Chapter 11. The present chapter provides only a brief outline of the management of spinal cord injury related to diving. In addition to the ABCs of trauma management, which include attention to the airway, breathing, and circulation, rescuers of victims of acute spinal cord injury caused by diving are faced with the problems of extrication from water and immobilization of the spine. The victim may have some alteration of consciousness or confusion and complain of numbness or tingling or neck pain. If breathing is impaired, use airway restoration measures, such as the jaw thrust or chin lift, that avoid neck motion. It is always helpful to recruit as many assistants as possible to help maintain spinal alignment and support the victim's body in the water until the body can be floated onto a flat surface or stretcher. Packs of towels or rolled magazines are helpful for neck immobilization during transport. Ensure that the patient is fixed firmly by straps or other means to avoid being dislodged by motion. A complete neurologic examination is performed after these acute resuscitative measures.

Imaging of the spinal cord injury is best accomplished with plain radiographs followed by magnetic resonance imaging, although computed tomography is also usually required. High doses of intravenously administered steroids are recommended as soon as possible after injury. Many patients require cervical traction for reduction, which is best performed with halo devices that can be converted to halo vest immobilization for short-term or long-term management. Operative decompression is required for patients with major compromise of the spinal canal, usually caused by indriven fractures of the vertebral body or disrupted disc. Surgical decompression may be indicated in incomplete injuries with persisting compression and is usually necessary for patients with progressive neurologic deterioration, such as a worsening paralysis or sensory loss in incomplete injuries or a rising neurologic level in complete injuries. Operative treatment may also be required for major instability of the vertebral column, which can be treated by anterior or posterior approaches often with various forms of internal fixation (9,16).

Spinal cord–injured patients require special measures for bladder and bowel management and continuing attention to avoidance of respiratory, skin, urinary tract, and thromboembolic complications. In general, both the acute and rehabilitation phases of care are best managed in spinal cord injury units with specialized equipment and experienced personnel (17).

DROWNING AND NEAR DROWNING

Drowning is defined as death from suffocation by immersion in water, and it is estimated that more than 10,000 drownings occur annually in North America. Three to five times as many suffer near drowning, which is defined as survival, at least temporarily, after suffocation by immersion in water (18,19).

In North America, approximately two-thirds of all drownings occur in inland waters, with swimming pools being the most common site. As noted earlier, in Canada, drowning is the leading cause of death in sport and recreation (1), with boating and fishing causing high numbers of fatalities. Small power boats and canoes are the most common craft involved in drownings. There are two high-risk groups, children of both sexes less than 5 years old and males 15 to 24 years of age, in whom alcohol is a significant contributing factor in 50% of deaths (20,21).

Although the pathophysiology of drowning and near drowning varies somewhat depending on whether freshwater or seawater is involved, the presence of cardiac damage, and whether the lungs are "wet" or "dry," the neurologic damage is due to hypoxemia and metabolic acidosis (18). Thus, treatment is directed toward rapid resuscitation with attention to airway, breathing, and circulation to restore normal blood gas values. Cardiopulmonary resuscitation at the water's edge is first accomplished by mouth-to-mouth ventilation, and when equipment or experienced personnel arrive, resuscitation continues with oxygen administration by face mask and bag or oropharyngeal airway or endotracheal intubation. These resuscitative maneuvers are performed without movement of the spine, because it is always safer to assume the concomitant presence of a spinal injury in all drowning or near-drowning victims. The prognosis for good neurologic recovery depends on the initial findings. In those with a spontaneous

pulse, even when the level of consciousness is decreased, recovery without neurologic sequelae almost always occurs (22). In those with incomplete return of function, consideration should be given to the need for treatment of cerebral edema or raised intracranial pressure, which occur as a result of the blood–brain barrier alterations caused by hypoxemia and metabolic acidosis (18). Neurologic sequelae can include prolonged coma, blindness (including cortical blindness), cerebral atrophy, and ventricular dilation. The use of intracranial pressure monitoring is controversial. For more information about management, the reader is referred to two excellent reviews of the management of near drowning (18,23).

PREVENTION

It is highly likely that almost all aquatic injuries and especially diving injuries are preventable. Knowledge of the epidemiology of these injuries allows targeting of several high-risk groups toward which prevention programs should be aimed. Prevention programs should begin at an early age because the 11- to 20-year-old decade is most frequently injured. Elementary schools are an excellent starting point for prevention programs, but because those in all age groups sustain these injuries, the message must also be directed at other age groups. In various countries, a coalition of groups are involved in these prevention programs, including the Royal Life Saving Society, the Red Cross, and the paraplegic and head injury associations. Think First, the National Prevention Program for Head and Spinal Cord Injuries organized by the main neurosurgic associations in the United States and Canada, is involved in the prevention of aquatic injuries in North America. The rising incidence of spinal injuries in private swimming areas, especially backyard pools (8), merits attention by these prevention programs.

Specific prevention materials are available for the prevention of diving injuries. For example, SportSmart Canada has created two videos that warn school-age children against the hazards of shallow-water diving. The first video, entitled "Dive Right," is aimed at children of elementary school age, and "Sudden Impact" is aimed at teenagers and comes with a leader's manual to be used by high school teachers during classroom presentation of the safe diving program. These videos are obtainable from local chapters or from the National Office of Think First (22 South Washington, Park Ridge, IL 60068).

Specific targets for drowning prevention programs include the parents of young children, who must be warned of the risks of leaving children unattended; children themselves; active young adult males, who are at the highest risk; and middle-aged males at risk in boating and fishing. High-risk recreational activities leading to drowning include those involving small power boats, canoes, and personal watercraft such as jet skis; sport fishing; unsupervised backyard pool or waterfront play; and snowmobiling on ice.

Boating and fishing injuries and fatalities can be significantly reduced by emphasizing two simple safety measures: use of life preservers and awareness of alcohol. Personal flotation devices can prevent most drownings that occur in sports and recreational aquatic activities, and major hazards are posed by the combination of alcohol consumption and recreational boating and fishing (24). The hazards of diving are similarly compounded by alcohol consumption (8).

Prevention strategies are enhanced by media participation in spreading the message about the hazards of shallow-water diving. Media campaigns should begin in the spring and continue throughout the summer in climates in which there is a major seasonal incidence of aquatic injuries (8). Radio, television, and newspaper warnings about the hazardous mixture of aquatic activities and alcohol consumption and the need to use personal flotation devices are to be encouraged in all countries.

There is an important role for governments in regulating certain aspects of aquatic activities. An obvious example is fencing around swimming pools. Other examples include regulations about water depth in both private and public pools, signage concerning diving prohibition or permission, and the use of personal flotation devices. It would be helpful to have specific signage agreed to by international convention warning against the hazards of diving into shallow water. These signs should be mandatory at all public pools and beaches and should be encouraged in all private swimming areas, especially backyard pools, which often have insufficient depth for diving. Everyone should be made aware that it takes almost double an individual's height in water depth to allow complete deceleration of the body (25). Prevention programs require the support of specific recreational organizations such as fishing and boating associations.

The medical profession can also play an important role in providing medical knowledge to groups involved with rescue and teaching methods of resuscitation. As well, warnings to patients at higher risk of drowning, such as epileptics (26), can be effective prevention.

Acknowledgment

The author wishes to acknowledge the assistance of the Ontario Ministry of Culture, Tourism and Recreation in providing research funds for collection of much of the data described in this chapter. The technical assistance of Virginia Edmonds, B.A., R.N., and Linda Rickards, R.N., is gratefully acknowledged.

REFERENCES

1. Tator CH, Edmonds VE, Duncan EG, Tator IB. Danger upstream: catastrophic sports and recreational injury in Ontario. *Ontario Med Rev* 1988;55:7–12.
2. Tator CH, Edmonds VE. Sports and recreation are a rising cause of spinal cord injury. *Phys Sports Med* 1986;14:157–167.
3. Tator CH, Duncan EG, Edmonds VE, Lapczak LI, Andrews DF. Changes in epidemiology of acute spinal cord injury from 1947 to 1981. *Surg Neurol* 1993;40: 207–215.
4. Kurtzke JF. Epidemiology of spinal cord injury. *Exp Neurol* 1975;48:163–236.
5. Kewalramini LS, Taylor RG. Injuries to the cervical spine from diving accidents. *J Trauma* 1975;15: 130–142.
6. Tator CH, Edmonds VE. Acute spinal cord injury: analysis of epidemiological factors. *Can J Surg* 1979;22: 575–578.
7. Tator CH, Edmonds VE, New ML. Diving: a frequent and potentially preventable cause of spinal cord injury. *Can Med Assoc J* 1981;124:1323–1324.
8. Tator CH, Palm J. Spinal injuries in diving: incidence high and rising. *Ontario Med Rev* 1981;48:628–631.
9. Bailes JE, Herman JM, Quigley MR, Cerullo LJ, Meyer PR Jr. Diving injuries of the cervical spine. *Surg Neurol* 1990;34:155–158.

10. Mennen U. A survey of spinal injuries from diving. *S Afr Med J* 1981;59:788–790.

11. Scher AT. Diving injuries to the cervical spinal cord. *S Afr Med J* 1981;59:603–605.

12. Silver JR. Spinal injuries in sports in the UK. *Br J Sports Med* 1993;27:115–120.

13. Good RP, Nickel VL. Cervical spine injuries resulting from water sports. *Spine* 1980;5:502–506.

14. Cheng CL, Wolf AL, Mirvis A, Robinson WL. Body surfing accidents resulting in cervical spine injuries. *Spine* 1992;17:257–260.

15. Frankel HL, Montero FA, Penny PT. Spinal cord injuries due to diving. *Paraplegia* 1980;18:118–122.

16. Tator CH, Duncan EG, Edmonds VE, Lapczak LI, Andrews DF. Comparison of surgical and conservative management in 208 patients with acute spinal cord injury. *Can J Neurol Sci* 1987;14:60–69.

17. Tator CH, Duncan EG, Edmonds VE, Lapczak LI, Andrews DF. Neurological recovery, mortality and length of stay after acute spinal cord injury associated with changes in management. *Paraplegia* 1995;33: 254–262.

18. Levin DL, Morriss FC, Toro LO, Brick LW, Turner GR. Drowning and near-drowning. *Pediatr Clin North Am* 1993;40:321–336.

19. Modell JH. Drowning vs. near drowning—a discussion of definitions. *Crit Care Med* 1981;9:351–352.

20. Harries MG. Drowning in man. *Crit Care Med* 1981;9:407–408.

21. Lacey G. Near drowning. *Emerg Prehosp Med* 1990;4:14–18.

22. Oakes DD, Sherck JP, Maloney JR, et al. Prognosis and management of victims of near drowning. *J Trauma* 1982;22:544–549.

23. Olshaker JS. Near drowning. *Emerg Med Clin North Amer* 1992;10:339–350.

24. Plueckhahn VD. Alcohol and accidental drowning: a 25 year study. *Med J Aust* 1984;141:22–25.

25. Albrand OW, Walter J. Underwater decelerator curves in relation to injuries from diving. *Surg Neurol* 1975;4: 461–464.

26. Ryan CA, Dowling G. Drowning deaths in people with epilepsy. *Can Med Assoc J* 1993;148:781–784.

Sports Neurology, Second Edition,
edited by Barry D. Jordan.
Lippincott–Raven Publishers, Philadelphia © 1998.

31

Equestrian Sports

William H. Brooks and *Doris M. Bixby-Hammett

*Neurosurgical Associates, 1401 Harrodsburg Road, Suite B 485,
Lexington, Kentucky 40504;
103 Surrey Road, Waynesville, North Carolina 28786

The varieties of equestrian sports extend from pleasure riding through fields and along trails to the excitement of racing; from the elegant formality of dressage to rodeos; from the exhibition of schooled airs above the ground to steeplechase.

When compared with other sporting events, those that involve the horse require special consideration. In no other sport are the partners or members of a "team" composed of two different species. Consequently, the rider must always be aware of his or her separation from as well as interdependence with the horse. The unexpected "decision" of the horse frequently results in accidents that would not occur in sports that depend entirely on human choice or anticipated failure of machinery. This is further compounded by the large potential energies that are involved in equestrian events: horses may weigh as much as 500 kg and are capable of moving at speeds of 65 km/hr. Further, a rider whose head may be as high as 3 m from the ground would be expected to sustain considerable impact forces if he or she falls or is thrown from the horse. It is the interrelation of the unpredictability of the horse–rider combination and the significant physical forces achievable that results in sport-related injuries.

EPIDEMIOLOGY

Horses are part of American life. There are 6.6 million equines in the United States, with 10,000 sanctioned horse shows and thousands of local unsanctioned events. In 1992 there were 245,824 youths involved in 4-H horse programs and over 12,000 youths active in the United States Pony Clubs. However, most horse-related activity is in recreational activities. Studies of horse-related sports show that the population at greatest risk are adolescent females (1). The largest increase in injuries is seen in people over 24 years of age (2) and most of the neurologic injuries occur during recreational activities (3).

Equestrian sports are associated with significant risk of participant morbidity and mortality (4). The rate of injury is estimated at 0.5 injury per 1000 riding hours. To underscore this risk, over 100 deaths directly related to equestrian activities are projected annually for the nation. In a study of horse-related fatalities, 65.8% were from falls from or with the horse and 34.2% of those who died were not mounted when the fatal injury occurred (5).

Experience and knowledge are different factors in injury. The number of years riding does not correlate with decrease in injury, but knowledge and proficiency do (6,7). A rider who has one accident is at greater risk of having a second accident (8); over two-thirds of all riders report more than one horse-related injury (9). Nine percent of Western-style riders sustained a second injury within 3 months of the first (10). The risks involved in any phase of horseback riding, including reinjury, cannot be overemphasized.

TYPES OF INJURY

Although most equestrian-related injuries involve the extremities, the most catastrophic injuries are to the central or peripheral nervous system (11,12) and spine. At least one-third of all injuries that arise from horseback riding involve the nervous system and/or spine (13). Head injuries, which account for over 90% of neurologic injuries, are usually concussions or cerebral contusions associated with minimal deficit (Glasgow Coma Scale >13). Severe cerebral injury may be observed in approximately 10% of cases (Glasgow Coma Scale <8). As many as 5% of patients with head injuries may also have spinal injuries; approximately 40% of individuals with spinal injuries have concurrent head injuries

Skull fractures, linear, basal, or depressed, are frequently seen in those who do not wear protective headgear (>40%) but rarely occur in those adequately protected. Intracranial hematoma (e.g., epidural, subdural, or intercerebral) may be found in about 15% of those requiring hospitalization and surgery. Injury to the spine may be expected in over of 10% of riders who sustain neurologic injury. These include injury confined to the spinal column (14%) as well as the spinal cord (6%). Most occur in the lumbar and/or thoracic vertebral column (55%); the cervical spine is less frequently injured (30%). These fractures are frequently associated with injury to the spinal cord, nerve root, or cauda equina. Brachial plexus and peripheral nerve injuries are infrequent and usually arise from chronic injury (e.g., carpal tunnel syndrome).

Although the actual occurrence of neurologic injuries is unknown because deaths from craniospinal injury or mild neurologic injury (grade 1 concussion) are frequently not reported, neurosurgery services can anticipate one to two equestrian-related injuries per month per 1,000,000 population referred. As the popularity of horseback riding increases, the numbers of people at risk for neurologic injury also increases. It is important to identify the mechanisms involved in these injuries, determine how they may be lessened or prevented, and thereby enhance the enjoyment of all who ride.

MECHANISMS OF INJURY

The mechanisms of injury fall into broad categories, occurring while the horse is being at-

tended or resulting from the rider being thrown or falling. Neurologic injury may occur in stabling areas, such as an unexpected kick or crushing or trampling by the horse. These injuries generally occur during horse management (feeding, grooming, saddling, loading, training, shoeing, breeding, or foaling) or when the horse is startled by an unexpected event.

The number of craniospinal injuries that occur in a sport is reflected in the degree of head-forward stance adopted. This position frequently arises in equestrian sports and thus ensures that head and/or spinal injury will accompany many riding accidents. Most injuries result from falls or being thrown. When this is associated with subsequent trampling of the rider by a falling or undirected horse, the risk of catastrophic injury increases greatly. Indeed, the mechanism of these injuries is potentially one of the most lethal of all sports-related accidents (Fig. 1). Unexpected falls have various causes related to both rider and horse. For example, an experienced rider may be thrown by a less experienced mount refusing to negotiate a complex jump. Alternatively, a less experienced rider may fall when a well-schooled horse takes a jump for which the rider is unprepared. In addition, the horse may lose its footing and fall while turning suddenly and thereby pin or crush the rider beneath it. Another source of potential injury is the rider's foot becoming caught in the stirrup or the rider holding or being entangled in reins after an unexpected dismount and being dragged, with repeated injury to the head, spine, or peripheral nerves.

Head injury accounts for most neurologic injuries related to equestrian sports. The mechanisms by which these cerebral injuries occur include dynamic loading (impact and impulsive) as well as static in accidents involving crush injury.

Most occur after dynamic loading, which includes the head striking the ground or another object (e.g., fence, jump rail, tree), in addition to the impulsion imparted by sudden acceleration–deceleration concurrent with the rider falling through the air. These forces in combination would be expected to result in both focal and diffuse cerebral injury as frequently observed in head-injured riders (Fig. 2, and see Fig. 1). Concussion and other diffuse brain injuries may

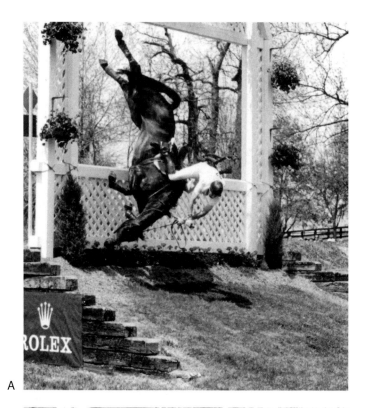

A

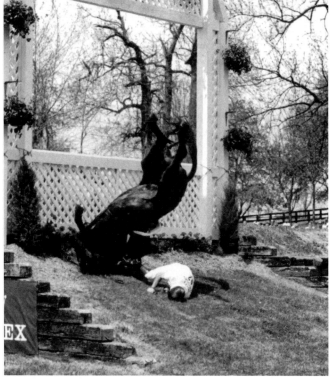

B

FIG. 1. This rider sustained diffuse cerebral injury in addition to fractured ribs, pneumothorax, and vertebral body fracture despite wearing a helmet and protective vest.

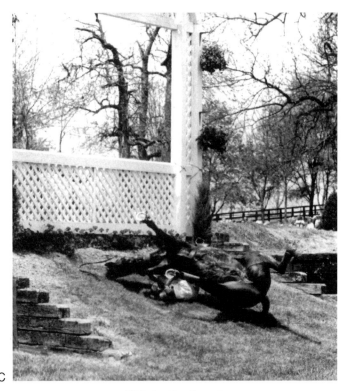

C

FIG. 1. *Continued.*

not be associated with skull fracture in riders who wear protective headgear, in contrast to the frequent fractures in riders with the same brain injuries who were not wearing protective headgear. Although the risk of sustaining linear or depressed skull fracture may be lessened by appropriate headgear, the injurious effects of rotational or angular and translational forces are not lessened or prevented. This observation explains why head injuries may be seen even in riders who routinely wear protective helmets.

Spinal injuries occur less frequently than head injuries and represent only 5% to 10% of all injuries to the nervous system. Fractures of the spine associated with equestrian sports are most frequently observed in the thoracolumbar region; those of the lumbar and cervical regions are less common. These fractures occur most commonly after being thrown and landing on the buttocks or in a flexed position. The addition of a rotational component to forced flexion increases the likelihood of instability and concurrent injury to the

cauda equina and/or nerve roots. Fracture of the cervical spine usually occurs when the rider's head strikes the ground with the neck in a flexed position. These fractures should be considered as unstable. Hence, any rider who sustains a fall should have proper evaluation before moving or remounting.

Frequently, the question of whether and how to remove the helmet of an unconscious rider may arise. Protective riding helmets are radiolucent; hence, it is not necessary to remove a helmet in order to obtain adequate radiographs of the skull or, particularly, the cervical spine. Moreover, riding helmets currently available do not limit access to the face, mouth, or nose and do not prevent free access to the airway. Therefore, there is little reason to remove these helmets before radiography to rule out the presence of cervical spine fracture or before full evaluation by a health care giver. Indeed, the helmet of an unconscious rider should *not* be removed until appropriate radiographs have been obtained

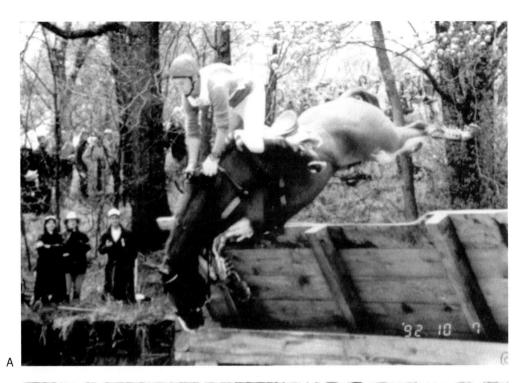

A

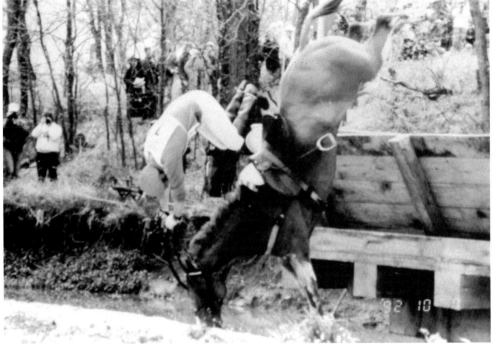

B

FIG. 2. Although this rider wore protective headgear, he sustained a traumatic subarachnoid hemorrhage, diffuse cerebral contusions, and concussion resulting from the combination of impact and inertial forces incurred during this fall. Note rotation of head during this fall.

and the presence of a cervical fracture is completely eliminated.

Cervical fracture arising from axial loading has not been observed. This is probably because the falling or thrown rider tends to fall with the neck extended or, most commonly, with both neck (cervical spine) and arms extended in attempting to lessen the impact (Fig. 2). This maneuver explains the large numbers of upper extremity fractures occurring in horseback riding.

Injury to the peripheral nervous system is generally confined to the brachial plexus. These injuries occur as the fallen rider attempts to maintain a firm grip on the reins or saddle (Fig. 3). They may be further complicated if the rider pulls the horse down on himself or herself because of not releasing the reins to allow the horse to regain its balance. These injuries are stretch injuries and generally improve with varying degrees of recovery in 3 to 6 months. Cervical root avulsion has not been reported. Chronic injury to the median nerve is commonly observed in riders involved in an equestrian discipline that requires holding the reins with the wrist in a flexed

position. Although this would not be expected to occur in beginning riders or those involved in a discipline not requiring such a posture, these complaints are common among older riders and those involved in activities such as dressage.

PREVENTION

Although certain biomechanical factors that produce neurologic injury are inherent to equestrian sport, the overall risk associated with these injuries may be lessened by: (a) identifying individuals who should not ride; (b) requiring the use of fitted, secured protective headgear of the highest standard (e.g., ASTM F1163) and other protective equipment as it is demonstrated to improve safety and becomes available; and (c) developing criteria for allowing resumption of riding after accidents. There are specific conditions that absolutely contraindicate equestrian sport participation: These include any symptomatic (neurologic or pain-producing) abnormalities or spinal anomalies with potential instability that render the spinal cord vulnerable to

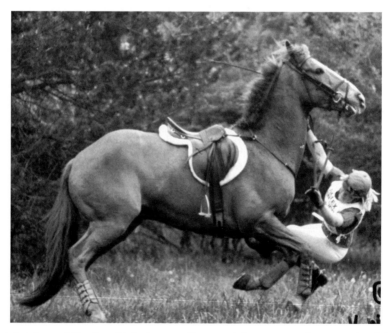

FIG. 3. Stretch injury of the brachial plexus with complete recovery in approximately 12 weeks occurred as a result of this injury.

injury (e.g., congenital absence of the odontoid process or significant previous cervical fracture or dislocation); temporary quadriplegia, paraplegia, or paralysis of any etiology; permanent cerebral sequelae of head injury (e.g., seizures, peripheral field deficits, or dementia); and repeated painful injury to the cervical or lumbar spine, particularly with radiographic evidence or severe degenerative osteoarthritis. Idiopathic epilepsy that is well controlled should not interfere with participation in equestrian sports. Posttraumatic seizures, however, suggest that competitive riding be eliminated. Exceptions to these criteria may be considered for those who wish to enjoy horseback riding in a noncompetitive manner. The hazards of riding, however, should be fully discussed with the prospective rider and, if necessary, with his or her parents or guardian. Frequently, injuries occur during leisurely trail rides or while the rider is being instructed, so the hazards of horseback riding cannot be treated lightly (14).

For competitive riders who sustain neurologic injuries, thorough evaluation is strongly recommended before resumption of competition. Conditions requiring such evaluation include brachial plexus injury producing significant (temporary or permanent) neurologic impairment, herniated intervertebral disc with or without surgical treatment, prolonged or repeated postconcussive syndrome, any intracranial condition requiring operation, and recurrent cervical or lumbar musculoligamentous injuries.

Repeated concussion should be carefully evaluated in relation to the factors involved. These injuries may result from lack of protective headgear, inexperienced riders attempting feats that are beyond their capabilities, and the use of horses that are incapable of performing in a specific phase of an equestrian sports. Repeated concussion has been shown to cause problems in attention, concentration, memory, judgment, and the speed of the thinking process with a resultant lowering of the IQ; hence these injuries must not be dealt with passively. Although these factors strongly suggest that competitive riding be curtailed, each case must be evaluated individually.

Guidelines for resuming horseback riding after head injury are identical to those well known and established for other sporting endeavors that are associated with cerebral injury (e.g., contact sports). Individuals should not be allowed to ride without resolution of all symptoms attributable to concussion. Headache, vertigo, memory loss, and any alteration of cognitive function precludes safe horseback riding. It should be underscored that recurrent head injury occurs in approximately 30% of horseback riders within 1 to 2 months of an initial concussion. Thus, care should be exercised in advising resumption of equestrian sports following a cerebral concussion without neurologic evaluation and consent. Any question regarding a safe return to equestrian-related activities should be referred to a neurologist or neurosurgeon.

Particular attention should be directed to protective headgear after a rider sustains a head injury or any contact to the head. The helmet should be examined carefully for cracks and/or alterations in the liner and hard shell. Any suspicion of a defect warrants closer examination by the manufacturer before using this particular helmet again. Remember, do not mount a horse without wearing a fitted, secure protective helmet. The purchase of a new helmet is advisable after involvement in a riding accident resulting in contact of the head.

The occurrence of spinal cord injury generally precludes horseback riding because of neurologic defects that render riding difficult if not impossible. Individuals who sustain an injury to the spinal cord that does not result in permanent neurologic deficits are more problematic. In general, although pleasure riding may be permissible, it is prudent to advise cessation of competitive equestrian activities in individuals who have sustained any form of spinal cord injury. Individuals who sustain vertebral fractures, ligament injuries possibility associated with instability, and/or a shallow spinal canal resulting from advanced degenerative arthritis or of congenital origin should be evaluated by a neurosurgeon before resuming any form of horseback riding.

Tradition is strong in equestrian events, and the hat is proper attire in all types of riding (Table 1). Nothing has done more to limit the number of severe neurologic injuries than use of appropriate protective headgear in all phases of riding.

TABLE 1. *American Society for Testing and Materials equestrian standard Safety Equipment Institute–certified helmet*

Type	Advantages	Disadvantages
English	Meet rules for English show tack New models lighter weight	Black velvet shows wear and age Generally more expensive
Schooling	Hard outer shell durable and practical Can use different helmet covers Most models vented for coolness Visor can be removed for versatility Less expensive than other styles Microthin shells lightest weight	Requires black velvet cover for English show classes Ultralightweight less durable than hard shell models Venting prevents use for watering horse using helmet in place of bucket
Western	Traditional Western style required for show classes Wide brim for sun protection Available in felt and straw	Most expensive of equestrian hats[a] Heavier than microthin shell helmets Harness not yet accepted by some judges despite AHSA rules forbidding them to penalize riders for wearing protective headgear

[a] When compared with premium Western felt hats without protection, average price.

Riding helmets were independently tested from 1981 to 1986 using parts of the United States Polo Association (USPA) 1979 standard on National Operating Committee on Standards for Athletic Equipment (NOCSAE) test systems. The improved American Society for Testing and Materials (ASTM) standard F116388 helmets were first available in 1989 (Fig. 4).

Standards require that helmets provide adequate protection against penetration by blunt or sharp objects as well as pass rigorous testing to ensure the proper redistribution of impact forces that are capable of resulting in brain injury (concussion or contusion). A suspension system that can prevent loss from the head is mandatory. This is an important feature of any riding helmet, because head injuries may occur when the helmet is lost from the head in an accident. Testing measures the amount of stretch of the system at the moment of impact.

Although a riding hat may meet all requirements of the testing organization, it is not fully protective unless it fits the rider's head properly. It should fit as snugly as possible, yet be comfortable. The retention system must always be fastened when mounted on the horse or preparing to mount. If present, the laces at the back of the hat must be tightened to prevent forward rotation. If a riding hat sustains a significant impact, it should be returned to the manufacturer for inspection or be replaced. All Safety Equipment Institute–certified ASTM standard riding hats must be identified on the permanent ASTM SEI label required in F1163. A current list of helmets that afford the highest protection against head injury is available from each state horse specialist, the United States Pony Clubs (4071 Iron Works Pike, Lexington, KY 40511), or the American Medical Equestrian Association (103 Surrey Road, Waynesville, NC 28786). Although a protective hat may reduce the neurologic consequences of a fall by decreasing the effects of direct impact, no equestrian helmet is capable of preventing diffuse axonal injury resulting from impulsive forces associated with a fall.

Safety features of other parts of riding tack and gear have been developed over the years. Safety release catches on the stirrup of the English saddle are designed to prevent a dislodged rider from being dragged by allowing the weight of the fallen rider to open a lever that releases the stirrup leathers from the saddle. This may be ineffective in riders (particularly children) whose weight is insufficient to open the release mechanism. For such riders, the catch should always be maintained in an open position. Safety stirrups are being developed, but, to date, none have been tested for effectiveness.

The use of protective vests has gained great popularity (Fig. 5) The effectiveness of these garments is primarily anecdotal; no investigations have established their ability to limit neu-

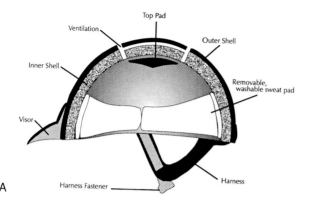

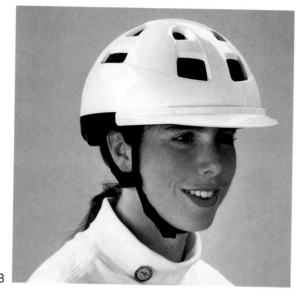

FIG. 4. A: Diagram of parts of an equestrian helmet. **B**: Schooling/trail ASTM (American Society for Testing and Materials) standard protective equestrian helmet. (International Riding Helmets "Prolite").

rologic injury. Although riders may receive fewer bruises and/or abrasions should they sustain a fall while wearing a padded garment, these vests are ineffective in limiting the motions of the spine involved in fracture and risk of neurologic injury. Moreover, they are insufficient to limit significantly crush injuries occurring when a fallen rider is rolled on by the horse (Fig. 1). Research into newer materials that may lessen the impact and thereby reduce injury is ongoing and, with the development of stricter standards, offers the hope that these injuries may be greatly reduced in the future.

Stretch injury to the lumbar plexus has been eliminated by the use of the heeled boot, which generally prevents a fallen rider from having his or her foot and leg caught in the stirrup of a fallen or runaway horse. The stirrup should be 2 to 3 cm wider than the boot, because if the stirrup is too small, the boot will become stuck and prevent the rider from voluntarily dismounting in the event of an emergency. Alternatively, if the stirrup is overly large, the foot may slip forward in a fall with the possibility of becoming fixed, which further increases the risk of injury. Because many accidents result from failure in the specialized equipment necessary for horseback riding, it is important for the rider to maintain and check all equipment (girth, saddle, and bridle) before each mounting. A break in the tack during a fast-moving event is sure to result in a fallen rider and the risk of neurologic injury.

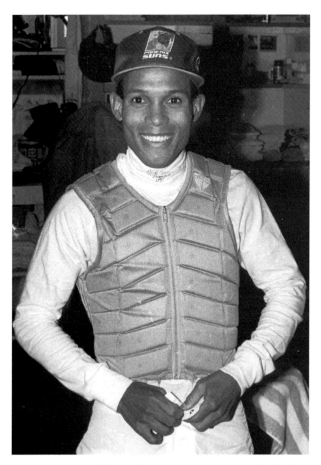

FIG. 5. The rider is wearing a vest. The value of protective vests in limiting injury to the chest, abdomen, and spine remains anecdotal.

In addition to the detailed attention to the rider and gear before horseback riding, there are considerations related to the rider's knowledge and the horse itself that must be dealt with to ensure a rider's safe participation. As equestrian sports gain popularity, the demand for schooled athletic horses has increased. Moreover, the coupling of an inexperienced rider with an overly aggressive, bold horse has become more frequent. This is to be condemned, as it greatly enhances the risk for serious injuries.

At present there are few, if any, guidelines that regulate competitive participation on the basis of the capabilities of a particular horse–rider combination. Appropriate direction can be found through equestrian organizations such as the United States Pony Clubs and the 4-H extension programs, which provide education in all aspects of horsemanship. The importance of proper instruction by a qualified teacher with certification from a recognized organization, such as the American Riding Instructor Certification Program, the Horsemanship Safety Association, the Association for Horsemanship Safety and Education, and the North American Riding for the Handicapped Association, cannot be overemphasized. It is recommended that all beginning riders be initiated into riding through instructors certified by one of these organizations.

It is equally important that the horse be properly trained, ridden regularly, and conditioned for the particular phase of riding required. Moreover, the rider must be aware of the fact that the horse may become fatigued. Although the horse may be willing to perform as required, it may tire and be incapable of peak performance. One major cause of fallen horses and riders is failure to clear a jump, in which the fatigued horse does not lift its knees sufficiently high, strikes the front of a fence or wall, and upsets both itself and the rider.

Any activity with horses involves risk of neurologic injury. Leadership by the equestrian regulatory associations and the medical community through education of those involved in equestrian sports as well as those who simply enjoy the pleasure of horseback riding can prevent the major portion of catastrophic neurologic injuries attributable to equestrian events. This can be accomplished only by careful consideration of the risk involved, insistence on secured fitted approved protective headgear and other proper safety equipment, thorough instruction by those appropriately qualified, and consideration of the horse as a fellow athlete.

REFERENCES

1. Bixby Hammett DM. United States Pony Clubs 10 year accident study: *USPC News* 1992;51.

2. Brooks WH, Bixby Hammett DM. Prevention of neurologic injuries in equestrian sports. *Phys Sports Med* 1988:16;84–95.

3. Grossman JA, Kinland DM, Miller CW, Winn HR, Hodge RH Jr. Equestrian injuries; results of a prospective study. *JAMA* 1978:240;1881–1882.

4. American Horse Council 1994 Horse Industry Directory; 5.

5. Gleave JRW. *The impact of sports on a neurological unit.* Cambridge, England: Institute of Sports Medicine, 1975.

6. Mahaley MS, Seaber AV. Accident and safety consideration of horseback riding. In: Proceedings of the Eighteenth AMA Conference on the Medical Aspects of Sports, Dallas, June 1976.

7. *MMWR* 1990:39;329–332

8. National Center for Health Statistics. *Vital statistics of the United States.* Washington, DC: Government Printing Office, 1993.

9. National Electronic Injury Surveillance System reports. National Consumer Product Safety Commission, Washington, DC.

10. Nelson DE, Rivara FD, Condie C, Smith SM. Injuries in equestrian sports. *Phys Sports Med* 22:5360.

11. Ponder DJ. The grave yawns for the horseman. *Med J Aust* 1984:632–615

12. Williams LP, Remmerg EF, Huff SI, et al. The blue fly syndrome: horse associated accidents. Presented at the one hundred third annual American Public Health Association meeting, Chicago, Nov 17, 1975.

13. Wolfenden K, Lower T, Clarke L. *Horse related injury.* Taree, NSW: Australia Coastal Public Health Unit.

14. Hamilton MC, Tranmer BI. Nervous system injuries in horsebackriding accidents. *J Trauma* 34:2;227–232.

Sports Neurology, Second Edition,
edited by Barry D. Jordan.
Lippincott–Raven Publishers, Philadelphia © 1998.

32

Football

Steven B. Cohen, *Russell F. Warren, and †Ronnie P. Barnes

Robert Wood Johnson Medical School — University of Medicine and Dentistry of New Jersey,
*675 Hoes Lane, Piscataway, New Jersey 08903; *The Hospital for Special Surgery, 535 East 70th Street,*
New York, New York 10021; †Department of Sports Medicine, New York Football Giants,
East Rutherford, New Jersey 07073

For physicians working with athletes at all levels of play, from youth leagues to professionals, injury of the nervous system has been an area of great concern. Physicians evaluating players for neurologic injury will obviously rely on their specific type of training to treat these problems. Although many injuries require only the player's removal from a game and subsequent appropriate referral, injury to the nervous system may require prompt recognition and treatment, often by an individual not specifically trained in these problems. This chapter outlines various neurologic problems that may be encountered in football. The relative incidences of injury, the mechanisms of injury, aspects of recognition, emergency management, and the athlete's return to play are discussed.

CONCUSSION

Incidence

There appears to be some variation in the incidence rates of concussion among studies. In Clarke's study (1), National Athletic Injury Reporting Service (NAIRS) data demonstrated that college football had 6.1 concussions per 100 athletes during each full season (the NAIRS definition of concussion included any injury resulting in disorientation requiring cessation of play and evaluation). Clarke (1) also noted that significant concussion requiring the athlete to stop playing for 1 week represented about 10% of the patients. In a study of 3063 high school football players in Minnesota, Gerberich et al. (2) noted a loss of consciousness or awareness in 19 per 100 players.

Powell (unpublished data, 1995), in a report to the National Football League (NFL) owners, analyzed the patterns and frequency of concussions in the NFL from 1985 to 1994. A concussion was defined as a game-related head injury that caused a player to be restricted from play during that specific game. The absolute number of game-related concussions during the ten season span is shown in Fig. 1. It should be noted that 1987 was a strike season and may represent a statistical oddity. Over the ten-season period the average number of game-related concussions per season was 92.1. Even though the absolute number of concussions has fluctuated, the proportion of concussions among all reported game-related injuries has remained fairly constant at about 8.5%. During a five-season span (1989 to 1993) there were 0.3 concussions per game and 2.47 concussions per 1000 game plays. Although the data for the 1994 season showed slightly increased values (0.38 concussions per game and 3.10 concussions per 1000 game plays), it was concluded that the rate of sustaining a concussion in the 1994 season was not statistically different from that in any other season previously analyzed. During the period 1989 to 1993, 445 concussions were reported. Among these one game was lost in 4.7% of the players sustaining a concussion, whereas 94% of the reported concussions resulted in no lost games.

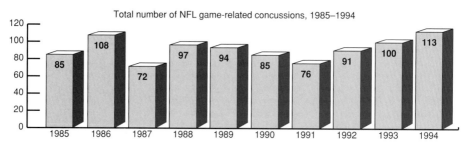

FIG. 1. Total number of NFL game-related concussions, 1985–1994. * 1987 represents data from a strike season

Concussion rates were also determined by the type of play. In comparing kickoffs and punts, over the ten-season period there was a greater likelihood of a sustaining a concussion during a kickoff than on a punt play. For each type of play, kickoff, punt, rushing, and passing, a concussion rate was determined per 1000 game plays. During the ten seasons studied from 1985 to 1994, concussions per 1000 kickoffs were consistently highest, ranging from 2.9 to 9.4 concussions per 1000 kickoffs. Passing (1.5 to 2.2), rushing (1.1 to 2.2), and punt (1.3 to 3.1) plays each maintained fairly consistent concussion rates per 1000 game plays. For the five seasons between 1989 and 1993, as expected, there was a higher frequency of concussions associated with tackling and being tackled than with blocking, being blocked, or other collisions.

Concussion analysis was done by position to determine the percentage over the ten-season period from 1985 to 1994 (Table 1). On offense, quarterbacks averaged 10.1% of the overall concussions (range: 8.2% to 11.7%), running backs averaged 8.5% (range: 3.2% to 10.6%), wide receivers averaged 13% (range: 4.7% to 19.7%), offensive linemen averaged 9.5% (range: 2.6% to 17.6%), and tight ends averaged 5.9% (range: 3.7% to 8.2%) over the ten seasons. On defense, defensive backs averaged 16.7% of the overall concussions (range: 11.8% to 25.0%). linebackers averaged 8.4% (range: 1.4% to 12.9%), and defensive linemen averaged 9.2% (range: 5.3% to 14.1%) over the ten-season period. The remaining 18.3% of the overall concussions (range: 9.7% to 23.1%) during the ten seasons occurred to special teams players. Based on the percentage of concussions by position, defensive backs, wide receivers, and special teams players are most associated with concussions, possibly indicating an increasing frequency because of the open-field nature of collisions at these positions. Powell's

TABLE 1. *Percentage of concussions in the National Football League by position*

Position	Year										Average
	1985	1986	1987	1988	1989	1990	1991	1992	1993	1994	
Offense											
Quarterback	8.2	11.1	9.7	11.3	11.7	11.8	7.9	9.9	10	9.7	10.1
Running back	10.6	9.3	8.3	10.3	3.2	3.5	9.2	9.9	10	10.6	8.5
Wide receiver	4.7	9.3	11.1	10.3	13.8	18.8	19.7	13.1	14	15	13
Offensive line	14.1	17.6	11.1	10.3	4.3	7.1	2.6	8.8	9	9.7	9.5
Tight end	8.2	3.7	4.2	4.1	7.4	4.7	6.6	5.5	9	5.3	5.9
Defense											
Defensive back	11.8	13.9	25	11.3	18.1	12.9	19.7	15.4	17	22.1	16.7
Linebacker	12.9	9.3	1.4	11.3	11.7	12.9	7.9	3.3	7	6.2	8.4
Defensive line	5.9	5.6	12.5	11.3	8.5	14.1	5.3	11	7	10.6	9.2
Special teams	22.4	20.4	16.7	18.6	21.3	14.1	19.7	23.1	17	9.7	18.3

analysis of concussion rates and frequencies demonstrated that the type of play, the type of activity, and the position group are critical in determining the injury scenario.

Alves et al. (3), in a report to the Ivy League team physicians regarding concussions in the league for 1983 to 1984, noted 154 concussions with approximately 50% occurring in games and 50% during practice. Overall, there was a random distribution for each quarter of a game. Offensive linemen and special teams players had a slightly increased incidence. Overall, approximately 95% fell into grade I ("ding"), with only 5.2% experiencing a loss of consciousness. Consciousness returned within 5 minutes in these players. Interestingly, although tackling accounted for 24% of the injuries, blocking resulted in 40%. Of the injured players, 61.8% missed the remainder of the game or practice, 70% resumed play within 5 days, and 82.4% returned by 10 days.

Zemper (4) noted that from 1988 to 1990, players with a history of cerebral concussion during the previous 5 years were six times as likely to incur an additional concussion than a player without a previous concussion. This is 1.5 times greater than the estimate of Gerberich et al. (2), who noted that a player having one episode of unconsciousness is at four times greater risk for a repeated episode than a player without a previous episode. In the NFL, 445 game-related concussions were reported by 341 players from 1989 to 1993, with 2 players incurring 5 or more concussions during the five seasons. These data demonstrate the repetitive incidence. Undoubtedly, there is considerable underreporting of incidents when a player experiences a transient "ding" but continues to participate. Alves et al. (3), in a prospective study, evaluated 2500 players who sustained a "minor head injury" and noted that 200 were reinjured.

Classification

We have found that for the purposes of dealing with athletic injuries, those encountered in football in particular, it is more useful to use four grades evaluating altered consciousness, confusion, and amnesia (Table 2).

TABLE 2. *Grading of concussions in athletics*

Grade	Symptoms
I	Altered consciousness; confused but no loss of consciousness; "ding" (stunned); no amnesia
II	Amnesia; no loss of consciousness
III	Loss of consciousness for less than 3 minutes
IV	Loss of consciousness for more than 3 minutes

The vast majority of episodes (95%) that occur in football are grade I, or a ding in players' vernacular. The player is often confused; the period of time varies, but the confusion may clear so rapidly that the physician is not called on to evaluate the player. Alternatively, teammates may state that the player's behavior is different several plays after the injury. In grade II there is amnesia without loss of consciousness. It is not uncommon for players in this state to make an outstanding play but to have no recollection of the event. The amnesia is generally anterograde, but a more serious type (retrograde) may on occasion be noted, implying a greater severity of the injury. Often, despite the player's full recovery, there is no recall for the specific injury producing event. In grade III there is a transient loss of consciousness by the time the physician arrives on the field to evaluate the player, so it may be difficult to ascertain whether there was in fact a period of unconsciousness. The player may be confused, anxious, and agitated, again making evaluation difficult. In grade IV the injured player experiences more than 3 minutes of unconsciousness. It is uncommon to see players truly unconscious for more than 3 minutes. In such a case, however, severe injury should be suspected and the player hospitalized immediately.

Evaluation and Management

In evaluating the player for concussive injury the physician needs to confirm immediately that the player is breathing and has a patent airway. If the player is awake, he should be asked to move his hands and feet. His neck should be checked for pain or localized tenderness, and he should be questioned regarding paresthesias in the feet or hands, which could indicate a cervical fracture or dislocation or transient quadriparesis. The helmet is left in place if there is concern about a possible neck injury. If the neck has not been injured, the helmet should be removed to aid medical evaluation. The player should be evaluated for orientation to time, location, and person. A brief neurologic examination, including evaluation for vision, speech, memory, strength coordination, and sensation, should follow. At this point the player may be assisted from the field.

If the player is unconscious, then extreme care should be taken to avoid neck movement. After checking the player for breathing and vital signs, a spineboard should be obtained. While one physician stabilizes the head with the helmet still on, the player may be rotated with the help of three to four assistants. Once the player is supine, the examination is repeated. The player should then be removed from the field with the aid of a spineboard and stretcher for a complete neurologic evaluation.

The following outline for evaluating players for return to play is based on more than 25 years of experience with high school, college, and professional teams. If the player has only been dinged (grade I) and does not experience loss of consciousness or amnesia, he may be considered for return to the game after 10 to 15 minutes. If he still feels disoriented or has any headache, vision change, or nausea, he should be kept out of the game. The player's memory should be assessed using recall testing for a series of objects or numbers, and his recollection of his responsibilities on specific plays should be tested. The mental status evaluation should also determine whether there are orientation, attention, or concentration deficits. If he passes these tests, he should be asked to run on the sidelines to determine that he has good balance and is free of any headache. Often, running produces a headache, precluding return to participation. Subsequent decisions regarding return to practice should be based on his progress and lack of a postconcussion syndrome. Magnetic resonance imaging (MRI) scans are not needed unless there was a distinct loss of consciousness (grades III and IV) or persistent neurologic symptoms.

In grade II concussions with amnesia for the event, time, or place, the player is removed from the game, observed, and evaluated neurologically. The level of amnesia may be anterograde or retrograde. The retrograde type represents a more severe degree of injury than the anterograde type. Often, when the player's confusion abates and memory returns, there is permanent loss of memory for the event. Generally, with amnesia the player sits out the remainder of the game. If his mental status returns to normal, with careful evaluation and no attention deficit or headaches, he may resume play later that week.

If the player has a second episode, a complete evaluation should be performed including MRI. The player is kept out of contact sports for 2 to 3 weeks and returns only if he is symptom-free while running. A third episode of a grade II injury generally precludes play for the remainder of that season.

In grade III, concussion with loss of consciousness, the player is removed from the game and subsequently admitted to the hospital for observation. Computed tomographic (CT) and MRI scans are obtained, as well as neurologic consultation. Roentgenograms of the cervical spine should be obtained if there is any indication of neck injury. The player may return to play within 2 weeks if the loss of consciousness was brief and if there is a complete return of mental function. Postconcussion syndrome or headache with exertion may develop. If a second, distinct episode of loss of consciousness occurs, consideration should be given to stopping play for the season or for 1 month.

In grade IV concussion with a true loss of consciousness for more than 3 minutes the player is kept out of play, often for the entire season, but at least 1 month. At the end of this time, if he is free of all symptoms and has a normal MRI scan, he may return, but a second episode precludes play.

A postconcussion syndrome is not uncommon after minor head injuries. Rimel et al. (5), in a study of "minor" head injuries among nonathletes, noted that at 3 months after injury 79% of the patients complained of headaches and 59% had problems with memory. Hugenholtz et al. (6) confirmed these results by using reaction time tests to show that even mild concussions (grades

I and II) can cause persistent posttraumatic symptoms of attentional and information processing impairment for more than a month after the injury. Headache, dizziness, and difficulty with memory often disappear over the next 2 weeks, but if they persist the player should not return to play until the complaints completely clear. If premature return is allowed, a serious second injury may occur; this is termed the second impact syndrome (see Chapter 17). Kelly et al. (7) concluded that individuals who are symptomatic from a concussion are at significantly increased risk for developing diffuse brain swelling after a second impact to the head. In essence, malignant cerebral edema occurs that is often refractory to treatment, resulting in a high mortality rate (8).

Kelly (9) has also proposed that repeated concussions spaced distant in time can cause cumulative neurologic damage. This can be documented by neurologic decline in mental performance, atrophy on repeated neuroimaging studies, and the development of dementia. This is more often seen as a result of head trauma in boxing but may occur in football if repeated concussions continue.

Prevention

In theory, prevention of concussion is accomplished in two ways. The first is to create rules that decrease the use of the head in football. Although such rules to eliminate spearing techniques were initiated in 1976, there was no significant reduction in the concussion rate for 1975 to 1978 (1). The second method is to improve helmet design. Helmets work to deflect impact energy and to improve the distribution of the load, and some helmets were suspected of raising concussion rates. The NAIRS data for 1975 to 1977 show that no particular helmet significantly increased the incidence of concussion. However, Zemper (4) in a 5-year prospective study of a national sample of college football teams studied the concussion frequency in the ten most commonly used models of football helmets for 1986 to 1990. The results indicated that when normalized to athletic exposures there was a significantly lower than expected frequency of concussions with the

Riddell M155 model helmet and a significantly greater than expected number of concussions with the Bike Air Power model. The remaining eight models all performed within expectation for concussion frequency.

During the 1995 owners' meeting, the National Football League's competition committee expanded the rules to protect "virtually helpless players," for example, quarterbacks who have released the ball and wide receivers who go into the air for a pass. The new guidelines prohibit players from using the face mask or "hairline" portion of the helmet to strike a defenseless player. This is a revision of the previous rule, which prohibited players from using the "crown" of the helmet as a weapon.

In attempting to decrease the incidence of concussion injuries or their recurrence, the player's helmet should be evaluated for proper fit; when the player holds his face mask the helmet should not slip on flexion, extension, or rotation of the head. At times an air-filled helmet may be substituted for a regular helmet. If an air-filled helmet is already being used, its pressure should be checked frequently. Recently, an external helmet device has been introduced (a lightweight polyurethane "ProCap" shell), but preliminary studies have been inconclusive regarding its role in the reduction of concussions, and whether it may result in increased neck injuries if the forces are not deflected. Finally, it may also be helpful to discuss with the coach the avoidance of spearing techniques in blocking and tackling.

CERVICAL SPINE INJURIES

Incidence

Injuries to the cervical spine with fracture or dislocation resulting in permanent quadriplegia are the most devastating injuries associated with football. There has been a reversal of the increasing incidence of these injuries that was noted in the 1970s. Torg and associates (10) created the National Football Head and Neck Injury Registry in 1975 to study football-related cervical spine injuries. Initially they collected data retrospectively from 1971 to 1975 and compared these with Schneider's data (11) from 1959 to 1963. Scheider reported the incidence of cervical spine fractures or dislocations in this population as 1.4 cases per 100,000 players, with 0.7 cases per 100,000 players resulting in quadriplegia. In contrast, Torg and colleagues (10,12) noted an increase in the number of cervical fractures and dislocations to 4.1 cases per 100,000, resulting in 1.58 cases per 100,000 of cervical quadriplegia. Overall, Torg noted a decrease in the number of deaths secondary to intracranial hemorrhage and an increase in the number for cervical quadriplegia. These changes were attributed to the improvements in the helmet and face mask instituted during the 1960s. The improvements appeared to result in increased use of the head to originate contact in tackling and blocking (i.e., spearing). It was also noted that defensive backs in particular were injured (college, 73%; high school, 52%).

With these findings the National Collegiate Athletic Association and the National Federation of State High School Athletic Associations created rule changes that preclude a player from intentionally striking another player with the top of his helmet and from deliberately ramming or butting an opponent. These changes have resulted in a significant decrease in the incidence of cervical spine fractures and dislocation as well as cervical quadriplegia in both high school and college football. There has been a drop in the number of cervical fractures and dislocations (13). Cantu and Mueller (14) have reported that since 1977, there has been an annual incidence of less than ten cases per year of permanent injury to the cervical cord from football.

Mechanism of Injury

Burstein et al. (13) have noted that the mechanism of injury is one of axial loading of the cervical spine and not hyperflexion or hyperextension. Some investigators have cited the face mask as being responsible for hyperextension resulting in the back of the helmet striking the neck, but film analysis of cervical injuries has demonstrated that this is not the case. When the spine is straight an axial load passes through the spine as in a segmented column. In tackling the neck is positioned between the head, which has decelerated rapidly, and the advancing trunk. When the load is excessive the spine fails in a flexion mode, resulting in fractures or facet dislocation (unilateral or bilateral). Much of the confusion regarding the mechanism of cervical spine injury appears to have resulted from the fact that the cervical spine is normally in mild lordosis (i.e., extension). Thus, when the neck flexes to about 30°, the cervical spine becomes straight. A load applied to the top of the helmet passes down the straightened cervical spine, creating an axial load.

Torg and colleagues have investigated the effect of axial loading on the cervical spine. They found that 51 of 55 cases of an anteroinferior cervical vertebral body fracture or "teardrop" (or "burst") fracture were the result of axial compression on the cervical spine (15). This fracture most often occurred (73%) when players attempting to make a tackle initiated contact with the crown of the helmet. The majority of teardrop fractures (74%) occurred at the level of the fifth cervical vertebra. Of the two types described by Torg, the less severe is the isolated fracture, compared with the three-part, two-plane fracture (anteroinferior corner fracture fragment, sagittal vertebral body fracture, fracture of posterior neural arch), which is associated with permanent neurologic sequelae, specifically quadriplegia (87%). Roentgenographic determination of the teardrop fracture is done with anteroposterior and lateral views as well as CT. In another study by Torg et al. (16) 25 patients were found to have traumatic C3-4 injuries from an axial load while playing football. Torg suggested that traumatic cervical spine lesions could be classified into upper (C1-2), middle (C3-4), and lower (C5-7) segments. The majority of injuries at the middle cervical level do not involve fracture but rather disc herniation, C3-4 subluxation, or facet dislocation. They concluded that middle-level energy inputs differ from those involving upper and lower cervical segments and that these lesions are very difficult to affect and maintain reduction. They recommend early aggressive treatment for these types of middle-segment injuries.

Evaluation and Management

In dealing with players with a head injury or any arm or leg weakness or paresthesia, there should be a high index of suspicion concerning an injury to the cervical spine. Management of such a player should be predicated on the assumption that there is a fractured cervical spine until the player is carefully examined. See the chapter on emergency management of cervical spine injuries for a detailed discussion of emergency management in this setting.

During the past decade physicians dealing with football players have become increasingly aware of a condition termed transient quadriparesis of the cervical spinal cord (see chapter on transient quadriparesis). This condition, which appears to occur most commonly in football, is the result of a blow to the head with sudden cervical flexion or extension. This is followed by a variable period of weakness or numbness in the arms, hands, or legs. Weakness may last for a few seconds up to 10 to 15 minutes, or it may clear with a residual numbness persisting for 1 to 2 days. Torg et al. (17) have speculated that the condition represents a transient neurapraxia of the cervical spinal cord.

Depending on the degree of clinical findings, two other diagnoses should be considered: acute disc herniation and anterior spinal cord injury (18). If there are significant findings of weakness that persist, an acute disc herniation may have occurred. However, the symptoms may also be transient in an acute disc herniation. In addition, cervical stenosis may be present and aggravate the symptoms. In anterior cord syndrome there is acute paralysis of all four extremities with loss of pain and temperature sensation up to the level of the lesion but preservation of position sense and vibratory and light touch (which are transmitted along the posterior column). In these patients myelograms and MRI scans are helpful in evaluating for an acute disc herniation and for the degree of stenosis.

In 1986 Ladd and Scranton (19) described two football players who had congenital cervical stenosis presenting as transient quedriparesis. One was injured in flexion, and one had a vertical and lateral blow. These players' myelograms demonstrated significant compression on the spinal cord that was not obvious from standard films, CT scans, or MRI evaluation. These investigators recommended that a metrizamide-enhanced myelogram should be followed by a CT scan to improve the diagnosis.

If a localized stenosis as opposed to a diffuse stenosis is noted, the patient should be counseled to give up contact sports unless the condition can be corrected. In addition, those with any degree of cervical instability should discontinue play. In contrast, patients with an episode of transient quadriparesis in whom a diffuse cervical spine stenosis has been identified may be allowed to return to play. Torg et al. (17) noted that of six players with diffuse injury three had a recurrence of transient quadriparesis but three continued to play without problems. Warren treated one player at the professional level who had two episodes of transient quadriparesis about 4 weeks apart and who, after 6 weeks rest, returned to play. This player experienced a mild recurrent episode 2 years later and continued to play for an additional 6 years. (R. F. Warren, *personal communication*, 1995).

The true incidence of cervical narrowing in football players, as defined by Pavlov's criteria, is unknown. In reviewing 60 professional football players with various cervical complaints but no known transient quadriparesis, Galinat and Warren (20) found that approximately 30% of the patients had ratios of less than 0.8, with some as low as 0.5.

Torg et al. (21) did an epidemiologic study to determine the significance and implications of developmental cervical spinal narrowing (stenosis) and reversible and irreversible cord injury. Four populations of football players (group 1, asymptomatic collegiate players; group 2, asymptomatic professional players; group 3, players with at least one episode of transient neurapraxia, group 4, players rendered quadriplegic as a result of a football injury) and a control group of nonathletes were studied. The study found that 41% of all asymptomatic college and professional players had a mean spinal canal/vertebral body ratio of 0.80 or less. Similarly in a study by Galinat and Warren (20) presented at the National Football League Team Physician Meeting in 1989 of 60 professional and 200 graduating asymptomatic football players, it was found that some ratios were below 0.8 and as low as 0.6 at one or more levels. A conclusion was made that this asymptomatic group may have a ratio of 0.80

or less without true canal narrowing because of their large vertebral bodies and that this ratio should not be used as a screening method for participation in contact activities (20,21). Analysis of group 3 in Torg's study showed that 93% of players who suffered at least one episode of transient neurapraxia had a mean ration of 0.80 or less but that none have gone on to permanent neurologic injury. Of the 177 quadriplegics interviewed in group 4, none had a previous transient episode before their major injury, suggesting that those experiencing a transient episode are not predisposed to permanent injury. Group 4 was also found to have a mean ratio of 0.95, which indicated that permanent neurologic loss occurred from the injury mechanism (axial loading of the cervical spine), resulting in failure from unstable fractures and/or dislocation rather than congenital cervical stenosis. In conclusion, Torg et al. (21) found no correlation between cervical stenosis and irreversible neurologic sequelae.

In football, with high loads being applied to the head and neck, players frequently note stiffness or discomfort about the neck. Often these are attributed to prior strains. Albright et al. (22), in a study of 75 college freshman football players, noted a 32% incidence of radiographic changes including compression fractures, narrowed disc spaces, neural arch fractures, and altered motion. Interestingly, players with a prior history of neck injury had only a 50% incidence of radiographic changes, and 19 of the 24 players with abnormal radiographs gave no history of significant neck pain. Thus, in evaluating players with cervical problems, preexisting conditions may or may not be related to new complaints. A case can therefore be made for obtaining lateral neck films of players when they enter a college or professional football program regardless of the presence of prior symptoms.

LUMBAR SPINE INJURIES

A variety of lumbar spine injuries may result from participation in football. Some of the more common injuries are transverse process fractures, spondylolysis–spondylolithesis, herniated nucleus pulposus, and lumbar spine contusions (43).

A transverse process fracture may result from direct trauma (such as by a helmet), rotation from

a violent muscle contraction, or both. Associated injuries that rarely accompany a transverse process fracture are visceral injuries and neurologic complications. In a study by Tewes et al. (23), there were 28 lumbar transverse process fractures in professional football players over a 9-year period, an average of more than 3 per year. All were unilateral, most commonly involving one vertebral level, either L-3 or L-4. The injury was caused by direct contact predominantly while tackling during a game (76%). Over half (55%) occurred in ball handlers. Diagnosis was made primarily from radiographs, although MRI or CT may be useful. Transverse process fracture complications were rare, with one player experiencing thigh numbness and one player receiving a kidney contusion. Recommended treatment for such an injury was rest. The average time to return to play was 24.5 days. Although return to play was slightly over 3 weeks in professional athletes, adequate healing of the fractured transverse process must be obtained before a player may be cleared to participate.

Spondylolysis, a defect in the pars interarticularis portion of a vertebra, and spondylolithesis, forward slippage of one vertebra on another due to a bilateral or unilateral defect in the pars interarticularis, are injuries that may also commonly occur in football. Although more common in gymnasts (24) spondylolysis and/or spondylolithesis may result from repeated rapid back extension against weight such as frequently occurs in offensive lineman or wide receivers hyperextending themselves while catching a pass. These type of injuries may also result from improper weight-lifting technique in the weight room in preparation for activity. Most athletes acquire the isthmic type of spondylolithesis (25) which is acquired and becomes symptomatic during adolescence. Spondylolithesis most commonly occurs with forward slippage of L-5 on S-1. Diagnosis may be made by radiography, and MRI, CT, or bone scan may also be helpful. If a player is diagnosed with spondylolysis, the physician needs to determine whether the defect is recent or recurrent, whether the fragment is unstable, whether it resulted from trauma, and whether it could develop into spondylolithesis (26). The most progressive forward vertebral displacement occurs between ages 9 and 14, and displacement usually terminates around age 20. Spondylolithe-sis is graded on the basis of the forward displacement of the top vertebra on the level below. A grade I spondylolithesis is slippage less than 25% displacement over the edge, grade II is between 25% and 50%, grade III is displacement between 50% and 75%, and grade IV is greater than 75% displacement over the edge. Grade I and II injuries are most often treated conservatively with activity restriction, nonsteroidal antiinflammatory drugs (NSAIDs), and/or bracing, unless there is a neurologic deficit or postural deformity. Grade III injuries or higher are usually treated surgically. A player with spondylolysis or spondylolithesis may return to play when symptoms subside.

A third common lumbar spine injury in football is a herniated nucleus pulposus resulting from a bulge or tear in the annulus fibrosus of a vertebral disc. This may occur in the skeletally immature athlete with vertebral abnormalities such a partial sacralization of L-5, facet tropism, and displacement of the ring apoplysis of a vertebra (26). In skeletally mature athletes, discogenic problems may result from degeneration of the annulus fibrosus allowing herniation of the nucleus pulposus as a result of repetitive trauma. Initial treatment is conservative with rest and NSAIDs. Patients who remain symptomatic for over 12 weeks may be treated surgically. A player may return to activity when asymptomatic and without any sign of neurologic deficit.

Sudden or repeated blows to the lumbar spine area may produce contusion or rib fracture. Players with trauma to the lumbar spine must be evaluated for visceral and/or neurologic complications as well as musculoskeletal complications.

BRACHIAL PLEXUS INJURIES

Incidence

Brachial plexus injuries (Table 3) are probably the most common injuries to neurologic tissues encountered in football. Robertson et al. (27) noted that approximately 50% of the players at the University of Wisconsin suffered a suspected injury of the plexus during their career. Clarke (1) noted that the incidence of plexus injury as reported by NAIRS did not change form 1975 to

TABLE 3. *Characteristics of brachial plexus injury*

Mechanism	Lateral neck flexion—initial injury (spearing subsequently aggravates the problem) Compression at Erb's point
Symptoms	Pain and paresthesia into arm
Findings	Weakness, particularly in the deltoid, biceps, and external rotators
Recovery	Frequently transient symptoms (1 to 5 minutes)
Return to play	Dependent on (1) neck range of motion, (2) full strength, (3) no pain, (4) no prior episodes in the game, (5) cervical neck roll.

1978, averaging approximately 2.2 cases per 100 players. The total incidence of these injuries did not change despite the rule change in 1976 that was instituted to decrease neck injuries by eliminating spear-tackling techniques. During this period, there was a 38% to 45% decrease in brachial plexus injuries while tackling. Meyer et al. (28) reported the incidence of brachial plexopathy of the stinger syndrome at the University of Iowa as approximately 15%. This incidence rate was increased by three times for players diagnosed with cervical spinal stenosis. In working with a professional team, we have noted an incidence of plexus injury during the season similar to that noted at the University of Wisconsin. In addition, we have found an association with a decreased Pavlov ratio and burners. The Pavlov ratio is measurement of the ratio of the vertebral canal diameter to the vertebral body size. However, it appears to be related to increased vertebral size rather than a decrease in the canal size. The Pavlov ratio has a high sensitivity index but low positive predictive value and should not be used as a screening tool for participation.

Mechanism of Injury

Brachial plexus injury was originally termed a nerve pinch syndrome. Chrisman et al. (29), in a study performed in 1965, described the initial injury as resulting from lateral flexion of the neck away from a blow. Subsequent flexion to either side or direct compression could cause a recurrence. Markey et al. (30) reported that a more common mechanism among intramural and varsity football players at West Point was compression of the fixed brachial plexus between the shoulder pad and superior medial scapula. This occurred when the most superficial aspect of Erb's point was compressed. Levitz et al. (31) found that the predominant mechanism (83%) of cervical nerve root neurapraxia in professional and collegiate football players was extension combined with ipsilateral compression. Most players initially complain of pain with paresthesias shooting down the arm toward the thumb, index finger, or ulnar side of the hand. In the acute injury, patients describe a burning pain down the affected extremity with decreased sensation. In patients with chronic brachial plexopathy, Markey et al. (30) described repeated acute stinger episodes increasing in frequency with no area of numbness. No muscle weakness is found distal to the elbow but there may often be a dropped shoulder with atrophy in the shoulder girdle. Generally, there is weakness in the arm lasting 1 to 2 minutes with initial prompt recovery. In some patients weakness may persist for 6 to 12 months, even after one episode. Speer and Bassett (32) described "the prolonged burner syndrome" with muscular weakness at 72 hours after injury, which correlated with positive electrodiagnostic testing at 4 weeks after injury. Generally, the prognosis for motor recovery is good, although permanent paralysis can occur.

Brachial plexus injury has been classified by Clancy (33) using Seddon's definition of nerve injury (Table 4). A grade I injury indicates a neurapraxia to the plexus in which a physiologic interruption of nerve function has occurred without anatomic damage. Generally there is a transient loss of motor and sensory function. The pain radiates down the arm and often into the hand with associated paresthesia. Motor function usually returns within minutes. In grade II injury there is anatomic injury to the brachial plexus; this is an axonotmesis. In this injury there is significant motor and sensory loss that may take 6 weeks to 4 months to recover. Electromyelographic (EMG) evaluation after 2 to 3 weeks demonstrates fibrillation potentials, particularly in the upper trunk of the brachial plexus. In addition, no alteration should be noted in the paraspinal mus-

TABLE 4. *Grading of brachial plexus injuries*

Grade	Symptoms
I	Neurapraxia; transient loss of motor and sensory sensation
II	Axonotmesis; significant motor and sensory loss; recovery time 6 weeks to 4 months
III	Neurotmesis; permanent damage to nerves; may be mixed lesion—axonotmesis and neurtomesis

culature; absence of such alteration places the lesion distal to the cervical foramen. Grade III lesions of the plexus are a neurotmesis in which there has been permanent damage to the nerves. These lesions may be mixed: a component may improve (axonotmesis) while residual damage persists in some nerves (neurotmesis). In general, permanent weakness is an uncommon end result of brachial plexus injuries in football.

Evaluation and Management

In evaluating players with brachial plexus injury, a careful examination for motor and sensory alteration is important, Weakness will most commonly be in the C5-6 distribution (deltoid, biceps, supraspinatus, and infraspinatus), with weak arm elevation and external rotation. The C5-6 nerve segments are generally more vulnerable to a traction injury and are most commonly involved. In C6-7 injury the strength of the triceps and intrinsics of the hand may be diminished. Paresthesia and weakness in the contralateral arm or legs raises the possibility of transient quadriparesis, anterior cord syndrome, or more severe cervical injury. In addition, it should be determined whether this is the player's first episode or one of many. Roentgenograms should be obtained if there is any significant neck pain, limited neck range of motion, or weakness or for an initial injury. Films should include anteroposterior, lateral, and oblique views as well as subsequent lateral views in flexion and extension if there is no fracture present.

If neck pain is a persistent component, the player should not resume play. If, however, there are no neck complaints, if cervical motion is full, and if the arm complaints have cleared with no residual weakness, the player may return to play wearing a neck roll or an orthosis. Upon return to play the player must be followed closely. Re-examination should be done after the game and again for the next several weeks, as weaknesses may become apparent several weeks following the injury (34). If the injury recurs, the player should be kept out of the game until a more complete workup can be obtained. Levitz et al. (31) concluded that players presenting with chronic burner syndrome may suffer from nerve root compression in the intervertebral foramina secondary to disc disease or cervical canal stenosis. If arm weakness persists, cervical films are obtained and EMGs performed 2 to 3 weeks after the injury. Kimura (35) and Hershman (34) suggest delaying EMG tests for approximately 3 weeks from initial injury to allow wallerian degeneration to occur or nondegenerative lesions to recover spontaneously. Robertson et al. (27) noted fibrillation potentials and positive sharp waves in at least one muscle in all their patients. Bergfield (36) performed a follow-up study of patients with this injury and noted that a high percentage of patients had persistent EMG changes several years later. Speer and Bassett (32) confirmed this in noting electrodiagnostic differences even though normal symmetric strength was found; thus, waiting for the EMG to return to normal before allowing a player to return to play is inappropriate. Instead, the decision should be based clinically on the absence of weakness, pain, and recurrence.

There are players, particularly those who initiate contact with their head (spearing), who once having had this injury develop a series of recurrences. This poses several problems to the player and physician. Undoubtedly, there is some risk of permanent nerve injury in these patients, but generally the weakness clears over several minutes only to recur with another episode. On occasion there is a slow period of recovery requiring 6 to 12 months.

In managing these players the coaches need to insist on proper blocking and tackling techniques. In addition, the trainers need to work on strengthening neck and shoulder musculature. The use of high shoulder pads and a soft cervical neck roll may decrease the recurrence rate. Markey et al.

(30) showed that a custom orthosis to protect brachial plexus compression may also decrease the recurrence rate. In the past some players have utilized straps from the helmet to the shoulder pads to decrease the degree of lateral flexion. In general, it is probably best to avoid these straps and in particular to avoid straps that restrict the neck from flexing or extending. If the player finds that, despite technique alterations, a collar, and exercises, he is still having repeated transient episodes, then a season away from contact sports may allow him to return at a later date.

PERIPHERAL NERVE INJURIES

Peripheral nerve injuries in football (Table 5) are relatively uncommon as isolated events. Injury to the axillary nerve associated with an anterior dislocation may occur as a direct result of the dislocation or secondary to excessive traction during a reduction maneuver. In general, if a dislocation occurs during a game and if it is the initial event, a brief attempt at reduction may be made by an experienced physician. If this is performed immediately, before excessive muscle spasm has occurred, a reduction may be successful.

On evaluation there may be motor injury without sensory loss, so that both functions need to be assessed. If the dislocation is an initial event, the shoulder should be protected for a period of 5 to 6 weeks. The nerve injury should be followed up by EMG examination at 2 to 3 weeks. In general, the prognosis for recovery is good. If the dislo-

TABLE 5. *Peripheral nerve injuries*

Nerve	Mechanism
Axillary	Anterior shoulder dislocation, direct blow
Peroneal	Knee dislocation, direct ice application, severe ankle sprain
Ulnar	Direct ice application, subluxation from movement or direct contact
Long thoracic	Direct blow
Suprascapular	Direct blow
Spinal accessory	Direct blow
Musculocutaneous	Brachial plexus injury or acute shoulder dislocation

cation has been one of many, then subsequent stabilization of the shoulder after recovery of the nerve injury should be considered, particularly if the athlete desires to return to play.

Although most often associated with anterior dislocation, isolated axillary nerve palsy may be secondary to a direct blow on the lateral aspect of the shoulder. Kessler and Uribe (37) reported on six professional and college football players (all interior linemen) with complete axillary nerve palsy resulting from a direct blow on the shoulder from a helmet. The average time to return to competitive sports was 9 months with maximal recovery greater than 1 year. We have seen one professional linebacker on preseason physical examination with a complete absence of deltoid function. The actual injury had occurred several years before, and he had been able to compensate with his rotator cuff. Although most players are able to return to the same functional level, time of return may be extended as a result of prolonged inactivity of the deltoid.

Nerve injuries may also be seen in association with knee injuries in which there is extensive damage to the lateral side of the knee resulting in gross instability and stretching of the peroneal nerve. In patients with knee dislocation there is a 14% to 40% incidence of neurovascular injury (38,39). These are traction-type lesions with a relatively poor prognosis for recovery (<50%) despite exploration and subsequent repair or nerve grafting. In evaluating patients with a knee dislocation or lateral instability, the neurovascular status is assessed initially with subsequent prompt reduction of the dislocation. If there is marked opening laterally, the examiner should be careful to avoid opening the lateral side excessively or repeatedly stressing the knee because injury to the nerve could be aggravated. Peroneal nerve injury can also occur when ice is placed directly on the knee after any type of knee injury. The injury that this causes to the nerve is generally transient and clears over 1 to 2 days, but recovery can be prolonged. Obviously, this injury can be avoided by not placing ice directly on the nerve but instead placing a pad between the knee and the ice.

Peroneal nerve injury may occur after an ankle sprain in which there has been sudden, violent, internal rotation applied to the lower leg com-

bined with inversion of the ankle, thus stressing the knee. In this setting, injury to the peroneal nerve may result in an epineural hematoma. The patient may complain of progressive weakness associated with pain and paresthesia. If suspected and explored early, release of the epineural hematoma may prevent scarring and permanent loss of nerve function.

Injury to the ulnar nerve may also result from the use of ice for elbow injuries. Again it is best avoided by proper placement of the ice with a wrap over the elbow. If motor loss occurs, recovery may be immediate or prolonged for up to 6 weeks, as we have seen in one quarterback. Subluxation of the ulnar nerve, reported by Childress (40) as occurring to 16.2% of the population, may present as paresthesia and pain as a result of repeated movement of the nerve or direct contact. If it is persistent, anterior transposition of the nerve may be required.

Peripheral nerve injury may also occur secondary to direct blows to the long thoracic nerve (serratus anterior), suprascapular nerve (supraspinatus and infraspinatus), and spinal accessory nerves (trapezius). Entrapment of the suprascapular nerve may be seen as ganglia over the suprascapular or spinoglenoid notch. Careful muscle evaluation about the shoulder detects these injuries, and followup EMG evaluation should be done at 2 to 3 weeks. These are generally of a neurapraxia type, with weakness improving over 2 to 6 weeks. Isolated injury to the musculocutaneous nerve (biceps) is rare, but it may be associated with a brachial plexus injury or an acute shoulder dislocation. This lesion usually resolves spontaneously with termination of strenuous exercise, and the prognosis is favorable.

CONCLUSION

The physician responsible for covering football games needs to keep a wide range of neurologic conditions in mind. This chapter mentions only the most common problems. Intracranial bleeds, including subdural and epidural hematoma as well as contusions, may occur. Chapter 17 on head injuries provides a discussion of these types of injuries.

REFERENCES

1. Clarke KS. Prevention: an epidemiologic view. In: Torg JS, ed. *Athletic injuries to the head, neck, and face.* Philadelphia: Lea & Febiger, 1982:15–26.

2. Gerberich, SG, Priest SD, Boen JR, et al. Concussion incidence and severity in secondary school varsity football players. *Am J Public Health* 1983;73:1370–1375.

3. Alves WM, Rimel RW, Nelson WE. University of Virginia prospective study of football-induced minor head injury: status report. *Clin Sports Med* 1987;6:211–218.

4. Zemper ED. Analysis of cerebral concussion frequency with the most commonly sued models of football helmets. *J Athletic Training* 1994;20:44–50.

5. Rimel RW, Giordani B, Barth JT, et al. Disability caused by minor head injury. *Neurosurgery* 1981;9:221–228.

6. Hugenholtz H, Stuss DT, Stethem LL, et al. How long does it take to recover from a mild concussion? *Neurosurgery* 1988;22:853–858.

7. Kelly JP, Nichols JS, Filley CM, et al. Concussion in sports: guidelines for the prevention of catastrophic outcome. *JAMA* 1991;266:2867–2869.

8. Cantu RC. Guidelines for return to contact sports after a cerebral concussion. *Phys Sports Med* 1986;14:75–83.

9. Kelly JP. Concussion. In: Torg JS, Shephard RJ, eds. *Current therapy in sports medicine,* 3rd ed. St. Louis: Mosby, 1995:21–24.

10. Torg JS, Quendenfeld TC, Burstein A, et al. National Football Head and Neck Injury Registry: report on cervical quadriplegia. 1971–1975. *Am J Sports Med* 1979; 2:127–132.

11. Schneider RC. Serious and fatal neurosurgical football injuries. *Clin Neurosurg* 1966;12:226–236.

12. Torg JS, Vesgo JJ, Sennett B, et al. The National Football Head and Neck Injury Registry: 14-year report on cervical quadriplegia, 1971 through 1984. *JAMA* 1985;254:3439–3443.

13. Burstein AA, Otis JC, Torg JS. Mechanisms and pathomechanics of athletic injuries to the cervical spine. In: Torg JS, ed. *Athletic injuries to the head, neck, and face.* Philadelphia: Lea & Febiger, 1982:139–142.

14. Cantu RC, Mueller FO. Catastrophic spine injuries in football. *J Spinal Disord* 1990;3:227–231.

15. Torg JS, Pavlov H, O'Neill MJ, et al. The axial teardrop fracture: a biomechanical, clinical, and roentgenographic analysis. *Am J Sports Med* 1991;19:355–364.

16. Torg JS, Sennett B, Vegso JJ, et al. Axial loading injuries to the middle cervical spine segment: an analysis and classification of twenty-five cases. *Am J Sports Med* 1991;19:6–20.

17. Torg JS, Pavlov H, Genuario SE, et al. Neurapraxia of the cervical spinal cord with transient quadriplegia. *J Bone Joint Surg Am* 1986;68A:1354–1370.

18. Schneider RC. A syndrome in acute cervical injuries for which early operation is indicated. *J Neurosurg* 1951; 8:360.

19. Ladd AL, Scranton PE. Congenital cervical stenosis presenting as transient quadriplegia in athletes. *J Bone Joint Surg Am* 1986;68A:1371–1374.

20. Galinat BJ, Warren, RF. Presented at the National Football League Team Physician Meeting, Indianapolis, IN, Feb 1989.

21. Torg JS, Naranja RJ Jr, Pavlov H, et al. The relationship of developmental narrowing of the cervical spinal canal to reversible and irreversible injury of the cervical spinal cord in football players: an epidemiologic study. *J Bone Joint Surg Am* 1996;78A:1308–1314.

22. Albright JP, Moses JM, Feldick HG, et al. Nonfatal cervical spine injuries in interscholastic football. *JAMA* 1976;236:1243–1245.

23. Tewes DP, Fischer DA, Quick DC, et al. Lumbar transverse process fractures in professional football players. *Am J Sports Med* 1995;23:507–509.

24. Jackson DW, Wiltse LL, Cirincione RJ. Spondylolysis in female gymnasts. *Clin Orthop* 1976;117:68–73.

25. Nuber GW, Bowen MK, Schafer MF. Diagnosis and treatment of lumbar and thoracic spine injuries. In: Nicholas JA and Hershman EB, eds. *Lower extremity and spine,* 2nd ed. St. Louis: Mosby, 1995:1153–1170.

26. Kraus DR, Shapiro D. The symptomatic lumbar spine in the athlete. *Clin Sports Med* 1989;8(1):59–69.

27. Robertson WC Jr, Eichman PL, Clancy WC. Upper trunk brachial plexopathy in football players. *JAMA* 1979;241: 1480–1482.

28. Meyer SA, Schulte KR, Callaghan JJ, et al. Cervical spinal stenosis and stingers in collegiate football players. *Am J Sports Med* 1994;22:158–166.

29. Chrisman OD, Snook GA, Stanitis JM, et al. Lateral-flexion neck injuries in athletics. *JAMA* 1965;192: 117–119.

30. Markey KL, Di Benedetto M, Curl WW. Upper trunk brachial plexopathy: the stinger syndrome. *Am J Sports Med.* 1993;21:650–655.

31. Levitz CL, Reily PJ, Torg JS. The pathomechanics of chronic recurrent cervical root neurapraxia ("burner syndrome"): a revised concept. Presented at AAOS, Orlando, FL, Feb 16–21, 1995.

32. Speer KP, Bassett FH. The prolonged burner syndrome. *Am J Sports Med* 1990;18:591–594.

33. Clancy WG Jr. Brachial plexus and upper extremity peripheral nerve injuries. In: Torg JS, ed. *Athletic injuries to the head, neck, and face.* Philadelphia: Lea & Febiger, 1982:215–220.

34. Hershman EB: Brachial plexus injuries. *Clin Sports Med* 1990;9(2):311–329.

35. Kimura J. *Electrodiagnosis in diseases of nerve and muscle.* Philadelphia: FA Davis Co, 1989:452–454.

36. Bergfield J. Brachial plexus injuries. Presented at the American Assosociation of Orthopaedic Surgeons Winter Sports Injuries Course, Steamboat Springs, CO, Mar 27, 1987.

37. Kessler KJ, Uribe JW. Complete isolated axillary nerve palsy in college and professional football players: a report of six cases. *Clin J Sports Med* 1994;4:272–274.

38. Reckling FW, Peltier LF. Acute knee dislocations and their complications. *J Trauma* 1969;9:181–191.

39. Sisto DJ, Warren RF. Complete knee dislocation: a follow-up study of operative treatment. *Clin Orthop* 1991;263:200–205.

40. Childress HM. Recurrent ulnar-nerve dislocation at the elbow. *Clin Orthop* 1975;108:168–173.

41. Mendoza FX, Main K. Peripheral nerve injuries of the shoulder in the athlete. *Clin Sports Med* 1990;9(2): 331–342.

42. Symonds CP. Concussion and its sequelae. *Lancet* 1962;l:1–5.

43. Watkins RG, Dillin WH. Lumbar spine injury in the athlete. *Clin Sports Med* 1990;9:419–70.

Sports Neurology, Second Edition,
edited by Barry D. Jordan.
Lippincott–Raven Publishers, Philadelphia © 1998.

33

Ice Hockey

Susan Goodwin Gerberich, *Janny Dwyer Brust,
†Sheldon Robert Burns, and ‡Beth Johnson

*University of Minnesota School of Public Health, Box 807 UMHC, 420 Delaware Street S.E.,
Minneapolis, Minnesota 55455; *Allina Health System, Public Affairs Department,
5601 Smetana Drive, P.O. Box 9310, Minneapolis, Minnesota 55440;
†Minneapolis Sports Medicine Center, 720 Washington Avenue South, Edina, Minnesota 55435;
and ‡Minneapolis, Minnesota 55409*

There are multiple theories on the origins of hockey; however, there is general agreement that it commenced in the British Isles and France and was subsequently introduced to Canada with eventual introduction into the United States in the late 1800s. Participation in ice hockey has increased dramatically not only in the United States but also throughout Canada and Europe (1). Reasons for this increase include heightened media coverage of hockey at all levels from youth to Olympic competition; the expansion of hockey to warm climates, particularly in the southern United States, where hockey has not been played traditionally; and the growth of women's hockey.

USA Hockey, Inc. is the national governing body for the sport of ice hockey in the United States and is the official representative to the United States Olympic Committee (USOC) and the International Ice Hockey Federation (IIHF). It is responsible for organizing and training teams for international competitions, and it is also involved in coordinating activities with other national ice hockey federations around the world as well as with the National Hockey League (NHL) and the National Collegiate Athletic Association (NCAA) (2).

Professional ice hockey has spread rapidly across the United States and Europe. The expansion into southern U.S. locations has particularly broadened appeal of this activity. In the 1995 to 1996 season, 11 professional teams were located in warm climates in the United States.

In 1993 to 1994, 21,150 teams, involving youth 8 years of age and younger through those classified as seniors, were registered by USA Hockey Inc.; this was nearly double the number 10 years before and seven times greater than that in the first documented year of activity in 1968 to 1969 (2). These teams account for more than 300,000 participants (3) and are located in 11 regions throughout the country, with 8% located in the Pacific District and 2% in the Southeastern District. Approximately 2% of all teams in 1993 to 1994 were designated as girls' or women's teams (2).

At the intercollegiate level, more than 40 schools offer women's ice hockey, either club or varsity level. In 1993 to 1994, the Eastern Collegiate Athletic Association started the first intercollegiate women's ice hockey league in the nation, with 12 member schools.

Interscholastic hockey programs at the secondary school level, which are under the jurisdiction of the National Federation of State High School Leagues (NFSHSL), reported a registration of 22,032 male participants among 935 teams in 15 states during the season 1993 to 1994; a total of 194 female participants, who played on teams with males, were registered among 39 teams in

10 states (NFSHSL, personal communication, 1995).

In 1998, women's ice hockey was played for the first time as a medal sport in the Winter Olympics in Nagano, Japan. However, it is reported that women, as well as men, have played on organized hockey teams since the late 1800s. Nevertheless, membership on teams at the youth, high school, and college levels has exploded. This explosion in membership is a reflection of girls' and women's interest in participation in the sport with accompanied efforts to increase their access to the sport. On March 23, 1994, these efforts led to Minnesota becoming the first state in the United States to sanction ice hockey at the high school level for girls. In 1995, Minnesota held its first state high school tournament for female hockey players, while male players celebrated their 51st year. From 1992–1993 to 1994–1995, Minnesota experienced a fourfold increase in girls' teams at the Squirt and Peewee levels from 15 to 75 teams. This increase prompted Minnesota legislation (MN S.F. 2913, Chapter 632) that requires all publicly funded indoor ice rinks (approximately 180) to set aside prime ice time for female skaters at the following rate: 1994 to 1995, 15%; 1995 to 1996, 30%; and 1996 to 1997, 50% (M. Witchger, personal communication, April 1995).

In general, the environment of ice hockey games is conducive to injury, given the nature of the game (frequent collisions), its tools (hockey sticks, pucks, and skate blades), the surrounding ice surface, goal posts, and unyielding boards of the hockey arena. As a result of the forces generated among the players in this environment, a wide variety of types and severities of injuries may occur (3).

A comprehensive approach to understanding the mechanical forces implicated in ice hockey injuries is essential to the development of a knowledge base that can aid in reducing the frequency of these injuries and controlling their severity (4). The potential for injury in ice hockey is inherent in the fact that skating velocities generated during play may range between 20 mph for young hockey players (12 to 14 years of age) to 30 mph for senior amateur players. Speeds of 15 mph, while a player is sliding on the ice, have also been documented (5). Collisions

with the goal posts, boards, pucks, or other persons are common events.

On the basis of cinematographic analysis (5), speeds of the hard rubber puck propelled by the curved, bladed stick used in this sport may range from 50 mph for young players to 90 mph for senior amateur players to more than 120 mph for professional players. The maximal impact force of the puck at its terminal velocity can be as much as 1250 pounds (force). A study of puck impact on various hockey face masks (72) revealed deformation of the masks with puck speeds as low as 50 mph. Deformation with facial contact occurred at speeds of about 60 mph. Together with the increasing skill levels, the use of precision-made curved sticks has enabled an increase in the forces generated and speeds attained. Given the range of puck speeds that may be attained (5), it is apparent that there is potentially a high risk of injury from this source.

EPIDEMIOLOGY

Frequency and Types of Injuries

Data relevant to injuries associated with ice hockey participation are extremely limited. As with other types of sports and recreational activities, there is no standardized system for reporting and recording mortality and morbidity (7). In addition, few studies have been conducted to determine the magnitude of the injury problem in this sport. On the basis of limited emergency department data collected on product-related injuries, there were an estimated 22,479 ice hockey–related injury cases in the United States in 1986. From data provided by the United States Consumer Product Safety Commission (USCPSC) for 1993, it is estimated that there were 27,352 product-related injuries associated with ice hockey (V. B. Leonard, USCPSC, personal communication, 1995). Between 1973 and 1980, 10 deaths attributed to hockey injuries were reported by Rutherford et al. (8). Over the 14-year period between 1980 and 1993 a total of 14 related deaths were reported. (V. B. Leonard, USCPSC, personal communication, 1995). Because there is no standard reporting or recording system, however, these figures are probably low; moreover, the deaths reflect actual numbers from a sample of emergency departments in the United States versus estimates that would reflect much higher numbers. In comparison with football, which is estimated to have approximately 40 times as many participants, particularly at the high school level, the risk of fatality and injury among hockey participants appears to be much greater (9).

Serious eye (10,11) and dental (12) injuries were identified as the primary injuries associated with hockey participation. In response to an apparent increase in permanent eye and dental injuries (10,13), full face masks were first required in Minnesota in 1975 for all secondary school interscholastic players. This measure was subsequently instituted at the national level as a recommendation during the seasons 1983 to 1984 and 1984 to 1985 and became a requirement for the 1985 to 1986 season (14). At the same time, an equipment standard for eye and facial protection was passed by the American Society of Testing and Materials (ASTM) and adopted by AHAUS (now USA Hockey) in 1977. Mandatory face mask legislation was implemented at the college level in 1979 by the Eastern Collegiate Athletic Association and by the National Collegiate Athletic Association (15) for the 1980 season. Protective headgear is now required at all levels, including the professional and international levels. Although face masks are not required at the professional level, they are required by the NCAA and the NFSHSL and are strongly recommended by USA Hockey at all player levels. In addition to eye and dental injuries that have been reported, serious head (16–18) and neck (19–21) injuries have been associated with hockey.

A documented increase in catastrophic spinal cord injuries appears to be a recent phenomenon in the history of ice hockey. Between 1976 and 1983, Tator and Edmonds and their colleagues (19–21) documented 42 spinal cord injuries among hockey participants in organized programs in Canada. These involved primarily the mechanism of axial loading applied to the head in neutral alignment with the neck and torso, or in slight flexion, as a result of head-first collisions into the boards (65%) or another player (10%) (22). On the basis of previous reports (19–21), this was considered an epidemic. Between 1982 and 1986, the numbers increased markedly; there were approxi-

mately 15 major spinal injuries documented each year (22). Evidence in 1981 of three cases involving fractured necks within a 3-week period among high school hockey players in a metropolitan area of Minnesota, where no surveillance system was in place, added further concern. Typical of reporting limitations, two of these cases were identified through the press (23) and the other was discovered inadvertently. In response to this finding, a 2-year comprehensive epidemiologic study (9) was initiated to determine the rates, types, and severities of injuries incurred by secondary school varsity hockey players in Minnesota between 1982 and 1984 and to identify factors potentially associated with these injuries, including the use of the face mask.

Using the definition from previous investigations (7,24–26), Gerberich et al. (9) defined an injury as an acute traumatic event that kept the athlete from participation on any performance day (practice or game) or from regular activity after the day of onset. Any concussion or dental injury, regardless of time lost, was also considered reportable. Among the 12 high school hockey teams that were selected for study within a 30-mile radius of a large metropolitan area, a total injury rate of 75 cases per 100 players was documented in the first year; this represented one or more injuries incurred by 41% of the 251 players on the teams. On the basis of the total potential hours of exposure, this amounted to a rate of 5.0 injuries per 1000 hours of play (9). In the second year of study, 33% of the 229 players had one or more injuries, amounting to a rate of 51 cases per 100 players. Head and neck injuries accounted for 22% and 25%, respectively, of the total injuries verified through follow-up investigations for the 2 years of the study (Fig. 1). A major finding in this study was a high rate of concussions, including loss of consciousness or amnesia or both, as a result of a blow to the head (27,28). Among the total players, 9% experienced a concussion, accounting for 12% of the total injuries in the first year and 8% in the second year (Fig. 2).

In a similar 2-year epidemiologic study conducted in Denmark in 1983 to 1984 among 210 adult elite players (mean age, 22.7 years), an overall injury rate of 90 cases per 100 players was documented; this accounted for a rate of 4.7 injuries per 1000 hours of exposure (29). Any

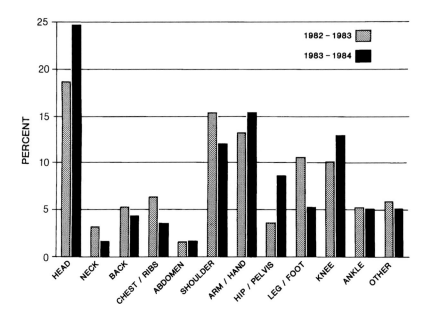

FIG. 1. Distribution, by body area, of injuries incurred by high school hockey players.

injury associated with hockey participation that curtailed or hindered a player's activity or required special treatment to enable the injured player to play was included in the study. Of the total injuries, 28% involved the head; concussions accounted for 14.3% of all injuries. No other injuries relevant to central nervous system trauma were identified. It was also reported that, although 63% of the total injuries were seen by a physician, only 8% of those identified as a concussion were seen by a physician; 55% were seen by a physiotherapist. The definition of concussion and the method of documenting the cases were not reported in the study, however.

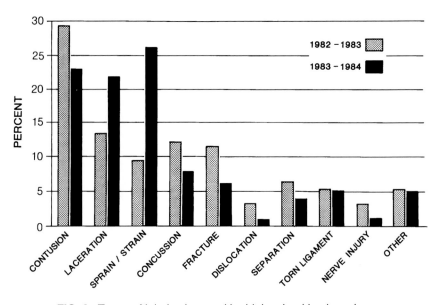

FIG. 2. Types of injuries incurred by high school hockey players.

Brust et al. (30) conducted a prospective study of injuries among nine Minnesota community hockey teams involving 150 male players, aged 9 to 15 years, during the 1990 to 1991 season. In addition to data collection on injury, information was collected on knowledge, attitudes, and behaviors from all participants. The injury definition used was "any ice hockey or ice hockey–related injury that resulted in a player not being able to continue to participate in a game or practice or that kept a player from participating in physical activities the following day." Among 52 documented injuries, 23% occurred to the head and neck.

Among the 27,352 product-related ice hockey injuries estimated by the USCPSC in 1993, 38% occurred to the head and neck. The types of injuries identified among the 14 deaths reported, between 1980 and 1993, were traumatic injuries to the brain (43%), heart (36%), and spinal cord (14%) and asphyxia (7%) from drowning (V. B. Leonard, USCPSC, personal communication, 1995).

Risk Factors

Analyses of characteristics between injured and noninjured hockey players in the study by Gerberich et al. (9) revealed statistically significant differences in age, height, and weight. In general, the older, taller, heavier player was injured most frequently; the only exception to this was the 14-year-old player, whose risk of concussion was found to be as great as that of the 17-year-old player. Injured players also had significantly greater playing experience than noninjured players (9.1 and 8.6 years, respectively). Significant differences between injured and noninjured players were also evident by position played, with defensemen and wings accounting for much greater percentages of injuries.

Injuries occurred primarily during competition (82%). Most player injuries were associated with situations involving breakout plays (20%), forechecking (17%), and backchecking (12%). Head injuries were most frequently associated with forechecking (31%) and breakout plays (27%).

Analyzed by activity, legal activities of body checking were associated with a large percentage of the injuries (38%), and illegal activities were associated with 26% of the injuries. Head injuries were primarily associated with players colliding with another player (45%), hitting the boards (34%), or being hit with a stick (22%).

In a 1985 to 1986 study in Quebec, Regnier et al. (31) compared injury rates between 28 PeeWee teams that allowed checking and 21 teams that had banned checking. The rate of fractures was 12 times greater among persons playing on the teams that allowed checking. Moreover, 88% of all fractures incurred were related to body checking. Players on the teams that allowed body checking compared with those that banned it had, on average, 12.4 and 9.1 penalties per game, respectively. Penalties were also assessed by type: instrumental penalties are those aimed at gaining a tactical advantage and involve little aggression such as tripping, holding, and interference; hostile penalties, such as charging, cross-checking, and roughing, are meant to intimidate or hurt an opponent. Although the number of instrumental penalties was not influenced by body checking, there were significantly more hostile penalties assessed to teams that allowed body checking.

In a substudy, Regnier et al. (31) also compared the ten smallest members of the Peewee teams with the ten largest members for grip strength measured by a hand dynamometer, maximum skating speed measured by photoelectric cells, and impact force and speed at impact measured by a force platform setup. On average, the larger Peewees were twice as heavy and 30 cm taller than the smaller members. Furthermore, the larger Peewees were able to exert an impact force 70% greater than that exerted by the smaller players. Yet, there were no differences in skating speed and speed at impact.

Fair-Play (32) is an approach intended to integrate sportsmanship into the game without changing the structure of the game. Under Fair-Play rules, one point is assessed to a team that ends a game with less than a preestablished number of penalties (six for Peewee and eight for Bantam level). This approach was instituted in some Canadian youth ice hockey leagues with the intent of reducing rule infractions and aggressive and violent behavior. During the 1989 to 1990 hockey season in Quebec, seven Peewee CC (competitive) and 16 Bantam CC teams playing under Fair-Play rules were compared with 16 Peewee CC and 16 Bantam CC teams not playing under those rules. The results of this analysis revealed that averages of 4.5 and 5.7 penalties per team per game were assessed, respectively, to Peewee teams playing under the Fair-Play rules compared with those who were not. Major penalties for the entire season were 1.3 and 6.3, respectively. Among the Bantam teams, there were fewer penalties for the teams that incorporated Fair-Play rules compared with those that did not (7.8 and 8.4, respectively); however, these latter results were not statistically significant.

Brust et al. (30) also identified numerous potential risk factors for injury in the study of Bantam players, 13 to 15 years of age. Average weight and height and the respective ranges were 53 kg (37 to 90) and 55 cm (133 to 188). Injured players had a mean weight of 51 kg, compared with a mean weight of 63 kg for uninjured players. Analysis of the activities involved revealed that legal checking (20%), illegal checking (39%), and violations (27%) accounted for 86% of the game-related injuries. Of 29 injuries resulting from illegal game activities, only four penalties were assessed; 15% of the injuries occurred during practice and the remaining 85% occurred during games, including regular season games, tournaments, or scrimmages. Although these players had an average of 7 years of experience playing on hockey teams (range, 2 to 11 years), only half (51%) reportedly knew that checking from behind could cause another player serious injury or death. Moreover, 26% of the players who stated they knew the seriousness of such activity said they would do it, if "angry" or "to get even." Among both Peewee and Bantam level players, 73% reported receiving instruction in "giving" and 69% in "taking" a check.

Data from the study in Denmark (29) indicated that 76% of the concussions occurred during matches and that 24% were associated with training, a finding similar to that from the Minnesota data (9). According to the classification system used in the study in Denmark, forward playing positions accounted for 52% of the injuries and defense positions accounted for 44%.

In response to the documented catastrophic spinal cord injuries in Canada (19–21), comprehensive biomechanical studies were conducted by Bishop et al. (33,34) to investigate the potential effect of the addition of the face mask on neck injury. Using an instrumented anthropometric head and neck fitted with a hockey helmet and face shield, these investigators studied the effect of a collision with the boards by a hockey player (33). Large axial forces occurred with the neck in neutral and flexion positions and a large shear force occurred with the neck in extension, indicating a risk of dislocation. It was concluded that, even if these types of collisions do not produce fractures, they can be expected to produce substantial muscle and ligament damage.

These investigators further hypothesized that the use of face masks gives players a feeling of invincibility, so that they take unwarranted risks during games and practices (34). Brust et al. (30) reported that 55% of 129 youth players believed their helmets and face masks protected them from all head and neck injuries; no significant differences were evident by playing level. Evidence from the 2-year comprehensive epidemiologic investigation by Gerberich et al. (9) indicated not only an apparent increase in aggressive behavior with the introduction of the face mask but also an increased risk of concussions and all types of injuries among players who reported that the face mask allowed them to be more aggressive in play. Players who reported that the face mask blocked their vision in any direction had a risk of concussion 3.4 times that of players who did not report this as a problem (Table 1).

Among players in this study who identified that their primary reason (either first, second, or third of eight reasons) for playing hockey was to get rid of aggressions and tensions, the risk of incurring a concussion during the season was 2.5 times greater than for players who identified other reasons (9). Waller (35,36) cited another study that also found differing motivational levels among players. Players who played hockey "for the joy of it" were not influenced by movies showing what was described as aggressive hockey. In contrast, the players who were interested primarily in winning showed a significant increase in aggressive behavior during their next game after watching the movies. In the study by Brust et al. (30), 34% of the games that involved injuries were de-

TABLE 1. *Relationship between the proportion of high school hockey players who perceived face mask interference with vision and the proportion of those who incurred a concussion, 1982–1983 (9) and 1983–1984 seasons*

Concussion	Perception of face mask blocking ability to see in any direction		
	Yes	No	Total
Yes	15	17	32
No	91	352	443
Total	106	369	475

Odds ratio = 3.41; 95% C.I. = 1.70 – 6.85; $P < .001$.

scribed as hostile; these included environments in which players called each other names, which involved fighting, or in which parents exhibited anger or referee calls were disputed.

Although studies have not focused specifically on potential gender differences in injury rates experienced in hockey, a study of eight matched men's and women's intercollegiate varsity teams (37) that were studied prospectively for 1 year found no differences for any of the sports with the exception of gymnastics. Basketball, fencing, swimming, tennis, indoor track, outdoor track, and volleyball were the other sports included in this study. It was found that when men and women compete in sports that are technically similar, the injury rates are comparable; in sports that are technically different, the rates would not be expected to be the same. A preliminary study of injuries experienced by boys and girls participating in ice hockey tournaments showed that males experienced a higher rate of injuries than females (7.7 and 3.1 per 100 players) and more serious injuries (i.e., fractures and concussions versus bruises) (38). At the present time, women's rules in ice hockey do not usually allow checking. Should these rules change, injury rates would be expected to be more comparable to those documented for men.

Another potential risk factor for ice hockey participants is the activity of in-line dry-land skating. This activity was first popularized in Minnesota in 1980 (39) to enable out-of-season training for hockey on dry land. It was estimated to have over 12 million participants in 1993 with an annual growth of 34% to 51% between 1988 and 1993. This sport, which includes ice hockey players who

participate to maintain their skill levels throughout the year and those who are involved either competitively or strictly for recreation, has its own unique set of potential risk factors that have not been well studied and will not be elaborated upon in this forum. However, it is important to recognize the potential for both positive outcomes as well as injury consequences to ice hockey participants who participate in in-line skating and to investigate this through future study.

NEUROLOGIC INJURIES

Head Injuries

As shown in Table 2, there have been a number of efforts to document the magnitude of the problem of hockey-related injuries. In addition to the great variations in the geographic locations of these studies, there are large differences in their methodologies. Although head injury appears to be a significant problem, the classification of head injury typically encompasses various injuries ranging from lacerations to fractures and affecting any area of the head. With the exception of the two epidemiologic studies described above (9,29), there has apparently been little effort to identify the incidence of brain injury, including concussion, through population-based investigations.

According to Bishop et al. (40), head injuries in hockey usually occur in one of two ways: the player is struck on the head with a stick or puck traveling at high speed (low mass–high velocity impact) or the player collides with the boards, the goal post, the ice surface, or another

TABLE 2. *Location, by body site, of hockey related injuries*

Body Site	Study[a]										
	1	2	3	4	5	6	7	8	9	10	11
					Percentage of Total Injuries						
Head	36.7	42.0	45.1	7.0	28.0	18.7	24.8	6.0 (head and concussion)	13.5	10.0 (head and face)	6.3
Concussion	—	—	—	—	14.3	12.0	8.0		—		
Scalp	—	—	—	—	45.9	—	—	15.0 (other head injuries)			
Eye	—	—	—	2.6	—	—	—	—	—	—	—
Neck	0.4	—	9.2 (neck and shoulders)	—	—	3.2	1.7	3.0	9.7	—	—
Back	—	—	—	—	7.0	5.3	4.3	6.0	23.1	—	15.8
Trunk	5.0	—	12.2	—	—	11.7	13.6	5.5	17.4	13.0 (trunk and inguinal)	—
Upper extremities	21.9	18.0	7.9	10.7	19.0	28.9	27.4	35.0	19.3	55.0	24.2 (upper limb)
Lower extremities	35.7	21.0	25.6	30.0	27.0	26.2	23.0	26.0	17.3	19.0	53.7 (lower limb)
Multiple injuries	0.3	—	—	—	—	—	—	—	—	—	—
Other	—	19.0	—	3.8	19.0	5.9	5.1	3.5	—	—	—
Total	100.0	100.0	100.0	100.0	100.0	99.9	99.9	100.0	100.3	97.0	100.0

[a] Study 1 (65), Czechoslovakia, 1967–1968, 65,881 players (data from insurance records, injuries requiring more than 14 days of treatment); study 2 (66), Switzerland, 1967–1972, 2680 injuries (data from insurance records); study 3 (67, 68), United States and Canada, 1970–1971 (9 American and 21 Canadian collegiate teams); study 4 (69), United States, 1974–1975, player ages 5 years to adult (357 Minor Leage Hockey Association players, 350 junior amateur players, 207 secondary school players, 17 professional players); study 5 (29), Denmark, 1983–1984 (14 teams, 210 elite adult players); study 6 (9), United States, 1982–1983 (12 teams, 251 secondary school interscholastic players); study 7 (9), United States, 1983–1984 (12 teams, 229 secondary school interscholastic players); study 8, AHAUS, 1983–1984 (data from 393 insurance claims for 4579 teams); study 9 (30), United States, 1990–1991 (9 teams—Squirts, Peewees, and Bantams, 150 players—ages 9 to 15); study 10 (70), Finland, 1990–1991 (54 teams, 1437 players, ages 9 to 18 years); study 11 (71), Sweden, 1982–1985 (elite team, 3-year study, 24 to 25 players per year).

person (high mass–low velocity impact). From the fatality data identified by the USCPSC for 1980 to 1993, 6 of the 14 cases involved brain injuries that occurred as a result of being hit by a stick or a puck or as a result of a collision with another player; in at least two of these cases, it was noted that helmets were worn (V. B. Leonard, USCPSC, personal communication, 1995).

During the late 1960s and early 1970s, morbidity and mortality from head injuries incurred in hockey activities became an area of major concern (40–42). In concert with this concern was the question about the effectiveness of the ice hockey helmet (10). Bishop et al. (40) embarked on a series of laboratory impact studies to test five different helmets that were designed to meet the Canadian Standards Association (CSA) standard for the manufacture of helmets (43). Although these investigators found that the performance of the helmets was not uniform among models or within models at different test points on the helmets, the critical concussive threshold value was apparently not exceeded. Further investigation of this problem continues.

Some of the most serious brain injuries occur without any evidence of skull fracture (27). Reid and Reid (44) found that head injury is dependent on the magnitude and direction of impact, the structural features and physical reactions of the skull, and the position of the head at the moment of impact. Thus, any blow to the head may be injurious.

The finding of the 2-year study of high school hockey participants (9) showed a high incidence not only of brain concussion but also of neurologic symptoms after a blow to the head, neck, or back; these mechanisms require further investigation. In addition to the documented concussions, additional symptoms of blurred vision, double vision, and incoordination after a blow to the head or neck were identified by the players (Fig. 3). Furthermore, among the players with concussions, 36% had previously experienced a loss of consciousness; this amounted to a risk two times greater than that of players who had never previously experienced a loss of consciousness (Table 3). These findings are similar to those reported in a comprehensive epidemiologic study of more than 3000 high school football players that used a similar methodology (7,25).

Although most of the reported concussions were classified as being of mild severity, this classification is disputed because of evidence of residual effects. Jennett (45) discussed the fact that mild concussion has a legacy of permanent brain damage because effects of repeated concussion are cumulative (46). An example of this

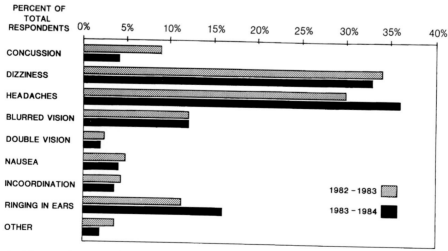

FIG. 3. Incidence of concussions and concussion symptoms among high school hockey players, 1982–1983, 1983–1984 seasons.

TABLE 3. *Relationship between the proportion of high school hockey players who previously incurred a loss of consciousness and the proportion of those who incurred a concussion during hockey season participation, 1982 to 1983 (9) and 1983 to 1984*

Concussion during hockey season participation	Previous loss of consciousness		
	Yes	No	Total
Yes	11	20	31
No	91	356	447
Total	102	376	478

Odds ratio = 2.15; 95% C.I. = 1.01–4.59; $P < .05$.

has been demonstrated in boxers who sustain repeated concussions (47). Even brief unconsciousness is associated with some degree of brain damage, traces of which are permanent. The association between head injury and dementia of the Alzheimer type, as demonstrated in a case-control study by French et al. (48) and others (6,49), is also of concern. Evidence of the effects of brain injury on college academic performance reported by Gerberich et al. (50) further suggests a need to consider the long-term effects not only of the severe cases but also of the mild cases.

Data collected by Brust et al. (30) in the study of 150 players (Peewees, Bantams, and Squirts), aged 9 to 15 years, revealed that 69% reported receiving at least one blow to the head, neck, or back sometime during the season. Among the Peewee and Bantam level players who are in body-checking leagues, 83% reported incurring at least one hard hit to the head, neck, or back during the season. The most frequently associated symptoms were headaches, dizziness, and neck pain.

Cervical Spine Injuries

According to Torg (51), injuries to the cervical spine that involve quadriplegia occur most commonly as a result of axial loading. In hockey, when the player is pushed into the boards head first, the cervical spine is compressed between the rapidly decelerated head and the continued momentum of the body, providing a dominant load on vertebral bodies C-5 and C-6 (34).

Cervical spine injuries were not recognized as a problem among hockey players until the first cluster of cases was documented between 1974 and 1981 by Tator et al. (21,52); five of the six identified cases were treated in two Toronto hospitals within a 13-month period (1980 to 1981). All cases involved cervical vertebral body burst fractures and associated neurologic sequelae. Furthermore, the mechanism of injury in five cases involved collisions into the boards (or another player, in one case) by helmeted players with accompanying axial loading of the flexed neck. Initial striking of the boards with the neck in extension may have prevented serious spinal cord injury in one of the players.

Because there had been no reports of acute spinal cord injuries among hockey players treated in these Toronto hospitals between 1948 and 1973, with the exception of one reported in 1966 (22), a country-wide investigation was initiated in cooperation with the Canadian Committee on Prevention of Spinal Injuries associated with hockey (20). As a result of this endeavor, 117 injuries among individuals between 11 and 47 years of age were reported; 109 were associated with the cervical spine, and these were most frequently burst fractures or fracture dislocations. Of the 73 spinal cord injuries reported, 29 resulted in complete motor and sensory loss to the individual and 9 resulted in complete motor and incomplete sensory loss; 5 players were known to have died as a result of their injuries. Nearly all of the injuries resulted from collision of the players head first into the boards or another player with their head in neutral alignment with the neck and torso or in slight flexion; 31 of the 49 players who had been pushed or checked were struck from behind. "Almost all the players in this series were wearing helmets, and more than two-thirds were wearing face masks" (22).

Although there were limitations in the data, the number of reported injuries over the 21-year period studied (1966 to 1987) increased from 2 in 1979 to approximately 15 per year between 1982 and 1986. With possible limitations in the ability to detect all cases and the lack of data relevant to the populations at risk over this period, interpretation of these data is problematic. The relative absence of cases before 1974 (one case was reported in 1966), however, suggests a significant problem. Moreover, the number of cases has apparently continued to increase.

It is believed that a situation analogous to that of football (53) also exists in hockey, whereby the mandatory addition of the helmet in the 1970s and further addition of the face mask are believed to have altered the nature of the game (34,54,55). Initial epidemiologic (9,29) and biomechanical studies (33,34,56) have only begun to address this extremely complex problem. However, in 1988, the American College Hockey Coaches Association meeting came to a unanimous agreement that face masks promoted rough and violent hockey play. In response to this agreement, they called for the approval of a half-shield or visor-type of mask to decrease the violent play (57).

Although three cases involving cervical fractures that occurred within a 3-week period precipitated an investigation in Minnesota, only a small proportion (3%) of the injuries documented in the 2 year epidemiologic study (9) were associated with the neck. The incidence of symptoms after a blow to the head, neck, or back (together with percentages of residual symptoms at the time of the study) is identified in Table 4. Among the players who experienced symptoms during the hockey season, a large proportion reported persistent residual symptoms or problems at the time of the study. Furthermore, players who had previous symptoms and reported neck pain, back pain, or upper extremity symptoms (numbness, tingling, or weakness) after a blow to the head, neck, or back were at significantly greater risk of experiencing these symptoms than players who did not have previous symptoms (9).

Neck symptoms should be a cause for concern when associated with contact sports or activities

(58). Moreover, individuals younger than 18 to 21 years of age are especially susceptible to neck injury because development of the vertebrae and adjoining cartilage is not complete until that time (59). Although the symptoms documented in this study, in isolation from other techniques of physical examination and radiographic studies, are not diagnostic, some of these players may have had associated pathology. Thus, each case must be considered with regard to potential long-term effects.

CRITERIA FOR RETURN TO PLAY

An injury can be compounded and recovery delayed by failure to recognize its occurrence in the first place or as a result of not accessing appropriate diagnostic and therapeutic resources. A comprehensive epidemiologic study documented that a large percentage of potentially severe athletic injuries, including trauma to the head and neck, either were not recognized as potentially dangerous or were not managed appropriately (7,24,25). Because many individuals with such injuries may not initially come to the attention of a trained sports medicine provider, it is essential to implement a system that prohibits injured players from returning to competition before they can be thoroughly evaluated by a health care professional. Players incurring a head or neck injury should have an initial evaluation and a repeated examination, if necessary, before receiving permission to return to play. Before participation, the person must be free of any symptoms and have return of full strength, full range of motion, and normal function in the body areas relevant to the injury. It is also imperative that the athlete be psychologically prepared and ready to return.

Appropriate management of cases involving head and/or neck injuries is paramount. During the assessment process, both the head and neck must always be examined carefully; one must always assume that there could have been a concomitant cervical spine injury. Initial stabilization of the injured athlete is of utmost importance. Triage is determined by the severity of the injury. Utilization of the three-level severity classification scheme for brain injury is useful in the initial management and follow-up of such cases. However, proper

TABLE 4. *Incidence of symptoms after a blow to the head, neck, or back among high school hockey players 1982 to 1983 (9) and 1983 to 1984 seasons*

| | Incidence (%) | | | |
| | 1982–1983 | | 1983–1984 | |
Symptoms	Symptoms	Residual symptoms[a]	Symptoms	Residual symptoms[a]
Neck pain	9.2	26.0	10.9	23.0
Tingling, burning, or numbness in upper extremities	6.4	0.0	3.5	50.0
Tingling, burning, or numbness in lower extremities	4.8	0.0	3.9	22.2
Back pain	15.1	39.5	12.7	55.2
Reduced strength in upper extremities	10.4	19.2	5.2	25.0
Reduced strength in lower extremities	6.4	6.3	7.0	50.0

[a] Residual symptoms among those players who had symptoms during the season

classification depends entirely on thorough history taking and clinical evaluation.

The person with a mild (grade I) concussion involving brief symptoms of headache, ringing in the ears, incoordination of body movements, or mental confusion and no loss of consciousness should be removed from the activity for at least several minutes. Under no circumstances should the player be permitted to resume contact or regular activity until he or she can move with usual dexterity and speed (27,28) and is completely asymptomatic both at rest and on exertion (60). More important, athletes must not return to play until they can answer questions appropriately about what they were doing just before the head injury (e.g., "What was the last play you just made?" "What were you assigned to do on the field?" "What game were you just playing?") (61). Furthermore, the individual must be watched closely for signs of changing orientation, fatigue, and inappropriate behavior (27). Because amnesia may occur 10 to 20 minutes after a blow to the head, continuous assessment of players is important. Potential complications include intracranial hematomas and cerebral contusions. Such complications must be suspected in any individual complaining of acute or chronic headaches (28) or persistent neurologic symptoms.

Persons with a moderate concussion (28) (grade II) involving loss of consciousness with recovery in less than 5 minutes, or more than 30 minutes of posttraumatic amnesia (28), must be removed from activity and, according to the Colorado Medical Society Guidelines for the Management of Concussion in Sports, should not be permitted to participate until they are asymtomatic for at least two weeks (62). Typically, the individual cannot remember what happened just before loss of consciousness. Symptoms of headache, visual disturbances, hallucinations, ringing in the ears, drowsiness, nausea, and dizziness may be experienced in various combinations. Evaluation and observation in an acute care setting, capable of handling a situation that could deteriorate, is mandatory for at least 24 hours; frequent checks must be made for any changes in neurologic status. Furthermore, the player must not be permitted to return to athletics or regular activities if any of these symptoms or other neurologic abnormality (e.g., weakness, numbness, tingling or burning of the extremities, or behavioral changes) persists.

The person with a severe concussion (grade III) who is unconscious for 5 minutes or more, or has significant neurologic dysfunction, or has had 24 hours or more of posttraumatic amnesia (60) should be hospitalized immediately (27) and examined by a neurologist and/or a neurosurgeon; transport must be managed from the field by ambulance with cervical spine immobilization. Return to activity must not be allowed until a physician has conducted a thorough neurologic examination and given permission to resume play.

Cumulative effects of concussions can be severe. It has been recognized that an individual who has experienced two moderate concussions should be referred to a neurologist or neurosurgeon for consultation, with serious consideration given to limiting activity to noncontact sports (28). Appropriate judgment of each case is required, however. In the case of a single severe head injury in which structural damage is evidenced by clinical examination or specialized techniques, total restriction from contact sports may be warranted (28). Kelly et al. (62) reported a concern, based on clinical evidence, that individuals who are symptomatic from a concussion even without loss of consciousness are at risk of developing diffuse brain swelling after a second impact to the head. Thus, it is imperative to examine such individuals thoroughly and restrict their participation from activities that could result in such consequences.

Guidelines for return to contact sports for the individual who has experienced transient quadriplegia have been suggested by Cantu (63). "Return after a first episode of transient quadriplegia is deemed acceptable if the athlete has complete resolution of symptoms, full range of motion, and normal curvature of the cervical spine, as well as no evidence of spinal stenosis on magnetic resonance imaging (MRI), contrast-enhanced computerized tomography (CT) or myelography. . . . Cervical spinal stenosis is known to increase the risk of permanent neurological injury." (See Chapter 14.)

PREVENTION AND CONTROL OF NEUROLOGIC INJURIES

In contrast to data reported earlier (10–13), serious eye and dental injuries do not currently appear to be a major problem among hockey players who wear eye and dental protection, including face masks (63). Substitution of these injuries for more severe and potentially catastrophic injuries must not be permitted, however. In view of the risks of brain and spinal cord injuries and symptoms identified among the players in the 2 year epidemiologic study conducted in Minnesota (9), in concert with other evidence (7,24,25,27,45,46,50), it is imperative that vigorous preseason screening and post-injury evaluation through comprehensive history taking and examination be initiated. In addition, players must be informed of potential risks associated with collision forces to the head and neck(54). Intensive educational programs involving coaches, players, and parents (when appropriate) to facilitate understanding of these risks must be an integral part of any sports activity in which there is a potential for such injuries (54). The potential prophylactic use of neck muscle conditioning programs should also be considered (19).

In particular, the findings suggest a need to investigate further the relevant equipment, to ensure its proper fit, and to use equipment that appropriately dissipates impact forces; this is especially crucial for the helmet (33,34,40,56). Clearly, the use of protective equipment, such as the face mask, and how it appears to have changed the game need to be further evaluated.

In view of the large percentage of injuries associated with collisions into the boards, changes in the material composition of the boards to facilitate energy absorption need to be investigated. The national and international use of breakaway goal posts, already in place in most locations (9), seems to be extremely important in reducing collision forces. The addition of material to the goal frame to disseminate forces must also be considered through future study. It has also been recommended that hockey organizations avoid using small rinks because of the increased likelihood of player–player and player–board collisions (19).

On the basis of evidence (9), there also is a need to improve rule enforcement by coaches and officials to prevent use of illegal techniques that result in injury. Before the 1970s, body checking was allowed only in the defensive zone in high school interscholastic games. This strategy is used in the young player leagues as well as in "over 40" leagues and requires further investigation. Rule changes to limit or eliminate body checking can be expected to facilitate a reduction in injuries. A Canadian study comparing three Peewee leagues, two that allowed body checking and one in which body checking was banned, showed that players in one of the leagues that allowed body checking were 12 times more likely to suffer a fracture during the course of a game than players in the league where body checking was banned (31).

Determining the true magnitude of the injury problem in hockey requires a system that facilitates ongoing surveillance not only of injuries involving short-term disability and activity limitation but also of those that may result in long-term disability or death. Comprehensive recording and reporting systems are essential to the identification of variables associated with the injury events and should be incorporated in every program (64). In this manner, realistic strategies for the prevention and control of injuries may be developed.

Acknowledgments

Support, in part, for this effort was provided by the Regional Injury Prevention Research Center, Division of Environmental and Occupational Health, School of Public Health, University of Minnesota, Minneapolis. The authors appreciate the assistance and information provided by Vicky B. Leonard, Technical Information Specialist, National Injury Information Clearing House, U.S. Consumer Product Safety Commission, Washington, DC; the National Federation of State High School Associations, Kansas City, Missouri; U.S.A. Hockey, Inc., Colorado Springs, Colorado; and Mitzi Witchger, Witchger and Associates, Gender Equity Consultants, Minneapolis, Minnesota.

REFERENCES

1. Orr F. *The story of hockey,* New York: Random House; 1971.
2. U.S.A. Hockey, Hockey Statistics, Colorado Springs, CO, 1995.
3. Sim FH, Simonet WT, Melton LJ III, et al. Ice hockey injuries. *Am J Sports Med* 1987;15:30–40.
4. Robertson LS. *Injuries: causes, control strategies, and public policy.* Lexington, MA: Lexington Books, 1984.
5. Sim FH, Chao EY. Injury potential in modern ice hockey. *Am J Sports Med* 1978;6:378–384.
6. Mortimer JA, Van Duijn CM, Chandra V, et al. Head trauma as a risk factor for Alzheimer's Disease: a collaborative re-analysis of case-control studies. *Int J Epidemiol* 1991;S28–S35.
7. Gerberich SG, Priest JD, Boen JR, et al. Concussion incidence and severity in secondary school varsity football players. *Am J Public Health* 1983;73:1370–1375.
8. Rutherford GW, Miles RB, Brown VR, et al. Cited in Kraus JF, Conroy C: Mortality and morbidity from injuries in sports and recreation. *Annu Rev Public Health* 1984;5:163–192.
9. Gerberich SG, Finke R, Madden M, et al. An epidemiological study of high school ice hockey injuries. *Child Nerv Syst* 1987;3:59–64.
10. Pashby TJ, Pashby RC, Chisholm LDJ, et al. Eye injuries in Canadian hockey. *Can Med Assoc J* 1975;113:663.
11. Vinger PF. Ocular injuries in hockey. *Arch Ophthalmol.* 1976;94:74.
12. Nadeau J. Special prosthesis. *J Prosthet Dent* 1968;20:62.
13. Rontal E, Rontal M, Wilson K, et al. Facial injuries in hockey players. *Laryngoscope* 1977;87:884–894.
14. Fawcett RG, (ed). *1983–84 Official high school hockey rules.* Kansas City, MO: National Federation of State High School Associations, 1983.
15. Reilly MF. The nature and causes of hockey injuries: a five-year study. *Athletic Train* 1982;3:88–90.
16. Feriencik K. Case report: depressed skull fracture in an ice hockey player wearing a helmet. *Phys Sports Med* 1979;7:107.
17. Feriencik K. Trends in ice hockey injuries: 1965 to 1977. *Phys Sports Med* 1979;7:81–84.
18. Gibbs RW. Unsafe headgear faulted in critical hockey injuries. *Phys Sports Med* 1974;2:39-42.
19. Tator CH, Edmonds VE. Acute spinal cord injury: analysis of epidemiological factors. *Can J Surg* 1979; 22: 575–578.
20. Tator CH, Edmonds VE. National survey of spinal injuries in hockey players. *Can Med Assoc J* 1984; 130:875–880.
21. Tator CH, Ekong CEU, Rowed DW, et al. Spinal injuries due to hockey. *Can J Neurol Sci* 1984;11:34–41.
22. Tator CH, Edmonds VE, Lapczak L, et al. Spinal injuries in ice hockey players, 1966–1987. *Can J Surg* 1991: 34:63–69.
23. Soucheray J. Two broken necks certify need for trainers. *Minneapolis Tribune.* 1981, Feb 20, p. 1D.
24. Gerberich SG, Priest JD, Boen JR, et al. Spinal trauma and symptoms in high school football players. *Phys Sports Med* 1983;11:122–139.
25. Gerberich SG. *Analysis of High School Football Injuries and Concomitant Health Care Provision.* Thesis, University of Minnesota, Minneapolis, 1980.
26. National Athletic Injury/Illness Reporting System. *NAIRS sports-related incidence charts, 1976–1979.* University Park, PA: Pennsylvania State University, 1980.
27. Gerberich SG, Priest JD, Grafft J, et al. Injuries to the brain and spinal cord: Assessment, emergency care, and prevention. *Minn Med* 1982;65:691–696.
28. Maroon JC, Steele PB, Berlin R. Football head and neck injuries: an update. *Clin Neurosurg* 1980;27:414.
29. Jorgensen V, Schmidt-Olsen S. The epidemiology of ice hockey injuries. *Br J Sports Med* 1986;20:7–9.
30. Brust JD, Leonard BJ, Pheley A, et al. Children's ice hockey injuries, *Am J Dis Child* 1992;146:741–747.
31. Regnier G, Boileau R, Marcotte G, et al. Effects of body-checking in the Pee-Wee (12 and 13 year old) Division in the Province of Quebec. In: *Safety in ice hockey.* Philadelphia: ASTM; 1989:84–103.
32. Marcotte G, Simard D. Fair-play: an approach to hockey for the 1990s. In: Castaldi CR, Bishop PJ, Hoerner EF, eds. *Safety in ice hockey.* Philadelphia: American Society for Testing and Materials, 1993.
33. Bishop PI, Norman RW, Wells RP. A study of selected mechanical factors involved in neck injuries in ice hockey. *Proceedings of the Ninth International Congress of Biomechanics,* Waterloo, Canada, Aug 1983. Champagne, IL: Human Kinetics Publishers, 1985:167–171.
34. Bishop PT, Norman RW, Wells RP, et al. Changes in the center of mass and moment of inertia of a headform induced by a hockey helmet and face shield. *Can J Appl Sport Sci* 1983;8:19–25.
35. Waller J. *Injury control.* Lexington, MA: Lexington Books, 1985.
36. Ryan T. Study assessed influence of movies on hockey players. *Burlington, VT: Free Press.* 1982, 20 January, 1D.
37. Lanese RR, Strauss RH, Leizman DJ, Rotondi AM. Injury and disability in matched men's and women's intercollegiate sports. *AJPH* 1990;80:1459–1462.
38. Brust JD, Leonard BJ, Roberts WO, et al. Hockey injuries at tournaments: are girls different from boys?

Abstracts: American Public Health Association, 122nd Annual Meeting, Washington, DC, Oct 30–Nov 3, 1994.

39. Chen AD. Rec.sport.skating.inline frequently asked questions (FAQ). Usenet rec.sport.skating.inline, available via anonymous www:http://garnet.acns.fsu.edu/~adchen/rec.skate.html 1995.

40. Bishop PJ, Norman RW, Pierrynowski M, et al. The ice hockey helmet: how effective is it? *Phys Sports Med* 1979;7:97–106.

41. Bolitho N. Head injuries in amateur ice hockey. *Natl Safety Congr Trans* 1969;27:20–28.

42. Fekete JF. Severe brain injury and death following minor hockey accidents—the effectiveness of the safety helmets of amateur hockey players. *Can Med Assoc J* 1968; 99:1234–1239.

43. Canadian Standards Association. *Hockey helmets* CSA Preliminary Standard Z262.1, 1973.

44. Reid SE, Reid SE Jr. Football neck muscles and head impact. *Surg Gynecol Obstet* 1978;147–513.

45. Jennett B. Assessment of the severity of head injury. *J Neurol Neurosurg Psychiatry* 1976;39:647–655.

46. Gronwall D, Wrightson P. Memory and information processing capacity after closed head injury. *J Neurol Neurosurg Psychiatry* 1981;44:889–895.

47. Corsellis JAN, Bruxton CJ, Freeman-Browne D. The aftermath of boxing. *Psychol Med* 1973;3:270–303.

48. French LR, Schuman LM, Mortimer JA, et al. A case-control study of dementia of the Alzheimer type. *Am J Epidemiol* 1985;121:414–421.

49. Graves AB, White E, Koepsell TD, et al. The association between head trauma and Alzheimer's Disease. *Am J Epidemiol* 1990;491–501.

50. Gerberich SG, Gibson RW, Fife D, et al. Effects of brain injury on college academic performance. *Neuroepidemiology* 1997;16:1–14.

51. Torg JS. Epidemiology, pathomechanics and prevention of athletic injuries to the cervical spine. *Med Sci Sports Exerc* 1985;17-295–303.

52. Tator CH. Neck injuries in ice hockey: a recent, unsolved problem with many contributing factors. *Clin Sport Med.* 1987;6:101–115.

53. Schneider RC. *Head and neck injuries in football: mechanisms, treatment, and prevention.* Baltimore: Williams & Wilkins, 1983.

54. Gerberich SG. School sports injuries. In: Association of Trial Lawyers of America, Johns Hopkins Injury Prevention Center, *Good sports: preventing recreational injuries,* 1993.

55. Reynen PD, Clancy WG. Cervical spine injury, hockey helmets, and face masks. *Am J Sports Med* 1994; 22:167–170.

56. Smith AW, Bishop PJ, Wells RP. Alterations in head dynamics with the addition of a hockey helmet and face shield under inertial loading. *Can J Appl Sports Sci,* 1985; 10: 68–74.

57. Walsh S. A proposal for the use of the half face, clear plastic visor for National Collegiate Athletic Association hockey. In: Castaldi CR, Bishop PJ, Hoerner EF, eds. *Safety in ice hockey.* Philadelphia: American Society for Testing and Materials, 1993.

58. Funk FF, Wells RE. Injuries of the cervical spine in football. *Clin Orthop* 1975;109: 50–58.

59. Feldick HG, Albright JP. Football survey reveals "missed" neck injuries. *Phys Sports Med* 1976;4:77–81.

60. Cantu RC. Guidelines for return to contact sports after a cerebral concussion. *Phys Sports Med* 1986;14:75-83.

61. Yarnell PR, Lynch S. The ding amnestic states in football trauma. *Neurology.* 1973;23:1967.

62. Kelly JP, Nichols JS, Filley CM, Lillehei KO, Rubinstein D, Kleinschmidt-DeMasters BK. Concussion in sports: guidelines for the prevention of catastrophic outcome. *JAMA* 1991,266:2867–2869.

63. Cantu RV, Cantu RC. Guidelines for return to contact sports after transient quadriplegia [Letter to the editor]. *J Neurosurg* 1994;80:592-594.

64. Gerberich SG. Sports injuries: implications for prevention. *Public Health Rep* 1985;100:570–571.

65. Hornof Z, Napravnik C. Analysis of various accident rate factors in ice hockey. *Med Sci Sports* 1973;5:283–286.

66. Biener K, Muller P. Les accidents du hockey sur glace. *Can Med* 1973;14:959–962.

67. Hayes D. *The Nature, Incidence, Location and Causes of Injury in Intercollegiate Ice Hockey.* Thesis. University of Waterloo, Ontario, Canada, 1972.

68. Hayes E. Hockey injuries: how, why, where and when. *Phys Sports Med* 1975;3:61–65.

69. Sutherland GW. Fire on ice. *Am J Sports Med.* 1976; 4:264–269.

70. Björkenheim J-M, Syvähuoko I, Rosenberg PH. Injuries in competitive junior ice-hockey. *Acta Orthop Scand* 1993;64:459–461.

71. Lorentzon R, Wedrèn H, Pietilä T. A three-year prospective study of a Swedish elite ice hockey team. *Am J Sports Med* 1988;16:392–396.

72. Norman RW, Bishop PJ, Pierrynowski MR. Puck impact response of ice hockey face masks. *Can J Appl Sports Sci* 1980;5:208–214.

Sports Neurology, Second Edition,
edited by Barry D. Jordan.
Lippincott–Raven Publishers, Philadelphia © 1998.

34

Martial Arts

Richard D. Birrer

Family Medicine/Emergency Medicine, Catholic Medical Center of Brooklyn and Queens,
88-25 153rd Street, Jamaica, New York, 11432

The martial arts are broadly defined as the fighting systems derived from Asia. Familiar examples include judo, aikido, jujitsu, karate, tae kwon do, kempo, and kung fu. Each system emphasizes certain techniques (i.e., kicks, punches, throws, or grabs) and strategies (i.e., use of the opponent's momentum or offensive posturing). There are many styles or variations within each school. The number of participants in the sport is now more than 8,000,000 nationally (1). An estimated 75,000,000 individuals train internationally, and the number continues to grow. New schools and styles within a system spring up on a regular basis, so that it is no longer possible to view the sport as organized under a central body of rules and regulations. As a result, it is virtually impossible to enforce existing guidelines and recommendations. Nonetheless, the Amateur Athletic Union and the U.S. Olympic Committee have developed and established rules and regulations governing tournament conditions. Judo has been a regular part of the Olympic Games for more than three decades now, and tae kwon do had a premier demonstration in the 1988 games.

EPIDEMIOLOGY

Little research has been done investigating the profile of the martial arts athlete, injury type and extent, or merits of one style over another. Because of the historical and political development of the martial arts, it has been difficult to collect accurate data on the type, frequency, extent, predisposing risk factors for, and prevention of injuries. For the most part, data have usually been derived from retrospective surveys, observations at tournaments and training halls, and the analysis of hospital emergency department records. Since 1976 approximately 54,000 martial arts injuries have been catalogued by a number of national and international survey (2–6). In addition 245,000 injuries have been estimated for the same period on the basis of electronic surveillance data (7).

When the data are broken down into actual injuries, approximately 17,500 athletes with a 4:1 male/female distribution have been involved (5,7). Approximately 30% of the injuries occurred in tournament or competitive situations, with the remaining 70% occurring in nontournament or training situations. The total actual data represent approximately 24,000 martial arts years. Overall, there were 1.71 injuries per athlete-year. Tournament or competitive conditions were characterized by a greater injury rate and more severe injuries. Males experienced significantly higher injury rates and severity compared with females. The distribution of injuries by type was contusions, 43%; sprains and strains, 34%; lacerations and abrasions, 15%; and fracture-dislocations, 6%. When classified by anatomic site, the lower extremity was involved approximately 31% of the time, and the neck was injured least often (2%). Injuries to the remaining portions of the body occurred between the two extremes. Most injures were mild to moderate in extent, with less than 5% considered severe or very severe. However, although

11% of all injuries occurred to the face and head, such injuries were ranked as most severe; the hospitalization rate was 0.32 per 100,000 participants per year (7). There were 28 deaths recorded. Rarer, serious injuries have been reported in the medical literature (8–20).

In terms of specific neurologic trauma, the survey data are not sufficient to make general comments on or predictions of injury in this sport. Nonetheless, sporadic neurologic injuries have been reported. Most of the reported deaths in the martial arts have involved neurologic damage to the head and neck.

TYPES OF NEUROLOGIC INJURIES

Craniocerebral Injuries

It is unclear from the literature whether judo or karate causes more craniocerebral injuries (21); however, it does appear that judo causes more serious craniocerebral injuries when they occur (22) (Table 1). The usual mechanism of injury in judo is an impact from a throwing technique. Craniocerebral injury in karate is most commonly due to an erroneous kick, although less frequently it has followed a missed fall or inappropriate punch (20).

Most cases of martial arts head trauma involve contusions of the soft tissues of the face and scalp. Lacerations, abrasions, nasal hemorrhage, fractures of the teeth, and orbital injuries are common in karate. Orbital blowout fractures have been noted in erroneous straight punches

TABLE 1. *Craniocerebral injuries in the martial arts*

Cranial
Soft tissue contusion
Lacerations
Abrasions
Nasal hemorrhage
Tooth fractures
Eye injuries (including retinal detachment)
Skull fracture
Cerebral
Concussion
Cerebral contusion
Cerebral infarction
Subdural hematoma
Intracerebral hemorrhage
Subarachnoid hemorrhage

and roundhouse kicks. Blind spinning back kicks have led to fracture of the zygoma process and maxilla. Concussions typically follow a missed fall or excessive blow from either a foot or a fist in noncontact tournament conditions (23). Most concussions are grade I, with the athletes being "dinged" or "out on their feet." Recovery is usually prompt and complete in most cases. However, there may be delayed recovery in some individuals, placing them at risk for the "second impact" syndrome (24).

More serious head injuries have included skull fracture, retinal detachment, cerebral contusions, cerebral infarction, subdural and intracerebral hemorrhages, and rupture of a berry aneurysm. At least 19 cases of skull fracture, most of which involved the facial bones, were recorded. Of these, 63% recovered fully, but the remainder had permanent sequelae such as partial field or unilateral blindness, posttraumatic epilepsy, or cosmetic deformity. Two cases of nonfatal cerebral infarction followed excessive karate blows to the head (25,26). There have been three cases of acute subdural hematomas recorded in judo from missed falls (27). There were nine deaths due to head injury: intracerebral hemorrhage (four), subdural hemorrhage (three), ruptured berry aneurysm (one), and massive cerebral contusions (one). Seven of these injuries followed missed falls in judo in which the athlete landed on his or her head, particularly the temporoparietal and occipital portion of the skull (28,29). The case of the ruptured berry aneurysm also occurred during judo but was not associated with a throwing technique. There were two deaths in karate, both of which appeared to have followed an excessive blow to the head from a spinning back kick and roundhouse kick (20,28). Long-term sequelae, such as the "punch drunk" syndrome seen in boxers, have been reported in the sport (30,31). Strangle or "sleeper" holds in judo may cause clinically significant anoxic injury by reduction of blood flow to the brain (32,33).

Neck Injuries

Neck injuries in the martial arts may be secondary to a forceful blow to the head or a fall on the head or neck. Blind spinning back kicks or inappropriately excessive front or roundhouse kicks have been noted to produce cervical fracture-dislocations. There have been at least 17 deaths in judo and karate due to cervical fracture-dislocations, with most occurring in judo (29). One case was associated with a preexisting cervical anomaly of congenital stenosis of the spinal canal (34). The usual mechanism of injury consists of a beginner who is thrown and lands on the front of the head or the back of the neck (35). The soft tissues of the neck may also be injured from a direct karate blow or the judo technique of strangling (i.e., "sleeper" hold) (36). At least two cases of extracranial artery trauma have resulted from the use of such techniques (37,38). One case involved thrombosis with laryngeal fracture and the other vertebral artery dissection.

Back Injuries

The lower spine is vulnerable to injury when the defending player forcibly resists the attacking player, striking at the waist. The use of a biased throwing technique in judo can lead to spondylolysis (28). Any lifting or throwing technique with violent twisting of the body can result in a fracture of the pars interarticularis. A 2-mm rotation of a vertebral body can greatly impinge on the neural foramina, resulting in pain. If the injury is not carefully managed with appropriate rehabilitative exercises and a lumbar corset to allow healing, which often takes 6 to 9 months, spondylolisthesis and chronic pain result. Although cases of grade II and III spondylolisthesis have been successfully managed in the sport of martial arts, significant amounts of pain and disability frequently accompany the condition. A modification of training techniques, choosing an alternative martial art such as tai chi, and surgery should be considered for grade III and IV slippages.

Peripheral Nerve Injuries

Damage to peripheral nerves in the martial arts is uncommon. Nonetheless, a focused direct or indirect blow can cause neural contusion and, rarely, rupture (Table 2). A blow to the upper outer arm from a roundhouse kick as occurs in sparring has been noted to lead to radial nerve contusion. This

TABLE 2. *Peripheral nerves that have been injured in the martial arts*

Radial nerve
Ulnar nerve
Peroneal nerve
Axillary nerve
Long thoracic nerve
Spinal accessory nerve
Interdigital nerve of the foot
Dorsal scapular nerve

injury is characterized by weakness of wrist and/or finger extension and paresthesias in the distribution of the radial pulsary branch.

A blow to or a fall on the posterior elbow has caused contusion to the ulnar nerve in its groove along the medial epicondyle of the humerus. Similarly, the repeated practice of an incorrectly executed knife hand strike on a hard surface has led to contusion and fibrosis of the peripheral branch of the ulnar nerve. Paresis, paresthesias, and even atrophy of the ulnar side of the hand were noted in one case (39).

Peroneal nerve injury has also been documented in martial arts (40). Although strikes and kicks below the belt are not allowed during competitive training, a blocked crescent kick or a side kick to the lateral aspect of the knee has been noted to contuse the peroneal nerve, leading to paresis, pain, and/or paresthesias. Usually the "electrical shock" or tingling that shoots through the distribution of the nerve to the lateral side of the leg and dorsal foot lasts seconds to minutes, unless actual damage to the nerve has resulted. More significant injury with hemorrhage into the nerve sheath or actual crash of the nerve itself can result in weakness of ankle dorsiflexion and potential foot paralysis.

Repeated irritation of the ball of the foot (from kicks or stances), particularly in the area of the third and fourth toes, has produced or aggravated a Morton's neuroma (39). Click associated with numbness of the adjacent sides of the two involved toes is typically present and is commonly associated with a tingling sensation or electric shock feeling that runs down into the same toes.

Contusions of the anterior portion of the shoulder resulting from direct kicks or punches or a missed fall have produced trauma to the axillary, long thoracic, and dorsal scapular nerves (41). A direct blow striking just between the coracoid and the head of the humerus may contuse the axillary nerve. Severe numbing pain in the arm may occur, which causes the athlete to feel that the arm is useless. There may be sensory loss and dysfunction of the muscles of the upper arm. There has been one case of persistent deltoid paralysis with an area of hypesthesia in the circumflex distribution of the axillary nerve (39).

Due to a sharp blow to the base of the neck, damage to the long thoracic nerve may result in scapula winging alata (42). Such an injury results in loss of scapular fixation to the chest wall; if the arm is pulled forward, the vertebral border of the scapula swings outward.

The spinal accessory nerve, which is located somewhat superficially near the surface of the trapezius muscle, has been injured by direct blows to that area from inappropriate karate chops and kicks (39). The athlete usually has difficulty in elevating the shoulder toward the ear and may show scapula winging with an abduction. There may be severe aching pain as well. Symptomatic therapy has usually sufficed. Injuries to the other long nerves of the body (i.e., median, sciatic, and obturator) have thus far not been reported in the martial arts.

RETURN TO PLAY

The athlete can return to training or competition following an acute injury as long as the physical examination is normal and there are no complaints of paresthesias, pain, or weakness. Significantly, there should be full active and passive range of motion and normal strength, mental status, station, and gait, including the ability to cut and do figure-of-eights. In addition, an individual who has suffered a concussion irrespective of the grade should refrain from further activity until cleared neurologically. Individuals who have a chronic neurologic injury should be assessed for disability based on sensory, motor, and mental deficits. Any deficits that impair the athlete's coordination, strength, or orientation prohibit competition. Training within the limits of pain and disability is acceptable as long as it does not lead to further injury or disability.

PREVENTION

In general, despite the difficulties in obtaining raw data on injuries and making valid comparisons among different studies, it can be said that the risk of neurologic injury is small in the martial arts. Nevertheless, when neurologic trauma does occur, it is more severe than injuries to other organ systems. Approximately 80% of deaths recorded in the martial arts are due to neurologic injury. Prevention of these potentially devastating injuries, therefore, is of paramount importance (5,43) (Table 3).

As already noted, the major risk factors include direct and indirect blows to the head and cervical spine, with most of these occurring in a nonsupervised or poorly supervised setting (44). Prevention, therefore, consists of safe instruction from a qualified trainer (45). In many instances it is difficult to determine the qualifications of the trainer because of the differences in certification among martial arts styles and systems. Often an interview with the instructor, observation of actual teaching methods, and informal talks with students and other trainers are the sole criteria for a student's decision about the safety of the instruction. Certainly, a training hall with functional equipment, clean mats, and a set of rules or guidelines that are enforced are reliable indicators of a safety-conscious environment. On the other hand, unhygienic locker rooms, absence of or lack of enforcement of regulations in the training hall, and poor upkeep of equipment indicate a low concern for the safety of the athletes. At a minimum, the training hall rules or guidelines should instill a solid sense of confidence through discipline. Excessive force or contact and unsporting conduct are unacceptable in a training hall situation and should be dealt with firmly. The early introduction of sparring and advanced techniques such as jumps, sweeps, and throws

TABLE 3. *Prevention of neurologic injury in the martial arts*

Supervision by trained personnel certified in first aid and basic cardiac life support
Safe conditioning and training
Regular use of protective equipment
Appropriate medical supervision at competitions and tournaments

without an effective period of conditioning and training is equally unacceptable because of the potential for serious injury.

Use of protective gear is of secondary preventive importance. The currently available headgear does not protect the cervical spine. Head injury caused by direct or indirect blows in the training hall situation is for the most part uncommon. In such situations training partners usually know one another well, and techniques are controlled by the instructor. It has also been argued that headgear is clumsy and reduces peripheral vision, but there have been no prospective or retrospective studies done to determine whether this is the case. The use of headgear should be reserved for tournament situations irrespective of the amount of contact allowed. Although most tournaments in the United States are noncontact, the stresses of the competitive situation and the varied enforcement of regulations often lead to inadvertent contact to the head and ancillary structures. The use of other protective gear is regularly recommended for the prevention of other organ system injuries. At this time it is not possible to make any substantive comments about whether such gear will have a favorable impact on the reduction of peripheral neurologic injuries.

Finally, competitive situations such as tournaments should be supervised by a licensed physician. McLatchie and Morris (46) have shown that trained medical officers can significantly reduce the number and severity of injuries in the sport. Many tournaments are not supervised by a physician; rather, a health paraprofessional such as an emergency medical technician, nurse, physician assistant, or trainer provides coverage. Such individuals as well as the tournament sponsors take significant risks of litigation.

REFERENCES

1. *The Perrier study of fitness in america.* New York: Lewis & Harris Associates, 1979.
2. Birrer RB, Birrer CD. Martial arts injuries. *Phys Sports Med* 1982;10:103–108.
3. Birrer RB, Birrer CD. Unreported injuries in the martial arts. *Br J Sports Med* 1983;17;131–134.
4. Birrer RB, Halbrook SP. Martial arts injuries: the results of a five-year national survey. *Am J Sports Med* 1988; 16;408–410.
5. Birrer RB. Injury epidemiology in the martial arts. *Am J Sports Med* 1996;24:72–79.
6. McLatchie GR. Analysis of karate injuries sustained in 295 contests. *Injury* 1976;8:132–134.
7. U.S. Consumer Product Safety Commission. *Martial arts: National Electronic Injury Surveillance System (NEISS), 1979–1994,* vols 2–18. Washington, DC: National Injury Information Clearing House.
8. Saito K. Sports in orthopaedic surgery. *J Jpn Orthop Assoc* 1934;9:540–544.
9. Kurland H. A short study of tournament injuries. *Karate Illus* 1981;3;32–36.
10. Dvorine W. Kendo: a safer martial art. *Phys Sports Med* 1979;7:87–89.
11. Birrer RB, Birrer CD, Son DS, et al. Injuries in tae kwon do. *Phys Sports Med* 1981;9;97–103.
12. Stricevic MV, Patel MR. Okazaki T, et al. Karate: historical perspective on injuries sustained in national and international tournament competitions. *Am J Sports Med* 1983;11:320–324.
13. McLatchie GR. Surgical and orthopaedic problems in sport karate. *Medisport* 1979;1:40–44.
14. Kurland H. Injuries in karate. *Phys Sports Med* 1983;10: 80–85.
15. Cantwell JD, King JT. Karate chops and liver lacerations. *JAMA* 1973;224:1424.
16. McLatchie GR, Davies JE, Caulley JH. Injuries in karate: a case for medical control. *J Trauma* 1980; 20: 956–958.
17. Hirata K. Injuries of karate in all Japan. *Jpn Educ Med* 1967;3;123–124.
18. Kodama T. Sports injury. *Jpn J Phys Fitness* 1962; 3;45–49.
19. Birrer RB, Robinson T. Pelvic fracture following karate kick. *N Y State Med J* 1991;91:503.
20. Oler M, Tomson W, Pepe H, et al. Morbidity and mortality in the martial arts: a warning. *J. Trauma* 1991; 31:251–253.
21. Hirakawa K, Hashizume K, Nakamura N, et al. Head injuries in sports. *Brain Nerve Inj* 1971;3:579 (Japanese).
22. Jackson F, Earle KM, Beamer Y, et al. Blunt head injuries incurred by Marine recruits in hand-to-hand combat (judo training). *Milit Med* 1967;132:803–808.
23. Zemper ED, Pieter W. Cerebral concussions in tae kwon do athletes. In: Hoerner EF, ed. *Head and neck injuries in sports.* ASTM STP 1229. Philadelphia: ASTM, 1994.
24. Gronwall D, Wrightson P. Delayed recovery of intellectual function after minor head injury. *Lancet* 1974: 2:605–609.
25. Almer S. Westerberg CE. Discussion of the panorama of injuries associated with karate; potential risks need new attention; brain infarction in an 18-year-old boy after a karate blow. *Lakarditningen* 1985;82:2886–2888.
26. Almer S, Westerberg CE. Cerebral infarction following a karate fight. *Presse Med* 1985:14:2299.
27. DeVera-Reyes JA. Three cases of chronic subdural hematoma caused by the practice of judo. *Acta Luso Esp Neurol Psiquiatr* 1970;29:53–56.
28. Nakamura N. Judo and karate—do. In: Schneider RD, Kennedy JC, Plant ML, eds. *Sports injuries; mechanisms, prevention and treatment.* Baltimore: Williams & Wilkins, 1985:417–430.
29. Koiwai EK. Fatalities associated with judo. *Phys Sports Med* 1981;9:61–66.
30. Stiller JW, Weinberger BR. Boxing and chronic brain damage. *Psychiatr Clin North Am* 1985;8:339–356.

31. Birrer RB, Robinson T. Pelvic fracture following karate kick. *N.Y State Med J* 1991;91:503.

32. Owens RG, Ghadiali EJ. Judo as a possible cause of anoxic brain damage. A case report. *J Sports Med Phys Fitness* 1991;31:627–628.

33. Rodriguez G, Francione S, Gardella M, et al. Judo and choking: EEG and regional cerebral blood flow findings. *J Sports Med Phys Fitness* 1991;31:605–610.

34. Godt P, Vogelsang H. Uncommon judo injuries: cervical disk herniation and acute high cervical cord damage associated with congenital stenosis of the cervical spinal canal. *Unfallheikunde* 1979;82:215–218.

35. Torg JA. Epidemiology, pathomechanics, and prevention of athletic injuries to the cervical spine. *Med Sci Sports Exerc* 1985;17:295–303.

36. Koiwai EK. Deaths allegedly caused by the use of "choke holds" (Shime-Waza). *J Forensic Sci* 1987; 32:419–432.

37. Lannuzel A, Moulin T, Amsallem D, et al. Vertebral-artery dissection following a judo session: a case report. *Neuropediatrics* 1994;25(2):106–108.

38. Wos W, Puzio J, Opala G. Traumatic internal carotid artery thrombosis following karate blow. *Pol Przegl Chir* 1977;9:1271–1273.

39. Nieman EA, Swan PG. Karate injuries. *Br Med J* 1971;1:233–235.

40. Cossa JF, Evrard D, Poilleux R. Un des inconvenients du judo: Luxation isolee del'articulation peroneo-tibiale superiuvre. *Rev Chir Ortho Reparatrice Appareil Moteur* 1968;54(2):211–214.

41. Jerosch J, Castro WH, Geske B. Damage of the long thoracic and dorsal scapular nerve after traumatic shoulder dislocation: case report and review of the literature. *Acta Orthop Belg* 1990;56(3–4):625–627.

42. Bjerrum L. Scapula alta induced by karate. *Ugeskr Laeger* 1984;146:202.

43. Kodama T. Sport injuries and their prevention. Proceedings of the International Congress of Sports Science. Basel, Switzerland, 1964.

44. McLatchie GR. Recommendations for medical officers attending karate competitions. *Br J Sports Med* 1979; 13:36–37.

45. Hirano K, Seto M. Dangers of karate. *JAMA* 1973; 226:1118–1119.

46. McLatchie GR, Morris EW. Prevention of karate injuries—a progress report. *Br J Sports Med* 1977; 11:78–82.

Sports Neurology, Second Edition,
edited by Barry D. Jordan.
Lippincott–Raven Publishers, Philadelphia © 1998.

35

Mountain Climbing

Edward G. Hixon

Adirondack Surgical Group, RFD Box 410 B, Lake Colby Drive, Lake Saranac, New York 12983

Mountaineering is an individual sport. Its informality is an attraction, with personal goals that are hard to define. Adaptation to the often hostile wilderness mountain environment is basic. The sport is protean and not subject to empirical analysis. The neurologic complications of mountaineering medical problems account for the greatest morbidity and mortality.

The popularity of mountaineering is increasing. The American Alpine Club has estimated that there are more than 100,000 active climbers in the United States (1). Grand Teton National Park records more than 8000 climbs yearly (2). Joshua Tree National Monument estimates 4000 climbers daily on big weekends and 300,000 climber days yearly. Very high altitude is reached by more than 5000 climbers and trekkers in the Himalaya each year (3). As more people become involved, medical problems increase. Climbing is a hazardous sport. Risks enhance the excitement and become an attraction for some. Most climbs are accomplished by small groups and are unrecorded. Rates of injury and illness are difficult to determine. At best, they are extrapolations or rough estimates. Knowledge of mountaineering medical problems is based on anecdotal evidence. Indeed, many altitude research data are collected under extreme conditions. This does not detract from the validity of observations but provides the context for reaching conclusions from data that are incomplete or subjective.

As most of the world's highest summits have been attained, climbers have sought to achieve different goals. Climbing "by fair means" (without supplemental oxygen) has replaced a preoccupation with oxygen apparatus design and use for extreme altitude. Rock walls that once were climbed with the use of artificial direct aids (pitons, bolts, and so forth) are now climbed solo and "clean," in a fraction of the time previously required. The mountaineer's goal has become ascent of the most difficult route, use of the simplest and least amount of equipment, and choice of the most difficult time (winter). Involvement with the environment is passionately sought without violating it in any way. "Take only pictures. Leave only footsteps." As attractive as these philosophical approaches are, the potential for injury and illness may be increased. The ultimate accomplishment, "by fair means," was Reinhold Messner's and Peter Habelar's ascent of Mt. Everest without supplemental oxygen in 1978 (4). Since that time Messner has climbed all 14 of the world's highest peaks (over 8000 m) solo and without supplemental oxygen. This accomplishment is a particularly important milestone because many members of the scientific community felt that it was impossible. It was believed that the hypoxia of extreme altitude would result in permanent neurologic injury or death. Although Messner, Habelar, and several additional climbers (including Larry Nielson, United States, 1983) have attained the summit of Everest (29,028 feet) without supplemental oxygen and have no ill effects, concern remains. There is increasing evidence of neurologic complications. Subtle neurologic and neuropsychologic long-term deficits have been reported (5,6). Neuropsychologic changes are described by virtually all climbers who ascend to extreme altitude. Residual neurobehavioral impairment has been described in 58% of extreme altitude climbers, all of whom had a normal neurologic examination. Structural abnormalities were documented by magnetic resonance imaging (MRI) in 48% (7). Transient and permanent neurologic complications secondary to altitude illness are established. These range from impairment of cognitive function to hemiplegia (8–15). Neuromuscular problems have been attributed to peripheral hypoxic effects on the muscle fiber as well as central effects (16). The risk of permanent neurologic deficit following exposure to altitude, with or without illness, cannot be ignored.

Included are avalanche, weather, lightning, rock and icefall, altitude, and earthquake. Subjective hazards are under the climber's control. Included are accidents due to inexperience, skill and ability deficits, poor conditioning, misuse of equipment, and group dynamic problems. The climber must maximize avoidance of objective hazard and control of subjective hazard. Messner has stated that the secret to survival on 8000 m peaks is the ability to avoid objective hazard. He did not say how; this appears to be largely due to experience and instinct. In North America, where there are more inexperienced climbers, there are more accidents related to subjective hazards. The ratio of subjective to objective is 3:1. In the Himalaya, the domain of the experienced, objective hazard predominates (ratio reversed).

MOUNTAINEERING HAZARD

The danger involved in mountaineering is inherent. From 1921 to 1979, 77 climbers reached the summit of Mt. Everest (29,028 feet or 8,848 m). There were 17 expeditions successful in placing climbers on the summit (17). Out of 43 expeditions, 44 known deaths occurred (4).

Mountaineering hazard may be categorized as objective or subjective. Objective hazard is independent of the climber's control and due to the environment or weather for the most part. Accidents due to objective hazard are "acts of God."

ALTITUDE

Altitude is best described in terms of its effect on the climber (Fig. 1). High altitude is from 5000 feet (1500 m) to 11,500 feet (3500 m). At high altitude, most healthy climbers experience mild symptoms but rapidly become able to tolerate them. The risk of severe altitude illness is low. Very high altitude is from 11,500 feet (3500 m) to 18,000 feet (5500 m). Here climbers are able to function by acclimatization. The risk of severe altitude illness is increased. Extreme altitude is above 18,000 feet (5500 m). It is survivable only

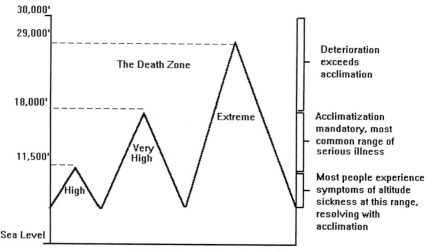

FIG. 1. The climber at altitude.

by allowing for acclimati-zation by slow ascent. This is the death zone. Deterioration takes place faster than the benefits of acclimatization. The risk of serious altitude illness is high (18). Rapid ascent to extreme altitude is likely to be fatal. This was learned in 1875 by the occupants of the balloon Zenith, which ascended to above 25,000 feet. Two of three survived (19). Messner's and Habelar's ascent of Mt. Everest (29,028 feet) in 1978 was possible only by superb acclimatization. The difference is in the rate of ascent, hours versus weeks.

Slow ascent (weeks) allows acclimatization. A good rule is to limit ascent to 2000 feet a day above 5000 feet (20). Acclimatization is necessary for comfort at high altitude, health and function at very high altitude, and survival at extreme altitude.

The percentage of oxygen in the air is constant at 20.93% regardless of altitude. As altitude increases, the barometric pressure (the sum of the partial pressures of all gases of the atmosphere) decreases. In proportion to the decrease in barometric pressure, the partial pressure of oxygen decreases. As the partial pressure of oxygen in ambient air decreases, the pressure of oxygen in the body decreases the arterial P_{O_2}. The necessity of acclimatization has been well demonstrated. The stimulus for acclimatization is hypoxia, practically speaking at about 10,000 feet or 3000 m. The climber's aerobic power or maximum oxygen uptake (MV_{O_2} max) is not improved by acclimatization and is dependent on the oxygen tension in the ambient air and the blood. The MV_{O_2} max decreases at a rate of 3% per 1000 feet gain in altitude. (18, p. 8; 19, p. 227). Acclimatization increases the climber's capacity for work, given the limitation of decreased aerobic capacity that is obligate with increasing altitude.

The process of acclimatization is complex and affects the whole body. Hyperventilation occurs in response to hypoxia producing respiratory alkalosis. This causes an increase in alveolar oxygen by forcing more oxygen into the lungs with a corresponding decrease in carbon dioxide. The kidney increases excretion of bicarbonate to offset alkalosis and maintain a more normal pH. The body is therefore able to maintain its hemoglobin saturation with oxygen in a hypoxic environment (O_2sat). O_2sat is maintained in the 90%

to 70% range with increasing altitude by acclimatization up to extreme heights. Above 18,000 feet (5500 m), O_2sat falls rapidly with increasing altitude to levels of about 55% at 29,000 feet (9000 m), lower with exercise. At levels of 20,000 feet, on a cellular level, oxygen transport is "maxed out," and no further oxygen is extracted (21). The cardiorespiratory changes mentioned take approximately 3 weeks to become maximal for most individuals.

Erythropoiesis is stimulated by hypoxia. Blood hemoglobin increases to over 20 g/100 mL, hematocrit above 60%. Above this level the viscosity of the blood dramatically increases, and the benefit of increased carrying capacity of oxygen is decreased. The opitmum hematocrit is 50% to 60% (19,p.182;22). Higher hemoglobin and hematocrit are associated with thromboembolic disease and are maladaptive. Hematologic acclimatization takes about 6 weeks.

Acclimatized climbers on the summit of Mt. Everest without supplemental oxygen are near death. The atmospheric pressure is 253 torr (23). In 1981, Dr. Chris Pizzo obtained alveolar samples of himself on the summit of Mt. Everest. He was not using oxygen. From these samples, the arterial P_{O_2} was calculated to be 30 torr and the P_{CO_2} was 6 torr (23). The O_2sat was calculated to be from 73% to 63.4%, possibly lower with exercise at this altitude (29,028 feet). Life is barely sustained.

Acclimatization is accompanied by many complex changes on a cellular level, as well as at a system level. Despite acclimatization, hypoxia persists and progresses to severe levels. Neurologic symptoms are universal; the extreme altitude mountaineer is in a state of chronic neurologic deficiency. The hypocapnea of hyperventilation (cerebral vasoconstriction) is overridden by hypoxic vasodilation. Increased cerebral blood flow (CBF) results. At 5430 m an increase of 67% has been described (24). Neurologic problems have previously been described. Neurobehavioral changes such as paranoia, obsessiveness, depression, and anxiety have been described with changes in the Minnesota Multiphasic Personality Inventory (25,26).

Additional changes occur at altitude. Temperature decreases 6.5°C with every 1000 m increase in altitude. Wind velocity is dramatically increased at altitude. The increase in the wind chill index increases the risk of cold injury, hypothermia, and frostbite. Thin air increases the ultraviolet irradiation, which is magnified by reflection from snow and ice. Sunburn, snowblindness, and even heat injury can occur. The humidity of the air is low. With hyperventilation, the result is dramatic pulmonary water loss. Mental status changes and other neurologic symptoms are protopathic to these conditions. The neurologic problems of altitude are thus expanded by other coexisting conditions such as hypothermia and dehydration.

ALTITUDE ILLNESS

Mountaineers risk altitude illness at extreme, very high, and high altitude. The syndromes of altitude sickness are discussed separately but all have in common the etiology, altitude hypoxia. There may be a progression of symptoms form mild to severe. These may include symptoms from one or all of the major syndromes, or one symptom may predominate and present acutely with no warning. In most altitude illness, neurologic symptoms are present or dominate.

Altitude in excess of 10,000 feet (3000 m) is usually required for illness to develop. Good physical condition offers no protection from altitude illness but is of obvious benefit to mountaineers in general. Illness is most likely to affect those who climb too fast, climb too high, work too hard, and stay too long. An attitude of immortality, underestimation of the effects of altitude, enthusiasm, impatience, and excessive goal orientation are predisposing personality traits. Good conditioning, strength, and endurance, when combined with these traits, are characteristic of but not confined to youth. Highly motivated young mountaineers are more likely to develop mountain illness unless thorough knowledge and a prophylactic strategy are incorporated in their climbing plan. Anaerobic exercise early in an ascent is more detrimental than aerobic. Acclimatization is the best way to avoid sickness; it is under the control of the climber. Slow ascent with adequate rest is the key. Ascents may be categorized: rapid—hours, fast—days, and slow—weeks. Ascending at rates of 1000 to 2000 feet daily at altitude above 5000 feet is optimal with rest days interspersed (19,20). The climbers' dictum "climb high but sleep low" is good advice. Acclimatization usually takes as long as 3 to 6 weeks for those going to extreme altitude. For lower altitudes, less time is required. (Three weeks is a good estimate for optimal performance and enjoyment of altitude.) There is a popular approach among climbers to climb extremely fast and return before developing symptoms. This is dangerous unless preceded by a necessary acclimatization period (3 to 6 weeks) at a high base camp (10,000 to 15,000 feet). Again, there are no acclimatization benefits of altitudes below 10,000 feet. (lack of sufficient hypoxic stimulus) or of altitudes above 20,000 feet (deterioration exceeds acclimatization benefits).

ACUTE MOUNTAIN SICKNESS

From 8000 to 9000 feet, 12% may be expected to develop acute mountain sickness (AMS) (Table 1) (27). At 14,000 feet, 52.5% are afflicted (28). After 24 to 48 hours of exposure to altitude, symptoms of AMS may develop. Shortness of breath, weakness, malaise, anorexia, headache, insomnia, nausea, and vomiting are included to variable degrees. Sleep may be accompanied or disturbed by Cheyne-Stokes respiration. Symptoms are often worse at the end of the day and at night. The degree of severity ranges from mild, where the climber can "bite the bullet" and continue, to severe, where one is totally incapacitated. AMS is self-limited and usually resolves in a few more days; a few cases progress to more severe altitude illness.

AMS is a neurologic symptom complex with headache dominant. Edema is a common occurrence in all altitude illness. Fluid retention is noticed by puffy facies, tight rings, ankle swelling, and elevation of blood pressure. Prior to the development of hyperventilation (previously described as a key element of acclimatization), hypercapnea is present. This produces cerebral vasodilation. Increased cerebral blood flow (CBF), vasodilation, hypertension, and generalized edema occur before the compensation of acclimatization. AMS develops, especially headache. This headache is relieved by oxygen and forced hyperventilation temporarily.

TABLE 1. *Altitude illness*

Syndrome	Incidence	Onset	Hallmark symptoms	Treatment	Sequelae
Acute mountain sickness (AMS)	12% 8000–9000 ft (27)	1–2 days	Headache, malaise, anorexia	Acetazolamide (descent unnecessary)	None
High-altitude pulmonary edema (HAPE)	0.5% 11,500 ft (35)	2–3 days	Dyspnea, cough, frothy sputum, cyanosis	Descent mandatory, diuresis, furosemide, oxygen, pressurization	Survivors experience none
High-altitude cerebral edema (HACE)	0.02% (1.8% of AMS experience HACE) above 12,000 ft (27)	2–3 days	Ataxia, severe headache, altered mental status	Descent mandatory, dexamethasone, acetazolamide, oxygen, pressurization	Survivors may experience severe neurological deficit
High-altitude retinal hemorrhage (HARH)	56% 17,000 ft and above (39)	Unknown	None	None	None (rare scotoma)
High-altitude cachexia (HAC)	100% above 18,600 ft for extended periods (weeks)	Gradual	Weight loss, weakness, loss of vigor	High caloric Intake, high-carbohydrate diet	None

It is aggravated by anaerobic exercise (hypertension producing).

As the disease is nonfatal and self-limited, treatment other than time is not necessary. Descent is necessary only for severe cases. The symptoms are ameliorated by the use of acetazolamide (Diamox). Acetazolamide is a carbonic anhydrase inhibitor that causes hyperventilation and hypocapnea. It is also a mild diuretic and diminishes fluid retention. For treatment, doses of 250 to 500 mg twice daily are usually adequate. A degree of prophylaxis can be obtained by starting several days prior to ascent. The side effects of numbness and tingling of the hands and feet are relieved by dose reduction. The mechanism is much more complex, but simplistically it may be considered to simulate acclimatization. Other medications have been suggested, such as ibuprofen, steroids, sumatripan, and nifedipine, among many others. My personal preference is acetazolamide as it is simple, safe, effective, and inexpensive. It appears to address the physiologic need. If headache is not relieved, I prefer ibuprofen, 400 mg. This usually works well in spite of a tendency to aggravate fluid retention. I believe it best to avoid "sleeping pills" at altitude and favor acetazolamide for sleep disturbance.

Descent is rarely necessary. It is appropriate for the small number (2%) who are severely incapacitated and are likely to progress to more severe altitude illness. In many ways, AMS is similar to seasickness—"You're not going to die but you wish you would."

HIGH-ALTITUDE PULMONARY EDEMA

High-altitude pulmonary edema (HAPE) was first described by Houston in 1960 (Table 1) (29). It can occur at high altitude but is most often seen very high. Symptoms usually appear after 2 to 3 days. Dyspnea is severe and progresses from cough to frank pulmonary edema with frothy, bloody sputum. The outpouring of edema fluid is rapid and may progress to death in hours; victims drown in their own edema. The fluid is a transudate but it occurs in the absence of right heart failure. There are similarities to adult respiratory distress syndrome. Cyanosis is dramatic and may be accentuated by the hemoconcentration at alti-

tude. Pulmonary hypertension is present, along with increased permeability, generalized edema, and decreased oxygen transport.

Treatment with diuretics such as furosamide (Lasix) has been recommended. In the mountain environment, climbers are often dehydrated and hypotension is a risk. Morphine, recommended for cardiac edema, risks respiratory depression. HAPE occurs in individuals whose respiratory response to altitude is diminished (30). The calcium channel blocker nifedipine, in doses of 20 mg sublingually followed by 20 mg of sustained-release formulation, has been shown to be successful in treating HAPE and may be the drug of choice (31). Prophylactic use has been recommended (32). The drug treatment of HAPE is sophisticated and requires a knowledgeable and experienced physician. It is inappropriate for untrained personnel to carry dangerous medications in a kit and use them in a cookbook fashion.

The concept of treatment of HAPE by pressurized chambers is not new and is effective. Previously, the equipment was too cumbersome to be of benefit to the mountaineer. Pressurized bags are now available. The concept is to bring the victim to a lower altitude artificially by enclosing the victim in a pressurized bag. The Gamow and Certex bags are pressurized by foot pumps to 140 and 220 mbar, respectively (altitude reduction equivalents of 1500 and 2500 m, respectively). The benefits of hyperbaric treatment can by dramatic. Perfection of the techniques and equipment is continuing (33). These devices may be particularly appropriate for expeditions supported by lay personnel.

Hospital treatment of HAPE includes artificial ventilation and endotracheal intubation. Oxygenation may require supplementation with positive end-expiratory pressure (PEEP). The usual risks of hypotension and barotrauma (pneumothorax) are to be considered. An additional hazard in HAPE is the aggravation of associated cerebral edema leading to coma by impedance of venous return by PEEP.

The treatment which is most often lifesaving, is descent. It must be as rapid as possible beginning with the earliest symptom. A few thousand feet may be all that is necessary. It is observed that recovery is rapid. It is also said that following recovery the victim may resume climbing. This, although possible, is rarely practical and, from personal experience, a bad idea. Drug administration, if sophisticated, may be advantageous but even in the best of circumstances should not delay descent. Oxygen is beneficial and can be given during descent. HAPE has been noted in well-conditioned, well-acclimatized experienced climbers. An incidence ranging from 0.5% to 15.5% could be anticipated (34). It is highest in young adolescents. In the Himalaya an incidence of 0.5% of those going to 3500 m has been recorded (35). In Peru, an incidence of 0.6% has been reported for those going to 3750 m (36).

HIGH-ALTITUDE CEREBRAL EDEMA

High-altitude cerebral edema (HACE) is encountered at altitudes usually above 12,000 feet (Table 1). It was first described in 1975 by Houston and Dickinson (37). Two or three days pass prior to development of symptoms. The predominant symptom is severe headache. Changes in mental status follow: decreased cognitive ability, ataxia, hallucinations, stupor, and coma, with rapid progression to death. HAPE and HACE are dangerous and the mortality rate is in the range of 50% if descent is impossible (38). Pathologic findings are diffuse edema, petechiae, and hemorrhages. Increased CBF with cerebral vasodilation is present. Hypercapnea resulting from hypoventilation aggravates HACE, as does hypertension. The generalized fluid retention and edema of altitude contribute. The etiology is the hypoxia of altitude. Papilledema signifying increased intracranial pressure is usually found. The increased pressure confined within the skull leads to cerebral hypoxia and death.

Treatment is aimed at reducing intracranial pressure and edema. Rest, upright position, and oxygen are indicated. Hyperbaric bags may give dramatic improvement. Steroids such as dexamethasone (Decadron) 12 mg, or betamethasone, 4 mg every 6 hours, are beneficial. Acetazolamide is beneficial (500 mg every 6 hours). These medications may be given orally in conscious patients.

Intravenous administration is required in coma. The treatment of choice is descent as fast as possible and as early as possible.

Progression from severe AMS to HACE is seen in 1.8% (27). HACE may suddenly appear without warning in fit, well-acclimatized mountaineers at extreme altitude.

HIGH-ALTITUDE RETINAL HEMORRHAGE

Retinal hemorrhages are commonly seen at altitude. At 5360 m, high-altitude retinal hemorrhage (HARH) was seen in 56% (Table 1) (39). If HARH occurs in the macula, a permanent scotoma or blind spot may result. Functional vision is unlikely to affected. The etiology is felt to be increased vascular permeability. Descent is not thought to be mandatory.

HIGH-ALTITUDE CACHEXIA

High-altitude cachexia (HAC), occurs to all who remain at extreme altitudes for extended periods (at least weeks) (Table 1). No permanent human habitation has persisted above 17,000 feet. At very high and extreme altitude, the body's rate of deterioration exceeds the benefits of acclimatization (19, p. 80). This is the limit of the body's ability to compensate for hypoxia, and the ability to transport oxygen maximally from the lungs to the blood is maxed out. This is the death zone.

HAC is similar to starvation. There is loss of vigor, strength, and weight. Climbers on a 3-month expedition to the Himalaya often report loss of as much as 25% of their body weight. Weight loss at altitude is approximately half from fat loss and half from muscle loss. One should not "bulk up" in anticipation of weight loss. Those who start with the lowest body fat are the least affected. Sherpa typically have 10% to 12% body fat and do not lose weight until extreme altitude (40).

HAC is minimized by a high-carbohydrate diet. Fat produces the highest amount of energy per unit weight; its metabolism, however, requires oxygen. Protein metabolism requires water in a dehydrating environment. Carbohydrate is the most efficient. It is said that a high-carbohydrate diet effectively reduces summit elevation by 2000 feet.

There is evidence that HAC is preventable during a 3-month expedition by increased fluids, increased calories, and a high-carbohydrate diet (5 liters per person per day and 6000 kcal per person per day, 35% calories from carbohydrate) (40,41).

Adequate rest is important and rest days should follow hard climbing days. This fact is known to distance athletes and trainers; without adequate rest, performance decreases and overtraining results. Climbing strategy should minimize exposure to extreme altitude.

The 1983 German–American Everest expedition was able to minimize HAC by these measures. One climber achieved the summit of Mt. Everest with no weight loss.

THROMBOEMBOLIC DISEASE

Increased erythropoesis secondary to hypoxia commonly produces hemoglobin concentrations greater than 20 g/dL with hematocrits above 60%. This requires 3 to 6 weeks or longer at very high or extreme altitude. The increased carrying capacity of oxygen is offset by increased viscosity and decreased delivery capacity due to sludging at hematocrits above 60%. Above this level viscosity increases dramatically, Virchow's triad (hypercoagulable state, stasis, and injury) is well known. The predisposition to thromboembolic disease at altitude is confirmed by an increased incidence of peripheral thrombophlebitis, pulmonary emboli, and cerebral thrombosis. Chest pain and hemoptysis in a mountaineer at very high or extreme altitude are likely to be due to a pulmonary embolus. Treatment with heparin empirically or even prophylaxis with aspirin runs a theoretical risk of blindness by aggravation of HARH. Intracranial bleeding is also a risk. Identification of those at risk is possible (many hemoglobin meters stop at 20 g/dL). Exposure to extreme altitude should be minimized. The major controllable way to limit thromboembolic disease is to avoid dehydration. Keep the urine dilute with a light yellow color on the snow.

TRAUMA

Trauma is the major cause of mortality and morbidity at all altitudes. Neurologic trauma is frequent and often the most significant. Estimates of injury rates can be obtained from regulated climbing areas such as Grand Teton National Park. At this site over a 10-year period (1970 to 1980) 71,655 climbs were registered; 144 accidents occurred and 30 climbers were killed. An injury rate of 2 per 1000 climber-days is not excessive (2). Alpine skiing rates are reported as 3.4 to 7.4 cases per 1000 skier-days (42,43). Rates for cross-country skiing (not perceived as dangerous) are reported to be 1.5 to 2 cases per 1000 skier-days (44). In the Grand Teton study, head injury accounted for 22% and neck and back injuries accounted for 6%. Multiple injuries were seen in 14% (2). By far, subjective hazards accounted for the greatest number of accidents (82% nonfatal, 72% fatal) (2). Prevention of accidents is through education and experience. Failure of properly used equipment is an uncommon cause of injury. The statement "equipment in 1980 does not fail" remains true (P. Ershler, Head Guide, Rainier Mountaineering, summit climber Mt. Everest, 1984).

One way to prevent or reduce the severity of head injury is to use a helmet. A helmet should be worn for all rock and ice climbing. Many varieties are available. The best rule of thumb for purchase is, "Buy a $20 helmet only if you have a $20 head." Novice climbers should seek the advice of an authority before any equipment acquisition. Novice use of high-technology equipment without proper instruction amounts to "outdriving one's lights."

Technical mountaineering rescue is a complex subject. The problems an elite climber can encounter require an elite rescue. Basic mountaineering texts provide an introduction to technical rescue. All mountaineers should have knowledge of rescue, evacuation, and first aid commensurate with the difficulty of the ascent or the remoteness of the climbing area. All expeditions need a high degree of self-rescue ability. Several aspects of neurologic trauma that relate to mountaineering deserve additional reading and emphasis. The reader is referred to literature for further information about the care and transport of those with a neurologic injury (45,46).

Head Injury

Airway maintenance is the first principle in treating head injury. The major preventable cause of death is hypoxia resulting from obstruction or aspiration. For all those with head injuries with unconsciousness, the presence of unstable cervical spine injury should be assumed until ruled out radiographically. Shock occurring with head injury is almost always due to coexistent other injury such as abdominal or chest injury, which must be sought and treated. Head injury alone rarely causes shock. Although severe head injury requires neurologic evaluation and possible surgery by specialists, immobilization, airway maintenance, and supportive care are within the ability of all physicians and rescue personnel. The rapid evacuation and transport of a patient to a medical center should not involve sacrifice of the basic principles of trauma life support.

In 1978, a Sherpa with a skull fracture and intracranial bleeding was saved by the skilled surgery of an Austrian surgeon in the Khumbu ice fall (Mt. Everest, Nepal). I have included instruments for skull decompression in the medical kit for three expeditions to Mt. Everest. It is, however, more important to be prepared to maintain an airway and support and evacuate than to intervene surgically under less than adequate conditions. The latter is required only in remote areas devoid of medical, transport, and rescue facilities.

Spine Injury

It cannot be overemphasized: assume unstable cervical spine injuries until ruled out. In the unconscious patient who has had a mechanism of injury sufficient to fracture the spine, immobilization must be instituted until fracture is ruled out with proper radiographs. In a reliable conscious patient, a trained rescuer or physician may be able to do this on clinical grounds, history, and physical examination. The latter is extremely important in the mountain environment. The logistics of evacuation are difficult if all individuals with sufficient trauma are assumed to have unstable spines. The immobilization necessary not only makes evacuation difficult but also delays care of other injuries and may endanger the life of the injured and rescuers. If cervical spine injury is to be ruled out on clinical grounds, it *requires* (a) a reliable patient (mental status must be normal and not clouded by injury, shock, alcohol, drugs, etc.; the pain-masking effect of the autonomic response to injury must be considered) and (b) a normal physical examination. This must include careful "skin on skin" palpation of the spine from the occiput to the sacrum with no tenderness, swelling, deformity, or other signs of injury. Distal neurologic examination and function must be normal. If these criteria are satisfied, immobilization is unnecessary. This is in contrast to the urban situation, in which immobilization is routine in all possible circumstances and evacuation is easily accomplished, usually within 1 hour, to a medical facility without technical difficulty.

When an airway problem exists with a suspected cervical spine injury, the rescuer must *not* hyperextend or flex the neck. Chin lift or jaw thrust techniques can usually be utilized with immobilization. Oral or nasopharyngeal airways are often useful. The former is to be avoided in conscious patients as it is tolerated poorly and may induce vomiting with insertion. Blind nasotracheal intubation is a good technique as it need not interfere with immobilization. However, the patient must be breathing to perform this. The anxious hyperpneic patient is often easier to intubate in this manner. For apneic patients who are unconscious, an oral tracheal airway, if it can be inserted without compromise of immobilization, is preferred; however, a surgical airway may be necessary. For adults an emergency cricothyroidotomy is the procedure of choice. Tracheostomy is an alternative and is preferred in infants and small children. These techniques should all be in the armamentarium of expedition physicians.

Rigid immobilization is required for all suspected spine injuries. Collars are available and should be considered as useful in extrication and adjuncts to rapid immobilization. Firm fixation to a backboard immobilizing the spine from occiput to feet is optimal. The cervical spine may be adequately immobilized from occiput to sacrum (short backboard) with legs and arms free if this makes extrication and evacuation safer. Complete immobilization is optimal. For spine injuries without associated injuries, even with associated neurologic deficit, the adequacy of immobilization and gentle evacuation is more important than speed. Spinal shock following distal vasodilation with neurologic deficit will usually respond to measures such as Trendelenburg position, antishock pneumatic compression trousers (compatible with and possible aids to immobilization), and intravenous fluids. If shock does not respond, one *must* consider blunt abdominal trauma or pelvic injury as a source of occult bleeding. These injuries are masked by anesthesia or hypesthesia distal to spinal cord injury. In such circumstances, additional occult injuries should be suspected and evacuation expedited.

An additional comment is appropriate with respect to high and extreme altitude. Experienced mountaineers in the Himalaya feel that speed is safety, allowing the fit mountaineer to decrease exposure to objective hazard. For the injured, speed is also important. There is increased pressure on rescuers and medical personnel to be able to act appropriately but rapidly. Evacuations must be as fast as possible without compromise of immobilization or principles. The rule is: no nonessentials and make maximum use of all resources.

CONCLUSION

This discussion has been broad. The problems described are germain to mountaineering. Neurologic problems are frequent and cause the greatest mortality and morbidity. No other sport makes greater demands. Physical and mental strength and endurance must be maximal. The climber operates in one of the world's most hostile environments. Knowledge of the sport's high-technology equipment and techniques is required. Knowledge of weather, geology, physics, altitude physiology, and medicine is required. The climber and climbing team are the first line of defense against illness and injury.

Those who adopt this sport cannot afford to rely on rescue teams and helicopter evacuation (which are often lifesaving). Mountaineers must take responsibility for themselves and their companions.

REFERENCES

1. *Accidents in North American mountaineering.* New York: The American Alpine Club, 1979.
2. Schusman, LC, Lutz LJ. Mountaineering and rock climbing accidents. *Phys Sports Med* 1982;10(6):52–61
3. Houston CS. Altitude Illness. *Emerg Med Clin North Am* 1984;2:503–512.
4. Messner R. *Everest, expedition to the ultimate.* London: Kage and Ward, 1979.
5. Cavaletti G, Tredici G. Long-lasting neuropsychological changes after a single high altitude climb. *Acta Neurol Scand* 1993;87:103–105.
6. Hamilton AJ, Trad LA, Cymerman A. Alterations in human upper extremity motor function during exposure to extreme altitude. *Aviat Space Environ Med* 1991:62:759–764.
7. Garrido E, Castello A, Ventura JL, Capdevila A, Rodriguez FA. Cortical atrophy and other brain magnetic sesonance imaging (MRI) changes after extremely high altitude climbs without oxygen. *Int J Sports Med* 1993;14:232–234.
8. Regard M, Landis T, Casey J, Maggiorini M, Oelz O. Cognitive changes at high altitude in healthy climbers and in climbers developing acute mountain sickness. *Aviat Space Environ Med* 1991;62:291–295.
9. Clark CF, Heaton RK, Weins A. Neuropsychological functioning after prolonged high altitude exposure in mountaineering. *Aviat Space Environ Med* 1983;54:202.
10. Hornbein TF, Townes BD, Schoene RB, Sutton JR, Houston CS. The cost to the central nervous system of climbing to extremely high altitude. *N Engl J Med* 1989; 321:1714–1719.
11. Jason GW, Pajurkova EM, Lee RG. High-altitude mountaineering and brain function: neuropsychological testing of members of a Mount Everest expedition. *Aviat Space Environ Med* 1989;60:170–173.
12. Kennedy RS, Dunlapp WP, Bandaret LE, Smith MG, Houston CS. Cognitive performance deficits in a simulated climb at Mount Everest: Operation Everest II. *Aviat Space Environ Med* 1989;60:99–104.
13. Regard M, Oelz O, Bruggar P, Landis T. Persistent cognitive impairment in climbers after repeated exposure to extreme altitude. *Neurology* 1989;39:210–213.
14. Townes BD, Hornbein TF, Schoene RD, Sarnquist FH, Grant I. Human cerebral function at extreme altitude. In: West JB, Lahiri S, eds. *High altitude and man.* Bethesda, MD: American Physiological Society, 1984:31–36.
15. Sharma A, Sharma PD, Malhotra HS, Kaul J, Pal LS, Das Guptra DJ. Hemiplegia as a manifestation of acute mountain sickness. *J Assoc Physicians India* 1990; 38:662–663.
16. Garner SH, Sutton JR, Burse RL, McComas AT, Cymerman A, Houston, CS. Operation Everest II: neuromuscular performance under conditions of extreme simulated altitude. *J App Physiol* 1990;68:1167–1172.

17. Unsworth W. *Everest, a mountaineering history* (Appendix 4-5). Boston: Houghton Mifflin, 1981.

18. Auerbach PS, Geehr EC, eds. *Management of wilderness and environmental emergencies.* St. Louis: Mosby 1989: Chapter 1:1–35.

19. Houston CS. *Going higher, the story of man and altitude.* Burlington VT:Charles S. Houston, MD, 1987.

20. Houston CS. Trekking at high altitudes. *Postgrad Med* 1990;88(1):56–69.

21. Sutton JR, Reeves JT, Wagner PD, et al. Operation Everest II: oxygen transport during exercise at extreme simulated altitude. *J. Appl Physiol* 1988;64:1309–1321.

22. Sutton JR. Mountain sickness. *Neurol Clin* 1992;10: 1015–1029.

23. West JB, Lahiri S. Barometric pressure at extreme altitudes on Mt. Everest: physiologic significance. *J. Appl Physiol* 1983:54:166–194.

24. Baumgartner W, Bartsch P, Maggrini M, Waber U, Oelz O. Enhanced cerebral blood flow in acute mountain sickness. *Aviat Space Environ Med* 1994:65: 726–729.

25. Nelson M. Psychological testing at high altitudes. *Aviat Space Environ Med* 1982:53:122–126.

26. Flynn CF, Thompson TL. Effects of acute increases in altitude on mental status. *Psychosomatics* 1990;31(2): 146–152.

27. Hackett PH, et al. The incidence, importance, and prophylaxis of acute mountain sickness. *Lancet* 1976; 2:1149–1155.

28. Foulke G. Altitude related illness. *J Exp Med* 1985; 3(3): 217–276.

29. Houston CS. Acute pulmonary edema of high altitude. *N Engl J Med* 1960;260:478–480.

30. Hackett PH, Rennie D, Hofmeister SE, et.al. Fluid retention and hypoventilation in acute mountain sickness. *Respiration* 1982;45:321–329.

31. Oelz O. A case of high altitude pulmonary edema treated with nifedipine. *JAMA* 1987;257;780.

32. Bartsch P, Maggiorini M, Ritter M, et al. Prevention of high altitude pulmonary edema with nifedipine. *N Engl J Med* 1991:325;1284–1289.

33. Bartsch P. Treatment of high altitude diseases without drugs. *Int J Sports Med* 1992;13:51.

34. Schoene RB. Pulmonary edema at high altitude, review, pathophysiology and update. *Clin Chest Med* 1985;6; 491–507.

35. Menon MD. High altitude pulmonary edema a clinical study. *N Engl J Med* 1965;273:66.

36 Hultgren HN. Markova FA. High altitude pulmonary edema; epidemiologic observations in Peru. *Chest* 1978: 74:372.

37. Houston CS, Dickinson J. Cerebral form of high altitude illness. *Lancet* 1975;2:758.

38. Lobenhoffer HP, Zink RA, Brendel W. High altitude pulmonary edema: analysis of 166 cases. In: Brendel W, Zink RA, eds. *High altitude physiology and medicine.* New York: Springer-Verlag, 1982: 219–231.

39. McFadden PM, Houston CS, Sutton JD. High altitude retinopathy. *JAMA* 1981;245:581–586.

40. Hixson EG. Unpublished recorded observations, China-Everest 1982, 1983 German American Everest Expedition, and China-Everest 1984.

41. Minutes of 1982 China-Everest Nutritional Symposium. San Francisco: Shaklee Inc., 1981.

42. Gutman J, Weisbach J, Wolf M. Ski injuries in 1972–74. *JAMA* 1974:230:1423–1425.

43. Earl AS, Moritz JR, et al. Ski injuries. *JAMA* 1962:180: 285–287.

44. Garrick JG. Epidemiology of ski injuries. *Minn Med* 1971;54:17–21.

45. *Emergency care and transportation of the sick and injured.* Chicago: The American Academy of Orthopedic Surgeons, 1971 (and updates).

46. *Advanced trauma life support course.* Chicago: The American College of Surgeons Committee on Trauma, 1984 (and updates).

Sports Neurology, Second Edition,
edited by Barry D. Jordan.
Lippincott–Raven Publishers, Philadelphia © 1998.

36

Rugby and Australian Rules Football

Paul McCrory

*Department of Neurology, University of Melbourne, Austin & Repatriation Medical Centre,
Studley Road, Heidelberg, Victoria, Australia 3084*

Rugby union, rugby league, and Australian rules football are spectacular and often brutal collision sports. These sports are fast, exciting, and extremely popular as spectator sports. Rugby football is currently played in over 104 countries throughout the world, whereas Australian rules football (ARF) is unique to the Australian subcontinent. Rugby football is separated into two broad divisions: the more popular amateur game, rugby union (RU), and the professional game, rugby league (RL). The vast majority of participants are male; however, a small but increasing number of women are now actively involved in organized team competitions (1,2).

Although the potential for catastrophic brain injury exists in these sports, it is fortunately rare. In contrast, concussion is commonly seen at all levels of participation. From a neurologic standpoint, the injuries seen in these sports are largely dominated by head and neck trauma. Other neurologic problems such as focal nerve entrapments, peripheral nerve trauma, eye injuries, headache, and epilepsy occur less frequently.

HISTORY AND NATURE OF THE GAMES

The game of rugby can trace its origins to the Rugby School in England, where in 1823, a schoolboy named William Webb Ellis *"first took the ball in his arms and ran with it,"* thus establishing the basis of the modern game (3). There are many remarkable resemblances to other forms of football played in the British Isles, such as Irish hurling, and even in Roman times, the game of harpastum. From these historical games, various local contests developed throughout England, the most famous being the football games played traditionally on Shrove Tuesday and Ash Wednesday in Chester and Ashborne. It is said somewhat apocryphally that the first ball ever used was in fact the head of a captured Danish warrior! From these gladiatorial beginnings, the early ad hoc rules became codified and the game of rugby union as we know it today was created. Other codes of football, such as gridiron, rugby league, and perhaps ARF, may owe their origins to the original game of rugby.

Rugby Union

Rugby union, sometimes called rugger, is played between two teams of 15 players. The game is played on a rectangular pitch, similar to an American football pitch, approximately 100 m by 70 m. Play is divided into two nonstop 40-minute halves plus injury time. There are no time-outs or player substitutions (except for injury). The ball is oval shaped and slightly larger than an American football. The object of the game is to carry or kick the ball across the opposition goal line. The players are allowed only to carry the ball forward, kick downfield, or pass the ball by hand backward to other teammates. Tackling the ball carrier is permitted, but no blocking or obstruction of other players is allowed. Players do not usually wear protective equipment. The game is fast, action packed, and entertaining, making it a popular spectator sport. A central referee controls the play with assistant referees (called "touch judges") along the sidelines.

Neurologic injuries are usually related to specific aspects of the game (3). Tackles account for approximately one-third of all injuries and the injuries are evenly divided between the tackler and the ball carrier. Head injuries such as facial lacerations and concussive brain injuries are often seen in this context. When the play is restarted in certain situations, a "scrum" forms, where the forwards come together as a tight mass and struggle to gain possession of the ball. About one-fifth of all injuries occur in this situation, with cervical spine injuries being the major concern. A "ruck" is said to occur when one or more players from each team close around the ball when it is loose on the ground between them. About one-fifth of all injuries occur during rucking, and head and neck injuries are the major neurologic problems seen. Injuries occurring in open play account for about one-tenth of all injuries, with musculoskeletal injuries predominating.

Points are scored, called a "try," when the offensive player places the ball over the opposition goal line. Field goals may also score points when the ball is kicked over the goal posts.

Worldwide, this is the most popular form of rugby football. It is played in over 100 countries and international "test" matches are watched by a television audience of millions. The game had remained staunchly amateur in status until recently, when professional players were allowed to compete. In England, Australia, South Africa, and New Zealand it is played mostly in private schools and universities, whereas in Europe, South America, and the Pacific Islands it is more of a popular sport.

Rugby League

Rugby league is the professional version of the game of rugby and is played by two teams of 13 players with up to 6 interchange players allowed. It is played on a rectangular pitch in two 40-minute nonstop halves. Each team is allowed a maximum of six tackles with the ball, and if no score has occurred, the opposing team is allowed

six tackles and so on. The ball must be either carried forward or kicked downfield and cannot be thrown or knocked forward. Scoring is the same as for rugby union. A central referee controls the play with other assistant referees along the sidelines. The players use minimal protective equipment. As in RU, tackles and scrums account for the majority of neurologic injuries.

The game traces its origins to the northern working class areas of England and Wales and to the eastern states of Australia and New Zealand, where it is the major form of rugby played. It is also played internationally, where fierce rivalry exists between these countries.

Australian Rules Football

ARF is unique to Australia. It is a fast, exciting game played by 18 players per team with three substitutes who can interchange at any time. The game is played on an oval field approximately 180 m by 140 m. The game is played in four 25-minute quarters with time added on for stoppages.

The ball, which is oval, may be carried forward by an offensive player but must be bounced every 15 m. The ball may be disposed of by kicking, which is done with great accuracy over distances of up to 90 m, or by "handballing," in which the ball is held in the palm and struck by the clenched fist of the other hand. After the ball is kicked, it is "marked" or caught, which then gives the player the opportunity to take an unhindered or "free" kick. The most spectacular aspect of the game is the high marks taken by the players, who use an opponent's back or shoulders to propel them high into the air to mark the ball. Players in possession of the ball may be tackled or bumped. The absence of protective padding often surprises North American viewers, given the degree and vigorous nature of the physical contact that occurs. The object of the game is to score as many points as possible. This is achieved by scoring goals (worth six points) or single points.

Because of the speed and intensity of the sport, the game is controlled by three central umpires, who each control one-third of the ground. These are assisted by two boundary umpires and a goal umpire at each end.

The game was first played in Melbourne, Australia in 1858. The current national competition was initially established as a local suburban competition in 1896. At present, there are 16 national teams, which compete to play off in the Grand Final held in Melbourne on the last week in September of each year. The game is a spectacular sport attracting crowds of up to 100,000 to regular season games.

The mechanisms of the neurologic injuries that occur have been studied and are fairly equally divided into those that occur in tackles (25%), marking contests (25%), and collisions (25%) (4,5). There is a small group of injuries that are a result of illegal plays (5%). Concussive brain injuries are a significant injury, accounting for approximately 4% of the total injuries; however, catastrophic head and neck injuries are extremely rare. Other neurologic injuries including headache, epilepsy, and focal nerve entrapments are seen infrequently.

EPIDEMIOLOGY OF NEUROLOGIC INJURIES

Comprehensive data collection of neurologic injuries in these codes of football is limited. Although many retrospective injury surveys have been published, only few prospective studies have been attempted. The best of these studies is by Seward et al. (4) in which the injury data were contemporaneously collected using common injury definitions and assessments from codes of football in Australia during the 1992 season. This included the injuries seen in elite and junior RU, RL, and ARF teams throughout Australia. The relative comparative risk of all forms of injury at elite level competition is set out in Table 1.

Concussive Brain Injuries

Prospective Studies

With regard to the specific neurologic injuries seen, there was wide variation between the differ-

ent codes. Head and neck injuries accounted for 28.5% of all injuries seen in RU, 37.3% in RL and 14.4% in ARF. The vast majority of these, however, were head and facial lacerations. The prevalence of concussion in the different sports is shown in Table 2. It is worth emphasizing that these concussions were significant enough to have the attention of the team physician drawn to them. It is likely that most minor concussive episodes or "dings" go unnoticed by medical or training staff.

In sequential injury surveys performed in elite ARF, the concussion rate has gradually increased from 2.2 to 4.7 concussions per 1000 player-hours over the past 5 years (4–7). (See Table 3.) The reason for this increase in not clear, but it may represent rule changes to increase the pace of the game.

One area of concern that was revealed in these studies was that junior (younger than 18 years) competitive football has concussion rates in excess of those of the senior levels of competition. It has been postulated that junior players may not have fully developed the necessary evasive strategies to avoid elements of the game such as collisions that may put them at risk of brain injury. If this postulate is correct, then it may indicate a need for particular preventive strategies to be developed and continued skill development to be considered mandatory for junior footballers.

TABLE 1. *Injury risk by football code*

	Rugby union	Rugby league	Australian rules football
Total injury rate per 1000 player-hours	62	173	68

TABLE 2. *Concussion prevalence by football code (% of total injuries)*

	Rugby union	Rugby league	Australian rules football
Concussion	5.3%	8.5%	3.6%

TABLE 3. *Incidence of concussion in Australian rules football (injury rate per 1000 player hours)*

Year	Concussion rate	
	Elite	Junior
1992	2.2	4.3
1993	2.0	5.4
1994	3.0	4.3
1995	4.1	—
1996	4.3	—
1997	4.7	—

In RL this has not been shown to be the case, as the players under 21 years old have a concussion rate similar to that at the senior level (4). The reason for this discrepancy between the junior levels of ARF and RL is not known.

The issue of concussion rates over time has not been adequately addressed in injury surveys in either RU or RL. Apart from the survey mentioned above, no comprehensive prospective database is being attempted at present. However, a number of smaller individual club- or school-based surveys have been published.

In addition to the studies on concussion prevalence, there have been a number of prospective studies investigating the specific complications of concussion, namely concussive convulsions, tonic posturing, and righting reflexes. These studies have demonstrated the benign nature of these dramatic events (8–10).

Retrospective Studies

Some of the difficulties that arise in interpreting different injury studies include different methodologies, different injury definitions, and different athlete populations. These in turn lead to wide variations in injury incidence. This makes the studies difficult to evaluate and of limited benefit, apart from their role as anecdotal observations. Most of the surveys are for elite professional competition, but school and other nonprofessional competitive matches are often included. (See Table 4.)

Catastrophic Head Injuries

Catastrophic injuries of the head and neck are fortunately rare in these sports. In these studies, none were recorded (4–7,11,12). Although described

TABLE 4. *Concussion incidence in different codes of football*

Code	Reference	Population[a]	Total injuries	Total concussions	Concussion incidence (% of total injuries)
Rugby union	46	E/N	1944	108	5.5
	47	N	1000	21	2.1
	48	S	556	2	0.4
	49	E	151	3	2.0
	50	E	88	5	5.7
	51	E	271	24	8.9
	52	S	574	48	8.4
	53	S	772	49	6.3
	54	S	1444	16	1.1
	1	N	103	21	4.9
	55	N	84	3	4.0
Rugby league	56	E	204	13	6.4
	57	E	187	16	8.5
	29	E	83	5	6.0
	58	E	1214	103	8.5
	30	E	83	5	6.0
	59	E	492	35	7.1
Australian rules football	60	E	792	21	2.7
	61	N	774	42	5.4
	62	E	531	30	5.6
	63	N	91	8	9.0
	5	E	2638	106	4.0
	64	E	146	5	3.4
	65	E	61	2	1.5
	58	E	941	34	3.6
	12	E	3031	115	3.8
	6	E	3133	91	2.9
	11	E	3587	81	2.2

[a] E, elite competition; N, nonprofessional competition; S, schoolboy competition.

in the American football and sporting literature, no cases of the so-called *second impact syndrome* have been reported from any of the football codes in this country (13–16). Unpublished studies by the author, in conjunction with the Victorian state coroner's office, reviewing all cases of death in Australian football between 1965 and 1997, did not reveal any case that would be attributable to the *second impact syndrome*.

Cervical Injuries

There have been many studies documenting the risk of cervical spinal injuries in rugby from all parts of the world (17–23). Of interest from the standpoint of neck injuries is the fact that a study of cervical cord injuries in Australia had highlighted particular aspects of RU in which the players were at high risk of spinal injury (22). This study analysed all spinal cord injuries from all codes of football throughout Australia over a 25-year period. A total of 107 spinal injuries (101 in the cervical region) were found from RU, RL, and ARF. The injuries by football code are set out in Table 5. When relative rates of injury are considered, it is important to take into account participation rates. ARF has a participation rate three times that of both rugby codes and RL twice that of RU. This means that RU is the most dangerous game from the standpoint of spinal cord injuries, particularly for schoolboys. The study also highlighted that collision at scrum engagement, not scrum collapse, was the way in which the majority of these injuries were sustained. As a result of this study, a number of rule changes were made and education programs instituted. These would appear to have been successful and have reduced the frequency of cata-strophic spinal cord injury significantly since that time (4,24).

Although much understandable concern has been directed to the acute spinal cord injuries, other acute and chronic noncord cervical injuries may actually contribute to significant long-term player morbidity. The most common acute cervical spine injury reported in some studies has been cervical facet joint irritation (2). Furthermore, early degenerative changes have been reported in the cervical spine in current and former rugby players (21,25). Front-row forwards seem to be the players most at risk of these cervical spine problems. When the mechanics of scrum play are considered, this type of injury is hardly surprising.

Within the scrum, there is a constantly left-directed force on all front-row forwards, which is maximal during the pushing phase of the scrum (26). The cervical spine is forward flexed and laterally flexed to the left by the force of binding with an opponent. The cervical spine is then rotated as the player strains to see the incoming ball. In such positions, the cervical spine is vulnerable to acute cord injuries as well as chronic damage to the facet joints, ligaments, and intervertebral discs.

Eye Injuries

Sport-related eye injuries are not only costly to the community through medical and hospital costs but can have a profound effect on the individual. Most eye injuries can be prevented by the correct supervision of play, enforcement of rules, and, in some sports, the use of eye protection devices. None of the codes of football under discussion utilize helmets or other forms of head protection on a routine basis. Team physicians need to have a high index of suspicion for the type and mechanism of injuries that predispose to eye damage. Ideally opthalmologic screening should be performed in all players with fractures of the facial skeleton, as the overall incidence of ocular damage is almost 5% (27,28). In practice, an even higher suspicion of ocular damage must be maintained when the fracture involves the orbital wall.

The most common ocular injuries seen with facial fractures are hyphema and corneoscleral

TABLE 5. *Total number of spinal cord injuries in rugby and Australian rules footballers, 1960 to 1985*

Football code	Adults	Schoolboys
Rugby union	26	11
Rugby league	42	6
Australian rules football	16	1

Adapted from ref. 22.

abrasions with anterior segment injuries. Retinal tears and hemorrhages occur with posterior segment damage. Penetrating globe injury is fortunately rare in all codes of football.

When the football code at risk of such injuries was studied, ARF was the most common sport seen. In a study of 137 consecutive facial fractures over a 3-year period, ARF accounted for 53% of the injuries, rugby for 6%, and soccer for 6% (28). Other sports such as cricket and horse riding accounted for most of the remainder. This study probably underrepresents the risk of eye injury in rugby, as the study was performed in an area where rugby is not commonly played.

Other Neurologic Injuries

In all codes, other neurologic injuries are rare. When taken across all codes these include brachial plexus–root injuries or "burners" (approximately 2% of total injuries), fractures of the facial skeleton (1.2% of total injuries), lumbar and cervical disc prolapses (0.6% of total injuries), eye injuries (0.4% of total injuries) and vertebral fractures without cord damage (0.2% of total injuries) (24,27,29,30). Ongoing research projects by the author into football-related central nervous system injuries in Australia have identified anecdotal reports of other conditions such as posttraumatic migrainous cortical blindness (one case) and traumatic quadraparesis (three cases).

MANAGEMENT CONSIDERATIONS

The acute management of head and neck injuries is discussed elsewhere in this book. This chapter attempts to outline some of the underlying management strategies that may superficially seem to differ from those employed in sports such as American football. Decisions regarding return to play after head injury are often controversial and rely on good clinical judgment rather than proscriptive guidelines. The underlying principle should always be to do no harm and to consider the player's welfare above any team consideration. A "safety first" approach should be seen as common sense in what can be a difficult management dilemma for a team physician.

Concussive Brain Injury

Indicative of the lack of consensus on the definition and classification of concussion is the abundance of classification systems that have been proposed in order to grade the severity of the injury. These classifications reflect anecdotal experience rather than scientifically validated schemes. Furthermore, they are sport specific. The spectrum of head injury seen, for example, in gridiron football is different from that in rugby and ARF. For these sports, there is a necessity to have a more detailed understanding and grading at the "mild" end of the concussion spectrum, whereas in gridiron the whole range of head injuries needs to be encompassed. Schemes such as those proposed by Cantu, Ommaya et al., Kelly, or Torg may be useful in sports such as gridiron but all have their limitations in the practical field situation for other sports such as rugby and ARF (31–35).

The recent classification system proposed by the American Academy of Neurology highlights this problem (36). Not only is the underlying basis of the structure nonscientific, but the grading system is impractical for team physicians, thus adding to rather than resolving this difficult issue.

Various studies have highlighted the role of neuropsychologic (NP) parameters in the assessment of players with concussive injury (37–44). The consolidation of clinical data and psychometric performance into a unified grading scheme has been attempted in ARF. All players have baseline NP testing at the start of the season and if they are concussed during the season, their NP performance can be serially measured until they have returned to their baseline level of performance. As experience is gained with this technique and normative reference data ranges are established, the role of baseline testing becomes less critical. The major NP parameters tested include memory as well as measures of speed of information processing, which have been shown to be sensitive markers of brain impairment following head injury (41). Specific tests such as the Digit Symbol Substitution Test and Choice Reaction Time are used routinely in this assessment. Other measures tested in different sports including Paced Auditory Serial Addition Task have been found to be impractical to administer in ARF. Based on clinical and NP evidence of recovery, it has been established that the majority of cases of concussion in ARF are mild and recover within days of the event (43–45). This is further supported by the data on missed matches after concussive brain injury. In the 1997 season, a total of 81 concussive injuries were recorded, yet only 12 missed matches resulted (11). Unpublished data on ARF players who have sustained several concussive injuries over a season and sporting career have shown no decrement in cognitive or clinical performance given that they have had a full recovery after each episode of concussion. This type of neurocognitive assessment has been used in ARF for the routine management of concussion since 1985 with great success.

With the ability to assess cognitive performance accurately utilizing these types of NP tests, the rationale for a mandatory exclusion policy becomes redundant. Although exclusion policies are still utilized in rugby, it should be seen in the setting of sports in which medical coverage is not universal and access to these NP tests is not easily available. In ARF, all teams have physicians managing the overall medical care of the players. These physicians attend all training sessions as well as all competitive matches and are readily available to immediately assess concussed players and administer NP tests if required.

It is important to emphasize that these tests are not used to diagnose concussion or as a substitute for a carefully performed neurologic examination. As catastrophic head injury can mimic concussion in the early stages, a full and detailed physical examination is mandatory. The NP tests may then be used to confirm clinical recovery and return to baseline level of functioning. Clearly, this is a role for experienced medically trained sports physicians. Unfortunately, there is no simple key upon which nonmedical personnel can diagnose or manage brain injuries.

Prevention of head and brain injury has been seen as a priority for all codes. Regulating authorities responding to medical and public pressure have been vigorous in enforcing correct play and removing particular plays that predispose to head injury, such as spear tackles. In addition, education campaigns in rugby and the development of modified rules for children to emphasize correct skill development have been instrumental in changing the culture of the sport toward safety for all participants.

Spinal Cord Injury

As scrums were found to be the most common situation in which cervical spinal injuries occur, it seems logical that attention was first directed at this aspect of the game. Changes in rules have already occurred in response to medical concerns. The most significant change in RU concerns the serum engagement, where there is now a "crouch-pause-engagement" sequence. This was introduced at senior level in 1988 after several years of testing at junior levels. These rule changes have depowered the scrum by reducing the speed and momentum generated at engagement and hence lessened the risk of injury. In RL, scrum play is relatively deemphasized in comparison with RU and hence is less of a problem in the causation of spinal cord injuries. The controlling bodies for rugby should be commended for this responsible stand.

Rule changes have also affected tackles. An example of this is the banning of "spear tackles." These are different from spear tackles in American football, in which the tackling player uses his head to ram or "spear" the opposing player. In RU, it implies a tackle in which the ball carrier is upended and driven head first into the ground. Correct tackling techniques such as the "eyes open and head up" approach are taught by coaching staff and continued skill development is emphasized for junior players. Videos of coaching tactics are widely available through national sports medicine bodies, schools, and the various rugby organizations.

Another preventive mechanism for players is the development and strengthening of neck muscles as an inbuilt "splinting" mechanism to protect the neck from some types of injury. This may have only a limited role in preventing cord injury, where axial loading is the major mechanism and muscular strength would not be expected to protect the neck significantly in this position, but it may reduce hyperextension-type injuries. This remains to be scientifically proved.

SUMMARY

In conclusion, the major neurologic problems facing these sports are mild concussive brain injury in both rugby and ARF with cervical cord injuries being a problem in rugby only. Significant advances in the prevention of spinal cord injuries have led to reductions in these types of catastrophic injury. Mild head injury is the subject of continuing research, and the use of neuropsychologic testing has led to new understanding in the management and recovery of concussive brain injury. Much needs to be done worldwide, including the development of national and international databases with common injury definitions. Only then will a full understanding of the risks inherent in these spectacular and exciting sports be evident.

REFERENCES

1. Havkins SB. Head, neck, face and shoulder Injuries in female and male rugby players. *Phys Sports Med* 1986; 14: 111–118.
2. Hazard H. Rugby league: incidence of head and neck injuries. In: Committee NHaMRCE, ed. *Football injuries of the head and neck.* Canberra: Australian Government Publishing Service, 1994:78–79.
3. Collinson D. Rugby injuries. *Australian Family Physician* 1984; 13: 565–569.
4. Seward H, Orchard J, Hazard H, Collinson D. Football injuries in Australia at the elite level. *Med J Aust* 1993; 159: 298–301.
5. Seward H, Patrick J. *A three year survey of Victorian football league injuries.* Melbourne: Victorian Football League Medical Officer's Association, 1986:1–20.
6. Orchard J. *AFL 1996 injury report.* Melbourne: Australian Football League Medical Officer's Association, 1996:6–8.
7. Orchard J, Wood T, Seward H. *AFL and VSFL Injuries— 1994 Report.* Melbourne: Australian Football League Medical Officers Association, 1995:7–8.
8. McCrory P. *Videoanalysis of the acute clinical manifestations of concussion in Australian rules football.* SMA/ACSP Annual Scientific Conference. Canberra: SMA, 1996:214–215.
9. McCrory P, Berkovic S. Concussive convulsions: incidence in sport and treatment recommendations. *Sports Medicine* 1998; 25: 131–136.
10. McCrory P, Bladin P, Berkovic S. Retrospective study of concussive convulsions in elite Australian rules and rugby league footballers: phenomenology, aetiology and outcome. *Br Med J* 1997; 314: 171–174.
11. Orchard J. *AFL injuries—Season 1997.* Melbourne: Australian Football League Medical Officer's Association, 1997:5–10.
12. Orchard J, Wood T, Seward H. *AFL 1995 Injury report.* Melbourne: Australian Football League, 1995:8.
13. Cantu RC. Second impact syndrome: immediate management. *Phys Sports Med* 1992; 20: 55–66.
14. Cantu RC, Voy R. Second impact syndrome: a risk in any contact sport. *Phys Sports Med* 1995; 23: 27–34.
15. McCrory P, Berkovic S. Second impact syndrome: a critical review. *Neurology* 1998;50:677–683.
16. Saunders RL, Harbaugh RE. The second impact in catastrophic contact-sports head trauma. *J Am Med Assoc* 1984; 252: 538–539.
17. Burry HC, Gowland II. Cervical spine injury in rugby football. *Br J Sports Med* 1981; 15: 15–19.
18. Micheli LJ, Riseborough EM. The incidence of injuries in rugby football. *J Sportsmed Phys Fitness* 1974; 2: 93–97.
19. Noakes T, Jakoet I. Spinal cord injuries in rugby union players. *Br Med J* 1995; 310: 1345–1346.
20. O'Carroll PF, Sheehan JM, Gregg TM. Cervical spine injuries in rugby league football. *Irish Med J* 1981; 74: 377–379.
21. Scher AT. Premature onset of degenerative disease of the cervical spine in rugby players. *South African Med J* 1990; 77: 557–558.
22. Taylor TK, Coolican MR. Spinal cord injuries in Australian footballers 1960–1985. *Med J Aust* 1987; 147: 112–118.
23. Williams JP, McKibbin B. Cervical spine injuries in rugby union football. *Br Med J* 1978; 2: 23–30.
24. NH&MRC. *Football Injuries of the Head and Neck.* Canberra: National Health & Medical Research Council of Australia, 1995.
25. Broughton II. Premature degeneration of the cervical spine in a rugby union player. *New Zealand Sports Medicine* 1993; 213: 48–49.
26. Milburn PD. Biomechanics of rugby union scrummaging. *Sports Medicine* 1993; 16: 168–179.
27. Crompton JL. Eye injuries. In: National Health and Medical Research Council Expert Committee, *Football injuries of the head and neck.* Canberra: Australian Government Publishing Service, 1994:34–35:
28. Crompton JL, Hammerton ME. Opthalmic injuries. In: David DJ, Simpson DA, eds. *Cranio-Facial-Maxillo Trauma.* Edinburgh:.Churchill-Livingstone, 1994:
29. Gibbs N. Injuries in professional rugby league. *Am J Sports Med* 1993; 21: 696–700.
30. Gibbs N. Common rugby league injuries. *Sports Medicine* 1994; 18: 438–450.
31. Cantu RC. Guidelines for return to contact sports after cerebral concussion. *Phys Sports Med* 1986; 14: 75–83.
32. Kelly JP, Nichols JS, Filley CM, Lillehei KO, Rubenstein D, Kleinschmidt-DeMasters BK. Concussion in sports: guidelines for the prevention of catastrophic outcome. *J Am Med Assoc* 1991; 266: 2867–2869.
33. Ommaya AK, Gennarelli TA. Cerebral concussion and traumatic unconsciousness: correlation of experimental and clinical observations on blunt head injury. *Brain* 1974; 97: 633–654.
34. Roos R. Guidelines for managing concussions in sports. *Phys Sports Med* 1996; 24: 67–74.
35. Torg JF, ed. *Athletic Injuries to the head, neck and face.* 2nd ed. St Louis: Mosby Year Book, 1991.

36. Kelly J, Rosenberg J. Diagnosis and management of concussion in sports. *Neurology* 1997; 48: 575–580.

37. Alves WM, Rimel RW, Nelson WE. University of Virginia prospective study of football induced minor head injury: status report. *Clin Sports Med* 1987; 6: 211–218.

38. Barth JT, Alves WM, Ryan TV, et al. Mild head injury in sports: neuropsychological sequelae and recovery of function. In: Levin HS, Eisenberg HM, Benton AL, eds. *Mild Head Injury*. New York: Oxford University Press, 1989:257–275.

39. Barth JT, Macciocchi SN, Giordani B, Rimel RW, Jane JA, Boll T. Neuropsychological sequelae of minor head injury. *Neurosurgery* 1983; 13: 529–533.

40. Gronwall D. Paced auditory serial addition task: a measure of recovery from concussion. *Perceptual & Motor Skills* 1977; 44: 367–373.

41. Gronwall D, Sampson H. *The psychological effects of concussion*. Auckland: Oxford University Press, 1974.

42. Gronwall D, Wrightson P. Cumulative effects of concussion. *Lancet* 1975; ii: 995–997.

43. Maddocks DL. Neuropsychological recovery after concussion in Australian rules footballers [PhD thesis]. Melbourne: University of Melbourne, 1995.

44. Maddocks DL, Dicker GD, Saling MM. The assessment of orientation following concussion in athletes. *Clin J Sports Med* 1995; 5: 32–35.

45. Maddocks D, Dicker G. An objective measure of recovery from concussion in Australian rules footballers. *Sport Health* 1989; 7: 6–7.

46. Weightman D, Browne R: Injuries in association and rugby football. *Br J Sports Med* 1974; 8: 183–187.

47. Adams ID. Rugby football injuries. *Br J Sports Med* 1977; 11: 4–6.

48. Davidson R, Kennedy M, Kennedy J, Vanderfield G. Casualty room presentations and schoolboy rugby union. *Med J Aust* 1978; 1: 247–249.

49. Davies JE, Gibson T. Injuries in rugby union football. *Br Med J* 1978; 2: 1759–1761.

50. Durkin TE. A survey of injuries in a first class rugby union football club from 1972–1976. *Br J Sports Med* 1977; 11: 7–11.

51. Myers PT. Injuries presenting from rugby union football. *Med J Aust* 1980; 2: 17–20.

52. Sugarman S. Injuries in an Australian schools rugby union season. *Aust J Sports Med Ex Sci* 1983; 15: 5–14.

53. Sparks JP. Rugby football injuries, 1980–1983. *Br J Sports Med* 1985; 19: 71–75.

54. Davidson RM. Schoolboy rugby union injuries, 1969–1986. *Med J Aust* 1987; 147:119–120.

55. Addley K, Farren J. Irish rugby union survey: Dungannon football club 1986–7. *Br J Sports Med* 1988; 22: 22–24.

56. Alexander D, Kennedy M, Kennedy J. Injuries in rugby league football. *Med J Aust* 1979; ii: 341–342.

57. Alexander D, Kennedy M, Kennedy J. Rugby league football injuries over two competition seasons [letter to the editor]. *Med J Aust* 1980; ii: 334–335.

58. Seward H, Patrick J. A three year survey of Victorian football league injuries. *Aust J Sci Med Sport* 1992; 24: 51–54.

59. Gissane C, Jennings D, Cumine A, Stephenson S, White J. Differences in the incidence of injury between rugby league forwards and backs. *Aust J Sci Med Sport* 1997; 29: 91–94.

60. Ferguson AS. Injuries in Australian rules football. *Ann Gen Practice* 1965; 10: 155–161.

61. Quinn N. Australian rules football injuries. *Aust Fam Physician* 1984; 12: 691–694.

62. Sali A, McColl D, Dicker GD. The extent of injuries in VFL footballers. *Aust Fam Physician* 1981; 10: 169–172.

63. Hoy G, Kennedy D. A survey of Victorian football association injuries in season 1981. *Sport Health* 1984; 2: 23–26.

64. Brukner P. Australian rules football injuries. In: Hermans G, ed. *Sports, Medicine and Health*. Amsterdam: Elsevier, 1990: 142–146.

65. Brukner P, Miran-Khan K, Carlisle J. Comparison of significant injuries in AFL players and umpires. *Aust J Sci Med Sport* 1991; 23: 21–23.

Sports Neurology, Second Edition,
edited by Barry D. Jordan.
Lippincott–Raven Publishers, Philadelphia © 1998.

37

Scuba Diving

Hugh D. Greer III

Santa Barbara Medical Foundation Clinic,
P.O. Box 1200, Santa Barbara, California 93102

Interest in sport diving increased greatly in the 1970s. About 250,000 new divers are certified annually by the various training agencies, and 2.5 to 3 million people dive with compressed air yearly. Certainly the great appeal of diving has to do with the adventure-filled and foreign environment that is denied to most air-breathing creatures. That environment, however, imposes stern restrictions, and the technology that enables divers to use it also exposes them to unusual hazards. The use of compressed air at depth introduces physiologic challenges that occur nowhere else and may cause injuries that occur under no other conditions. The breath-hold diver may drown and experiences problems with ear clearing and cold. The scuba diver faces the same hazards but must avoid the additional hazards of pulmonary overpressure injuries and decompression sickness (1,2).

EPIDEMIOLOGY OF DIVING-RELATED INJURY

Data on serious diving-related illness and injury come from several sources. The U.S. Navy reports a 0.1% incidence of decompression sickness in all fleet dives. There is a similar incidence (0.15%) of air embolism and pulmonary barotrauma. These figures include training, operational, and special warfare diving, both scuba and surface supplied. Navy diving is rigidly controlled and meticulously recorded. Most of it is also at shallow depth, and few repetitive dives are made. These data do not extrapolate well to the civilian population (3).

Data are available from National Underwater Accident Data Center (NUADC) at the University of Rhode Island from 1970 onward (4). This agency receives government support as well as data from various government agencies, including the Coast Guard, local authorities, health department reports, and the news media. NUADC reported 110 fatalities in 1970, 144 in 1974, and 130 in 1979.

The Divers Alert Network, an institution created in 1981 by the Commerce Department, National Oceanic and Atmospheric Administration, maintains a 24-hour watch to give assistance in diving injuries. Their initial data on 876 cases of diving injury country-wide indicate that most accidents occur among young and inexperienced divers, one-quarter of whom lack basic scuba certification and three-quarters of whom have only basic training. Nevertheless, a fair number of experienced sport divers undergo serious decompression sickness (5).

The Wrigley Marine Science Center, a campus of the University of Southern California, maintains a recompression chamber for the treatment of diving casualties. In the decade 1974 to 1985, the facility received 375 patients for the treatment of diving accidents. These were about equally divided between air embolism, serious decompression sickness, and type 1 (or pain only) decompression sickness. Some required repetitive treatment. There were 506 chamber treatments and 579 treatment evaluations in 10 years. This amounts to about 50 casualties per year, more than 1 per week during the summer and fall and fewer in the winter (6).

Catalina Island is the center of intense sport diving activity in California. The Catalina Decompression Chamber data are based on hundreds of thousands of scuba dives made every year within a radius of more than 100 miles; the data are probably fairly representative of civilian sport diving experience. Some of the data in the Catalina figures, however, and some of the more serious cases come from the commercial abalone and sea urchin fishing industry, whose members often violate safe diving practices. The commercial diving industry, excluding the diving fishermen, has relatively few accidents, but the ones that occur tend to be serious. This work often involves deep dives, long and complex saturation dives, mixed gas dives, and prolonged exposure to cold.

Figures based on partial data can certainly be misleading. Nevertheless, if one accepts an annual fatality figure of 150 for all diving-related causes and assumes conservatively that there are 1 million active divers (undertaking one or more dives per year) in the same reporting area, this produces a fatality rate for sport diving of 0.015% per active diver per year. The actual mortality rate is far less than that. Taken another way, there are less than a dozen sport diving deaths in California each year; compared to the highway toll on a holiday weekend, this number seems insignificant (2,4).

Certainly many diving injuries go unreported and untreated. For example, the western region of the Divers Alert Network fields about 3 calls a week, perhaps 150 to 200 per year. Less than half of these require recompression treatment.

PHYSICS, PHYSIOLOGY, AND THE UNDERWATER ENVIRONMENT

The problems unique to diving are governed by the physical laws of hydrostatic pressure and gas solubility. These immutable physical principles include Boyle's law, which states that the product of pressure times volume is constant or that the volume of a gas varies inversely with pressure; Charles' law, which states that the pressure-volume constant varies directly with absolute temperature; Dalton's law, which states that the total pressure of a gas is the sum of the partial pressures of each of the gases admixed; and Henry's law, which states that the amount of gas dissolved in a fluid is directly proportional to the partial pressure of that gas. Boyle's law and Charles' law are commonly expressed together as the general gas law.

There is one atmosphere of pressure at sea level. At a depth of 33 feet the pressure is doubled, and at 100 feet it increases fourfold. The application of Boyle's law is clear. If one takes a breath and dives to 33 feet, the volume of one's chest must be compressed by half. It happens just this way and is quite apparent when one observes breath-hold divers at 30 feet (they look remarkably skinny). If on the other hand one takes a full breath from a compressed air tank at 30 feet, holds it, and ascends to the surface, one's chest arrives at the surface twice as big. This is terribly dangerous and is the cause of pulmonary overpressure and arterial gas embolism, the most serious casualty in diving.

During every dive nitrogen is absorbed into tissue. Because nitrogen is an inert gas, the body tolerates this quite nicely at depths but pays for it on ascent. If the diver ascends more rapidly than the rate at which the nitrogen can be exhausted by diffusion, the nitrogen bubbles out of solution in the bloodstream and in tissues, causing decompression sickness. The dissolved gas itself can exert an anesthetic affect and cause nitrogen narcosis.

Simple compression of gas in the middle ear on descent may cause ear "squeeze," which is often a painful nuisance and occasionally the cause of permanent hearing loss.

Finally, the diver must deal with the physical demands of swimming (particularly on the surface), the energy requirements of cold water and hypothermia, and, not infrequently, seasickness. The marine environment is unforgiving, and a simple error of judgment that could be overlooked on the playing field or compensated for on a bicycle ride can be fatal at depth. For example, a player who becomes exhausted on the tennis court can interrupt a match to rest; an exhausted diver may drown.

The neurologist sees a common denominator in diving injuries because the nervous system is the principal target in almost every instance. Drowning, near drowning, and hypothermia cause hypoxia and metabolic encephalopathy. Arterial gas embolism targets the brain and brainstem, and decompression sickness principally affects the spinal cord. Nitrogen narcosis and oxygen toxicity cause transient encephalopathy.

TYPES OF DIVING INJURIES

Barotrauma

Barotrauma refers to physical injury produced by the expansion and compression of gas within body cavities. The term encompasses the changes of descent, in which gases are compressed and tissue is "squeezed," and those of ascent, in which gases expand and distend body cavities.

Barotrauma of Descent

"Squeeze" occurs when external pressure increases as the diver descends and the pressure of gas-filled spaces within the body cannot be equalized. Such occurs when the diver neglects to vent air through the nose to equalize the pressure inside the mask. On descent the mask is forced tightly against the face, and the facial tissue (including the eyes) tries to fill up the cavity. Petechial hemorrhages under the skin or conjunctiva may result. The ostia of sinus cavities are sometimes closed by mucus plugs, and on descent there may be sinus pain, edema, and hemorrhage into the sinus cavity. Gas in the gastrointestinal tract compresses without incident. In breath-hold divers, the chest cavity is greatly compressed. Well-conditioned breath-hold divers can take a full breath at the surface and dive to 100 feet without incurring pulmonary damage. The chest cavity is well able to tolerate this much compression, and even deeper dives have been done without chest trauma.

The ear suffers most from barotrauma of descent. Painful pressure on the eardrum and rupture can occur even at shallow depth if the diver does not equalize the pressure in the middle ear on descent. A more serious event is oval window rupture, which is caused by overly vigorous attempts to clear the ears. The resultant endolymph leak may cause permanent damage to the labyrinth and permanent hearing loss. In many cases the hearing loss is not immediately apparent but is recognized after the diver awakens the next morning, having slept with the injured ear dependent. Fluid leaks out of the labyrinth, and there is measurable, sometimes total and permanent, sensory neural loss (7,8).

Barotrauma of Ascent

Pulmonary overpressure is the most dangerous aspect of barotrauma of ascent and is the major cause of fatality in scuba diving (2,4,9,10). The basic mechanism is a straightforward violation of Boyle's law. A breath-hold diver's chest compresses on descent and expands on ascent (Fig. 1). The scuba diver, however, dives breathing all the way. On descent the air regulator continues to deliver air at an increasing pressure corresponding to depth. At 33 feet, the diver breathes air at a pressure of 2 atm. The lung volume remains the same, but at each breath the lungs contain twice the mass of air (twice the number of molecules) as at sea level. On ascent the diver continues to breathe, the air regulator providing air at gradually decreasing pressure matching the depth.

If the diver fills the lungs at 33 feet and then holds his or her breath for the ascent, a dangerous change takes place. The ambient pressure decreases, and the lungs swell. If the breath is held all the way to the surface, the lungs expand to accommodate the increased mass of air inside the chest. The chest cannot expand that much, and the lung ruptures (Fig. 2).

When pulmonary rupture occurs, a series of events may take place. Air may rupture into the pleural cavity with resultant pneumothorax, which itself increases in volume as the diver ascends. Air may dissect into the mediastinum, rise to the supraclavicular space where it presents as subcutaneous emphysema, or rupture into the pericardium. Both cause striking physical findings but little danger. Air that enters the pulmonary capillaries, however, may reach the pulmonary vein and the left heart and be pumped into the arterial circulation (Fig. 3). These emboli are distributed preferentially to the vessels serving the brain.

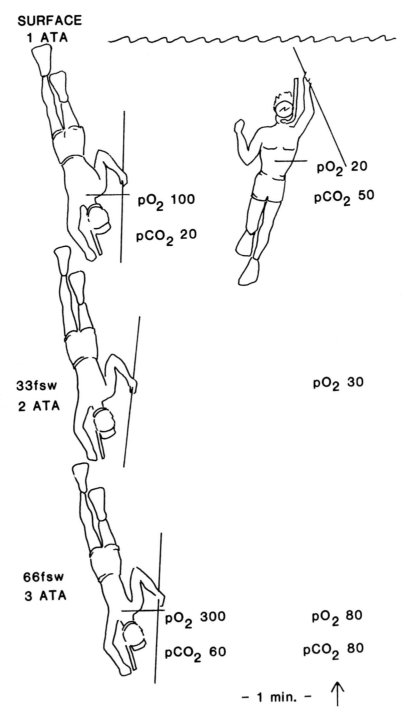

FIG. 1. Breath-hold diver. The chest compresses with descent and expands with ascent. The partial pressure of oxygen (pO_2) increases with depth. It is adequate when the diver leaves the bottom at 1 minute but decreases rapidly on ascent. The partial pressure of carbon dioxide (pCO_2) increases throughout the dive.

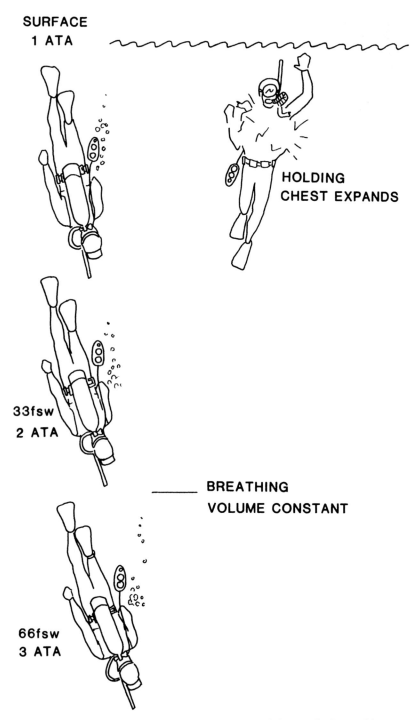

SURFACE
1 ATA

HOLDING
CHEST EXPANDS

33fsw
2 ATA

BREATHING
VOLUME CONSTANT

66fsw
3 ATA

FIG. 2. Scuba diver. The chest volume remains constant as air is supplied at ambient pressure. If the breath is held on ascent, the lungs are overpressured and rupture.

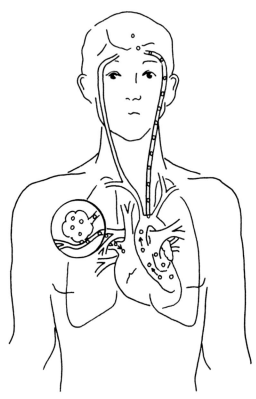

FIG. 3. Pulmonary overpressure accident. Air from ruptured alveoli may enter the pleural space (pneumothorax), the pericardium (pneumopericardium), or the mediastinum (pneumomediastinum and subcutaneous emphysema). If it dissects into the alveolar capillary bed, bubbles may be carried to the left atrium and pumped directly into the arterial circulation.

These are the first large vessels encountered after leaving the heart, and because the diver is ordinarily ascending head upward gravity plays a part (11,12). Emboli several millimeters long are found in vessels as small as 50 to 100 μm. Both carotid and vertebral basilar circulation receive the emboli.

Obstructive pulmonary disease, particularly asthma, is dangerous, because it may cause localized air trapping, which is quite beyond the diver's control (12,13).

Barotrauma from pulmonary overpressure presents immediately on surfacing. The diver commonly feels pain in the chest and shortness of breath and occasionally has bloody cough. The symptoms are those of an acute cerebral event.

The diver may lose consciousness immediately on surfacing, aspirate, sink, and drown. The diver may collapse immediately on climbing into the boat, complain of headache, lose consciousness, and convulse. Neurologic symptoms characteristic of cortical injury such as seizures, hemiparesis, quadriparesis, hemianesthesia, and cortical blindness are common. Cardiorespiratory arrest occurs often (13). The mortality rate is high, and the need for immediate recompression treatment is great.

Remarkably, many patients recover spontaneously and completely. Positive response to recompression treatment is often prompt and dramatic. Among patients who survive, recovery is generally good. The emboli occlude small arterioles rather than large trunks, and air emboli, unlike platelet emboli, eventually dissolve (14,15).

Pulmonary overpressure accidents occur most often among inexperienced divers. Training exercises in buoyant ascent, free ascent, buddy-breathing, and other maneuvers designed to deal with loss of air supply have accounted for many such cases. An emergency ascent from an out-of-air situation is often panicky, and with the desire to reach the surface the diver may simply neglect to exhale.

Decompression Sickness

Decompression sickness was the first of the diving maladies to come to medical attention. Bridge and tunnel workers on both sides of the Atlantic developed "bends" and "caisson disease" working under pressure in the construction of the Thames tunnels and the Brooklyn Bridge. The clinical features of decompression sickness and its natural history were well known in the 19th century, but the pathophysiology was not well defined until the 1970s (16,17).

Decompression sickness occurs when divers dive too deep, stay down too long, and ascend too quickly. Nitrogen is absorbed into tissue in accordance with Henry's law. The greater the pressure, the greater the amount of gas absorbed. If the diver stays at a given pressure long enough, all the tissues reach equilibrium with ambient gas pressure. When the diver, viewed as a complex tissue system, ascends, gas must come out of the tissues and be released again into the atmosphere. The problem of decompression sickness arises when ascent is too rapid, or tissue perfusion inadequate, and gas comes out of solution and into gas phase within tissues, producing bubbles. The bubbles account for all the manifestations of decompression sickness. The amount of bubbles produced depends on the depth of the dive, the length of the dive, and the rapidity of the ascent. Rapid decompression, called "blow-up," represents the most extreme form of decompression sickness and rarely if ever occurs in scuba divers. When it does occur, in deepsea divers making accidental rapid ascent from great depth, it is usually fatal.

The clinical spectrum of decompression sickness is commonly classified as type I and type II. Type I decompression sickness, the most benign form, is also called "pain-only bends" and describes pain in a single joint, bone, or tendon without other findings. Cutaneous bends or "niggles" causes itching of the skin, perhaps accompanied by an hemorrhagic rash (marmoratus cutis). Type I decompression sickness may occur shortly after surfacing or be delayed for many hours. In general, the sooner the symptoms appear, the greater the bubble population and the more ominous the event. These symptoms may presage more serious findings.

Type II decompression sickness, also called serious or neurologic decompression sickness, includes bilateral joint pain, weakness, sensory loss, paraplegia, loss of bowel and bladder control, girdle-like pain around the waist, vertigo, tinnitus, visual disturbance, headache, confusion, and nearly everything else that might be explained by bubbles acting as emboli in the central nervous system.

This may seem to be a crude classification, but it has practical application. In general, the greater the exposure and the greater the violation of decompression procedure, the more abundant the bubbles and the more serious the clinical illness. There is good correlation between the magnitude of bubble flow, detected by ultrasonography over the decompressing diver's vena cava, and the occurrence of decompression sickness.

The predilection of decompression sickness for the nervous system, and particularly for the spinal cord, is well known, although the cause is not obvious. Cerebral events such as seizure, hemiparesis, cortical blindness, hemisensory loss, and dysphasia are rare. Experimental decompression sickness in goats, dogs, and other animals has provided similar information. Animals subjected to decompression sickness develop paraplegia, as do humans. Their spinal cords show multiple intraspinal hemorrhages, both venous and arterial, particularly in the thoracic and lumbar cord. Palmer et al. (18) demonstrated that goats with clinical type I decompression sickness showed widespread intraspinal lesions and cortical lesions. The particular vulnerability of the thoracolumbar spinal cord was explained by Hallenbeck et al. (19), who induced decompression sickness in anesthetized dogs and observed the development of decompression sickness in the spinal cord under an operating microscope and with cinematography. These investigators found that the caudal–rostral flow of venous blood through the paravertebral venous plexus in the thoracolumbar region is affected by respiration, moving in a to-and-fro fashion that favors the accumulation of bubbles. As bubbles first begin to appear, they coalesce into larger and larger bubble masses, producing a froth that altogether impedes the venous return, resulting in venous infarction throughout the cord, particularly in the thoracic and lumbar regions (20) (Fig. 4).

There are other variables. Some tissues such as fat have a greater affinity for nitrogen, accepting it readily and holding large stores. Some tissues are better perfused and can accept and release gas more readily. For instance, blood is frequently exposed to the cappillary–gas interface in the lungs and exchanges gas rapidly. Venous blood, which is under lower pressure than arterial blood, bubbles earlier. Saturation and desaturation of the body is nonlinear and nonuniform.

It is an oversimplification to view decompression sickness simply as a matter of bubbles and mechanical obstruction. The bubbles of nitrogen act in a thrombin-like manner and cause platelet aggregation. This compounds the problem by introducing a second sort of circulating microembolus. Electron micrography demonstrates diffusion of gas into platelets and surface action of the

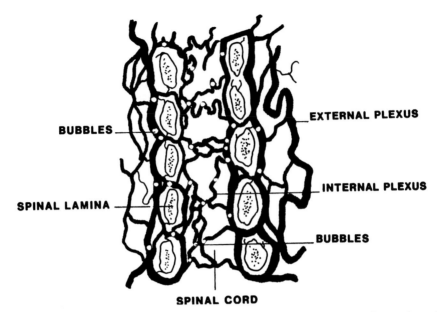

FIG. 4. Batson's plexus. The paravertebral venous plexus is a tortuous system of vessels and venous lakes surrounding the spinal cord within the canal and encircling the vertebrae: In decompression sickness, the entire system may be filled with a froth of bubbles.

bubbles themselves, which causes platelets to clump around them (21,22). The platelet aggregation phenomenon can be shown in vitro to deplete platelet-rich plasma. This platelet depletion effect can be prevented by platelet antagonists, such as theophylline, which increase the release of cyclic adenosine monophosphate. Drugs that affect a prostaglandin–thromboxane pathway, such as aspirin and indomethacin, have no effect (23,24).

These variables are taken into account in the design of decompression tables. Early investigators worked from the theoretical picture of the body as a series of tissues or compartments that accept and release gas at different rates, and decompression tables are designed to allow a diver to surface at a rate compatible with the slowest tissue for the depth and duration of the dive (17). These tables, which are based on theoretical and empirical-data, define safe diving practice. The U.S. Navy Air Decompression Tables, and similar tables used by other navies and by the commercial industry, are also the standard for most sport divers (8). They are not infallible, however. The U.S. Navy reports a bends incidence of 0.5% with strict adherence to tables. More conserva-

tive decompression schedules such as the "No Bubble Table," which is based on the absence of bubbles on Doppler sampling, provide an added margin of safety (25).

Adherence to diving tables is harder than it sounds. The US Navy tables were designed for use by surface-supplied divers, who are tethered to the ship by an umbilical that supplies air, communication, and a pneumofathometer (depth gauge). The tender on deck knows exactly how deep the diver is all the time and how long the diver has been there. The scuba diver, on the other hand, has no communication with surface and has to keep track of depth and bottom time.

These factors are critical. For instance, the U.S. Navy 60/60 No Decompression Table allows the diver to dive to 60 feet for 60 minutes. The diver who goes deeper or stays longer incurs a decompression debt and must stop at a given point for a given time on the way up. When the diver surfaces, he or she must keep track of the time spent on the surface if another dive is planned (26). Finally, the diver must ascend at a rate not to exceed 30 feet/min. A diver who violates any of these strictures or makes a mistake in addition has "omitted decompression" and runs the risk of decompression sickness. All these factors are easy to consider at one's desk, harder in the cold, in an open boat, or underwater. Self-discipline is difficult to maintain. Divers are tempted to "push the tables" to get the deeper lobster, the last abalone, or the most out of a diving weekend. Luck certainly plays a part. Many divers get away with gross violations of the tables time after time, and others are tempted to follow their example.

Working divers, both commercial and military, using air-filled scuba observe a depth limit of 130 feet. The scuba tank has a finite air supply and, at 130 feet, leaves little margin for safe decompression on ascent. It is possible for a scuba diver with a single 72–cubic foot bottle to dive to 150 feet and to incur a decompression debt that cannot be repaid with the remaining air supply.

The long-term consequences of decompression sickness are serious. Patients with type I decompression sickness who are treated promptly seem to have little residual effects, and even patients with serious decompression sickness sometimes respond dramatically to prompt recompression therapy. Many, however, are left with persistent neurologic findings, and some do not recover at all (27). Postmortem findings in patients with previous episodes of spinal decompression sickness have shown significant evidence of infarction, scarring, and nerve fiber loss even though they had made substantial clinical recovery. On the basis of this information, the consensus of opinion of medical diving experts precludes return to diving in patients who have had serious (type II) decompression sickness if they have any residual symptoms or findings after conventional primary treatment. Specifically, a diver who is entirely symptom free and has a normal neurologic examination after a single recompression treatment may return to diving after 1 month. A diver who has any residual symptoms or neurologic findings or has required extended or repeated treatment may not return at all. These strictures have great economic significance for the commercial diver, whose career is at an end. For the sports diver, the strictures lack authority but have the same meaning for the health of the spinal cord (27–29).

Nitrogen Narcosis and Oxygen Toxicity

Scuba divers breathe compressed air, which is a mixture containing 79% nitrogen, 20% oxygen, a tiny fraction of carbon dioxide, and a variable amount of water vapor. Oxygen is required to sustain life. It is actively transported and exchanged for carbon dioxide by hemoglobin. Nitrogen takes no part in metabolism and behaves as an inert gas. Both have toxic properties under pressure.

Nitrogen Narcosis

Physiologically nearly inert at sea level, nitrogen has narcotic properties under pressure. It has an affinity for fat, and therefore for brain tissue, and has about half the narcotic potency of nitrous oxide (30). Similar to the effect of alcohol, the narcotic effect of nitrogen begins with giddiness, tingling of the face and lips, dulling of mentation, and failure of judgment. There is some variation in individual susceptibility, just as there is to alcohol. Some experience a feeling of euphoria at 100 feet, and nearly all divers are affected at 150 feet.

It is the narcotic property of nitrogen, rather than decompression sickness, that limits the depth of air diving. In the commercial and military sectors, a mixture of helium and oxygen (heliox) is used for all dives below 170 to 180 feet to avoid narcosis. Helium has some problems of its own. Its solubility in fat, and therefore its narcotic effect, is only one-fourth that of nitrogen, but it conducts heat seven times as fast as nitrogen, so that divers breathing heliox require greater thermal protection. Helium is expensive and requires special equipment, but it enables divers to work at great depth without drunkenness.

Nitrogen, like alcohol, potentiates the sedative effect of other drugs (31). This includes not only tranquilizers and sedatives but also antihistamines and anti–motion sickness preparations. In one instance, an experienced diver using a transdermal scopolamine preparation for seasickness became confused and disoriented at only 60 feet (32).

Oxygen Toxicity

Pure oxygen is not suitable for diving because it has toxic effects on both the brain and the lung. These effects are time and depth dependent and determine the selection of gas mixtures and decompression schedules for working divers. Scuba divers breathe air, but the limitations of oxygen toxicity still have some bearing.

Oxygen under high pressure causes seizures. Nearly everyone can tolerate 100% oxygen at sea level, but about 1% of normal subjects convulse at 60 feet (2.8 atm) when breathing oxygen for 30 minutes. This is part of the standard oxygen tolerance test given to diving candidates in the U.S. Navy. A few convulse at lesser depths, and all who convulse are deemed unsuitable for diving (3). Oxygen at high pressure inhibits glutamic acid decarboxylase and causes a measurable decrease in brain γ-aminobutyric acid. This decrease accompanies convulsions in a number of species.

Pure oxygen has two advantages for clandestine military diving. Used in a closed-circuit rebreathing set, it makes no bubbles, and because all the gas is consumed a small bottle of compressed oxygen provides great endurance. The cost of a convulsion under water is great, however, and depth is accordingly curtailed. The U.S. Navy limits oxygen diving to 25 feet, with deeper excursions permitted only under exceptional circumstances (33,34).

For noncombat, nonemergency conditions, an upper limit of oxygen partial pressure of 1.6 atm is observed to avoid central nervous system oxygen toxicity. This limit is reached in air diving at 231 feet. Because nitrogen narcosis limits air diving to 170 feet, the scuba diver should not encounter this problem. It may come up in another context, however. The scuba diver under treatment for decompression sickness or air embolism is treated with 100% oxygen at 60 feet for prolonged periods. Standard treatment schedules provide for pure oxygen breathing periods of 20 or 30 minutes interrupted by air breaks of 5 or 10 minutes to lessen the likelihood of oxygen convulsions (3,34).

Prolonged exposure to hyperbaric oxygen causes lung damage as well. There are oxidative changes to pulmonary capillary endothelium and alveolar linings, which cause reduced vital capacity and loss of pulmonary compliance. This determines the upper limit of oxygen for long-saturation dives (0.5 atm) and the lower limit, which is necessary to support metabolism (0.16 atm). Pulmonary oxygen toxicity also limits the length and depth of treatment for decompression sickness and arterial gas embolism (35).

Hypoxia, Hyperventilation, and Breath-Hold Diving

Hypoxia is surely the major threat to a diver's life. Scuba gear supports life only for a predetermined time; the diver who exceeds that designed capacity before surfacing, will drown. This happens most often not because of equipment failure but because of fundamental operator error. Breath-hold divers may become hypoxic, lose consciousness, and drown simply because they hold their breath too long. (See Fig. 1.)

Hypothermia

Hypothermia is a constant part of the diver's life. As with air supply, thermal protection is designed to sustain the diver only for the planned duration of the dive. The time it takes for the diver's body to reach the ambient temperature is determined by an equation whose variables are the temperature gradient, heat supply, and insulation.

The diver must maintain a body temperature of 37°C against a heat sink that may vary from 0° to about 30°. These limits are extreme, and sport scuba divers rarely dive in water colder than 7°C (45°F). In tropical regions the water temperature is rarely lower than 24°C (75°F) but even with these temperatures the water is colder than the diver. Maximum survival time in water of 20°C (68°F) in ordinary clothes is 5 to 6 hours. A diver's wetsuit extends this to 36 hours. The colder the water, the more protection required and the shorter the survival time (36).

Heat production is not an important factor. Exercise increases heat production through muscle activity, but at the same time calories are consumed, and peripheral vasodilation conducts heat to the water more rapidly. Swimmers lost at sea are advised to be as still as possible to prolong survival. Shivering, an involuntary response to falling core temperature, increases heat production, but its usefulness is limited to a narrow range. Working divers at depth are commonly provided with an external heat source, usually a hot water suit supplied from the surface. Electrical heaters are used as well. The scuba diver must depend on passive insulation, most commonly a Neoprene wetsuit. These are effective in moderately cold water, down to about 10°C. For colder water, drysuits are needed (37).

Shivering heralds the onset of hypothermia. It begins at a core temperature of about 36°C and can be voluntarily suppressed until the core temperature reaches 35°C. At this point, shivering is uncontrollable and generalized. It has by this time produced a fourfold increase in heat production and at the same time a fourfold increase in energy consumption. Oxygen consumption is 2.5 to 5 times the resting level.

The limit of voluntary exposure for most divers is 35°C. With this loss of only 2° from the core temperature, even highly conditioned subjects become confused and unreliable, lose their will to carry out tasks, want nothing else than to get warm, and have a decreased will to survive. At 34°C there is amnesia, speech is dysarthric, and coordination is greatly impaired, and when core temperature reaches 33°C there is 50% mortality. Cardiac dysrhythmia begins at 32°C, response to pain and consciousness is lost between 30° and 29°C, and death from ventricular fibrillation may occur at any lower temperature (37,38).

The neurologic response to cold is both central and spinal. The hypothalamus responds to falling core temperature by shunting arterial circulation to the body core. The spinal reflex between cold receptors in the skin, at segmental levels, is involuntary but can be suppressed up to a point by voluntary muscle work. When shivering begins, there is an increase in resting muscle tone with a discharge frequency of 5 to 12 Hz. It is not centrally synchronized, and different frequencies may occur in different muscles at the same time. Muscles shivering at the same frequency are not synchronized. Amplitude of shivering varies greatly, and heat production varies accordingly. Shivering of such low amplitude that it is discernible only by electromyelography still produces heat.

Rate of heat loss alters the protective response. Divers who are well insulated and lose heat slowly over a long period of time may not have vasoconstriction or shivering or be much aware of cold until their core temperature is well below 35°C. The same is true of well-acclimated athletes such as breath-hold divers and surfers. This variation of tolerance, however, is only about 0.5° to 1.0° on either side of 35°C. Below that, loss of calories cannot be compensated by any means (39).

The treatment of hypothermia is rewarming. The conscious patient should be warmed as quickly as possible with whatever means are at hand. A hot bath or shower, radiant heat from a fire, a hot water hose inside the wetsuit, and hot beverages (if the diver is alert enough to swallow) are all effective. Care must be taken not to cause burns. Heated air or breathing gas is quite effective and is particularly appropriate in diving situations.

The patient with this level of hypothermia recovers promptly and completely. Deep hypothermia, with core temperature at 30° or less, is a much more critical problem. Cardiac dysrhythmia is an important cause of death in profound hypothermia. The myocardium at these temperatures is refractory to cardioversion, so that profoundly hypothermic patients should not be rewarmed until it can be done in a critical care unit by experienced personnel. The comatose hypothermic patient should be protected from further heat loss by blankets and should be provided with warm, moist oxygen if possible while under transport to the hospital. If ventricular fibrillation occurs, it will be necessary to continue cardiopulmonary resuscitation until the patient is delivered to critical care (38,40).

Although chronic hypothermia may come on slowly as the result of an insidious drain of energy, acute hypothermia is dramatic. As core temperature falls, an enthusiastic and efficient diver may become a stumbling, helpless patient in a matter of minutes.

Prevention of hypothermia is essential and elementary:

1. Divers must wear thermal protection in all but the warmest tropical water.
2. Don insulation first. Many calories have been lost by the time the diver begins to feel chilled.
3. The wetsuit should include boots, gloves, and, most important, a hood. The head is a disproportionate heat radiator because scalp and neck vessels have little vasoconstrictive ability.
4. The person in charge of a dive party must anticipate hypothermia and have a rewarming plan.

EMERGENCY MANAGEMENT AND TREATMENT OF DIVING-RELATED INJURIES

The diving casualty may not see a neurologist until long after the injury, but the neurologic outcome may be largely determined by effective early management. Trauma, hypothermia, asphyxiation, and water aspiration are problems sufficient unto themselves, but when they are complicated by the unique problems of the underwater environment unique treatment is required.

Diagnosis

When an injured diver is rescued from the water, the diagnostic algorithm proceeds as follows.

Population at Risk

Breath-hold divers may drown or nearly drown, may undergo ear and sinus "squeeze" and ruptured eardrums, and, rarely, may experience lung "squeeze" with pulmonary edema and hemorrhage. Scuba divers or any divers breathing from a compressed air source beneath the surface are subject to these same problems but may also have decompression sickness or pulmonary overpressure accidents, including arterial gas embolism. If the diver was not breathing from a compressed air source, decompression sickness and arterial gas embolism will not be present, and recompression treatment will not be required.

Timing

If the diver developed pulmonary or cerebral symptoms on reaching the surface or immediately after leaving the water, he or she should be assumed to have pulmonary overpressure injury. If cerebral symptoms are present, air embolism must be assumed, and recompression treatment will be required. If symptoms are delayed several minutes or even hours after surfacing, decompression sickness is an important consideration. Prompt recompression treatment may also be required, but the more delayed the onset of symptoms, the less compelling the emergency.

Dive Profile

The depth and duration of each dive, the time spent on the surface between dives, the total number of dives, the rate of ascent and the conditions of ascent from each dive, and the diving history on preceding days all have a bearing on the likelihood and severity of decompression sickness. As with all such analyses, however, useful conclusions must be based on good data. There is frequently a problem here. The diver may have only the most general idea of the depth and duration of the dives, surface intervals, and ascent rate. The diver may report a benign and trouble-free dive profile and still have decompression sickness. As noted earlier, time keeping and data collection underwater is not easy and may be given short shrift by divers who have other problems on their minds. Nevertheless, a dive history that includes several repetitive deep dives, or long dives below 50 feet, should be viewed with suspicion even if it is not clearly in violation of decompression protocol. In truth, there are ways to "get bent" even if one adheres to the U.S. Navy tables, particularly by doing many repetitive dives in the same day. Attention should be paid to what the diver was doing on the bottom and whether there was a panicky or out-of-air ascent. Rapid ascents increase the likelihood of both arterial gas embolism and decompression sickness. Recording and analyzing the dive profile takes some time. If there are obvious injuries or serious symptoms, treatment should not be delayed.

Physical Findings of Neurologic Injury

Physical findings of cerebral injury such as convulsion, hemiparesis, dysphasia, and blindness are presumptive evidence of air embolism. Weakness of the lower extremities, bilateral sensory loss, and bilateral limb pain are equally compelling evidence for serious decompression sickness. The sensory examination should not be neglected because the findings in spinal decompression sickness are often limited to patches of decreased sensation on the limbs or trunk.

On-Site Treatment

Once established, the presumptive diagnosis of diving injury, be it decompression sickness or arterial gas embolism, demands immediate treatment. If there is cardiorespiratory arrest, the need for resuscitation is obvious. Short of that, the patient, whether alert or in coma, should be placed in Trendelenburg's position (trunk down, legs up and tilted 30° to the left side). This position encourages bubbles to follow the inside curve of the aorta rather than enter the cerebral arteries.

The most important part of on-site treatment is administration of 100% oxygen. The damaging lesion is nitrogen bubbles within tissue, interrupting blood flow and damaging neural structures. At surface these bubbles have a calculated nitrogen pressure of 633 torr. Alveolar air has a pressure of about 573 torr, so that the off-gassing gradient, breathing air at sea level, is 60 torr. If the patient breathes pure oxygen, the alveolar nitrogen pressure becomes 0 torr and the gradient 633 torr, which represents a tenfold increase. This enormous treatment advantage, which Behnke and Shaw (41) called "the oxygen window" (Table 1) is the most important part of treatment of both arterial gas embolism and decompression sickness.

Even greater advantages are gained with treatment under pressure, but the availability of oxygen in the field for immediate treatment is of the utmost importance. Most sport dive boats carry oxygen; private individuals should do so as well. This is not as simple as it sounds, however. A small bottle of oxygen, with a plastic mask does not take up much room, but neither does it work well. The object is to exclude air and to deliver pure oxygen until the patient is placed in a recompression chamber. This means a close-fitting mask and a one-way circuit. If the injured diver breathes 20 L/min, he or she will quickly exhaust a small oxygen bottle. For treatment to be effective, the emergency kit must have a large oxygen supply, perhaps the size of a welding bottle.

Communication and Transport

Communication and transport often represent the weakest area in the handling of marine casualties. Diving injuries occur offshore, often at some distance from emergency medical treatment and at even greater distance from a recompression facility. If the person in charge of the dive does not have an evacuation plan, minutes and hours are lost. After first aid, cardiopulmonary resuscita-

TABLE 1. *The oxygen window*

Conditions	Nitrogen pressure (torr)		
	Bubble	Alveolar	Gradient
Surface			
Air	633	573	60
100% oxygen	633	0	633
60 feet			
Air	1772	1615	157
100% oxygen	1772	0	1772
165 feet			
Air	3796	3438	360
50% oxygen, 50% nitrogen	3796	1719	2019

tion, and administration of oxygen, the next concern is getting the patient to recompression as rapidly as possible. If the boat is an hour or so away from medical assistance, it should be got underway immediately. If the distance is greater, consideration must be given to obtaining outside help and air transport. Nevertheless, emergency evacuation is difficult, and reaction time is often determined by factors beyond the control of the responding agency. Forethought and advance planning are invaluable. Remarkably, those on the accident scene are, often so ill-prepared that they are unable to give the rescuers their position.

If air evacuation can be accomplished, it must be done at low altitude because ascent from sea level further complicates both decompression sickness and arterial gas embolism. Nonpressurized aircraft should observe a 500-foot limit, and pressurized aircraft should maintain sea level pressure. Many are not able to do so. Cabin pressure in most commercial jets is maintained at an equivalent altitude of 5000 to 6000 feet. Decompression to this extent aggravates decompression sickness already present and may precipitate decompression sickness in subjects with recent diving exposure (42).

The destination of the diving casualty is a competent recompression chamber. Planning is required here as well. Location of the nearest competent chamber should be in every diver's emergency plan.

Recompression Therapy

Definitive treatment for arterial gas embolism and decompression sickness is recompression. Administration of oxygen under pressure accomplishes the following three objectives:

1. *Reduction in bubble size.* Bubble volume decreases in direct proportion to absolute pressure. As pressure is doubled, bubble volume is halved. This allows bubbles in vessels to pass on to smaller vessels and relieves the distortion caused by bubbles crowding tissue. The pressure-volume relationship is inverse and linear, but the pressure-diameter ratio is not. Doubling the pressure halves the volume but not the diameter. Compression to 6 atm reduces volume by

6 and not quite halves the diameter. There is a practical limit here. Further compression to great depths reduces the bubble size by a fraction but increases and continues the absorption of nitrogen. For this reason, 6 atm (165 feet) is the maximal conventional treatment depth.

2. *Oxygen delivery to tissue.* At 2.8 atm (60 feet), air has a partial oxygen pressure of 428 torr. If the diver breathes pure oxygen, the partial pressure is 2141 torr, or 14 times the equivalent in surface air. This is excellent treatment for hypoxia. Oxygen under this pressure readily dissolves in tissue, even in the presence of arterial obstruction.

3. *Nitrogen washout.* Hyperbaric oxygen treatment increases the off-gassing gradient of nitrogen (see Table 1). This is the most important feature of the treatment. Beyond 6 atm (165 feet), which is the deepest treatment depth, efficiency of pure hyperbaric oxygen falls off because of central nervous system toxicity. Deep recompression reduces bubble size but cannot give much advantage in off-gassing. The body equilibrates at the treatment depth and saturates as it absorbs more nitrogen. Advantage can be gained at 165 feet with a mixture of 50% nitrogen and 50% oxygen. This provides enough oxygen to repair the off-gassing gradient but not so much as to risk convulsions (41,43).

Decompression generally follows the treatment schedules prescribed in the U.S. Navy Diving Manual. The minimal acceptable treatment for decompression sickness is U.S. Navy Table 6. This requires compression to 60 feet. The diver breathes pure oxygen, interrupted with air breaks, for 90 minutes. Pressure is then decreased to 30 feet over a period of 30 minutes, and the diver continues oxygen breathing for 2 more hours. The diver then ascends to the surface at 1 foot/min, still breathing oxygen. Total recompression time is 4 hours and 45 minutes.

For arterial gas embolism, reduction of bubble size is a more important objective. Table 6A begins with an initial compression to 6 atm (165 feet), where the diver remains for 30 minutes, then begins an ascent at 25 feet/min to 60 feet. The treatment then continues on a schedule similar to Table 6 (15).

The treatment schedules may be extended. If the diver improves during the initial treatments but the improvement is less than complete, additional oxygen breathing periods can be added at 60 feet and still more at 30 feet and the total recompression time extended to more than 12 hours. The fully extended Table 6 amounts to 8 oxygen breathing periods at 60 feet and 18 at 30 feet. This oxygen exposure produces symptoms of pulmonary oxygen toxicity with measurable decrease in vital capacity in many subjects. It is pulmonary oxygen toxicity that limits treatment.

Treatment outcome is principally determined by severity of the insult and by promptness of treatment. The initial treatment is definitive. Follow-up treatment on subsequent days is of dubious value (44).

NEUROLOGIC OUTCOME

Decompression illnesses (DCS and AGE) are similar to traumatic and ischemic models in that outcome is largely determined by the extent of acute injury and response to initial treatment. It is sometimes difficult to distinguish DCS and AGE, and both can occur together. Some basic differences exist. AGE causes strokelike cerebral disease. Persisting deficits may include dysphasia, cortical blindness, hemiparesis, and dementia. Recovery, however, is strikingly better than that observed after stroke in older people. AGE patients are generally much younger than stoke patients and most make a surprisingly good recovery, even from profound insults. Post-AGE epilepsy has not been reported.

DCS causes spinal cord disease. Myelopathy is the cause of nearly all long-term disability from diving injury. Although divers with acute DCS may have cerebral symptoms such as confusion, visual loss, and generalized fatigue; evidence of persisting injury is limited to the spinal cord. (27,44,48).

Barring specific events of injury, diving as a sport or occupation has not been shown to cause neurologic injury. That is, if one does not "get bent," there do not appear to be serious health consequences of occupational diving. Moderate hearing loss may be an exception (45–47).

REFERENCES

1. Cousteau JY. Dumas F. *The silent world.* New York: Harper & Row; 1953.
2. Edmonds C, Lowry C, Pennefather J. *Diving and subaquatic medicine.* 2nd ed. Sydney, Australia: Sydney Diving Medical Center, 1981.
3. *U.S. Navy diving manual* (NAVSEA 0994-LP-001-902D Revision I). Washington, DC: Department of the Navy; 1981.
4. McAniff JJ. *US underwater diving fatality statistics 1970–1978.* Washington, DC: Department of Commerce; 1980.
5. *DAN Report on diving accidents and fatalities* 1994. Durham: Duke University Medical Center.
6. Pilmanis A. *Personal communication, 1986.*
7. Farmer JC. Otologic and paranasal sinus problems in diving. In: Bennett PB, Elliot DH. eds. *The physiology and medicine of diving.* 3rd ed. London: Bailliere Tindall, 1982:507–536.
8. Molvaer OI. Lehmann EH. Hearing acuity in professional divers. *Undersea Biomed Res* 1985;12:333–339.
9. Schench HV, McAniff JJ. *United States underwater fatality statistics* 1972 (report URI 73-8, NOAA Grant 4-3—159-31). Providence. RI: University of Rhode Island, 1972.
10. Greene KM. Causes of death in submarine escape training casualties: analysis of cases and review of the literature. *Report: Admiralry Marine Technology Laboratory Alverstoke.* 1978;R:78–402.
11. Schaefer KE, McNulty MC, Carey CR, et al. Mechanism in development of interstitial emphysema and air embolism on decompression from depth. *J Appl Physiol* 1958;13:15–29.
12. James RE. Extra-alveolar air resulting from submarine escape training: a post-training roentgenographic study of 170 submariners. *US Nav Submarine Med Res Lab Rep* 550, 1968.
13. Linaweaver PG. In: Schilling CW, Carlston CB, Mathias RA, eds. The *physician's guide to diving medicine.* New York: Plenum, 1984:496–506.
14. Gorman DF, Brownining DM. Cerebral vasoreactivity and arterial gas embolism. *Undersea Biomed Res* 1986; 13:317–335.
15. Leitch DR, Greenbaum LJ Jr, Hallenbeck JM. Cerebral air embolism: is there benefit in beginning HBO treatment at 6 bar? *Undersea Biomed Res* 1984;11:221–235.
16. Bert P, Hitchcock MA, Hitchcock FA. trans. *La pression barometrique.* Columbus, OH: Columbus College Books, 1943:394.
17. Boycott AE, Damant GCC, Haldane JBS. The prevention of compressed air sickness. *J Hyg (Cambe)* 1908; 8:342.
18. Palmer AC, Blakemore WF, Payne JE, et al. Decompression sickness in the goat: nature of brain and spinal cord lesions at 48 hours. Undersea Biomed Res 1978;5:275–286.
19. Hallenbeck JM, Bove AA, Elliot JH. Mechanisms underlying spinal cord damage in decompression sickness. *Neurology* 1975;25:308–329.
20. Hallenbeck JM. Cinephotomicrography of dog spinal vessels during cord damage in decompression sickness. *Neurology* 1976;26:190–204.
21. Hallenbeck JM, Obrenovitch T, Kumaroo K, et al. Several new aspects of bubble-induced central nervous system injury. *Philos Trans R Soc London* 1984;304:177–184.

22. Thorsen T, Burbakk A, Oystedal T, et al. A method for the production of N2 microbubbles in platelet-rich plasma in the aggregometer-like apparatus and effects on the platelet density in vitro. *Undersea Biomed Res* 1986;13:271–288.

23. Thorsen T, Oystedal T, Verheide A, et al. Effects of platelet antagonists on reduction in platelet density caused by microbubbles in vitro. *Undersea Biomed Res* 1986;13:209–304.

24. Thorsen T, Dahlen H. Bjerkvig R, et al. Transmission and scanning electron microscopy of N2 microbubbles—activated human platelets in vitro. *Undersea Biomed Res* 1987;14:45–58.

25. Eatock BC. Correspondence between intravascular bubbles and symptoms of decompression sickness. *Undersea Biomed Res* 1984;13:320–329.

26. Buhlmann AA. Decompression after repeated dives. *Undersea Biomed Res* 1987;14:59–67.

27. Greer H. The natural history of decompression sickness. Bethesda, MD: *Undersea Medical Society;* 1984:7–20.

28. Palmer AC. Spinal cord lesions in a case of "recovered" spinal decompression sickness. *Br Med J* 1981;283:888–905.

29. Consensus recommendations. In: Davis JC, ed. The return to active diving after decompression sickness or arterial gas embolism. Bethesda, MD: *Undersea Medical Society;* 1980;8.

30. Fowler B, White PL, Wright GR, et al. Narcotic effects of N2O and compressed air on memory and auditory reception. *Undersea Biomed Res* 1980;7:35–46.

31. Fowler B, Hamilton K, Porlier G. The effect of ethanol and amphetamine on inert gas narcosis in humans. *Undersea Biomed Res* 1986;13:345–355.

32. Greer H. Personal communication, 1983.

33. Kaufmann BD, Owen SG, Lambertson CJ. Effects of brief interruption of pure oxygen breathing upon central nervous system tolerance to oxygen. *Fed Proc* 1956; 15:107.

34. Butler FK, Thalmann ED. Central nervous system oxygen toxicity in closed-circuit scuba divers: Part II. *Undersea Biomed Res* 1986;13:195–224.

35. Clark JM, Lamberton CJ. Pulmonary oxygen toxicity: a review. *Pharmacol Rev* 1971;23:37–133.

36. Golden F St C. Thoughts on immediate care: the immersion incident. *Anesthesia* 1975;30:364.

37. Webb P. *Thermal restraints in diving.* Wilmington. CA: Commercial Diving Center, 1977:20.

38. Revler JB. Hypothermia: pathophysiology, clinical settings, and management. *Ann Intern Med* 1978;89:519–554.

39. Park YS, Rahn H, Lee IS, et al. Patterns of wet suit diving in Korean women breathhold divers. *Undersea Biomed Res* 1983;10:203–212.

40. Lloyd EL. Hypothermia: the cause of death after rescue. *Alaska Med* 1984;26:74.

41. Behnke AR, Shaw LA. The use of oxygen in the treatment of compressed air illness. *US Nav Med Bull* 1937; 35:61–73.

42. Edel PO, Carroll JJ, Honaker RW, et al. Interval at sea level pressure required to prevent decompression sickness in humans who fly in commercial aircraft after diving. *Aerospace* Med 1969;40:1105–1110.

43. Leitch DR, Hallenbeck JM. Oxygen in the treatment of spinal cord decompression sickness. *Undersea Biomed Res* 1985;12:269–290.

44. Denison DM. In: Francis TJ, Smith DJ, eds. *Describing decompression illness.* Bethesda, MD: Undersea and Hyperbaric Medical Society, 1991.

45. Curley MD, Wallick MT, Amerson TL. Long-term health effects of US Navy Diving—Neuropsychology. In: *Long Term Health Effects of Diving an International Consensus Conference.* Bergen, Norway: Univ. of Bergen, 1994: 209–228.

46. Moon RE, Massey ELO. Long term complications of diving and their management. In: *Long Term Health Effects of Diving. An International Consensus Conference,* Bergen, Norway: Univ. of Bergen, 1994:81–103.

47. Nylland H, Todnem, K, Skaidsvoll H, et al. A 10 year experience in Norway. In: *Long Term Health Effects of Diving. An International Consensus Conference,* Bergen, Norway: Univ. of Bergen, 1994:125–130.

48. Palmer AC, Calder IM, Yates PO. Cerebral vasulopathy in divers. *Neuropathol Appl Neurolbiol* 1992;18:113.

Sports Neurology, Second Edition,
edited by Barry D. Jordan.
Lippincott–Raven Publishers, Philadelphia © 1998.

38

Soccer

Donald T. Kirkendall and *William E. Garrett, Jr.

*Departments of Orthopaedic Surgery and Physical/Occupational Therapy,
Duke University Medical Center, Box 3435, Durham, North Carolina 27710;
Department of Orthopaedics, UNC Hospitals, CB #7055, Chapel Hill, NC 27599-7055

Unquestionably, soccer is the most popular team sport in the world. The international governing body, the Fédération Internationale de Football Association (FIFA), has more members than does the United Nations. It is estimated that, around the world, there are over 60 million registered players and an equal number of unregistered players. The World Cup, contested every 4 years, commands a worldwide audience of 1.5 billion viewers. In the United States, soccer is less recognized, but is still the third most popular sport among children under 18 years of age, with over 1.4 million players registered with the U.S. Youth Soccer Association (1).

THE NATURE OF THE GAME

Two teams of 11 players each play two 45-minute periods with a 15-minute half-time. By international rules, two substitutions are permitted, but local leagues generally set their own rules on substitution (e.g., number of substitutes, when to substitute, free substitution). No time-outs are allowed, but the stoppages of play (ball out of play, fouls, etc.) are frequent enough that the total time the ball is in play is around 60 minutes, depending on a variety of factors such as the environment, tactics, and the nature of the opposition. Youth competitions use a smaller field,

ball, and shorter games with more liberal substitutions. Moderate contact occurs during the game. The rules are few and open to interpretation by the officials. The pendulum has swung toward a more strict interpretation of the rules, especially as concerns the so-called professional foul, that is, an intentional foul to stop a clear scoring opportunity.

The physical demands of the game are well documented (2,3). The typical professional adult player covers around 10 km during a game. About two-thirds of that distance is covered at the low intensities of a walk or jog. The other third is covered at a "cruise" (running with manifest purpose and effort) or a sprint. About 900 to 1000 discrete activities are performed in a game, meaning that there is a change in running speed or direction every 4 to 5 seconds. Fatigue later in the game reduces the volume and intensity of running in the second half. The intensity of effort averages about 75% of maximal capacity over the course of a game. A player may jump 16 times and fall 5 times during a game. A most unique aspect of soccer is the use of the head to advance the ball while the use of the arms is against the rules of the game. A player may head the ball five or six times during a game and an unknown amount in training. The use of the head has raised concern over the immediate and long-term effects of heading.

EPIDEMIOLOGY OF SOCCER INJURIES

The overall injury pattern of soccer must be appreciated to see where head and spinal injuries fit. Unfortunately, there are few well-controlled studies of the injury incidence in soccer. Most of the data comes from studies of large youth tournaments, emergency room reports, or insurance claims. The populations for these studies may be large, but there are inherent biases. The prospective studies of Ekstrand (4) and the National Collegiate Athletic Association (NCAA) Injury Surveillance System (5) are examples of more systematic reporting of soccer injuries.

The injury rate per 1000 hours for male players has been reported to range from a low of 1.7 (ref. 6; a large French recreational league) to 14.3 during games in players over 16 years of age (7) to 23 in a large Norwegian study (8). For women, the rate is reported as 1.1 (9) to 44 (8). In the NCAA survey, the rates are 7.8 and 7.9 for men and women, respectively (5).

The most frequently injured body part is, as expected, the lower extremity, with reports of over half to nearly 85% of injuries being to the legs (1,4,6–8,10). Injuries to the ankle account for about a quarter to a third of all injuries, and the knee accounts for just over 20% of all soccer injuries (1). Table 1 depicts the average incidence of injury by anatomic location. The percentages exceed 100 because of differences in reporting. The majority of injuries are sprains, contusions, and strains (Table 2).

Although direct comparisons between studies are not possible, Lohnes et al. (1) draw some

TABLE 1. *Relative incidence of soccer injuries by anatomic location*

Anatomic location	Percent of total injuries [a]
Lower extremity	65
Ankle	36
Knee	20
Thigh	16
Upper extremity	13
Foot	12
Head	9.8
Pelvis	9
Trunk	6

Compiled from ref. 1.
[a] Percentages exceed 100 because of differences in reporting definitions.

TABLE 2. *Relative frequency of injury type in soccer players*

Type of Soccer Injury	Percent of Total Injuries
Sprain	33
Contusion	24
Strain	19
Fracture	10.7
Concussion	3
Other injuries	10

Compiled from ref. 1.

basic conclusions about injuries from soccer. First, the severity and frequency of injury increase with age, level of competition, and number of games. Second, injuries in children under the age of 12 do not result in a significant loss of playing time. Third, younger girls are about twice as likely to be injured as are boys. This difference is not evident in older players. Fourth, central attackers and midfielders are most frequently injured. Goalkeepers are most likely to sustain an injury to the upper extremity. Fifth, half to two-thirds of all injuries are to the legs. Sixth, the majority of injuries are contusions, sprains, and strains. Finally, disabling injuries are rare, making up less than 0.1% of all injuries.

MECHANICS OF HEADING

There is concern on the part of many parents regarding the use of protective helmets for young players. As the incidence of head injuries is very small and the incidence of serious injuries of any type is also very small in youth, there might be some argument that headgear may actually increase the chances of injuries such as lacerations or contusions (1).

Heading a soccer ball is a well-timed, coordinated, active event. The ball should be struck at the hairline. Coaches continually stress that the *player* is to strike the ball, not the reverse. An initial extension of the trunk is coordinated with chin tucked in toward the chest. The forceful flexion of the trunk and thrust of the neck impart force to the ball. Heading during a stationary 2-foot jump, while running, while diving, or from a running jump only adds to the complexity of the skill. The arms are used for balance but may be forcefully drawn into the body during the entire motion to add more force to the act (Fig. 1).

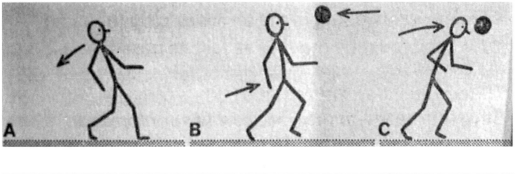

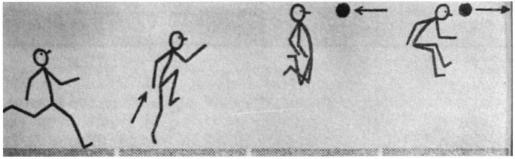

FIG. 1. Illustration of body mechanics used when (**top**) heading the ball from the ground or (**bottom**) heading the ball in the air. (From Wade A. *Soccer: guide to training and coaching.* Boston: Heinemann, 1997:69, 71.)

Three phases of heading are generally described: preparation, contact, and recovery. Preparation is dominated by the action of the trunk. Contact, 10 to 23 msec (11), results in deformation of the ball and rebound off the head. Coaches generally tell their charges to keep their eyes open while heading, but this is a challenge for players of all ages and abilities. The contact phase can also be divided into three phases. Ball contact and deformation are followed by the change of direction of the ball and finally the recoil of the ball off the head (12). The change in velocity of the ball during contact ultimately determines the impact on the head of the player.

An adult ball (size 5, 0.43 kg), kicked as hard as possible by a skilled player, can travel at over 100 km/h (13,14) with a resulting impact of 200 to 1200 newtons (12,14) according to ball velocity. Towend (15) reported that the linear acceleration of the head is on the order of 20 to 55 G with a head injury criterion (HIC) of 1.4 to 11 (12). In comparison, 2% of the population might experience a serious brain injury with an HIC of 500 and 15% with an HIC of 1000. Impact forces on the head vary according to the mass of the player. The smaller player (e.g., 55 kg) would be hit at 1.24 times body weight, whereas a 70-kg player would be struck at 1.0 times body weight. The smaller the player, the greater the impact. Thus, the use of the smaller ball for young players is obvious.

Burslem and Lees (11) noted that the linear deceleration of the head during heading is just under 200 rad/s^2. For comparison, the deceleration needed to induce head injury is estimated to be between 5000 and 9000 rad/s^2. The data on the impulsive blow to the head and the resulting deceleration show that heading is not a dangerous activity. Minor changes in the electroencephalogram (EEG) can be observed during heading (16). However, the importance of timing and skill performance when heading cannot be overemphasized because appropriate skill performance minimizes the deceleration of the head during heading (11).

INJURIES TO THE HEAD

Acute Injuries

The head, face and neck make up about 10% of the body surface area and also about 10% of all soccer injuries (12). The mechanism of injury has changed over the years. Prior to 1960, most injuries seemed to be due to player-to-ball contact. Since then, the use of waterproof balls has minimized the water saturation and subsequent weight gain of the ball and most injuries have been reported to be head-to-head or head-to-foot (Fig. 2) resulting in minor lacerations, abrasions, and concussions (17). Over an 8-year period, 96% of head and neck injuries were due to player-to-player contact (18). In spite of the lack of protective headgear and the opportunity for impact from heading, the incidence of concussions is reported to be 0.03 per 1000 hours of athlete exposure (5), with most injuries occurring during competition (19). Earlier data (20) showed 33 deaths while playing soccer between 1933 and 1959. Fourteen of these were due to head injuries such as a fractured skull ($n = 5$), subdural hematomas ($n = 5$), cerebral hemorrhage ($n = 2$), epidural hematoma ($n = 1$), and spinal cord transection ($n = 1$). Details on the mechanism of injury are incomplete in these older papers from Europe, but head-to-head collisions, accidental ball contact with the head, and a wet, heavy ball were mentioned. The older, leather balls could absorb water and nearly double in weight, which would result in a rather deadly projectile. The modern waterproof, molded synthetic leather covered with urethane effectively negates the effect of water on the mass of the ball.

In a review of 8640 soccer-related injuries, Sane and Ylipaavalniemi (21) noted that just over 6% of the injuries were to the teeth, alveolar processes, or the lower third of the skeleton of the face. Similar data were reported by Nysether (22). Over 95% of these injuries were to players older than 15 years. Obviously, both studies recommended the use of protective mouthgear. Dental guards, although not directly studied, may be appropriate for goalkeepers, players with orthodontic appliances, or other types of dental work. Dental guards are not mandatory but may be advisable.

Soccer ball induced eye injuries were reported by Burke and co-workers (23) and Orlando (24). All injuries involved hyphema and retinal damage from the impact of the ball to the eye. In addition, corneal abrasions, traumatic iritis, retinal tears, and retinal hemorrhage were observed. In no case was there any permanent impairment.

Chronic Injuries

Probably of greater concern than the results of one or a few episodes of heading impact, are the cumulative effects of a career of heading. The data on this are somewhat controversial.

Tysvaer et al. (25,26) studied 69 Division I Norwegian soccer players (mean age = 25 years) and showed that 35% had abnormal EEG tracings and one had an abnormal neurologic examination. The frequency of abnormal EEG tracing was greater in players under 25 (44%) years than in the older players (26%). There were abnormal EEG tracings in 13% of their control subjects. Over half the players had a significant head injury while playing soccer, with over 10% complaining of prolonged symptoms.

Retired soccer players (mean age = 49 years) were studied by computed tomography (CT) (27). Over 25% had central cerebral atrophy, widened lateral ventricles, cortical atrophy, and cysts of the septum pellucidum. These cysts, seen in only 1.5% of the population, are commonly seen in boxers. Psychologic profiles of the retired players were constructed and over 80% had mild to severe defects in attention, memory, concentration, and judgment (27). The effects of repeated minor head trauma were blamed for the defects. In contrast, Haglund and Eriksson (28) studied Swedish players compared with boxers and track and field athletes and found none of the responses described in Tysvaer's series of studies. The boxers had neurologic deficits from their career, but the soccer players were no different from the track athletes. The results of Haglund and Eriksson (28) argue against the effects of cumulative minor head trauma.

The data of Tysvaer and coworkers have been widely interpreted to suggest that repeated minor blows to the head, as seen during heading, can

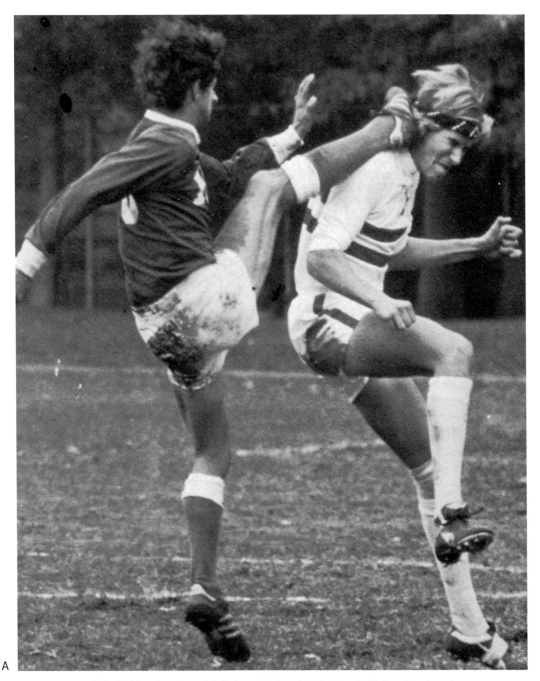

A

FIG. 2. Head and neck injuries: (**A**) head-to-foot and (**B**) head-to-head.

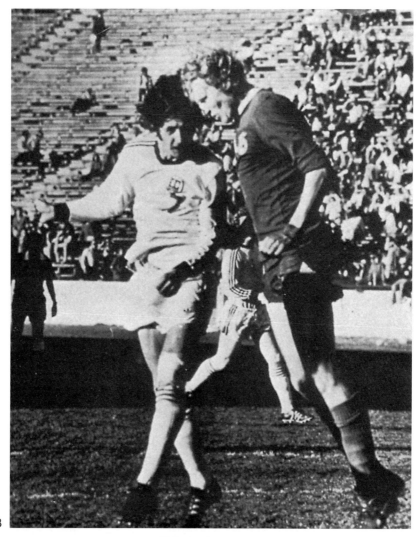

B

FIG. 2. *Continued.*

result in neurologic damage. One aspect that has been neglected is the incidence of head injuries from player-to-player or player-to-ground contact that are no doubt of more significance than heading a ball. Over half the active professionals reported a serious head injury during their career (26,29). Barnes (30) reported on a survey of elite youth participants in the U.S. National Sports Festival. In a total of 72 males, 74 concussions reported and numerous subconcussive collisions were reported. Jordan et al. (31) compared national team players from the United States with track athletes using MRI scans and a head injury symptom questionnaire. In the soccer players, symptoms and MRI findings were not correlated with age, experience, exposure, or estimated number of headers. However, there was a correlation between symptoms and prior concussive episodes, suggesting that acute head injuries, not repetitive heading, were responsible for evidence of encephalopathy. Thus, the neurologic findings reported from Norway have not been documented in the Swedish and American studies. In addition, even if there were more symptoms or objective involvement, it would be impossible to differentiate the cause as repetitive heading rather than the concussions most often due to head-to-head contact.

INJURIES TO THE SPINE

Cervical Spine

The Norwegian series of papers also looked at cervical spine injuries in retired players (27). They surveyed and performed radiographs on 43 former players and compared the results with those for age-matched controls. Nearly 60% of the former players had decreased neck range of motion and just over 20% complained of chronic neck pain or stiffness. There was radiographic evidence of healed compression fractures of the lateral masses in five players. Degenerative arthrosis at all levels of the cervical vertebrae was demonstrated in a majority of the players. Middle-aged Japanese players were examined for cervical symptoms (32). Of particular note was the presence of posterior vertebral spurs and ossicles between spinous processes and calcification of the nuchal ligament. They concluded from these radiologic findings that heading the ball places stress on the lower cervical vertebrae.

Lumbar Spine

Low back injuries have not been systematically documented in the literature, so one has to assume that the incidence of such injuries is minimal. The NCAA data (5) show that trunk injuries occur at a rate of 0.41 and 0.34 per 1000 athlete-exposures in men and women, respectively. In a recall of trunk injuries at a major university (33), injuries occurred to the lumbar spine, hip, thoracic spine, and abdomen. Most of the contusions, mild strains, and sprains did not need to be seen by a physician. Over 20 years of the survey, only one athlete needed surgery.

Clinically, spondylolysis has been observed in youth players. Stinson (34) summarized spondylolysis and reported an incidence rate of about 5% of the young population. The condition usually develops in children between 5 and 10 years of age. Typically, there is a bilateral fracture of the pars interarticularis on a single vertebra. In sports, spondylolysis may appear in athletes who place high rotation and extension demands on their back. Spondylolysis has been documented in gymnastics, diving, football, wrestling, and weight lifting. In soccer, there have been some

clinical observations of this pars interarticularis defect in high school boys. When the muscles stabilize the trunk, the rotation in kicking a ball places shear forces across the pars interarticularis (33). If the defect should occur, placing players in a molded rigid brace to limit hyperextension provides symptomatic relief and allows them to continue playing, when pain free (33), while the defect heals.

RETURN TO PLAY

A head injury must first be graded. Table 3 shows an algorithm for grading a concussion. The severity and frequency of concussions dictate when an athlete may return to play (Table 4). Given the frequency of subconcussive and concussive injuries suffered by soccer players, appropriate guidelines must be followed before allowing a player to return to activity. It must be emphasized that these guidelines are arbitrary.

PREVENTION

Heading per se is a safe activity. Barnes (30) noted that players reported symptoms related to heading only when the ball was headed improperly or when the ball was wet. Prevention of head and neck injuries involves five concepts. First, proper heading technique must be taught and continually stressed. Second, the use of a dry ball appropriate to the age and size of the player will reduce the impact forces on the head of younger and smaller players. Third, the periodic use of resistance exercises for the neck muscles will add strength that may add support for the neck. Fourth, improved skill and fitness should minimized the opportunities for player-to-player and player-to-ground contact, but these unfortunate occurrences may be unavoidable given the nature of the game.

TABLE 3. *Grading of the severity of concussion*

Grade	Loss of consciousness	Duration of posttraumatic amnesia
1 (mild)	None	< 30 min
2 (moderate)	< 5 min	.5 h to < 24 h
3 (severe)	> 5 min	≥ 24 h

From ref. 35.

TABLE 4. *Guidelines for return to play*

Grade	First concussion	Second concussion	Third concussion
1 (mild)	After 1 week if asymptomatic[a]	In 2 weeks if asymptomatic at that time for 1 week	Terminate season; may play next season if asymptomatic
2 (moderate)	After 1 week if asymptomatic	Minimum 1 month; may return if asymptomatic for 1 week; consider terminating season	Terminate season; may play next season if asymptomatic
3 (severe)	Minimum 1 month; may return to play if asymptomatic for 1 week	Terminate season; may play next season if asymptomatic	

From ref. 8, with permission.
[a] No headache, dizziness, or impaired orientation, concentration, or memory during rest or exertion.

A FINAL NOTE

Catastrophic injuries from soccer are indeed rare. However, according to the Centers for Disease Control, there have been 18 deaths over a 24-year period due to injuries sustained by a falling goalpost. Head injury was the cause in 14 of the deaths. The victims were children, mostly under 12 years of age, who were climbing on an unstable goalpost. These deaths did not occur during the game. The fifth method for the prevention of head injuries is to require that all goalposts should have a warning label advising against climbing and to ensure that all posts should be fixed permanently in the ground or stored face down and secured when not in use.

REFERENCES

1. Lohnes JH, Garrett WE, Monto RR. Soccer. In: UF, Stone DA, eds. *Sports injuries: mechanisms, prevention, treatment.* Baltimore: Williams & Wilkins, 1994:603–624.
2. Bangsbo, J. *Fitness training in football—a scientific approach.* Copenhagen: HO + Storm, 1994.
3. Reilly TR, Thomas V. A motion analysis of work-rate in different positional roles in professional football match play. *J Hum Movement Studies* 1976;2:87–97.
4. Ekstrand J, Gillquist J. Soccer injuries and their mechanisms: a prospective study. *Med Sci Sports Exerc* 1983;15:267–270.
5. National Collegiate Athletic Association: *Injury surveillance system: men's and women's soccer injury/exposure summaries, 1986–1987 to 1991–1992.* Overland Park, KS: NCAA, 1992.
6. Berger-Vachon C, Gabard G, Moyen B. Soccer accidents in the French Rhone–Alps Soccer Association. *Sports Med* 1981;3:69–77.
7. Nielson AB, Yde J. Epidemiology and traumatology of injuries in soccer. *Am J Sports Med* 1989;17:803–807.
8. Nilsson S, Roass A. Soccer injuries in adolescents. *Am J Sports Med* 1978;6:358–361.
9. Sullivan J, Gross R, Grana W, Garcia-Moral C. Evaluation of injuries in youth soccer. *Am J Sports Med* 1980;8:325–327.
10. Roaass A, Nilsson S. Major injuries in Norwegian football. *Br J Sports Med* 1979;13:3–5.
11. Burslem I, Lees A. Quantification of impact accelerations of the head during the heading of a football. In: Reilly T, Lees A, Davids K, et al., eds. *Science and football: Proceedings of the 1st World Congress of Science and Football.* London: E&FN Spon Ltd, 1987:243–248.
12. Lynch JM, Bauer JA. Acute head and neck injuries in soccer. Presented at the U.S. Soccer Symposium on the Sports Medicine of Soccer, Orlando, FL, 1994.
13. Aagaard P, Trolle M, Simonsen EB, Bangsbo J, Klausen K. High speed extension capacity of soccer players after different kinds of strength training. In: Reilly T, Clarys J, Stibbe A. eds. *Science and football: Proceedings of the 1st World Congress of Science and Football.* London: E&FN Spon Ltd, 1991:92–94.
14. Schneider K, Zernicke RF. Computer simulation of head impact: estimation of head injury risk during soccer heading. *Int J Sport Biomech* 1988;4:358–371.
15. Townend MS. Is head the ball a dangerous activity? In: Reilly T, Lees A, Davids K, et al., eds. *Science and football: Proceedings of the 1st World Congress of Science and Football.* London: E&FN Spon Ltd, 1987:237–242.
16. Aross T, Ohler K, Barolin GS. Cerebral trauma due to heading: computerized EEG analysis in football players. *Z EEG EMG* 1983;14:209–212.
17. Fields KB. Head injuries in soccer. *Phys Sports Med* 1989;17(1):69–73.
18. Frenguelli A, Ruscito P, Biccioo G, Rizzo S, Massarelli M. Head and neck trauma in sporting activities: review of 208 cases. *J Craniomaxillofacial Surg* 1991;19:178–181.
19. Maehlum S, Daljord OA. Acute sports injuries in Oslo: a one-year study. *Br J Sports Med* 1984;18:181–185.
20. Smodlaka, VN. Death on the soccer field and its prevention. *Phys Sports Med* 1981;9(8):101–104.

21. Sane J, Ylipaavalniemi P. Maxillofacial and dental soccer injuries in Finland. *Br J Oral Maxillofac Surg* 1987; 25:383–390.

22. Nysether S. Dental injuries among Norwegian soccer players. *Community Dent Oral Epidemiol* 1987;15(3): 141–143.

23. Burke MJ, Sanitato JJ, Vinger PF, Rayomond LA, Kulwin DR. Soccerball-induced eye injuries. *JAMA* 1983;249:2682–2685.

24. Orlando RG. Soccer-related eye injuries in children and adolescents. *Phys Sports Med* 1988;16(11):103–106.

25. Tysvaer AT, Lochen EI. Soccer injuries to the brain: a neuropsychologic study of former soccer players. *Am J Sports Med* 1991;19:56–60.

26. Tysvaer AT, Storil OV. Association football injuries to the brain; a preliminary report. *Br J Sports Med* 1981; 15:163–166.

27. Sortland O, Tysvaer AT. Brain damage in former association football players: an evaluation by cerebral computed tomography. *Neuroradiology* 1989;31:44–48.

28. Haglund Y, Eriksson E. Does amateur boxing lead to chronic brain damage? A review of some recent investigations. *Am J Sports Med* 1993;21:97–109.

29. Tysvaer AT, Storli OV. Soccer injuries to the brain: a neurologic and electroencophalographic study of active football players. *Am J Sports Med* 1989;17:573–578.

30. Barnes B, Cooper L, Kirkendall DT, McDermott TP, Jordan BD, Garrett WE. Concussion history in elite male and female soccer players. Am J Sports Med (*in press*).

31. Jordan SE, Green GA, Galanty HL, Mandelbaum BR, Jabour BA. Acute and chronic brain injuries in United States national team soccer players. *Am J Sports Med* 1996;24:205–210.

32. Kurosawa H, Nakashita K, Nakashita H, Sasaki S, Yamanoi T. Cervical spines of middle aged soccer players: radiographic findings and computer simulation. Presented at the U.S. Soccer Symposium on the Sports Medicine of Soccer, Orlando, FL, 1994.

33. McCarroll JR. Back and trunk injuries. In: Garrett WE, Kirkendall DT, Centiguglia. eds. *The U.S. Soccer Sports Medicine Book*. Baltimore: Williams & Wilkins, 1996.

34. Stinson JT. Spondylolysis and sondylolisthesis in the athlete. *Clin Sports Med* 1993;12:517–528.

35. Cantu RC: Cerebral concussion in sport management and prevention. *Sports Med* 1992;14:64–74.

Sports Neurology, Second Edition,
edited by Barry D. Jordan.
Lippincott–Raven Publishers, Philadelphia © 1998.

39

Winter Sports

Bradford A. Stephens

Bradford A. Stephens: P.O. Box 790 Lake Placid, New York 12946

Winter sports are enjoyed by millions of people around the world. Nature provides us with a wonderful, friction-free surface of snow and ice in the winter. We have developed a number of forms of sports to take advantage of this gift of nature. Usually this takes a form of sliding down a hill at high speeds. Although this is exciting and thrilling, it is also highly dangerous. The kinetic energy developed while hurtling downhill leads to the potential for high-energy trauma, which frequently includes neurologic injuries. In this chapter, we discuss neurologic injuries in Alpine skiing, cross-county skiing, freestyle skiing, ski jumping, freestyle aerial ski jumping, and snowboarding.

ALPINE SKIING

Alpine skiing is a very popular sport. In the United States over 50 million skier visits are recorded annually (1). Alpine skiing is generally a safe and healthy sport that is enjoyed by all ages. Most injuries are musculoskeletal in nature and not life threatening. However, there are also less common, but more serious, neurologic injuries in Alpine skiing.

Epidemiology

The incidence of injuries in Alpine skiing has been well documented in the literature (2–6). Fortunately, the overall rate of injuries has decreased from 10 injuries per 1000 skier-days in the 1950s and 1960s to 5 injuries per 1000 skier-days in the 1970s and now down to approxi-

mately 2.5 injuries per 1000 skier-days (4). The reduction in injury is due primarily to the improvement in equipment. The development of well-functioning release bindings and high, rigid boots has been effective in reducing injuries to the ankle and lower leg. Also, the replacement of ski straps by ski brakes has lowered the incidence of lacerations.

However, the improvement of skiing equipment has actually increased the rate of some injuries. This is most noted with knee injuries. With the stiff, rigid boots and the powerful carving skis, the rate of serious ligamentous injuries to the knee has increased steadily. Also, there is a definite increase in serious head and neck injuries (1,7). This seems to be directly related to the dramatic increase in skiing speed allowed by better equipment and better grooming techniques.

Injuries in skiing involving the head and spine are a relatively low percentage of the injuries incurred by skiers. In general, head injuries have been reported to be between 8% and 11% of skier injuries (3,4,8,9). Spinal injuries have been reported to be at 3%(4,9). Morrow et al. (10) studied 16 skier deaths reported in Vermont over 7 years between 1979 and 1986. Of the 16 deaths, 14 were a result of head and neck injuries. During the seven seasons, 24 million skier-days were logged for an estimated rate of 1 death per 1.5 million skier-days. Assuming that the overall injury rate for skiing is 2.5 injuries per 1000 skier-days, that would be 0.25 head injuries per 1000 skier-days and 0.075 spine injuries per 1000 skier-days.

Skiers suffering head and spine injuries have been noted to be relatively young and also predominantly male. Morrow et al. (10), in their study of fatalities in Vermont, noted that 61% were in the age group 15 to 25. Shealy (1), in his review of 71 fatalities from 1970 to 1991, found that the average age was 27. Also, Morrow et al. found that 81% of the fatalities in Vermont were male, and Shealy found 83% to be male.

Skiing at high speed and out of control is a major factor in serious ski injuries (1,7,10). Skiers with today's boots, skis, and well-groomed slopes can easily reach extreme speeds. Downhill racers exceed 80 mph and many recreational skiers frequently exceed 40 mph. At these speeds, tremendous kinetic energy develops and the injuries that occur are those of high-speed trauma as seen in automobile accidents. Many of us who practice near major ski areas have noted a definite increase in the number of injuries involving severe trauma in skiers (1,7). Morrow et al. (10) noted in the Vermont study that, of the 14 fatal accidents with neurologic causes, all the skiers were noted to be skiing out of control by witnesses. At the time of injury, 5 of the 14 were racing another skier and 2 were preparing for a ski race. Both Shealy (1,2) and Harris (7) in their reviews of head and neck injuries in skiing noted that high speed and loss of control were major factors in the injuries. They also noted that these skiers were usually advanced skiers or racers. This is dramatically opposite to other ski injuries, which usually involve inexperienced skiers.

The next most common cause of serious neurologic injuries in skiing is the skier's collision with a fixed object. This is most commonly a tree and then, in lesser frequency, a rock, a lift tower, or another skier. In the Vermont study, 14 of the 16 fatalities were caused by collision with a fixed object. In seven of the incidents, the skier fell and then slid into the object (10). Nine skiers struck trees, two struck rocks, two collided with metal towers, and one hit a drainage ditch. In Harris's (7) study of neurologic injuries in skiers in Lake Tahoe from 1975 to 1988, he found 347 neurologic injuries of which 171 were caused by collision; 67 struck other skiers, 25 struck boulders, 19 struck trees, and 13 struck lifts.

Improved grooming techniques have also been a major factor in skiing injuries. First, the improved grooming techniques allow the skier to ski much faster. Also, the groomed slopes frequently become hardened and icy and offer little deceleration to skiers once they fall. This lack of deceleration force is exacerbated by the development of new ski clothing made from synthetic fibers that are very slippery. In Lake Placid we have experienced a number of serious injuries to skiers who were skiing at slow speed, fell on steep slopes, actually accelerated after they fell, and were unable to self-arrest their slides. These skiers were seriously injured as they tumbled at high speed or slid into a fixed object, most commonly a tree.

Types of Injuries

Neurologic injuries in Alpine skiing vary according to the type and intensity of the trauma. Lindsjo et al. (8) reviewed 258 head injuries reported from 1979 to 1982 in Salen, Sweden (Table 1) (1). The most common injuries were

TABLE 1. *Head injuries*

Causes and types of injury	Injured skiers
Falls (n = 70)	
Head contusion with open wound	30
Head contusion without open wound	10
Concussion	24
Eye contusion	1
Tongue bite	1
Pain in cervical spine	1
Dental injury	2
Headache	1
Falls + blow from ski (n = 27)	
Head contusion with open wound	26
Head contusion without open wound	1
Ski pole blow (n = 19)	
Head contusion with open wound	15
Head contusion without open wound	2
Eye contusion	1
Tooth injury	1
Collision (n + 40)	
Head contusion with open wound	17
Head contusion without open wound	8
Eye contusion	2
Concussion	12
Skull base fracture, death	1

From ref. 8, with permission.

head contusions with open wounds (44%) and head contusions with concussions (33%). Of the 159 head injuries occurring while skiing, 36 were concussions. Of the 36 patients with concussions, 32 were hospitalized. There was one death from basal skull fracture. Harris (7), in his studies of patients hospitalized for neurologic injuries in Lake Tahoe from 1975 to 1988, found 347 neurologic injuries. In the 347 neurologic injuries, there were 82 skull fractures, with frontal fractures being most frequent, followed by basal fractures and then parietal fractures. There were combined head and neck injuries in 25% of the skiers studied. There were 34 cranial surgeries and 8 laminectomies, with or without fusion. Morrow's Vermont study noted that there were 13 skull fractures in the 16 deaths (see Table 2). There were seven occipital fractures in which there was noted a rapid demise of the patients. There were four parietotemporal and basal fractures. In these fractures, the patients survived a longer period of time before their deaths.

Spinal injuries have been surveyed by both Johnson and Tapper (see Table 3) with very similar percentages (11). These injuries are usually a result of falls versus collisions. Also, contusions

TABLE 2. *Lethal head injuries*

		Primary lesions		Secondary lesions	Approximate time from injury to death (h)
Case	Skull fracture	Hematomata	Other		
1	—	*Subdural[a] (100 cc)*	—	—	<1
2	Occipital, base	Subdural (20+cc)	*Contusions*	Swelling	<½
4	Facial, base	—	*Contusions*	—	2–3
5	Base	Epidural (drained)	—	*Edema, herniation infarct (PCA)[b]*	104
6	Base	Intraparechymal	Contusions	*Edema, herniation*	22
7	Dislocation occiput–C1–C2, orbit	— (Note: lethal chest injury also: *laceration of thoracic aorta*)	*Pons-med lac.[c]*	—	1–2
9	—	Subarachnoid subdural (small)	—	*Edema, herniation, encephalomalacia*	22
1	Head	—	—	—	
2	Head	Rib fracture (Fx)	Chest contusions	Atherosclerosis	
3	Chest	—	Lac., chin	Atherosclerosis	
4	Head	—	Contusion, leg	—	
5	Head	Scapular Fx	—	—	
6	Head	Tibia, fibula Fx	—	—	
7	Head–neck, chest (see "major")	Transection of aorta with hemothorax	Abrasions of hip	—	
8	Abdomen	Skull Fx (outer table, frontal sinus), pulmonary contusions	Contusion thumb	—	
9	Head	Rib Fx	Contusion, hip and leg	Bronchopneumonia, atherosclerosis, mild	

From ref. 10, with permission.
[a] Immediate cause of death is given in italics.
[b] PCA, posterior cerebral artery.
[c] Pons-med lac., pontine medullary laceration.

TABLE 3. *Prevalence of skiing injuries to the spine*

Injuries	Johnson (15) (1972–1980)	Tapper (9) (1939–1976)
Total injuries	2596 (100%)	10,120 (100%)
Total spinal injuries	75 (2.95%)	337 (3.17%)
Back sprain and contusion	42 (1.6%)	187 (1.8%)
Cervical sprain	20 (0.8%)	83 (0.8%)
Compression fracture	8 (0.3%)	26 (0.2%)
Sacrum and coccyx	4 (0.15%)	33 (0.3%)
Cervical fractures	0	8 (0.07%)
Thoracic fractures	1 (0.1%)	0

From ref. 11, with permission.

and sprains are much more frequent than fractures. Oh (12) reviewed 18 patients with cervical fracture dislocations hospitalized in Chur, Switzerland from 1978 to 1983. Twelve of these patients suffered head injuries along with the cervical injury and one patient died with complete fracture dislocation of C2-3 and a severe cerebral contusion. Four of the 18 underwent spinal stabilization for instability and persistent neurologic deficit.

Treatment of Neurologic Injuries in Alpine Skiing

It is essential that all ski areas and winter sports venues have in place a comprehensive treatment plan for the emergency management of severely injured skiers. Fortunately, the National Ski Patrol provides excellent on-hill emergency management of injuries. All personnel have been thoroughly trained in basic life support and are well trained to recognize the potential for neurologic injuries. They are equipped with specialized splints and head and neck braces to protect the skier during transfer to the base area.

Advanced life support is the next level of care essential to a comprehensive emergency care system at a ski area. Once the skier has been transported to a fixed first-aid area, advanced life support personnel with proper equipment should be available. This should include equipment for intravenous fluid resuscitation, maintenance of an airway including intubation equipment, electrocardiac monitoring and management, and emergency medication. Communication equipment, either phone or radio, must be available for direct communication with medical control at the supervising hospital and with neurologic consultants.

Once the patient is stabilized, an advanced life support transportation system must be available for the most effective and rapid transportation to the hospital. In many cases, this is best provided by helicopters.

Prevention

As in all areas of medicine, prevention of injury is the most effective form of treatment. In Alpine skiing, we must look at the known causes of injury to attempt to prevent them. Excessive speed is the dominant factor associated with severe neurologic injuries in Alpine skiing. Improved boot and ski technology, along with better grooming, has allowed the skier to ski much faster. However, it is the skier who, in the final analysis, determines the speed. Therefore, our energies must be directed toward educating skiers about the risks associated with skiing fast.

Collisions with fixed objects, trees, rocks, or lift towers are the next most common factor noted in serious neurologic injuries. This is a difficult situation, especially in the East, where most ski slopes have been cut through forested hillsides leaving the trails lined with trees. Protective safety nets are used effectively during Alpine racing. This type of protective equipment would be effective at ski areas where there is high speed terrain. Certainly, the lift towers need to be well padded.

Grooming is another area where ski areas can significantly affect skiing speeds. Not only do the hard smooth surfaces allow fast skiing, they also do little to slow the skier's speed once there is a fall. In some instances, on steep terrain, skiers actually accelerate after they fall. This problem is accentuated by the new synthetic clothes. This clothing is very slick, which becomes a serious problem, especially when inexperienced skiers are on steep slopes that they cannot handle. Ski areas need to look at this problem carefully and study grooming techniques that will help control skiers' speed while they ski and to help decelerate them once they fall. Also, it is extremely important that ski trails are well signed to keep inexperienced skiers off steep slopes.

Finally, the use of helmets in skiing should be examined carefully. Studies have shown a reduction in head injuries with the use of helmets in recreational skiers (13). Helmets are required in Alpine racing and have been effective in preventing neurologic injuries. The public has accepted the use of helmets in bicycling, and I believe there is a good case for their use in Alpine skiing. Helmets are certainly important for skiers who plan to ski at high speeds, on well-packed slopes, on steep terrain, or on narrow trails lined with trees.

Physicians who are responsible for emergency care of skiers at recreational ski areas or during Alpine races need to have a thorough understanding of the evaluation and treatment of neurologic emergencies. First, it is important to recognize that the ski patrol has the expertise in on-hill management and transportation of skiing injuries. Once the patient is transported to the base emergency facility, a rapid neurologic assessment is important. It may be necessary to intubate a patient with head injury and protect the cervical spine. As in other sports, an understanding of the level of concussion is important in advising the athlete. Certainly, the risk of second impact injury is important.

Interestingly, there was an apparent example of the second impact syndrome during the 1980 Olympics in Lake Placid. An 18-year-old downhill racer had suffered a "minor" head injury 2 weeks prior to the Olympics in a World Cup team race. While racing at Lake Placid, he was severely jarred as he struck a mogul. He did not fall. However, as he approached the finish line, he fell and slid across the line. He stood for a few minutes, then complained of dizziness and collapsed. He was found to have fixed, dilated pupils and was in deep coma with shallow respirations. He was immediately intubated and transferred by helicopter to the hospital. A computed tomographic (CT) scan revealed massive swelling of the left cerebral hemisphere. He remained in deep coma until his death (14).

CROSS-COUNTRY SKIING

Cross-country skiing is a sport enjoyed by millions of people wherever there is snow. Much cross-country skiing is done on prepared tracks for classic diagonal stride technique or on groomed trails for skating techniques. However, a great deal of cross-country skiing is done on unprepared trails, slopes, and fields. The mode of skiing varies greatly from ski "walkers" to racers, and the technique varies from traditional diagonal stride to skating technique. Also, in downhill situations either traditional Alpine techniques or telemark techniques are used.

Because of the varied type of skiing and the ubiquitous nature of cross-country skiing, it is difficult to ascertain the population at risk in order to study the incidence of injuries. However, many studies have been done estimating the population at risk. The results have shown injuries range from 0.2 injuries per 1000 skier-days to 1.5 injuries per 1000 skier-days (15,16). However, Boyle et al. (16) in Vermont did a prospective study in five cross-country ski centers for two seasons from 1989 to 1991. In the initial year, with poor conditions and low numbers of skiers, there were 1.5 injuries per 1000 skier-days, and in the second year, with better conditions and a higher number of skiers, there were 0.48 injuries per 1000 skier-days. This averaged out to 0.72 injuries per 1000 skier-days. Interestingly, most of the skiers who were injured were inexperienced and 88% of the injuries occurred when the skier was actually skiing downhill. Neurologic injuries in cross-country skiing are infrequent. This is primarily due to the fact that cross-country skiing is usually done at a relatively slow speed, which causes low-energy injuries. In contrast, Alpine skiing usually causes high-speed, high-energy injuries. When injuries do occur in cross-country skiing, it is usually in the downhill portion of the skiing.

Neurologic injuries in cross-country skiing are infrequent. Boyle et al. (16) noted that there was one concussion and one fractured sacrum. The mechanism of falling in cross-country skiing is often a seated fall, which can cause compression fractures. Another type of fall is in a downhill situation in which the skier falls forward. This can result from the narrow cross-country ski cutting into the snow and throwing the skier forward. Also, in the telemark turn, skiers have their weight forward, and when they fall they are usually thrown forward. This accounts for the many upper extremity injures noted in cross-country skiing. A patient in Lake Placid who suffered C-5, C-6, fracture subluxation with neurologic deficit that required decompression and fusion was an inexperienced skier who was on a steep, narrow trail and could not control his speed. He was skiing fast before the fall, in which he was thrown forward and somersaulted.

Cross-country skiing is a sport enjoyed by many skiers. It is usually quite safe. The most dangerous situation is in the downhill phase. This is extremely dangerous for inexperienced skier, as cross-country skis are difficult to turn and do not control speed well.

SKI JUMPING

Ski jumping is a beautiful and exciting sport that has potential for serious injuries. As opposed to Alpine and cross-country skiers, there are relatively few ski jumpers in the United States. Ski jumpers reach speeds of 60 mph on the in-run and travel 70 mph to 90 mph in the air. The ski jump has a steep in-run with a short takeoff portion, a fairly flat knoll over which ski jumpers fly, and then a steep landing hill. The ski jumper does not reach a great height over the terrain but travels in trajectory fairly parallel to the landing hill.

The most serious injuries occur when the jumper falls on the in-run. This usually causes the skier to slide down the in-run and then be thrown onto the knoll of the hill, which is fairly flat. If jumpers lose control and fall on the landing hill, they usually hit and slide, because the trajectory is nearly parallel to the landing hill.

The incidence of injuries in ski jumping has been looked at carefully in two major studies. First, Wright et al. (17) reviewed hospital records of injuries to ski jumpers in Lake Placid for 5 years and found 47 injured skiers. They found an injury rate of 4.3 injuries per 1000 skier-days

during non–World Cup and Olympic Games training and competitions and 1.2 injuries per 1000 skier-days during World Cups and Olympics. A study done in Sapporo, Japan from 1985 to 1990 found injuries in 7831 jumps (18). There were 71 falls and 43 injuries. This gave an injury rate of 5.5 injuries per 1000 jumps (18).

Injuries in ski jumpers are frequently to the upper extremities and to the head and neck. This is primarily because the skiers lean well forward to take advantage of the aerodynamic foil. Wright et al. (17) found a ratio of upper extremity to lower extremity injuries of 2:1. In this study seven concussions were found: five were mild and did not require hospitalization and two of the jumpers were hospitalized for short periods of time but did not have any residual disability (17). There was also one mild compression fracture of the thoracic spine. In the Sapporo study, there were 41 injuries overall: 5 of these were concussions and 9 were cervical strains (18).

Webster (19), in a review of serious disabling injuries in Norwegian ski jumpers from 1977 to 1981, found 14 injuries. He estimated that there were 5 million jumps during this period of time (19). Three of the 14 injuries were cervical fracture-dislocations with complete paraplegia. One of the injuries was an intracerebral hematoma.

Serious neurologic injures are a potential in ski jumping, but fortunately they are rare. The injuries have been related to snow and weather conditions. Soft snow is dangerous for landing because the skier can sink into the snow and be thrown forward. Also, gusty, variable winds are extremely dangerous as they can easily throw the jumper off while in the air. The overall rate of injury has decreased steadily with better facilities, grooming, and training.

FREESTYLE AERIAL SKI JUMPING

The aerial component of freestyle skiing is a spectacular sport in which a skier jumps over 30 feet in the air, does up to three backward somersaults and up to four twists, and then lands on a steep landing hill and skis off. There is obviously tremendous potential for serious neurologic injuries in this sport.

The U.S. Free Style Ski Team is one of our most successful national teams, winning many world titles. This sport is now an Olympic sport and is rapidly growing in popularity. Freestyle skiing began in the 1960s and 1970s with "hot dog" skiing. This led to many uncontrolled contests. Unfortunately, there was a high rate of serious cervical injuries. The United States Ski Association gained control of the sport and banned inverted aerial maneuvers in 1975. After the institution of strict control of contests and rigid training prerequisites before competing, aerial maneuvers were reinstated in 1980.

The incidence of injuries during the time when inverted maneuvers were banned was carefully studied by Dowling (20). During these five seasons, all injuries at the World Cup level were reported and analyzed. Over these five seasons, 3180 skiers were entered. They trained or competed for 10,188 skiing days. An injury was defined as an accident requiring at least 1 day of lost training or competition. Sixteen injuries were noted in the Aerial Ski Team, giving a rate of 4.7 injuries per 1000 skier-days. The average age was 16.2 and the rates of injuries among men and women were similar. Injuries to the head and spine made up 46% of these injuries. Interestingly, there were no injuries to the cervical spine. There were two compression fractures of the thoracolumbar spine, with only one requiring a short period of hospitalization. Also, there were five mild concussions without residuals.

Since 1980, when the aerial maneuvers were reinstated, careful control of competitions and training has been instituted. The athlete must perform an aerial maneuver at least 200 times in water facilities during the summer before being allowed to perform the maneuver on snow. The conditions of the jumps are controlled and the landing is kept soft by chopping the snow. Athletes are required to wear helmets. However, the design and type of helmet are not specified.

Despite the fact that these athletes are subjected to severe high-energy forces in their falls, they have been able to protect themselves from severe head and neck trauma. In reviewing the records of the U.S. Free Style Team over the past 3 years, I can find only three grade 1 concussions, which did not require hospitalization. Also, I can find only three reports of cervical strain, requiring an athlete to miss competition. One herniated cervical disc was found in an athlete this season, requiring an anterior discectomy and fusion.

There is, however, great concern about athletes who suffer repetitive mild head trauma resulting from "slap-backs." This is a situation in which the skier is doing a backward somersault and overrotates. The backs of the skis hit the snow and the athlete is thrown back against the back and head. This is a relatively common situation in this sport. The athletes are frequently dazed momentarily. Unfortunately, they frequently do not report their symptoms for fear of losing training and competition time. Mecham et al. (21) reported the incidence of slap-backs to be 16.2%. They instrumented the helmets and found that maximum head acceleration magnitude was relatively low during these slap-backs. This appears to explain why there have not been more severe concussions. However, the high number of head impacts in slap-backs raises concern about repetitive brain trauma and needs to be studied further. Also, the danger of "second impact" syndrome needs to be recognized by all involved in this sport. The athlete must be held from training and competition until any signs of mental dysfunction have completely cleared.

Freestyle aerial skiing is a unique and thrilling sport. It has come a long way in its short history as an organized sport in preventing injury. Further work on helmet design and further study of the effects of repetitive head impacts from slap-backs need to be done.

SNOWBOARDING

Snowboarding is a rapidly growing winter sport. It is thought that 10% of all the slope users are now snowboarders, and it is projected that this number will grow rapidly to 30%. Snowboarding is now an Olympic sport. It was initially the sport of young counterculture males, usually ex-skateboarders and surfers, but it is becoming more and more a sport enjoyed by both sexes and all ages.

The characteristics of snowboarding that affect injuries are primarily that both feet are fixed to one board and that no poles are used. The typical injury is one of impact, as the rider is thrown against the snow, striking with the upper body. Because of this, there is a higher rate of injuries to the upper body than in Alpine skiing. Also, the initial boot used was a soft boot with little support, and there was a much higher rate of ankle injuries in snowboarding than in Alpine skiing. Now, a transition to rigid boots is taking place. There are fewer injuries to ankles with these, but more tibia fractures and serious knee injuries. The overall rate of injury is difficult to ascertain because of the difficulty in controlling the population at risk. However, two studies that best gauge this show an injury rate of approximately 4 per 1000, which is higher than the accepted Alpine rate of injury of 2 per 1000 at this time (22,23).

Neurologic injuries are noted with different frequencies in the studies that have been done. Janes and Fincken (23) reviewed 937 injuries to snowboarders recorded in Vail, Colorado over three seasons from 1988 through 1991. Among these injuries there were 19 (2%) concussions and 10 vertebral fractures (1%). The severity of these injuries was not detailed. McLennan and McLennan (24) evaluated 460 snowboarding injuries from 1986 to 1990 and noted 2% head injuries and 4% spine injuries. However, they noted that there were no severe head or neck injuries in the study. Calle and Evans (25) reviewed records of 487 snowboarding injuries at six different Vermont ski areas from 1991 to 1993 and also the records of 568 snowboarding injuries recorded by the Consumer Product Safety Commission. There were 27 (5.5%) concussions and no deaths in the Vermont study. There were no concussions and five deaths (1.7%) in the national survey. The deaths were noted to be due to collisions with rocks and trees. We have also seen incidents of severe head and neck injuries in Lake Placid related to snowboarders skiing fast, out of control, and colliding with trees. Wambacher et al. (26) reviewed snowboarding injuries in Innsbruck between 1988 and 1995. In 124 injuries there were 47 (4%) head injuries and 33 (3%) severe spine injuries (26).

Neurologic injury in snowboarding, as in Alpine skiing, is related primarily to the snowboard rider's speed and control. As with Alpine skiing, educating riders about the dangers of collisions and encouraging the use of helmets would be the most helpful forms of prevention.

SUMMARY

Winter sports are enjoyed by millions of people around the world. Many athletes are drawn by the thrill of rapidly sliding on or flying over winter's frictionless world. However, the element of high speed in winter sports leads to the risk of high-energy trauma and neurologic injury. There is still much work to be done to protect winter athletes and prevent injury.

REFERENCES

1. Shealy JE. Death in downhill skiing. *Skiing trauma and safety: 5th International Symposium;* 349–357.
2. Shealy JE. Comparison of downhill ski injury patterns—1978–81 vs. 1988–90. *Skiing trauma and safety: Ninth International Symposium,* 23–32.
3. Young LR, Lee SM. Alpine injury pattern at Waterville Valley—1989 update. *Skiing trauma and safety: Eighth International Symposium,* 125–132.
4. Johnson RJ, Ettinger CF, Shealy JE. Skier injury trends—1972–1990. *Skiing trauma and safety: Ninth International Symposium,* 11–22.
5. Ekeland A, Holtmoen A, Lystad H. Alpine skiing injuries in Scandinavian skiers. *Skiing trauma and safety: Eighth International Symposium,* 144–156.
6. Johnson RJ, Incavo SJ. Alpine skiing injuries. In: Casey MJ, et al, eds. *Winter Sports Med* Philadelphia: FA Davis Co, 1990:351–358.
7. Harris JB. Neurologic injuries in skiing and winter sports in America. In Jordan BC, Tsairis P, Warren RF, eds. *Sports Neurol* Rockville: Aspen Publishers, 1989; 295–304.
8. Lindsjo U, Hellquist E, Engkuist O, Balkfors B. Head injuries in Alpine skiing. *Skiing trauma and safety: Fifth International Symposium,* 375–381.
9. Tapper EM. Ski injuries from 1936–1976: the Sun Valley experience. *Am J Sports Med* 1978;6:114.
10. Morrow PL, McQuillen EN, Eaton LA, Bernstein CJ. Downhill ski fatalities: the Vermont experience. *J Trauma* 1988;28(1):95–100.
11. Frymoyer J, Pope M, Kristiansen T. Skiing and spinal trauma. *Clin Sports Med* 1982;1:309–318.
12. Oh S. Cervical injury from skiing. *Int J Sports Med* 1984;5:268–271.
13. Ungerholm S, Gustavsson J. Skiing safety in children: a prospective study of downhill skiing injuries and their relation to the skier and his equipment. *Int J Sports Med* 1985;6:353–358.
14. McQuillen JB. Head injuries in winter sports. In: Casey MJ, et al, eds. *Winter Sports Med* Philadelphia: FA Davis Co, 1990;191–193.

15. Johnson RJ, Incavo SJ. Cross country ski injuries. In: Casey MJ, et al, eds. *Winter Sports Med* Philadelphia: FA Davis Co, 1990;302–307.

16. Boyle H, Johnson RJ, Pope MH, et al. Cross-country skiing injuries. *Skiing trauma and safety: Fifth International Symposium,* 411–422.

17. Wright JR, et al. Ski-jumping injuries. In: Casey MJ, et al, eds. *Winter Sports Med* Philadelphia: FA Davis Co, 1990;324–330.

18. Sugawara M, Serita K, Takada Y, Watanabe M, Kondo H. Analysis of skiing injuries in Sapporo, Japan during 1979 through 1984. In: Mote CD, Johson RJ, eds. *Skiing trauma and safety: Sixth International Syposium,* 1987:271–279.

19. Webster K. Serious ski jumping injuries in Norway. *Am J Sports Med* 1985;13:124–127.

20. Dowling PA. Prospective study of injuries in United States Ski Association freestyle skiing 1976–77 to 1979–80. *Am J Sports Med* 1982;10:268–275.

21. Mecham MD, Greenwald RM, Macintyre JG, Johnson SC. Incidence and severity of head impact during freestyle aerial ski jumping. Second World Congress on Sports Trauma, *AOSSM 22nd Annual Meeting,* June 18, 1996.

22. Bladin C, Giddings B, Robinson M. Australian snowboard injury data base study: a four-year prospective study. *Am J Sports Med* 1993; 21;701–704.

23. Janes PC, Fincken GT. Snowboarding injuries. *Skiing trauma and safety: Ninth International Symposium,* 255–261.

24. McLennan JC, McLennan JG. Snowboarding: what injuries to expect in this rapidly growing sport. *J Musculoskel Med* 1991; Nov: 75–89.

25. Calle SC, Evans JT. Snowboarding trauma. *J Pediatr Surg* 1995;30:791–794.

26. Wambacher M, Gabe M, Wiscatter R, Benedette KP. Pattern of snowboarding injuries. Second World Congress on Sports Trauma, *AAOSM 22nd Annual Meeting,* June 18, 1996.

Sports Neurology, Second Edition,
edited by Barry D. Jordan.
Lippincott–Raven Publishers, Philadelphia © 1998.

40

Neurologic Injuries in Other Sports

Barry D. Jordan

Reed Neurological Research Center, UCLA School of Medicine, 710 Westwood Plaza, Los Angeles, California 90095-1769

The frequency of neurologic injury in sports is often dictated by the nature of the sport. Obviously, contact sports such as boxing, football, rugby, and hockey are associated with a high frequency of head and cervical spine injuries. There are several sports not mentioned in the preceding chapters in which neurologic injuries are uncommon but nonetheless do occur. These sports, including baseball, lacrosse, weightlifting, and others, are briefly reviewed in this chapter.

BASEBALL

Both brain and peripheral nerve injuries have been reported in baseball. Garfinkel et al. (1), in a survey of medical problems affecting a baseball team, reported two cases of concussion out of a total of 382 injuries over a 2-year period. In a population-based survey of 2861 Little League baseball players, Pasternak et al. (2) noted two cases of closed head injury that were minor in nature and not associated with a catastrophic outcome. Despite the rarity of documented head trauma in baseball, an intracerebral hematoma has been reported in a 12-year-old Little Leaguer who was struck in the head with a pitched ball (3). Ulnar neuropathy in the throwing arm of pitchers has also been reported (4). Other peripheral nerve injuries encountered in baseball include the radical (5), suprascapular (6), and axillary nerves (7,8). Long et al. (9) described a clinical entity, "pitcher's arm," in which there are reduced sensory nerve action potentials in the throwing arm of pitchers. This is believed to

be secondary to a repetitive use injury to the brachial plexus. Although this electrodiagnostic finding does not affect pitching performance, it had clear implications in the interpretation of diagnostic testing. In softball, radial neuropathy has been reported secondary to "windmill" pitching (10). The pronator teres syndrome has also been reported in baseball (11).

BASKETBALL

Neurologic injuries are rarely reported in basketball. According to Zvijac and Thompson (12), concussion accounts for 0.19% to 3% of basketball injuries. Back injuries probably represent the most frequently encountered neurologic injuries in basketball. It has been reported that back injury represents 8.2% and 13.0% of women's and men's basketball injuries, respectively (13). Although catastrophic spine injuries have not been reported in the literature, noncatastrophic spine fractures may occur (14–16).

CANOEING AND KAYAKING

Competitive canoeists and kayakers often experience injuries to the lower back (17). Low back pain is most common during heavy training and in paddlers older than 25 years of age (17). Muscle strain injuries to the back are usually short-lived and can be prevented with preworkout stretching. Chronic low back pain and lumbar disc disease may require a standard low back exercise program to alleviate the pain, and surgery may occasionally be indicated. Median nerve entrapment in the carpal tunnel secondary to excessive wrist torque while canoeing may also be encountered.

FIELD SPORTS

Paley and Gillespie (18) described a 17-year-old female high jumper who experienced several episodes of transient neurologic dysfunction associated with flexion of the neck. These episodes were characterized by paresthesias and brief paralysis. Her neurologic examination was normal, and flexion–extension views of the cervical spine demonstrated anterior subluxation of C-5 or C-6. She was treated with a posterior cervical fusion of C-5 to C-6 and advised not to return to high jumping for at least 12 months. Although one episode of transient neurologic dysfunction occurred while she was high jumping, the investigators attributed her cervical spine instability to chronic flexion–rotation loading of the cervical spine secondary to an incorrect landing technique. Instead of landing on the back, shoulders, and base of the neck, this athlete landed almost vertically on her neck with the cervical spine hyperflexed and rotated. This injury could be prevented by proper training techniques.

GOLF

Low back pain is a common medical problem encountered in golf (19–23) and is typically related to the golf swing. During the golf swing there is rotation of the lumbar spine at the top of the back swing, with subsequent uncoiling and hyperextension through the down swing and follow through (22). These movements result in significant mechanical loads on the lumbar spine. Back pain in golfing may be associated with lumbar strains or sprains, disc degeneration with or without herniation, spondylolysis, or spondylosis (22).

In addition to lumbar spine pathology, golfers may develop thoracic spine injuries. Ekin and Sinaki (24) reported thoracic spine compression fractures that resulted from golfing in two women diagnosed with osteoporosis. Jamieson and Ballantyne (25) reported a case of thoracic spine disc prolapse that presented with a 10-year history of Lhermitte's symptom precipitated by a rotatory movement of the thoracic spine during the golf swing.

Besides spine injuries, serious head injury may rarely be encountered in golf. In a survey of patients with head injuries admitted to a neurosurgical unit in Glasgow, Lindsay et al. (26) reported 14 cases of head trauma resulting from golf. The majority of these injuries were depressed skull fractures caused by a golf club or a ball. Three cases were complicated by an intracranial contusion or hematoma. Overall, the recovery from these 14 cases of head trauma was good and not associated with significant disability.

Peripheral nerve injury at the elbow or wrist may also be encountered in golf. Ulnar nerve irritation can occur at the elbow and may be accompanied by medical epicondylitis (27). At the wrist, carpal tunnel syndrome can result from repetitive grasping and wrist motion (28). In golf, carpal tunnel syndrome may respond to conservative therapy (e.g., night splinting); however, refractory cases may require carpal tunnel steroid injection or carpal tunnel release.

A rather unusual neurologic condition unique to golf is called golfer's cramp or "yips"(29). In this condition, the golfer experiences a jerk, spasm, or freezing of movement while putting or chipping. Golfer's cramp represents a type of occupational cramp and can be classified as a focal task-specific dystonia (see Chapter 24 for more detail).

GYMNASTICS

Catastrophic injury to the nervous system in gymnastics is commonly associated with the trampoline. Torg and Das (30), in a review of the international literature, identified 114 cervical spine injuries with associated quadriplegia resulting from use of the trampoline and minitrampoline. The C5-6 vertebral level was the most common site of injury. Pathologic lesions included vertebral body compression-burst fractures and facet dislocations with intervertebral disc herniations. The "skilled performer" attempting difficult maneuvers and somersaults represented the type at risk for sustaining a cervical spine injury (30). In view of the potential dangers associated with the trampoline and minitrampoline, Torg and Das recommended that these activities have no place in recreational, educational, or competitive gymnastics. Short of banning, Rapp and Nicely (31) made several safety suggestions to prevent cervical spine injury in trampoline gymnasts. These safety precautions included proper trampoline instruction, a certification program for physical education teachers, and proper specifications for equipment. They also recommended that advanced maneuvers such as somersaults be performed only by experienced gymnasts.

Although less devastating than cervical spine injuries, lumbar spine injuries can occur in gymnastics (32–40). Garrick and Requa (32) noted that strains and sprains involving the lumbar spine area occurred more frequently in women's gymnastics than in most other interscholastic athletic activities. Mackie and Taunton (37) reported five cases of lumbar hyperextension syndrome in a group of 100 young female gymnasts during a 40-month period. In addition to acute and chronic lumbar sprains and strains, spondylolysis represents a relatively common lumbar spinal injury in gymnasts. Once a gymnast is diagnosed with spondylolysis, medical intervention should be implemented to prevent the progression of spondylolisthesis (36). Other less common lumbar spine injuries that can be encountered in gymnastics include lumbar disc degeneration or herniation and vertebral fractures (34). The most common mechanism of chronic low back pain in gymnasts is repeated hyperextension of the lumbar spine compounded by impact loading caused by tumbling and landing from a height (38). In young female gymnasts it has been hypothesized that problems of the lumbar spine are often associated with periods of rapid growth (33).

Traumatic brain injury is a rather uncommon consequence in gymnasts. Caine et al. (39) reported one case of concussion in an epidemiologic investigation of injuries affecting young competitive female gymnasts. This injury accounted for less than 1% of gymnastic injuries during the surveillance period. Despite the relatively low occurrence of brain trauma in gymnastics, it should be a medically anticipated injury because of its associated morbidity and mortality.

Peripheral nerve injuries represent another uncommon neurologic injury in gymnastics. Hirasawa and Sakakida (41) reported seven cases of peripheral nerve injury in gymnastics. These included ulnar nerve (two cases), and lateral femoral cutaneous nerve (one case) injury. Also of interest, there have been three case reports of femoral neuropathy associated with gymnastics (42–44). Traumatic femoral neuropathy may be associated with (43,44) or without (42) a hematoma of the iliacus muscle. An iliacus hematoma should be suspected as the cause of a femoral neuropathy when the onset of paralysis is delayed (44) and/or a tender mass is palpated in the iliac fossa (43). In cases without an iliacus hematoma, the mechanism of femoral nerve injury may be secondary to hemorrhage into the nerve sheath or stretching of the nerve (42). Femoral nerve injury secondary to an iliacus hematoma in gymnastics appears to be associated with sudden flexion or extension of the hips that involves a violent contraction of the iliacus muscle with resultant hemorrhage or avulsion of the muscle.

LACROSSE

Although neurologic complications of lacrosse are infrequent, head injuries should be anticipated. Kuland et al. (45), in a survey of 58 summer league lacrosse players, noted only three concussions. At the University of Virginia, 34 lacrosse players experienced a total of 78 injuries, one of which was a concussion (46). In a more comprehensive survey, Mueller and Blyth (47) observed six concussions among 586 collegiate lacrosse players from 20 National Collegiate Athletic Association teams. In addition to concussion, more serious traumatic brain injury can occur in lacrosse. For example, Rimel et al. (48) reported an epidural hematoma in a lacrosse player struck in the cranium with a lacrosse stick.

PARACHUTING AND SKYDIVING

Lumbar spine injuries are the second most common injury among parachutists and are usually caused by compression and torsion of the spine (49). Most of the compression fractures occur at the thoracolumbar junction between T-11 and L-2. Parachutists landing at high speeds while standing upright experience flexing of the lumbar spine. Because the thoracolumbar region is the least flexible area of the lumbar spine, it is the most susceptible to flexion injuries. This is further compounded if the parachutist twists his or her body on landing.

RODEO

Injuries to the head and neck in rodeo typically occur during the ride in rough stock events or during the dismount (50). According to Nebergall (50), tremendous forces are generated through the head and spine as the animal jumps, twists, kicks, and turns trying to dislodge the rider. These violent whipping motions can result in spinal sprain, strains, and intervertebral disc rupture. Concussions typically occur during the dismount when the rider sustains a blow to the head from the animal or lands on the head (50). Concussions account for 4.9% to 13.8% of rodeo injuries (50–53). Serious brain and spinal cord injuries have been associated with riding bulls in rodeo events in Lousiana from 1994 to 1995 (54). These injuries included a C-5 and C-6 vertebral fracture with incomplete spinal cord injury, a concussion associated with loss of consciousness, an incomplete T10-11 spinal cord injury, and a brain injury associated with unconsciousness for 5 days.

RUNNING AND JOGGING

Peripheral neuropathy and back pain are the most common neurologic injuries associated with running and jogging. Massey and Pleet (55) reported three types of nerve impairments thought to be directly attributable to running. These were peroneal entrapment neuropathy, meralgia paresthetica, and cervical radiculopathy. Moller and Kadin (56) described a case of bilateral common peroneal entrapment in a jogger who presented with a 2-year history of pain, superficial numbness, and coldness in the anterolateral aspect of both legs. Any case of peroneal neuropathy should be differentiated from the anterior tibial compartment syndrome. The anterior compartment syndrome is an ischemic myopathy associated with postexertional leg pain, swelling of the leg, footdrop, and diminished or absent dorsalis pedis pulses.

Gluten (57) reviewed 10 cases of herniated lumbar disc associated with running. All 10 runners experienced acute back and leg pain during or shortly after running, and all ran at least 20 miles per week. Treatment modalities included conservative treatment with bed rest and antiinflammatory drugs, traction, injections of epidural steroids, and laminectomy (three cases).

SHOOTING SPORTS

Low back pain probably represents the most common musculoskeletal complaint in rifle and pistol shooters. Prolonged rigid and static hyperextension and rotation of the spine create significant stress on the lower spine. In one study, 78% of shooters experienced back pain during competition and 63% experienced back pain after competition (58). Flexibility and biomechanical tests indicated that ilioband tightness correlated significantly with the development of low back pain.

Paralysis of the serratus anterior muscle secondary to a long thoracic neuropathy has also been reported in shooting (59). A 25-year-old world class marksman noticed right posterior shoulder pain over a 2-week period that was followed by weakness of the serratus anterior muscle and prominent winging of the scapula. Electromyographic testing confirmed a long thoracic neuropathy. It was hypothesized that traction on the long thoracic nerve produced by chronic and repetitive positional stress during shooting was responsible for the neuropathy.

SKATING

Skating sports (i.e., in-line skating, rollerskating, and skateboarding) may be associated with serious head injuries. Schieber et al. (60), in a survey of skating injuries identified by the National Electronic Injury Surveillance System (NEISS), reported 30,863 in-line skating injuries, 92,963 rollerskating injuries, and 34,938 skateboarding injuries in 1 year. Head injuries of any severity constituted 4.8% of injuries among in-line skaters, 3.8% among rollerskaters, and 6.9% among skateboarders. Concussion, blunt trauma, skull fracture, or closed head injuries accounted for 2% to 3% of skating injuries. Accordingly, it has been recommended that protective headgear be worn during participation in these activities (60).

TENNIS AND RACQUET SPORTS

Radial nerve entrapment or cervical radiculopathy should be considered in the differential diagnosis of "tennis elbow." Tennis elbow, also known as lateral epicondylitis, is a multifactorial syndrome characterized by lateral forearm pain with tenderness in the vicinity of the lateral epicondyle (61). Compression of the deep branch of the radial nerve (posterior interosseus nerve) as it passes dorsal to the fibrous edge of the supinator muscle can present as lateral forearm pain. This can be differentiated from true lateral epicondylitis in that deep palpation of the volar aspect of the radial head elicits more pain than does palpation of the lateral epicondyle (61). Also, in the radial tunnel entrapment syndrome, pain is more characteristically produced with isoresisted supination of the forearm as opposed to isoresisted extension of the wrist. Because the neurologic supply to the lateral forearm is derived from the C-5 through C-8 nerve roots, radicular involvement of these nerve roots can also elicit lateral forearm pain with or without neck pain. Accordingly, any patient presenting with lateral forearm pain should have cervical radiculopathy ruled out in the differential diagnosis.

In addition to radial neuropathy, other neuropathies that can be encountered in tennis include the ulnar (62), axillary (63), long thoracic (63), and suprascapular (63) nerves.

Low back pain represents a not uncommon condition among tennis players. Causes of low back pain in tennis players include lumbar strain, lumbar disc degeneration or herniation, facet impingement or arthropathy, and piriformis syndrome (64).

WEIGHT LIFTING AND TRAINING

Shea (65) described a 26-year-old weight trainer who developed acute quadriplegia minutes after using progressive resistance exercise machinery.

Cervical spine roentgenograms, computed tomographic (CT) scanning, and myelography were all unremarkable. A metrizamide CT scan performed 7 days after admission demonstrated a fusiform swelling of the cervical spine at C-4 and C-5 but was otherwise normal. The patient was diagnosed as having spinal apoplexy of unknown etiology. Whether the development of spinal apoplexy was causally related to the use of resistive exercise machinery or was an unrelated coincidence is totally speculative.

Ulnar neuropathy has also been reported in weight lifters. Dangles and Bilos (66) noted an ulnar neuritis in a 39-year-old competitive weight lifter that was attributed to compression, stretch, and friction of the nerve. This patient was treated with medial epicondylectomy and decompression of the ulnar nerve between the heads of the flexor carpi ulnaris.

In addition to the preceding injuries, acute cervical radiculopathy has been reported during weight lifting (67). The mechanism of acute cervical radiculopathy during weight lifting is probably secondary to a combination of forceful hyperextension and axial loading superimposed on degenerative changes of the cervical spine. The hyperextension increases neural foraminal encroachment by osteophytic spurs and the axial loading produces compressive forces on the disc, thus precipitating herniation.

WRESTLING

Injuries to the head and neck can be anticipated in both freestyle and Greco-Roman style wrestling. Cerebral concussions, although rare, may occur when both wrestlers' heads collide as they simultaneously try for a takedown or from a fall on the head (68). Neck injuries in wrestling can range in severity from a minor cervical sprain to a catastrophic cervical spine fracture. Neck injuries are potentially the most serious of all wrestling injuries but are uncommon because of neck strengthening exercises and the vigilance of the officials. (68) Neck sprains are usually secondary to a twisting maneuver such as a head lock, and compression fractures usually result from a direct fall on the head.

According to Estwanik et al. (69), brachial plexus injuries ("burners" or "pinched-nerve syndrome") account for 37% or all head and neck injuries in interscholastic wrestling. A brachial plexus injury is a stretch of the nerves produced when the wrestler's head goes sideways in one direction and the shoulder in the opposite (68). This can typically occur when a wrestler falls simultaneously on the shoulder and the side of the head (68). Treatment may consist of a cervical collar, physiotherapy with ultrasound, and intermittent cervical traction. Wrestlers with the pinched-nerve syndrome are usually advised to discontinue neck bridging exercises and to substitute isometric buddy-system resistance neck exercises (69). Further preventive measures can include coaching in offensive and defense maneuvers to protect the neck (68).

In addition to head and neck injuries in wrestling, back injuries can also be anticipated. In a survey of interscholastic wrestling injuries by Estwanik. et al (69), various back problems were encountered, but few were serious. The most common back injury was lumbosacral strain (59%), followed by spondylolysis or spondylolisthesis (25%). Back injuries have been reported to occur more frequently in Greco-Roman wrestling than in freestyle wrestling. (70).

An extremely rare and rather unexpected neurologic complication of wrestling has been stroke. Rogers and Sweeny (71) reported a case of brainstem stroke from compromised vertebral artery blood flow in a 17-year-old wrestler. This athlete developed acute vertigo, ataxia, and numbness with associated tingling of the face and body immediately after being placed into several neck holds (half-Nelson's) by his opponent. Vertebral angiography demonstrated a small right vertebral artery with no visualization beyond the second cervical vertebra. The mechanism of vertebral artery obstruction in this case was secondary to defective dens formation and excessive mobility of the second cervical vertebra. According to the investigators, it is important to recognize that vertebral ischemia complications can occur as a result of stressful neck extension and rotation positions during warm-up sessions and actual wrestling matches.

REFERENCES

1. Garfinkel D, Talbot AA, Clarizo M, et al. Medical problems on a professional baseball team. *Phys Sports Med* 1981;9:85–93.
2. Pasternak JS, Veenema KR, Callahan CM. Baseball injuries: a Little League survey. *Pediatrics* 1996;98: 445–448.
3. Hart EJ. Little League baseball and head injury. *Pediatrics* 1992;89:520–521.
4. Wotjys EM, Smith PA, Hankin FM. A cause of ulnar neuropathy in a baseball pitcher—a case report. *Am J Sports Med* 1986;14:422–424.
5. Bontempo E, Trager SL. Ball thrower's fracture of the humerus associated with radial nerve palsy. *Orthopaedics* 1996;19:537–540.
6. Ringel SP, Treihaft M, Carry M, et al. Suprascapular neuropathy in pitchers. *Am J Sports Med* 1990;18: 80–86.
7. Redler MR, Ruland LJ, McCul FC. Quadrilateral space syndrome in a throwing athlete. *Am J Sports Med* 1986;14:511–513.
8. Cormier PJ, Matalon TS, Wolin PM. Quadrilateral space syndrome: a rare cause of shoulder pain. *Radiology* 1988;167:797–798.
9. Long RR, Sargent JC, Pappos AM, et al. Pitcher's arm: an electrodiagnostic enigma. *Muscle Nerve* 1996;19: 1276–1281.
10. Sinson G, Zager EL, Kline DG. Windmill pitcher's radial neuropathy. *Neurosurgery* 1994;34:1087–1090.
11. Barnes DA, Tullos HS. An analysis of 100 symptomatic baseball players. *Am J Sports Med* 1978;6:62–67.
12. Zvijac J, Thompson W. Basketball. In: Caine DJ, Caine CG, Lindner KJ, eds. *Epidemiology of sports injuries,* Champaign, IL: Human Kinetics, 1996:86–97.
13. Zelisko JA, Noble HB, Porter M. A comparison of men's and women's professional basketball injuries. *Am J Sports Med* 1982;10:297–299.
14. Whiteside JA, Fleagle SB, Kalenak A. Fractures and refractures in intercollegiate athletes. An eleven-year experience. *Am J Sports Med* 1981;9:369–377.
15. Garth WP, Van Patten PK. Fractures of the lumbar lamina with epidural hematoma simulating herniation of a disc: a case report. *J Bone Joint Surg* 1989;71:771–772.
16. Clark JE. Apophyseal fracture of the lumbar spine in adolescence. *Orthop Rev* 1991;20:512–516.
17. Walsh M. Preventing injury in competitive canoeists. *Phys Sports Med* 1985;13:120–128.
18. Paley D, Gillespie R. Chronic repetitive unrecognized flexion injury of the cervical spine (high jumper's neck). *Am J Sports Med* 1986;14:92–95.
19. Burdorf A, Van Der Steenhoven GA, Tromp-Klaren EGM. A one-year prospective study on back pain among novice golfers. *Am J Sports Med* 1996;24:659–664.
20. McCarroll JR, Rettig AC, Shelbourne KD, et al. *Phys Sports Med* 1990;18(3):122–126.
21. McCarroll JR, Gioe TJ. Professional golfers and the price they pay. *Phys Sports Med* 1982;10(7):64–70.
22. Hosea TM, Gatt CJ. Back pain in golf. *Clin Sports Med* 1996;15(1):37–53.
23. McCarroll JR. The frequency of golf injuries. *Clin Sports Med* 1996;15(1):1–7.
24. Ekin JA, Sinaki M. Vertebral compression fractures sustained during golfing. *Mayo Clin Proc* 1993;68: 566–570.

25. Jamieson DRS, Ballantyne JP. Unique presentation of a prolapsed thoracic disc:Lhermitte's symptom in a golf layer. *Neurology* 1995;45:1219–1221.

26. Lindsay KW, McLatchie G, Jennett B. Serious head injury in sport. *BMJ* 1980;281:789–791.

27. Kohn HS. Prevention and treatment of elbow injuries in golf. *Clin Sports Med* 1996;15(1):65–83.

28. Murray PM, Cooney WP. Golf-induced injuries of the wrist. *Clin Sports Med* 1996;15(1):85–109.

29. Sachdev P. Golfer's cramp: clinical characteristics and evidence against it being an anxiety disorder. *Move Disord* 1992;7:326–332.

30. Torg JS, Das M. Trampoline-related quadriplegia: review of the literature and reflections on the American Academy of Pediatrics' position statement. *Pediatrics* 1984;74:804–812.

31. Rapp GF, Nicely PG. Trampoline injuries. *Am J Sports Med* 1978;6:269–271.

32. Garrick JG, Requa RK. Epidemiology of women's gymnastics injuries. *Am J Sports Med* 1980;8:261–264.

33. Caine DJ, Lidner KJ. Overuse injuries of growing bones: the young female gymnast at risk. *Phys. Sports Med* 1985;13:51–64.

34. Goldstein JP, Berger PE, Windler GE, Jackson DW. Spine injuries in gymnasts and swimmers. An epidemiologic investigation. *Am J Sports Med* 1991;19:463–468.

35. Dixon M, Frickler P. Injuries to elite gymnasts over 10 years. *Med Sci Sports Exerc* 1993;25:1322–1329.

36. Nattiv A, Mandelbaum BR. Injuries and special concerns in female gymnasts: detecting, treating, and preventing. *Phys Sports Med* 1993;21(7):66–82.

37. Mackie SJ, Taunton JE. Injuries in female gymnasts. Trends suggest prevention tactics. *Phys Sports Med* 1994;22(8):40–45.

38. Wadley GH, Albright JP. Women's intercollegiate gymnastics. Injury patterns and "permanent" medical disability. *Am J Sports Med* 1993;22:314–320.

39. Caine D, Cochrane B, Caine C, Zemper E. An epidemiologic investigation of injuries affecting young competitive female gymnasts. *Am J Sports Med* 1989;17:811–820.

40. Caine DJ, Lindner KJ, Mandelbaum BR, Sands WA. Gymnastics. In: Caine PJ, Caine CG, Lindner KJ, eds. *Epidemiology of sports injuries.* Champaign, IL: Human Kinetics, 1996:213–246.

41. Hirasawa Y, Sakakida K. Sports and peripheral nerve injury. *Am J Sports Med* 1983;11:420–426.

42. Brozin IH, Martlel J, Goldberg I, et al. Traumatic closed femoral nerve neuropathy. *J Trauma* 1982;22:158–160.

43. Takami H, Takahashi S, Ando M. Traumatic rupture of iliacus muscle with femoral nerve paralysis. *J Trauma* 1983;23:253–254.

44. Guiliani G, Poppi M, Acciarn N, et al. CT scan and surgical treatment of traumatic iliacus hematoma with femoral neuropathy: case report. *J Trauma* 1990;30:229–231.

45. Kuland DN, Schildwachter TL, McCue FC, et al. Lacrosse injuries. *Phys Sports Med* 1979;7:83–90.

46. Nelson WE, DePalma B, Gieck JH, et al. Intercollegiate lacrosse injuries. *Phys Sports Med* 1981;9:86–92.

47. Mueller FO, Blyth CS. A survey of 1981 college lacrosse injuries. *Phys Sports Med* 1982;10:87–93.

48. Rimel RW, Nelson WE, Persing JA, et al. Epidural hematoma in lacrosse. *Phys Sports Med* 1983;11:140–144.

49. Evenson L. Parachuting: high risk in free-flying sport. *Phys Sports Med* 1983;11:171–174.

50. Nebergall R. Rodeo. In:Caine PJ, Caine CG, Lindner KJ, eds. *Epidemiology of sports injuries.* Champaign, IL: Human Kinetics, 1996:350–356.

51. Griffin R, Peterson KD, Halseth JR, et al. Injuries in professional rodeo: an update. *Phys Sports Med* 1987; 15(2):104–115.

52. Meyers MC, Elledge JR, Sterling JC, et al. Injuries in intercollegiate rodeo athletes. *Am J Sports Med* 1990; 18:87–91.

53. Nebergall RW, Bauer JM, Eimen RM. Rough riders: how much risk in rodeo? *Phys Sports Med* 1992;20 (10):85–92.

54. Morbidity Mortality Weekly Report. Bull riding related brain and spinal cord injuries. Louisiana, 1994–1995.

55. Massey EW, Pleet AB. Neuropathy in joggers. *Am J Sports Med* 1978;6:209–211.

56. Moller BN, Kadin S. Entrapment of the common peroneal nerve. *Am J Sports Med* 1987;15:90–91.

57. Gluten G. Herniated lumbar disk associated with running: a review of 10 cases. *Am J Sports Med* 1981;9: 155–159.

58. Volski RV, Bourguignon GJ, Rodriguez HM. Lower spine screening in the shooting sports. *Phys Sports Med* 1986;14:101–106.

59. Woodhead AB. Paralysis of the serratus anterior in a world class marksman. *Am J Sports Med* 1985;13: 359–362.

60. Schieber RA, Branche-Dorsey CM, Ryan GW. Comparison of in-line skating injuries with rollerskating and skateboarding injuries. *JAMA* 1994;271;1856–1858.

61. Lee DG. Tennis elbow: a manual therapist's perspective. *J Orthop Sports Phys Ther* 1986;Sep:134–141.

62. Field LD, Altchek DW. Elbow injuries. *Clin Sports Med* 1995;14(1):59–78.

63. Kuhn JE, Hawkins RJ. Surgical treatment of shoulder injuries in tennis players. *Clin Sports Med* 1995;14(1): 139–161.

64. Hainline B. Low back injury. *Clin Sports Med* 1995; 14(1):241–265.

65. Shea JM. Acute quadriplegia following the use of progressive resistance exercise machinery. *Phys Sports Med* 1986;14:120–124.

66. Dangles CJ, Bilos ZJ. Ulnar nerve neuritis in a world champion weightlifter: a case report. *Am J Sports Med* 1980;8:443–445.

67. Jordan BD, Istrico R, Zimmerman RD, et al. Acute cervical radiculopathy in weightlifters. *Phys Sports Med* 1990;18(1):73–76.

68. Snook GA. A survey of wrestling injuries. *Am J Sports Med* 1980;8:450–453.

69. Estwanik JJ, Bergfild JA, Collins HR, et al. Injuries in interscholastic wrestling. *Phys Sports Med* 1980;8: 111–121.

70. Estwanik JJ, Bergfield J, Conty T. Report of injuries sustained during the United States Olympic wrestling trials. *Am J Sports Med* 1978;6:335–340.

71. Rogers L, Sweeny PJ. Stroke: a neurologic complication of wrestling: a case of brainstem stroke in a 17-year-old athlete. *Am J Sports Med* 1979;7:352–354.

Subject Index